Reference Manual for Magnetic Resonance Safety, Implants, and Devices: 2018 Edition

Frank G. Shellock, Ph.D.

Adjunct Clinical Professor of Radiology and Medicine
Keck School of Medicine
University of Southern California

Director of MRI Studies of Biomimetic MicroElectronic
Systems (BMES) Implants, National Science Foundation
BMES Engineering Research Center
University of Southern California

Adjunct Professor of Clinical Physical Therapy, Division of
Biokinesiology and Physical Therapy, School of Dentistry
University of Southern California

Founder
Institute for Magnetic Resonance
Safety, Education, and Research

President
Shellock R & D Services, Inc.
Playa Del Rey, CA

Alexandra M. Karacozoff, B.S. - Associate Editor
MRI Safety Specialist
University of California, Davis
Davis, CA

Biomedical Research Publishing Group
Los Angeles, CA

Made in the United States of America

Library of Congress Cataloging-in-Publication Data

Shellock, Frank G.

Reference Manual for Magnetic Resonance Safety, Implants, and Devices: 2018 Edition

Frank G. Shellock

p. cm.

Includes bibliographical references.

ISBN 978-0-9891632-5-5

1. Magnetic resonance imaging—Complications—Handbooks, manuals, etc. 2. Metals in medicine—Magnetic properties—Handbooks, manuals, etc. 3. Implants, Artificial—Magnetic properties—Handbooks, manuals, etc. I. Title.

[DNLM: 1. Magnetic Resonance Imaging—contraindications—handbooks. 2. Nuclear Magnetic Resonance—handbooks. 3. Metals—handbooks. 4. Implants]

Great care has been taken to assure the accuracy of the information contained in this textbook that is intended for educational and informational purposes, only. Neither the publisher nor the author assume responsibility for errors or for any consequences arising from the use of the information contained herein.

Disclaimer

This textbook was designed to provide a desk reference for radiologists, MRI technologists, facility managers, MRI physicists, MRI researchers, and others. The information is current through the publication date of this textbook. MRI professionals are advised to check with the manufacturer of a given implant or device to obtain the most recent information prior to performing an MRI procedure on a patient with the implant or device in question. The content of this book is designed for general informational purposes only and is not intended to be nor should it be construed to be technical or medical advice or opinion on any specific facts or circumstances.

The author and publisher of this work disclaim any liability for the acts of any physician, individual, group, or entity acting independently or on behalf of any organization that utilizes information for a medical procedure, activity, service, or other situation through the use of this textbook.

The content of this textbook makes no representations or warranties of any kind, expressed or implied, as to the information content, materials or products, included in this textbook. The author and publisher assume no responsibilities for errors or omissions that may include technical or other inaccuracies, or typographical errors. The author and publisher of this work specifically disclaim all representations and warranties of any kind, expressed or implied, as to the information, content, materials, or products included or referenced in this textbook.

The author and publisher disclaim responsibility for any injury and/or damage to persons or property from any of the methods, products, instructions, or ideas contained in this publication.

The author and publisher disclaim liability for any damages of any kind arising from the use of the book, including but not limited to direct, indirect, incidental, punitive and/or consequential damages.

The information and comments provided in this book are not intended to be technical or medical recommendations or advice for individuals or patients. The information and comments provided herein are of a general nature and should not be considered specific to an individual or patient, whether or not a specific patient is referenced by a physician, technologist, individual, group, or other entity seeking information.

The author and publisher assume no responsibility for the accuracy or validity of the information contained in this book nor the claims or statements of any manufacturer or website that is referenced. Manufacturers' product specifications are subject to change without notice. Always read the product labeling, instructions and warning statements thoroughly before using any medical product or similar device.

Regarding the MRI information for a given material, implant, device, or object that may be referenced herein, because of ongoing research, equipment modifications, and changes in governmental and other regulations, no suggested or otherwise presented product information should be used unless the reader has reviewed and evaluated the information provided with the product discussed, by reviewing the latest information provided by the manufacturer, or by reviewing the pertinent literature.

DEDICATION

To Jaana,

A truly extraordinary person,
a gentle soul, and kindred spirit.

Senza di te la mia vita non ha senso.

Contents

Acknowledgements xiii

Preface xiv

SECTION I
    **GUIDELINES AND RECOMMENDATIONS FOR MR
    SAFETY**

Bioeffects of Static Magnetic Fields 2

Bioeffects of Gradient Magnetic Fields 10

Bioeffects of Radiofrequency Fields 14

B_{1+RMS} The root-mean-square value of the MRI Effective
    Component of the RF Magnetic (B_1) Field 21

Acoustic Noise and MR Procedures 24

Body Piercing Jewelry 33

Claustrophobia, Anxiety, and Emotional Distress
    in the MR Environment 35

Epicardial Pacing Leads and Intracardiac Pacing Leads 43

Guidelines for the Management of Patients with Coronary
    Artery Stents Referred for MRI Procedures 47

Guidelines for the Management of Patients with Heart Valve
    Prostheses and Annuloplasty Rings Referred for MRI
    Procedures 51

Guidelines for the Management of the Post-Operative Patient
    Referred for a Magnetic Resonance Procedure 55

Guidelines for Screening Patients for MR Procedures and
    Individuals for the MR Environment 57

Guidelines to Prevent Excessive Heating and Burns
    Associated with Magnetic Resonance Procedures 70

Infection Control in the MRI Environment 76

Magnetic Resonance Imaging: Information for Patients 80

Metallic Foreign Bodies and Screening... 85

Metallic Orbital Foreign Bodies and Screening 87

Monitoring Patients in the MR Environment.................................... 91

Monitoring Body Temperature During MRI 105

MRI Contrast Agents: ACR–ASNR Position Statement.............. 112

MRI Contrast Agents and Adverse Reactions............................... 114

MRI Contrast Agents and Breast Feeding Mothers 120

MRI Contrast Agents: Intracranial Gadolinium Retention......... 123

MRI Contrast Agents and Pregnant Patients............................... 130

MRI Contrast Agents and Nephrogenic Systemic
    Fibrosis 134

Pregnant Patients and MR Procedures.. 142

Pregnant Technologists And Other Healthcare Workers
    in the MR Environment 150

Prevention of Missile Effect Accidents 152

Signs to Help Control Access to the MR Environment.................. 156

Spatial Gradient Magnetic Field: How This Information Is
    Applied to Labeling of Medical Implants and Devices 159

Tattoos, Permanent Cosmetics, and Other Cosmetics.................. 166

Terminology for Implants and Devices 171

The Joint Commission: Excerpts Pertaining to Requirements
    for MRI Safety 180

Using Ferromagnetic Detection Systems in the
    MRI Environment 182

SECTION II
MR PROCEDURES AND IMPLANTS, DEVICES,
AND MATERIALS

General Information... 187

3-Tesla MR Safety Information for Implants and Devices........... 195

ActiFlo Indwelling Bowel Catheter System 200

ActiPatch 201

Alsius Intravascular Temperature Management 202

Ambulatory Infusion Systems 204

Aneurysm Clips 205

Argus II Retinal Prosthesis System 217

Baha, Bone Conduction Implant 220

Biopsy Needles, Markers, and Devices 221

Bone Fusion Stimulator/Spinal Fusion Stimulator 223

Bravo pH Monitoring System 224

Breast Tissue Expanders and Implants 225

Cardiac Pacemakers and
    Implantable Cardioverter Defibrillators 229

Cardiac Pacemakers, Implantable Cardioverter Defibrillators, and
    Other Cardiac Devices: MR Conditional Versions –
    Abbott/St. Jude Medical 246

Cardiac Pacemakers, Implantable Cardioverter Defibrillators, and
    Other Cardiac Devices: MR Conditional Versions –
    Biotronik 247

Cardiac Pacemakers, Implantable Cardioverter Defibrillators, and
    Other Cardiac Devices: MR Conditional Versions –
    Boston Scientific 248

Cardiac Pacemakers, Implantable Cardioverter Defibrillators, and
    Other Cardiac Devices: MR Conditional Versions –
    Medtronic, Inc. 249

Cardiac Pacemakers, Implantable Cardioverter Defibrillators, and
    Other Cardiac Devices: MR Conditional Versions –
    Sorin/LivaNova 250

Cardiovascular Catheters and Accessories 251

Carotid Artery Vascular Clamps 254

Celsius Control System or Temperature Modulation Therapy ... 255

Cerebrospinal Fluid (CSF) Shunt Valves and Accessories 260

Cochlear Implants 270

Codman Microsensor ICP (Intracranial Pressure)
    Monitor Transducer 274

Coils, Stents, Filters, and Grafts 275

Dental Implants, Devices, and Materials 279

Diaphragms 282

Dressings Containing Silver and MRI Procedures 283

Dressings Containing Silver and MRI Procedures:
    Aquacel AG 287

Dressings Containing Silver and MRI Procedures:
    Mepilex Ag and Mepilex Border AG 288

ECG (EKG) Electrodes 289

EmpowerMR Contrast Injection System.................................... 290

Epidural Pump, ambIT Infusion Pumps 291

Essure Device.. 292

External Fixation Devices... 293

Foley Catheters With and Without Temperature Sensors........... 297

Glaucoma Drainage Implants (Shunt Tubes)................................ 301

Guidewires.. 303

Halo Vests and Cervical Fixation Devices 305

Hearing Aids and Other Hearing Systems................................... 311

Heart Valve Prostheses and Annuloplasty Rings 312

Hemostatic Clips, Other Clips, Fasteners, and Staples 315

InSound XT Series and Lyric Hearing Device 319

Insulin Pumps.. 320

Intrauterine Contraceptive Devices and Other Devices 325

IsoMed Implantable Constant-Flow Infusion Pump 327

MAGEC System, Nuvasive, Inc. 328

Magnetically-Activated Implants and Devices 330

Medivance Nasogastric Sump Tube with YSI Series 400
    Temperature Sensor 333

MedStream Programmable Infusion System 335

Miscellaneous Implants and Devices 336

Neurostimulation Systems: General Information 338

Neurostimulation Systems: Deep Brain Stimulation,
    Medtronic, Inc... 344

Neurostimulation System: EndoStim Lower Esophagus
Stimulation (LES) Stimulation System,
EndoStim BV 345

Neurostimulation System: Enterra Therapy,
Gastric Electrical Stimulation (GES), Medtronic, Inc. 347

Neurostimulation System: InterStim Therapy - Sacral Nerve
Stimulation (SNS) for Urinary Control, Medtronic, Inc. 348

Neurostimulation System: Pulsante SPG (Sphenopalatine
Ganglion) Microstimulator, Autonomic Technologies, Inc. ... 349

Neurostimulation System: Senza Spinal Cord Stimulation
System, Nevro Corporation 351

Neurostimulation System: RNS System,
Neuropace 352

Neurostimulation Systems: Spinal Cord Stimulation,
Boston Scientific 353

Neurostimulation Systems: Spinal Cord Stimulation,
St. Jude Medical 354

Neurostimulation Systems: Spinal Cord Stimulation,
Medtronic, Inc. 356

Neurostimulation System: Spinal Cord Stimulation,
Stimwave Technologies, Inc. 358

Neurostimulation System: Vagus Nerve Stimulation,
Cyberonics/LivaNova. 359

Ocular Implants, Lens Implants, and Devices 360

Orthopedic Implants, Materials, and Devices 362

Otologic Implants 367

Oxygen Tanks and Gas Cylinders 371

Palatal System Implant Assembly 373

Patent Ductus Arteriosus (PDA) Occluders,
Atrial Septal Defect (ASD) Occluders,
Ventricular Septal Defect (VSD) Occluders,
and Patent Foramen Ovale (PFO) Closure Devices 375

Pellets, Bullets, and Shrapnel 377

Penile Implants 380

Pessaries 381

PillCam Capsule Endoscopy Devices 382

Prometra Programmable Pumps 383

Reveal Plus Insertable Loop Recorder, Medtronic, Inc. 384

Reveal DX 9528 and Reveal XT 9529
    Insertable Cardiac Monitors, Medtronic, Inc. 385

Reveal LINQ Model LNQ11 Insertable Cardiac Monitor,
    Medtronic, Inc. 386

St. Jude Medical (SJM) Confirm,
    Implantable Cardiac Monitor, St. Jude Medical 387

SAM Sling 388

Scaffolds 389

Scleral Buckle (Scleral Buckling Procedure) 390

Sophono Alpha Magnetic Implant 391

Surgical Instruments and Devices 393

Sutures 395

SynchroMed, SynchroMed EL, and
    SynchroMed II Drug Infusion Systems, Medtronic, Inc. 396

TheraSeed Radioactive Seed Implant 397

Transdermal Medication Patches 398

Vascular Access Ports, Infusion Pumps, and Catheters 402

VeriChip Microtransponder 404

VOCARE Bladder System, Implantable Functional
    Neuromuscular Stimulator 405

The List: Information and Terminology 407

The List 416

    Aneurysm Clips 416

    Biopsy Needles, Markers, and Devices 446

    Breast Tissue Expanders and Implants 454

    Cardiac Pacemakers, ICDs, and Cardiac Monitors 457

    Cardiovascular Catheters and Accessories 464

    Carotid Artery Vascular Clamps 467

    Cerebrospinal Fluid (CSF) Shunt Valves and Accessories 467

Coils, Stents, Filters, and Grafts.. *475*

Dental Implants, Devices, and Materials.................................... *520*

ECG Electrodes *521*

Foley Catheters With and Without Temperature Sensors........... *523*

Halo Vests and Cervical Fixation Devices *525*

Heart Valve Prostheses and Annuloplasty Rings........................ *527*

Hemostatic Clips, Other Clips, Fasteners, and Staples.............. *548*

Miscellaneous *555*

Ocular Implants, Lens Implants, and Devices *628*

Orthopedic Implants, Materials, and Devices *635*

Otologic Implants, Cochlear Implants, and Others.................... *658*

Patent Ductus Arteriosus (PDA),
   Atrial Septal Defect (ASD),
   Ventricular Septal Defect (VSD) Occluders,
   and Patent Foramen Ovale (PFO) Closure Devices *675*

Pellets and Bullets *678*

Penile Implants *680*

Pessaries.. *682*

Sutures *684*

Vascular Access Ports, Infusion Pumps, and Catheters *686*

The List: References **702**

**Appendix I: Criteria for Significant Risk Investigations of
Magnetic Resonance Diagnostic Devices, Center for Devices
and Radiological Health, Food and Drug Administration** **710**

**Appendix II: Websites for MRI Safety, Bioeffects,
and Patient Management.** **714**

Appendix III: Websites for Biomedical Companies...................... **716**

**Appendix IV: Establishing Safety and Compatibility
of Passive Implants in the Magnetic Resonance (MR)
Environment**.. **721**

Biography, Frank G. Shellock, Ph.D. **722**

Acknowledgements

I am truly indebted to Sam Valencerina, B.S., R.T. (R)(MR), MRI Clinical Coordinator and Manager, University of Southern California, University Hospital, Los Angeles, CA for his exceptional MRI capabilities and professional assistance in the evaluation of implants and devices. Special thanks to Mr. Mark Bass for his talented contributions that permit the timely publication of this textbook each year and to Crystal Newton for the amazing cover design.

Preface

Magnetic resonance (MR) procedures continue to expand with regard to clinical applications and complexity. Patient management and safety issues, including those involving implants and devices are important aspects of this diagnostic modality. Because MRI technology continuously evolves, it is necessary to update, revise, and add to the safety topics in this textbook in consideration of the latest information.

This annually-revised textbook series provides a comprehensive, yet concise, resource that includes guidelines and recommendations for patient management and safety based on the peer-reviewed literature, labeling information from biomedical device manufacturers, as well as documents developed by various professional organizations and other entities.

Section I presents safety guidelines, recommendations, and information for patient management relative to the use of MRI technology. Similar to prior editions, the content for **Section I** was reviewed and updated, as needed, with additional peer-reviewed articles added to the references. **Section II** provides information for implants and devices tested for MRI issues. "**The List**" continues to grow and contains data for thousands of items. Notably, many additional MR Conditional "active" implants have been added to this edition. Because of the complexity of the labeling for these particular devices, MR healthcare professionals are directed to the respective manufacturer's websites or other resources so that the latest information may be obtained and carefully followed. To facilitate this task, please refer to **Appendix III, Websites for Biomedical Companies**.

On a personal note, it is my great pleasure and honor to be involved in the exciting field of MRI and to contribute to the many important endeavors that ensure the safe use of this important technology.

Frank G. Shellock, Ph.D., FACR, FISMRM, FACC

Celebrating More Than 30 Years of Service to the MRI Community

SECTION I

Guidelines and Recommendations for MR Safety

Bioeffects of Static Magnetic Fields

The introduction of magnetic resonance (MR) technology as a clinical imaging modality in the early 1980s is responsible for a substantial increase in human exposure to strong static magnetic fields. Most clinical MR systems in use today operate at fields ranging from 0.2- to 3-Tesla. According to guidance from the U.S. Food and Drug Administration, clinical MR systems using static magnetic fields above 8-Tesla for adult patients or above 4-Tesla for neonates and infants, aged one month or less, are considered a significant risk. The exposure of patients or research subjects to fields above these level requires approval by an Institutional Review Board and the informed consent of the individuals.

Presently, the most powerful MR system used for human subjects operates at 10.5-Tesla and there are plans to develop even higher field strength scanners (e.g., 20-Tesla) as suggested by Budinger, et al. (2016). Several investigations have described physiologic findings obtained in human subjects, including volunteers, patients, and workers relative to exposures to a 9.4-Tesla MR system. For the short-term exposures experienced by volunteers and patients, no readily demonstrated health risks were identified. However, a study conducted to evaluate sensory symptoms and vestibular function in workers exposed to the 9.4-Tesla scanner revealed that all participants noted sensory symptoms related to the exposure. The investigators concluded that, while the workers experienced sensory symptoms, it is unclear whether long-term vestibular damage or other changes occurred. The higher rates of vestibular changes may argue for improved worker surveillance and exposure control.

With respect to short-term exposures, the available information pertaining to the effects of static magnetic fields on biological tissues is extensive. Investigations include studies on alterations in cell growth and morphology, cell reproduction and teratogenicity, DNA structure, gene expression, pre- and post-natal reproduction and development, blood brain barrier permeability, nerve activity, cognitive function and behavior, cardiovascular dynamics, hematological indices, temperature regulation, circadian rhythms, immune responsiveness, neurological processing of visual and auditory information, and other biological processes. The majority of these studies concluded that exposures to static magnetic fields produce no harmful bioeffects. Although there have been reports of potentially injurious effects of static magnetic fields on isolated cells or organisms, no effect has been verified or firmly established as a scientific fact. The documented serious injuries and few fatalities that have occurred with MR system magnets were in association with the inadvertent introduction or presence of ferromagnetic objects (e.g., oxygen tanks, wheelchairs, hospital beds, aneurysm clips, etc.) into the scanner room.

Regarding the effects of long-term exposures to static magnetic fields, there are several physical mechanisms of interaction between tissues and static magnetic fields that could theoretically lead to pathological changes in human subjects. However, quantitative analysis of these mechanisms indicates that they are below the threshold of significance with respect to long-term, adverse bioeffects.

Presently, the peer-reviewed literature contains very few, carefully controlled studies that support the absolute safety of chronic exposures to powerful magnetic fields. In addition, although there is no evidence for risks associated with a cumulative effect of magnetic field exposures, further studies of various populations (e.g., MR healthcare professionals who experience repetitive exposures, patients that undergo repeat studies, interventional MR users, etc.) will help establish guidelines for occupational and patient exposures to powerful static magnetic fields. Recently, the findings from several investigations have been published that have addressed occupational exposures to MR systems including those operating at 1.5-, 3-, 7-Tesla, and 9.4-Tesla.

REFERENCES

Acri G, et al. Evaluation of occupational exposure in magnetic resonance sites. Radiol Med 2014;119:208-13.

Atkinson IC, et al. Safety of human MRI at static fields above the FDA 8 T guideline: Sodium imaging at 9.4 T does not affect vital signs or cognitive ability. J Magn Reson Imag 2007;26:1222-7.

Atkinson IC, et al. Vital signs and cognitive function are not affected by 23-sodium and 17-oxygen magnetic resonance imaging of the human brain at 9.4 T. J Magn Reson Imag 2010;32:82-7.

Batistatou E, et al. Personal exposure to static and time-varying magnetic fields during MRI procedures in clinical practice in the UK. Occup Environ Med 2016;73:779-786.

Besson J, et al. Cognitive evaluation following NMR imaging of the brain. Journal of Neurology, Neurosurgery, and Psychiatry 1984;47:314-316.

Bongers S, et al. Retrospective assessment of exposure to static magnetic fields during production and development of magnetic resonance imaging systems. Ann Occup Hyg 2014;58:85-102.

Bongers S, et al. Exposure to static magnetic fields and risk of accidents among a cohort of workers from a medical imaging device manufacturing facility. Magn Reson Med 2016;75:2165-74

Brockway J, Bream P. Does memory loss occur after MR imaging? J Magn Reson Imag 1992;2:721-728.

Brody A, et al. Induced alignment of flowing sickle erythrocytes in a magnetic field: A preliminary report. Investigative Radiology 1985;20:560-566.

Brody A, et al. Preservation of sickle cell blood flow pattern(s) during MR imaging: An *in vivo* study. Am J Roentgenol 1988;151:139-141.

Budinger TF. Nuclear magnetic resonance (NMR) *in vitro* studies: Known thresholds for health effects. J Comput Assisted Tomog 1981;5:800-811.

Budinger TF, et al. Toward 20 T magnetic resonance for human brain studies: Opportunities for discovery and neuroscience rationale. MAGMA. 2016;29:617-39.

Cavin ID, et al. Thresholds for perceiving metallic taste at high magnetic field. J Magn Reson Imag 2007;26:1357-61.

Chakeres DW, de Vocht F. Static magnetic field effects on human subjects related to magnetic resonance imaging. Prog Biophys Mol Biol 2005;87:255-265.

Cretti FR, Gambirasio A. Study of occupational exposure to magnetic fields among operators of magnetic resonance scanning at the Papa Giovanni XXIII Hospital (Bergamo). Med Lav 2015;106:3-16.

de Vocht F, et al. Acute neurobehavior effects of exposure, health complaints and cognitive performance among employees of an MRI scanners manufacturing department. J Magn Reson Imag 2006;23:197-204.

de Vocht F, et al. Acute neurobehavior effects of exposure to static magnetic fields: Analysis of exposure-response relations. J Magn Reson Imag 2006;23:291-297.

de Vocht F, et al. Cognitive effects of head-movements in stray fields generated by a 7 Tesla whole-body MRI magnet. Bioelectromagnetics 2007;28:247-55.

de Vocht F, et al. Transient health symptoms of MRI staff working with 1.5 and 3.0 Tesla scanners in the UK. Eur Radiol 2015;25:2718-26.

Feychting M. Health effects of static magnetic fields: A review of the epidemiological evidence. Prog Biophys Mol Biol 2005;87:241-6.

Franco G, et al. Focusing ethical dilemmas of evidence-based practice in SMF-exposed MRI-workers: A qualitative analysis. Int Arch Occup Environ Health 2010;83:417-21.

Friebe B, et al. Sensory perceptions of individuals exposed to the static field of a 7 T MRI: A controlled blinded study. J Magn Reson Imaging 2015;41:1675-81.

Fuentes MA, et al. Analysis and measurements of magnetic field exposures for healthcare workers in selected MR environments. IEEE Trans Biomed Eng 2008;55:1355-64.

Ghodbane S, et al. Bioeffects of static magnetic fields: Oxidative stress, genotoxic effects, and cancer studies. Biomed Res Int 2013;2013:602987.

Glover PM, et al. Magnetic-field-induced vertigo: A theoretical and experimental investigation. Bioelectromagnetics 2007;28:349-61.

Gorlin A, et al. Acute vertigo in an anesthesia provider during exposure to a 3T MRI scanner. Med Devices (Auckl) 2015;8:161-6.

Gungor HR, et al. Are there any adverse effects of static magnetic field from magnetic resonance imaging devices on bone health of workers? Eklem Hastalik Cerrahisi 2014;25:36-41.

Gungor HR, et al. Chronic exposure to static magnetic fields from magnetic resonance imaging devices deserves screening for osteoporosis and vitamin D levels: A rat model. Int J Environ Res Public Health 2015;12:8919-32.

Hansson Mild K, et al. Exposure classification of MRI workers in epidemiological studies. Bioelectromagnetics 2013;24:81-4.

Hartwig V, et al. Biological effects and safety in magnetic resonance imaging: A review. Int J Environ Res Public Health 2009;6:1778-98.

Hartwig V. Engineering for safety assurance in MRI: Analytical, numerical and experimental dosimetry. Magn Reson Imaging 2015;33:681-9.

Heinrich A, et al. Women are more strongly affected by dizziness in static magnetic fields of magnetic resonance imaging scanners. Neuroreport 2014;25:1081-4.

Heinrich A, et al. Effects of static magnetic fields on cognition, vital signs, and sensory perception: A meta-analysis. J Magn Reson Imag 2011;34:758–763.

Heinrich A, et al. Cognition and sensation in very high static magnetic fields: A randomized case-crossover study with different field strengths. Radiology 2013;266:236-45.

Heinrich A, et al. Women are more strongly affected by dizziness in static magnetic fields of magnetic resonance imaging scanners. Neuroreport 2014;25:1081-4.

Hong CZ, Shellock FG. Short-term exposure to a 1.5 Tesla static magnetic field does not effect somato-sensory evoked potentials in man. Magnetic Resonance Imaging 1989;8:65-69.

Hsieh CH, et al. Deleterious effects of MRI on chondrocytes. Osteoarthritis Cartilage. 2008;16:343-51.

Innis NK, et al. Behavioral effects of exposure to nuclear magnetic resonance imaging: II. Spatial memory tests. Magnetic Resonance Imaging 1986;4:281-284.

International Electrotechnical Commission (IEC), Medical Electrical Equipment, Particular requirements for the safety of magnetic resonance equipment for medical diagnosis, International Standard IEC 60601-2-33, 2002.

International Commission on Non-Ionizing Radiation Protection (ICNIRP) statement, medical magnetic resonance procedures: Protection of patients. Health Physics 2004;87:197-216.

Kangarlu A, et al. Cognitive, cardiac, and physiological safety studies in ultra high field magnetic resonance imaging. Magnetic Resonance Imaging 1999;17:1407-1416.

Kannala S, et al. Occupational exposure measurements of static and pulsed gradient magnetic fields in the vicinity of MRI scanners. Phys Med Biol 2009;54:2243-57.

Karpowicz J, et al. Exposure to static magnetic field and health hazards during the operation of magnetic resonance scanners. Med Pr. 2011;62:309-21.

Karpowicz J, et al. Measures of occupational exposure to time-varying low frequency magnetic fields of non-uniform spatial distribution in the light of international guidelines and electrodynamic exposure effects in the human body. Med Pr. 2012;63:317-28.

Karpowicz J, Gryz K. Health risk assessment of occupational exposure to a magnetic field from magnetic resonance imaging devices. Int J Occup Saf Ergon 2006;12:155-67.

Kay H, Herfkens R, Kay B. Effect on magnetic resonance imaging on Xenopus Laevis embryogenesis. Magnetic Resonance Imaging 1988;6:501-506.

Kim SJ, Kim KA. Safety issues and updates under MR environments. Eur J Radiol 2017;89:7-13.

Laszlo J, Gyires K. 3 T homogeneous static magnetic field of a clinical MR significantly inhibits pain in mice. Life Sci 2009;84:12-7.

McRobbie DW. Occupational exposure in MRI. Br J Radiol 2012;85:293-312.

Muller S, Hotz M. Human brainstem auditory evoked potentials (BAEP) before and after MR examinations. Magnetic Resonance in Medicine 1990;16:476-480.

Nojima I, et al. Static magnetic field can transiently alter the human intracortical inhibitory system. Clin Neurophysiol 2015;126:2314-9.

Ossenkopp KP, et al. Behavioral effects of exposure to nuclear magnetic resonance imaging: I. Open-field avoidance behavior an passive avoidance learning in rats. Magnetic Resonance Imaging 1986;4:275-280.

Patel M, et al. Pilot study investigating the effect of the static magnetic field from a 9.4-T MRI on the vestibular system. J Occup Environ Med 2008;50:576-83.

Pophof B, Brix G. Magnetic resonance imaging: Recent studies on biological effects of static magnetic and high-frequency electromagnetic fields. Radiologe 2017;57:563-568.

Prasad N, Wright D, Ford J, Thornby J. Safety of 4-T MR imaging: Study of effects on developing frog embryos. Radiology 1990;174:251-253.

Rauschenberg J, et al. Multicenter study of subjective acceptance during magnetic resonance imaging at 7 and 9.4 T. Invest Radiol 2014;49:249-59.

Reddig A, et al. Analysis of DNA double-strand breaks and cytotoxicity after 7 Tesla magnetic resonance imaging of isolated human lymphocytes. PLoS One 2015;10:1-14.

Sakurai T, Terashima S, Miyakoshi J. Effects of strong static magnetic fields used in magnetic resonance imaging on insulin-secreting cells. Bioelectromagnetics. Bioelectromagnetics 2009;30:1-8.

Schaap K, et al. Inventory of MRI applications and workers exposed to MRI-related electromagnetic fields in the Netherlands. Eur J Radiol 2013;82:2279-85.

Schaap K, et al. Exposure to static and time-varying magnetic fields from working in the static magnetic stray fields of MRI scanners: A comprehensive survey in the Netherlands. Ann Occup Hyg 2014;58:1094-1110.

Schaap K, et al. Occupational exposure of healthcare and research staff to static magnetic stray fields from 1.5-7 Tesla MRI scanners is associated with reporting of transient symptoms. Occup Environ Med 2014;71:423-9.

Schaap K, et al. Work-related factors associated with occupational exposure to static magnetic stray fields from MRI scanners. Magn Reson Med 2016;75:2141-55.

Schenck JF. Health effects and safety of static magnetic fields. In: Shellock FG, Editor. Magnetic Resonance Procedures: Health Effects and Safety. Boca Raton, FL: CRC Press, 2001; pp. 1-30.

Schenck JF. Safety of strong, static magnetic fields. J Magn Reson Imag 2000;12;2-19.

Schenck JF, et al. Human exposure to 4.0-Tesla magnetic fields in a whole-body scanner. Medical Physics 1992;19:1089-1098.

Schlamann M, et al. Exposure to high-field MRI does not affect cognitive function. J Magn Reson Imag 2010;31:1061-6.

Schlamann M, et al. Short term effects of magnetic resonance imaging on excitability of the motor cortex at 1.5T and 7T. Acad Radiol 2010;17:277-81.

Schwartz J, Crooks L. NMR imaging produces no observable mutations or cytotoxicity in mammalian cells. Am J Roentgenol 1982;139:583-585.

Schwenzer NF, et al. Do static or time-varying magnetic fields in magnetic resonance imaging (3.0 T) alter protein-gene expression?-A study on human embryonic lung fibroblasts. J Magn Reson Imag 2007;26:1210-5.

Schwenzer NF, et al. In vitro evaluation of magnetic resonance imaging at 3.0 Tesla on clonogenic ability, proliferation, and cell cycle in human embryonic lung fibroblasts. Invest Radiol 2007;42:212-217.

Shellock FG, Crues JV. MR procedures: Biologic effects, safety, and patient care. Radiology 2004;232:635-652.

Shellock FG, Schaefer DJ, Crues JV. Exposure to a 1.5 Tesla static magnetic field does not alter body and skin temperatures in man. Magnetic Resonance in Medicine 1989;1:371-375.

Shellock FG, Schaefer DJ, Gordon CJ. Effect of a 1.5 Tesla static magnetic field on body temperature of man. Magnetic Resonance in Medicine 1986;3:644-647.

Short W, et al. Alteration of human tumor cell adhesion by high-strength static magnetic fields. Investigative Radiology 1991;27:836-840.

Silva AK, Silva EL, Egito ES, Carrico AS. Safety concerns related to magnetic field exposure. Radiat Environ Biophys 2006;45:245-52.

Simmons A, Hakansson K. Magnetic resonance safety. Methods Mol Biol 2011;711:17-28.

Theysohn JM, et al. Vestibular effects of a 7 Tesla MRI examination compared to 1.5 T and 0 T in healthy volunteers. PLoS One 2014;9:e92104.

Tocchio S, et al. MRI evaluation and safety in the developing brain. Semin Perinatol 2015;39:73-104.

Tomasi DG, Wang R. Induced magnetic field gradients and forces in the human head in MRI. J Magn Reson Imag 2007;26:1340-5.

Toyomaki A, Yamamoto T. Observation of changes in neural activity due to the static magnetic field of an MRI scanner. J Magn Reson Imag 2007;26:1216-21.

U.S. Department of Health and Human Services, Food and Drug Administration, Center for Devices and Radiological Health, Criteria for Significant Risk Investigations of Magnetic Resonance Diagnostic Devices, Guidance for Industry and Food and Drug Administration Staff. June 20, 2014.

Valiron O, et al. Cellular disorders induced by high magnetic fields. J Magn Reson Imag 2005;22:334-340.

van Nierop LE, et al. Effects of magnetic stray fields from a 7 Tesla MRI scanner on neurocognition: A double-blind randomised crossover study. Occup Environ Med 2012;69:759-66.

van Nierop LE, et al. Acute cognitive effects of MRI related magnetic fields: The role of vestibular sensitivity. Occup Environ Med 2014;71 Suppl 1:A16.

van Nierop LE, et al. Simultaneous exposure to MRI-related static and low-frequency movement-induced time-varying magnetic fields affects neurocognitive performance: A double-blind randomized crossover study. Magn Reson Med 2015;74:840-9.

Vaughan T, et al. 9.4-T human MRI: Preliminary results. Magn Reson Med 2006;56:1274-1282.

Vecchia P, Hietanen M, et al. Guidelines on limits of exposure to static magnetic fields. International Commission on Non-Ionizing Radiation Protection. Health Physics 2009;96:504-14.

Versluis MJ, et al. Subject tolerance of 7 T MRI examinations. J Magn Reson Imaging 2013;38:722-5.

Vijayalaxmi, et al. Magnetic resonance imaging (MRI): A review of genetic damage investigations. Mutat Res Rev Mutat Res 2015;764:51-63.

Vogl T, et al. Influence of magnetic resonance imaging on evoked potentials and nerve conduction velocities in humans. Invest Radiol 1991;26:432-437.

Von Klitzing L. Do static magnetic fields of NMR influence biological signals? Clin Phys Physiol Meas 1986;7:157-160.

Ward BK, et al. Vestibular stimulation by magnetic fields. Ann N Y Acad Sci 2015;1343:69-79.

Weintraub MI, et al. Biologic effects of 3 Tesla (T) MR imaging comparing traditional 1.5-T and 0.6-T in 1,023 consecutive outpatients. J Neuroimaging 2007;17:241-5.

Weiss M, et al. Bioeffects of high magnetic fields: A study using a simple animal model. Magnetic Resonance Imaging 1992;10:689-694.

Yamaguchi-Sekino S, et al. Biological effects of electromagnetic fields and recently updated safety guidelines for strong static magnetic fields. Magn Reson Med Sci 2011;10:1-10.

Yamaguchi-Sekino S, et al. Occupational exposure levels of static magnetic field during routine MRI examination in 3 T MR system. Bioelectromagnetics 2014;35:70-5.

Yuh WTC, Ehrhardt JC, Fisher DJ, Shields RK, Shellock FG. Phantom limb pain induced in amputee by strong magnetic fields. J Magn Reson Imag 1992;2:221-223.

Zahedi Y, et al. Impact of repetitive exposure to strong static magnetic fields on pregnancy and embryonic development of mice. J Magn Reson Imaging 2014;39:691-9.

Zaremba LA. FDA guidance for magnetic resonance system safety and patient exposures: Current status and future considerations. In: Shellock FG, Editor. Magnetic Resonance Procedures: Health Effects and Safety. Boca Raton, FL: CRC Press, 2001; pp. 183-196.

Zaun G, et al. Repetitive exposure of mice to strong static magnetic fields in utero does not impair fertility in adulthood but may affect placental weight of offspring. J Magn Reson Imaging 2014;39:683-90.

Zilberti L, et al. Assessment of exposure to MRI motion-induced fields based on the International Commission on Non-Ionizing Radiation Protection (ICNIRP) guidelines. Magn Reson Med 2016;76:1291-300.

Bioeffects of Gradient Magnetic Fields

During magnetic resonance (MR) procedures, gradient or time-varying magnetic fields may stimulate nerves or muscles in patients by inducing electrical fields. This topic has been reviewed over the years by various experts including Bencsik, et al. (2007), Schaefer, et al. (2000), Nyenhuis, et al. (1997), and Bourland, et al. (1999). The potential for interactions between gradient magnetic fields and biological tissues is dependent on a variety of factors including the fundamental field frequency, the maximum flux density, the average flux density, the presence of harmonic frequencies, the waveform characteristics of the signal, the polarity of the signal, the current distribution in the body, the electrical properties, and the sensitivity of the cell membrane.

GRADIENT MAGNETIC FIELD-INDUCED STIMULATION

Several investigations have characterized MR system-related, gradient magnetic field-induced stimulation in human subjects, including adults and children. At sufficient exposure levels, peripheral nerve stimulation is perceptible as tingling tapping, or other sensations. At gradient magnetic field exposure levels from 50% to 100% above perception thresholds, patients undergoing MRI may become uncomfortable or experience pain. At extremely high levels, cardiac stimulation is a concern. However, the induction of cardiac stimulation requires exceedingly large gradient fields that are more than an order of magnitude greater than those used currently by commercial MR systems.

With regard to gradient magnetic fields, the U.S. Food and Drug Administration considers that MR procedures using rates of change (dB/dt) sufficient to produce severe discomfort or painful nerve stimulation to be a significant risk. These safety standards for gradient magnetic fields associated with present-day scanners appear to adequately protect patients from potential hazards or injuries.

Studies performed in human subjects have indicated that the anatomical sites experiencing peripheral nerve stimulation vary depending on the activation of a specific gradient (i.e. x-, y- or z-gradient). For example, stimulation sites for x-gradients included the bridge of the nose, left side of the thorax, iliac crest, left thigh, buttocks, and the lower back. Stimulation sites for y-gradients included the scapula, upper arms, shoulder, right side of the thorax, iliac crest, hip, hands, and upper back. Stimulation sites for z-gradients included the scapula, thorax, xyphoid, abdomen, iliac crest, and upper and lower back. Notably, peripheral nerve stimulation sites were typically found at bony prominences.

According to Schaefer, et al. (2000), since bone is less conductive than the surrounding tissue, it may increase current densities in narrow regions of tissue between the bone and the skin, resulting in lower nerve stimulation thresholds than expected. Modifying gradient hardware and pulse sequences may be useful strategies to avoid unpleasant peripheral nerve stimulation that occurs with certain MRI techniques, as suggested by Weinberg, et al. (2007).

REFERENCES

Abart J, et al. Peripheral nerve stimulation by time-varying magnetic fields. Journal of Computer Assisted Tomography 1997;21:532–538.

Andreuccetti D, et al. Weighted-peak assessment of occupational exposure due to MRI gradient fields and movements in a nonhomogeneous static magnetic field. Med Phys 2013;40:011910.

Batistatou E, et al. Personal exposure to static and time-varying magnetic fields during MRI procedures in clinical practice in the UK. Occup Environ Med 2016;73:779-78.

Bencsik M, Bowtell R, Bowley R. Electric fields induced in the human body by time-varying magnetic field gradients in MRI: Numerical calculations and correlation analysis. Phys Med Biol 2007;52:2337-53.

Bonutti F, et al. Measurement of the weighted peak level for occupational exposure to gradient magnetic fields for 1.5 and 3 Tesla MRI body scanners. Radiat Prot Dosimetry 2016;168:358-64.

Bourland JD, Nyenhuis JA, Schaefer DJ. Physiologic effects of intense MRI gradient fields. Neuroimaging Clin North Am 1999;9:363–377.

Budinger TF, et al. Physiological effects of fast oscillating magnetic field gradients. Journal of Computer Assisted Tomography 1991;15:609–614.

Cohen MS, Weisskoff R, Kantor H. Sensory stimulation by time varying magnetic fields. Magn Reson 1990;14:409–414.

de Vocht F, et al. Exposure to alternating electromagnetic fields and effects on the visual and visuomotor systems. Br J Radiol 2007;80:822-8.

Doherty J, Whitman G, Robinson M, et al. Changes in cardiac excitability and vulnerability in NMR fields. Invest Radiol 1985;20:129-135.

Ehrhardt JC, et al. Peripheral nerve stimulation in a whole-body echo-planar imaging system. J Magn Reson Imag 1997;7:405–409.

Feldman RE, et al. Experimental determination of human peripheral nerve stimulation thresholds in a 3-axis planar gradient system. Magn Reson Med 2009;62:763-70.

Fuentes MA, et al. Analysis and measurements of magnetic field exposures for healthcare workers in selected MR environments. IEEE Trans Biomed Eng 2008;55:1355-64.

Glover PM. Interaction of MRI field gradients with the human body. Phys Med Biol 2009;54:R99-R115.

Glover PM, et al. Measurement of visual evoked potential during and after periods of pulsed magnetic field exposure. J Magn Reson Imag 2007;26:1353-6.

Ham CLG, et al. Peripheral nerve stimulation during MRI: Effects of high gradient amplitudes and switching rates. J Magn Reson Imag 1997;7:933–937.

Hartwig V, et al. Biological effects and safety in magnetic resonance imaging: A review. Int J Environ Res Public Health. 2009;6:1778-98.

Iachininoto MG, et al. Effects of exposure to gradient magnetic fields emitted by nuclear magnetic resonance devices on clonogenic potential and proliferation of human hematopoietic stem cells. Bioelectromagnetics 2016;37:201-11.

Irnich W, Schmitt F. Magnetostimulation in MRI. Magn Reson Med 1995;33:619–623.

International Commission on Non-Ionizing Radiation Protection (ICNIRP) statement, medical magnetic resonance procedures: Protection of patients. Health Physics 2004;87:197-216.

Kangarlu A, Tang L, Ibrahim TS. Electric field measurements and computational modeling at ultrahigh-field MRI. Magnetic Resonance Imaging 2007;25:1222-1226.

Kannala S, et al. Occupational exposure measurements of static and pulsed gradient magnetic fields in the vicinity of MRI scanners. Phys Med Biol 2009;54:2243-57.

King KF, Schaefer DJ. Spiral scan peripheral nerve stimulation. J Magn Reson Imag 2000;12:164-170.

Li Y, et al. Numerically-simulated induced electric field and current density within a human model located close to a z-gradient coil. J Magn Reson Imag 2007;26:1286-95.

Mansfield P, Harvey PR. Limits to neural stimulation in echo-planar imaging. Magn Reson Med 1993;29:746–758.

Nyenhuis JA, et al. Health effects and safety of intense gradient fields. In: Shellock FG, Editor. Magnetic Resonance Procedures: Health Effects and Safety. Boca Raton, FL: CRC Press, 2001;31-54.

Nyenhuis JA, et al. Analysis from a stimulation perspective of magnetic field patterns of MR gradient coils. J Appl Phys 1997;81:4314–4316.

Reddig A, et al. Analysis of DNA double-strand breaks and cytotoxicity after 7 Tesla magnetic resonance imaging of isolated human lymphocytes. PLoS One 2015;10:1-14.

Samoudi AM, et al. Numerically simulated exposure of children and adults to pulsed gradient fields in MRI. J Magn Reson Imaging 2016;44:1360-1367.

Schaap K, et al. Exposure to static and time-varying magnetic fields from working in the static magnetic stray fields of MRI scanners: A comprehensive survey in the Netherlands. Ann Occup Hyg 2014;58:1094-1110.

Schaefer DJ, Bourland JD, Nyenhuis JA. Review of patient safety in time-varying gradient fields. J Magn Reson Imag 2000;12:20-29.

Schwenzer NF, et al. Do static or time-varying magnetic fields in magnetic resonance imaging (3.0 T) alter protein-gene expression? A study on human embryonic lung fibroblasts. J Magn Reson Imag 2007;26:1210-5.

Shellock FG, Crues JV. MR procedures: Biologic effects, safety, and patient care. Radiology 2004;232:635-652.

U.S. Department of Health and Human Services, Food and Drug Administration, Center for Devices and Radiological Health, Criteria for Significant Risk Investigations of Magnetic Resonance Diagnostic Devices, Guidance for Industry and Food and Drug Administration Staff. June 20, 2014.

van Nierop LE, et al. Simultaneous exposure to MRI-related static and low-frequency movement-induced time-varying magnetic fields affects neurocognitive performance: A double-blind randomized crossover study. Magn Reson Med 2015;74:840-9.

Vijayalaxmi, et al. Magnetic resonance imaging (MRI): A review of genetic damage investigations. Mutat Res Rev Mutat Res 2015;764:51-63.

Vogt FM, et al. Increased time rate of change of gradient fields: Effect on peripheral nerve stimulation at clinical MR imaging. Radiology 2004;233:548-554.

Weinberg IN, et al. Increasing the oscillation frequency of strong magnetic fields above 101 kHz significantly raises peripheral nerve excitation thresholds. Med Phys 2012;39:2578-83.

Weintraub MI, et al. Biologic effects of 3 Tesla (T) MR imaging comparing traditional 1.5-T and 0.6-T in 1,023 consecutive outpatients. J Neuroimaging 2007;17:241-5.

Bioeffects of Radiofrequency Fields

The majority of the radiofrequency (RF) power transmitted for MR imaging or spectroscopy procedures is transformed into heat within the patient's tissue as a result of resistive losses. Not surprisingly, the bioeffects associated with exposure to RF radiation are related to the thermogenic aspects of this electromagnetic field.

Prior to 1985, there were no reports concerning the thermophysiologic responses of human subjects exposed to RF radiation during MR procedures. Since then, many investigations have characterized the thermal effects of MR-related heating.

SPECIFIC ABSORPTION RATE

Thermoregulatory and other physiologic changes that a human subject exhibits in response to exposure to RF radiation are dependent on the amount of energy that is absorbed. The dosimetric term used to describe the absorption of RF radiation is the specific absorption rate (SAR). SAR is the mass normalized rate at which RF power is coupled to biological tissue and is typically indicated in units of watts per kilogram (W/kg). The relative amount of RF radiation that an individual encounters during an MR procedure is designated as the whole-body-averaged SAR. Other SAR levels relative to the body part exposed or peak SAR level (i.e. the amount in one gram of tissue) may also be reported by the MR system.

Measurements or estimates of SAR are not trivial, particularly in human subjects. There are several methods of determining this parameter for the purpose of RF energy dosimetry. The SAR that is produced during an MR procedure is a complex function of numerous variables including the frequency (i.e. determined by the strength of the static magnetic field of the MR system), the type of RF pulse used (e.g., 90° vs. 180° pulse), the repetition time, the type of transmit RF coil used, the volume of tissue contained within the transmit RF coil, the shape of the anatomical region exposed, as well as other factors.

With regard to RF energy, the U.S. Food and Drug Administration currently indicates that MR procedures that exceed certain SAR values may pose significant risks (please refer to **Appendix I** to review these values).

THERMOPHYSIOLOGIC RESPONSES TO MR PROCEDURE-RELATED HEATING

Thermophysiologic responses to MR procedure-related heating depend on multiple physiological, physical, and environmental factors. These include the duration of exposure, the rate at which energy is deposited, the response of the patient's thermoregulatory system, the presence of an underlying health condition, and the ambient conditions within the MR system.

In regards to temperature regulation in human subjects, when exposed to a thermal challenge, the human body loses heat by means of convection, conduction, radiation, and evaporation. Each mechanism is responsible to a varying degree for heat dissipation, as the body attempts to maintain thermal homeostasis. If the thermoregulatory effectors are incapable of dissipating the heat load, an accumulation of heat occurs along with an elevation in local and/or overall tissue temperatures.

Various health conditions may affect an individual's ability to tolerate a thermal challenge including cardiovascular disease, hypertension, diabetes, fever, old age, and obesity. In addition, medications such as diuretics, beta-blockers, calcium blockers, amphetamines, and sedatives can alter thermoregulatory responses to a heat load. In fact, certain medications have a synergistic effect with RF radiation with respect to tissue heating. The environmental conditions (i.e. ambient temperature, relative humidity, and airflow) that exist in the MR system will also affect tissue temperature changes associated with RF energy-induced heating.

The first study of human thermal responses to RF radiation-induced heating during an MR procedure was conducted by Schaefer, et al. Temperature changes and other physiologic parameters were assessed in volunteer subjects exposed to a relatively high, whole-body-averaged SAR (approximately 4.0-W/kg). The data indicated that there were no excessive temperature elevations or other deleterious physiologic consequences related to exposure to RF energy.

Several studies were subsequently conducted involving volunteer subjects and patients undergoing MR procedures with the intent of obtaining information that would be applicable to patients typically encountered in the clinical MR setting. These investigations demonstrated that changes in body temperatures were relatively minor (i.e. less than 0.6 degrees C).

While there was a tendency for statistically significant increases in skin temperatures to occur, these were of no serious physiological consequence.

Interestingly, various studies reported a poor correlation between body temperature and skin temperature changes versus whole-body-averaged SARs associated with clinical MR procedures. These findings are not surprising considering the range of thermophysiologic responses that are possible in human subjects relative to a given SAR level. For example, as previously indicated, an individual's thermoregulatory system can be greatly impacted by the presence of an underlying condition or medication that can impair the ability to dissipate heat.

An extensive investigation by Shellock, et al. (1994) was conducted in volunteer subjects exposed to MR examinations performed at a whole-body-averaged SAR of 6.0-W/kg. To date, this is the highest level of RF energy that human subjects have been exposed to in association with MR procedures. Tympanic membrane temperature, six different skin temperatures, heart rate, blood pressure, oxygen saturation, and skin blood flow were monitored. The findings indicated that an MR exam performed at a whole body averaged SAR of 6.0-W/kg can be physiologically tolerated by an individual with normal thermoregulatory function.

VERY-HIGH-FIELD MR SYSTEMS

Clinical MR systems now operate at a static magnetic field strength of 3-Tesla. Many research scanners operate at 4-Tesla and 7-Tesla, one is operating at 9.4-Tesla, and one at 10.5-Tesla. These very-high-field MR systems are capable of depositing RF power that exceed those associated with a 1.5-Tesla MR system. Therefore, investigations are needed to characterize thermal responses in human subjects to determine potential thermogenic hazards associated with the use of these powerful scanners, especially since frequency-related differences likely exist. To date, several reports have studied MR procedure-related heating associated with very-high-field MR systems utilizing modeling techniques as well as other experimental methods.

REFERENCES

Alon L, et al. Method for *in situ* characterization of radiofrequency heating in parallel transmit MRI. Magn Reson Med 2013;69:1457-65.

Atalar E. Radiofrequency safety for interventional MRI procedures. Acad Radiol 2005;12:1149-1157.

Bermingham JF, et al. A measurement and modeling study of temperature in living and fixed tissue during and after radiofrequency exposure. Bioelectromagnetics 2014;35:181-91.

Barber BJ, et al. Thermal effects of MR imaging: worst-case studies on sheep. Am J Roentgenol. 1990;155:1105-10.

Boss A, et al. Tissue warming and regulatory responses induced by radio frequency energy deposition on a whole-body 3-Tesla magnetic resonance imager. J Magn Reson Imag 2007;26:1334-9.

Bottomley PA. Turning up the heat on MRI. J Am Coll Radiol 2008;5:853.

Bottomley PA, Edelstein WA. Power deposition in whole body NMR imaging. Med Phys 1981;8: 510-512.

Budinger TF. Nuclear magnetic resonance (NMR) *in vitro* studies: Known thresholds for health effects. J Comput Assisted Tomog 1981;5:800-811.

Collins CM. Numerical field calculations considering the human subject for engineering and safety assurance in MRI. NMR Biomed 2009;22:919-26.

Collins CM, Wang Z. Calculation of radiofrequency electromagnetic fields and their effects in MRI of human subjects. Magn Reson Med 2011;65:1470-82.

de Greef M, et al. Specific absorption rate inter-subject variability in 7-T parallel transmit MRI of the head. Magn Reson Med 2013;69:1476-85.

Drinkwater BL, Horvath SM: Heat tolerance and aging. Med Sci Sport Exer 1979;11:49-55.

Fiedler TM, et al. SAR simulations & safety. Neuroimage 2017 (In press).

Gorny KR, et al. Calorimetric calibration of head coil SAR estimates displayed on a clinical MR scanner. Phys Med Biol 2008;53:2565-76.

Gowland PA, De Wilde J. Temperature increase in the fetus due to radio frequency exposure during magnetic resonance scanning. Phys Med Biol 2008;53:L15-8.

Graesslin I, et al. A specific absorption rate prediction concept for parallel transmission MR. Magn Reson Med 2012;68:1664-74.

Graesslin I, et al. Comprehensive RF safety concept for parallel transmission MR. Magn Reson Med 2015;74:589-998.

Hand JW, et al. Prediction of specific absorption rate in mother and fetus associated with MRI examinations during pregnancy. Magn Reson Med 2006;55:883-893.

Hand JW, et al. Numerical study of RF exposure and the resulting temperature rise in the foetus during a magnetic resonance procedure. Phys Med Biol 2010;55:913-30.

Hartwig V, et al. Biological effects and safety in magnetic resonance imaging: A review. Int J Environ Res Public Health 2009;6:1778-98.

International Commission on Non-Ionizing Radiation Protection (ICNIRP) statement, medical magnetic resonance procedures: Protection of patients. Health Physics 2004;87:197-216.

International Electrotechnical Commission (IEC), Medical Electrical Equipment, Particular requirements for the safety of magnetic resonance equipment for medical diagnosis, International Standard IEC 60601-2-33, 2002.

Israel M, et al. Electromagnetic field occupational exposure: Non-thermal vs. thermal effects. Electromagn Biol Med 2013;32:145-54.

Kangarlu A, Shellock FG, Chakeres D. 8.0-Tesla MR system: Temperature changes associated with radiofrequency-induced heating of a head phantom. J Magn Reson Imag 2003;17:220-226.

Kangarlu A, Ibrahim TS, Shellock FG. Effects of coil dimensions and field polarization on RF heating inside a head phantom. Magnetic Resonance Imaging 2005;23:53-60.

Kenny WL. Physiological correlates of heat intolerance. Sports Med 1985;2:279-286.

Kikuchi S, et al. Temperature elevation in the fetus from electromagnetic exposure during magnetic resonance imaging. Phys Med Biol 2010;55:2411-26.

Kim SJ, Kim KA. Safety issues and updates under MR environments. Eur J Radiol 2017;89:7-13.

Jauchem JR. Effects of drugs on thermal responses to microwaves. Gen Pharmacol 1985;16:307-310.

Murbach M, et al. Whole-body and local RF absorption in human models as a function of anatomy and position within 1.5T MR body coil. Magn Reson Med 2014;71:839-845.

Murbach M, et al. Thermal tissue damage model analyzed for different whole-body SAR and scan durations for standard MR body coils. Magn Reson Med 2014;71:421-31.

Neufeld E, et al. Analysis of the local worst-case SAR exposure caused by an MRI multi-transmit body coil in anatomical models of the human body. Phys Med Biol 2011;56:4649-59.

Oh S, et al. Experimental and numerical assessment of MRI-induced temperature change and SAR distributions in phantoms and *in vivo*. Magn Reson Med Magn Reson Med 2010;63:218-23.

Rowell LB. Cardiovascular aspects of human thermoregulation. Circ Res 1983;52:367-379.

Schaefer DJ. Health effects and safety of radiofrequency power deposition associated with magnetic resonance procedures. In: Shellock FG, Editor. Magnetic Resonance Procedures: Health Effects and Safety. Boca Raton, FL: CRC Press, 2001;55-74.

Shellock FG. Radiofrequency energy-induced heating during MR procedures: A review. J Magn Reson Imag 2000;12:30-36.

Shellock FG, Crues JV. MR procedures: Biologic effects, safety, and patient care. Radiology 2004;232:635-652.

Shellock FG, Crues JV. Temperature, heart rate, and blood pressure changes associated with clinical MR imaging at 1.5-T. Radiology 1987;163:259-262.

Shellock FG, Crues JV. Corneal temperature changes associated with high-field MR imaging using a head coil. Radiology 1988;167:809-811.

Shellock FG, Crues JV. Temperature changes caused by clinical MR imaging of the brain at 1.5 Tesla using a head coil. Am J Neuroradiol 1988;9:287-291.

Shellock FG, Rothman B, Sarti D. Heating of the scrotum by high-field-strength MR imaging. Am J Roentgenol 1990;154:1229-1232.

Shellock FG, Schatz CJ. Increases in corneal temperature caused by MR imaging of the eye with a dedicated local coil. Radiology 192;185:697-699.

Shellock FG, Schaefer DJ. Radiofrequency energy-induced heating during magnetic resonance procedures: Laboratory and clinical experiences In: Shellock FG, Editor. Magnetic Resonance Procedures: Health Effects and Safety. Boca Raton, FL: CRC Press, 2001;75-96.

Shellock FG, Schaefer DJ, Crues JV. Alterations in body and skin temperatures caused by MR imaging: Is the recommended exposure for radiofrequency radiation too conservative? Br J Radiol 1989;62:904-909.

Shellock FG, Schaefer DJ, Kanal E. Physiologic responses to MR imaging performed at an SAR level of 6.0 W/kg. Radiology 1994;192:865-868.

Shrivastava D, et al. Radiofrequency heating at 9.4T: *In vivo* temperature measurement results in swine. Magn Reson Med 2008;59:73-8.

Shrivastava D, et al. Radio frequency heating at 9.4T (400.2 MHz): *In vivo* thermoregulatory temperature response in swine. Magn Reson Med 2009;62:888 95.

Shrivastava D, et al. Radiofrequency heating in porcine models with a "large" 32 cm internal diameter, 7T (296 MHz) head coil. Magn Reson Med 2011;66:255-63.

Shrivastava D, et al. *In vivo* radiofrequency heating in swine in a 3T (123.2-MHz) birdcage whole body coil. Magn Reson Med 2014;72:1141-50.

Shuman WP, et al. Superficial and deep-tissue increases in anesthetized dogs during exposure to high specific absorption rates in a 1.5-T MR imager. Radiology 1988;167:551-554.

Stuchly MA, Abrishamkar H, Strydom ML. Numerical evaluation of radio frequency power deposition in human models during MRI. Conf Proc IEEE Eng Med Biol Soc. 2006;1:272-275.

Tiberi G, et al. Investigation of maximum local specific absorption rate in 7 T magnetic resonance with respect to load size by use of electromagnetic simulations. Bioelectromagnetics 2015;36:358-66.

U.S. Department of Health and Human Services, Food and Drug Administration, Center for Devices and Radiological Health, Criteria for Significant Risk Investigations of Magnetic Resonance Diagnostic Devices, Guidance for Industry and Food and Drug Administration Staff. June 20, 2014.

van Lier AL, et al. Radiofrequency heating induced by 7-T head MRI: Thermal assessment using discrete vasculature or Pennes' bioheat equation. J Magn Reson Imag 2012;35:795-803.

van Rhoon GC, et al. CEM43°C thermal dose thresholds: A potential guide for magnetic resonance radiofrequency exposure levels? Eur Radiol 2013;23:2215-27.

Voigt T, et al. Patient-individual local SAR determination: *In vivo* measurements and numerical validation. Magn Reson Med 2012;68:1117-26.

Wang Z, Lin JC, Vaughan JT, Collins CM. Consideration of physiological response in numerical models of temperature during MRI of the human head.J Magnetic Resonance Imaging 2008;28:1303-1308.

Wang J. Issues with radiofrequency heating in MRI. J Appl Clin Med Phys 2014;15:5064.

Weintraub MI, Khoury A, Cole SP. Biologic effects of 3 Tesla (T) MR imaging comparing traditional 1.5-T and 0.6-T in 1,023 consecutive outpatients. J Neuroimaging 2007;17:241-5.

Wolf S, et al. SAR simulations for high-field MRI: How much detail, effort, and accuracy is needed? Magn Reson Med 2013;69:1157-68.

Zhang X, et al. Quantitative prediction of radio frequency induced local heating derived from measured magnetic field maps in magnetic resonance imaging: A phantom validation at 7 T. Appl Phys Lett 2014;105:244101.

B_{1+RMS}, The root-mean-square value of the MRI Effective Component of the RF Magnetic (B_1) Field

When performing magnetic resonance imaging (MRI) examinations on patients with implants and devices, it is important to be aware of, and to control, the amount of radiofrequency (RF) power that is utilized in order to ensure patient safety. The metric typically presented in MR Conditional labeling that addresses this matter is the whole body averaged specific absorption rate (SAR).

SAR is the rate at which energy is absorbed by the body when exposed to the RF electromagnetic field (B_1) and is measured in units of Watts per kilogram (W/kg) of body weight. SAR is patient-dependent and varies depending on the patient's size and mass (weight). Of note is that there is no direct way to measure SAR prior to or during an MRI procedure. As a result, MR system manufacturers rely on numerical models to conservatively estimate the SAR for a particular scan sequence and each manufacturer uses conservative assumptions for their SAR models to ensure that no patient is exposed to RF energy that exceeds the specified SAR limits.

When active implants and devices are present in patients, the use of SAR appears to be an unreliable means of characterizing RF-induced heating. Therefore, it is potentially dangerous to use SAR in these cases, as reported by Baker, et al. (2004). A number of years ago, the Joint Working Group comprised of scientists and individuals affiliated with MR system and device manufacturers, along with the FDA, recommended that B_{1+RMS} be used as a metric for implant heating as opposed to using SAR.

B_{1+RMS} is the root-mean-square value of the MRI effective component of the RF magnetic (B_1) field or, in other words, the time-averaged RF magnetic field component relevant for creating an MR image that is generated by the MR system during a scan. B_{1+RMS} is measured in units of micro-Tesla (μT). The MR scanner measures the B_{1+} field (the positively rotating RF magnetic field produced by the scanner) needed for an imaging sequence and uses the time averaged B_{1+} field, or B_{1+RMS}, that will occur due to a particular imaging sequence. Thus, the B_{1+RMS} value is calibrated by the MR system's software during the "prep" or "pre-scan" phase or measurements of an MRI exam. An important characteristic of of B_{1+RMS} is that it is not an estimated value but it is a known quantity based on the pulse sequence and the associated parameters. Furthermore, B_{1+RMS} is not patient-dependent nor is it calculated differently based on a given MR system manufacturer, as is the case with specific absorption rate levels.

Understanding the importance of B_{1+RMS} as it pertains to MR Conditional labeling of active implants and devices necessitates an appreciation of basic MRI physics. When a patient enters the MR scanner, protons in the body align in the direction of the static magnetic field (B_0), similar to a compass aligning with the Earth's magnetic field. An MR imaging sequence is composed of a series of RF pulses that produce a magnetic field that interacts with these magnetically-aligned protons and rotates them through a specific angle commonly referred to as the "flip angle". The RF magnetic field produced by the scanner is called the "B_1" field of which only one part, known as the positively rotating or "+" component, is useful for "flipping" the magnetically-aligned protons and allows MR images to be created. The maximum 10-second, time-averaged B_{1+} field strength of the RF pulses in the imaging sequence is the root-mean-square or "RMS" B_{1+} value of the imaging sequence.

In 2013, the International Electrotechnical Commission (IEC) mandated that all MR systems manufactured going forward must display the B_{1+RMS}. Therefore, it is unlikely to see this B_{1+RMS} information on older scanners or those with software that has not been recently updated.

B_{1+RMS} in MR Conditional Labeling for Active Implants

Considering that B_{1+RMS} is a more precise RF exposure metric than SAR, device manufacturers have begun to use values for B_{1+RMS} that must not be exceeded when scanning patients with active implants. When following B_{1+RMS} as a condition of use, the SAR value is irrelevant, unless, of course, a particular operating mode is also specified. Using B_{1+RMS} tends to provide better performance for the MRI exam because it has fewer limitations vs. using whole body averaged SAR values for patients with implants and devices.

The parameters that an MR system operator uses to modify B_{1+RMS} will vary with the particular MR system. By way of example, parameters and options that can be adjusted to reduce B_{1+RMS} include, the following:

1) Increase the RF pulse duration

2) Utilize a "Low SAR" mode or other similar option

3) Increase the repetition time (TR)

4) Reduce the number of slices for a given TR

5) Reduce the Echo Train Length (ETL)

6) Reduce the refocusing angle (FSE sequences)

7) Reduce the flip angle (e.g., for gradient echo pulse sequences)

8) Use a GRE sequence instead of a spin echo or fast spin echo pulse sequence

Besides being a presumably more precise RF exposure metric than SAR, another advantage to using B_{1+RMS} as opposed to SAR is that, once you adjust a particular sequence to a desired B_{1+RMS} value, that information can be saved in your protocol library for future use. The B_{1+RMS} will then remain at that value for the next patient unless the scan parameters are changed.

In summary, B_{1+RMS} is being used by device manufactures in their MR Conditional labeling for active implants. Therefore, it is vital to understand B_{1+RMS} and, if needed, how to adjust MRI protocols to achieve an acceptable B_{1+RMS} value in order to ensure patient safety.

[Portions excerpted with permission from William Faulkner, B.S., R.T. (R)(MR)(CT), FSMRT, MRSO (MRSC), William Faulkner and Associates, LLC, www.t2star.com and Medtronic, Inc.]

REFERENCES

Baker KB, et al. Evaluation of specific absorption rate as a dosimeter of MRI-related implant heating. J Magn Reson Imaging. 2004;20:315-20.

International Electrotechnical Commission. IEC 60601-2-33:2010. Particular requirements for the basic safety and essential performance of magnetic resonance equipment for medical diagnosis.

www.ismrm.org/smrt/E-Signals/2016FEBRUARY/eSig_5_1_hot_2.htm

www.medtronic.com/mrisurescan-us/pdf/3t-labeling-b1+rms.pdf

Acoustic Noise
and MR Procedures

Various types of acoustic noise are produced during the operation of an MR system. Problems associated with acoustic noise for patients and healthcare professionals include annoyance, verbal communication difficulties, heightened anxiety, temporary hearing loss and, in extreme cases, the potential for permanent hearing impairment.

Acoustic noise may pose a particular problem to specific patient groups. For example, patients with psychiatric disorders may become confused or suffer from increased anxiety because of exposure to loud noise. Sedated patients may experience discomfort in association with high noise levels.

In addition, neonates may have adverse reactions to acoustic noise. Reeves, et al. (2010) conducted a study to address this issue. The findings suggested that exposure of the fetus to 1.5-T MR imaging during the second and third trimesters of pregnancy is not associated with an increased risk of substantial neonatal hearing impairment or cochlear injury.

HEARING AND THE IMPACT OF ACOUSTIC NOISE

The human ear is a highly sensitive wide-band receiver, with the typical frequency range for normal hearing being between 20-Hz to 20,000-Hz. The ear does not tend to judge sound powers in absolute terms, but assesses how much greater one power is than another. The logarithmic decibel scale, dB, is used when referring to sound power.

Noise is defined in terms of frequency spectrum (in Hz), intensity (in dB), and time duration. Noise can be steady-state, intermittent, impulsive, or explosive. Transient hearing loss may occur following exposure to loud noise, resulting in a temporary threshold shift (i.e. a shift in the audible threshold).

With regard to acoustic noise associated with MR imaging, Brummett, et al. (1988) reported temporary shifts in hearing thresholds in 43% of the patients scanned without ear protection or with improperly fitted earplugs. Interestingly, a recent study by Jin, et al. (2017) reported that a 3-T MR neuroimaging examination with the acoustic noise at equivalent sound pressure levels ranging from 103.5 to 111.3 dBA lasting 51 minutes caused temporary hearing threshold shifts in healthy volunteers with hearing protection.

Fortunately, recovery from the effects of noise occurs in a relatively short period of time. However, if the noise insult is particularly severe, full recovery can take up to several weeks. If the noise is sufficiently injurious, a permanent threshold shift at specific frequencies may occur.

MRI-RELATED ACOUSTIC NOISE

The gradient magnetic field is the main source of acoustic noise associated with an MR procedure. This noise occurs during the rapid alterations of currents within the gradient coils. These currents, in the presence of the strong static magnetic field of the MR system, produce significant Lorentz forces that act upon the gradient coils. Acoustic noise, manifested as loud tapping, knocking, chirping, squeaking sounds, or other sounds is produced when the forces cause motion or vibration of the gradient coils as they impact against their mountings which, in turn, flex and vibrate.

Alteration of the gradient output (rise time or amplitude) by modifying MR imaging parameters causes the acoustic noise to vary. Noise tends to be enhanced by decreases in section thickness, field of view, repetition time, and echo time. In addition to dependence on imaging parameters, acoustic noise is dependent on the MR system hardware, construction, and the surrounding environment. Furthermore, noise characteristics have a spatial dependence. For example, noise levels can vary by as much as 10-dB as a function of patient position within the bore of the MR system. The presence and size of the patient may also affect the level of acoustic noise.

CHARACTERISTICS OF MR SYSTEM-RELATED ACOUSTIC NOISE

Gradient magnetic field-induced noise levels have been measured during a variety of pulse sequences for MR systems with static magnetic field strengths ranging from 0.35- to 4-Tesla. For example, Hurwitz, et al. (1989) reported that the MR imaging-related sound levels varied from 82 to 93-dB on the A-weighted scale and from 84- to 103-dB on the linear scale.

Later studies performed using a variety of MR parameters including "worst-case" pulse sequences that applied multiple gradients simultaneously (e.g., three-dimensional, fast gradient echo techniques) reported that these are among the loudest sequences, with acoustic noise levels that ranged from 103- to 113-dB (peak) on the A-weighted scale.

Additional studies measured acoustic noise generated by echo planar imaging (EPI) and fast spin echo sequences. Echo planar sequences tend to have extremely fast gradient switching times and high gradient amplitudes. Shellock, et al. (1998) reported high levels of noise ranging from 114- to 115-dBA on two different 1.5-Tesla MR systems tested during EPI sequences with parameters selected to represent "worst-case" protocols. At 3-Tesla, Hattori, et al. (2007) recorded sound levels that ranged from 126- to 131-dB on a linear scale, recommending the use of both earplugs and headphones for ear protection relative to the use of 3-Tesla MR systems when certain pulse sequences are used.

ACOUSTIC NOISE AND PERMISSIBLE LIMITS

In general, acoustic noise levels recorded in the MR environment have been below the maximum limits permitted by the Occupational Safety and Health Administration of the United States, especially when one considers that the duration of exposure is an important factor that determines the effect of noise on hearing.

The guidelines from the U.S. Food and Drug Administration for acoustic noise levels that should not be exceeded in association with the operation of MR systems are, as follows:

Sound Pressure Level - Peak unweighted sound pressure level greater than 140-dB. A-weighted root mean square (rms) sound pressure level greater than 99-dBA with hearing protection in place.

While the acoustic noise levels recommended for patients undergoing MR procedures on an infrequent and short-term basis may appear to be somewhat conservative, they are deemed appropriate when one considers that individuals with underlying health conditions may have problems with noise at certain levels or frequencies. Acoustic noise produced during MR procedures represents a potential risk to such patients. As previously mentioned, the possibility exists that substantial gradient magnetic field-induced noise may produce hearing problems in patients who are susceptible to the damaging effects of loud noises.

The exposure of staff and other healthcare workers in the MR environment is also a concern (e.g., those involved in interventional MR procedures or who remain in the room for patient management reasons). Accordingly, if loud noises exist in the MR environment, staff members should routinely wear hearing protection if they remain in the room during the operation of the scanner. In the United Kingdom, guidelines issued by the Department of Health recommend hearing protection be worn by staff exposed to an average of 85-dB over an eight hour day.

ACOUSTIC NOISE CONTROL TECHNIQUES

Passive noise control. The simplest and least expensive means of preventing problems associated with acoustic noise during MR procedures is routinely to use disposable earplugs or headphones. Earplugs, when properly used, can abate noise by 10- to 30-dB, which is usually an adequate amount of sound attenuation for the MR environment. Properly worn foam earplugs typically provide a sufficient decrease in acoustic noise that, in turn, is capable of preventing hearing problems. Therefore, for MR systems that generate substantial acoustic noise, patients should be required to wear these protective devices.

Unfortunately, passive noise control methods suffer from a number of limitations. For example, these devices hamper verbal communication with patients during the operation of the MR system. Additionally, standard earplugs are often too large for the ear canal of adolescents, infants, and neonates. In these patient populations, other types of hearing protection must be used such as MiniMuffs Neonatal Noise Attenuators.

Importantly, passive noise control devices provide non-uniform noise attenuation over the hearing range. While high frequencies may be well attenuated, attenuation is often poor at low frequencies. This is problematic because, for certain pulse sequences, the low frequency range is where the peak MR imaging-related acoustic noise is generated.

Active Noise Control (ANC). A significant reduction in the level of acoustic noise caused by MR procedures has been accomplished using active noise cancellation. Controlling noise from a particular source by introducing "anti-phase noise" to interfere destructively with the noise source is not a new idea with regard to MR systems. For example, in 1989, Goldman, et al. combined passive noise control and an active noise control system (i.e. an active system built into a headphone) to achieve an average noise reduction of approximately 14-dB.

Advances in digital signal processing technology allow efficient active noise control systems to be realized at a moderate cost. The anti-noise system involves a continuous feedback loop with continuous sampling of the sounds in the noise environment so that the gradient magnetic field-induced noise is attenuated. It is possible to attenuate the pseudo-periodic scanner noise while allowing the transmission of vocal communication or music to be maintained.

"Quiet" Pulse Sequences. Several investigators have described the development of "quiet" pulse sequences which substantially decrease acoustic noise and are acceptable for MR imaging and functional MRI examinations. These techniques are particularly interesting insofar as they may be utilized with echo planar imaging and other pulse sequences.

Silent Scan. Recently, Alibek, et al. (2014) described the use of "Silent Scan" technology which uses decreased gradient excitation levels to minimize acoustic noise associated with MR imaging. The acoustic noise levels were reduced significantly using a "Silenz" sequence compared with a conventional pulse sequence, according to the investigators. In another study, Costagli, et al. (2016) reported that acoustic noise was dramatically reduced using "Silent" T1-weighted brain imaging at 7-Tesla compared with conventional imaging. Thus, new techniques now exist that reduce acoustic noise and improve patient comfort.

OTHER SOURCES OF MR SYSTEM-RELATED ACOUSTIC NOISE

RF hearing. When the human head is subjected to pulsed radiofrequency (RF) radiation at certain frequencies, an audible sound perceived as a click, buzz, chirp, or knocking noise may be heard. This acoustic phenomenon is referred to as "RF hearing", "RF sound" or "microwave hearing".

Thermoelastic expansion is believed to be responsible for the production of RF hearing, whereby there is absorption of RF energy that produces a minute temperature elevation (i.e. approximately 1×10^{-6} degrees C) over a brief time period in the tissues of the head causing a hearing sensation. Subsequently, a pressure wave is induced that is sensed by the hair cells of the cochlea via bone conduction. In this manner, a pulse of RF energy is transferred into an acoustic wave within the human head and sensed by the hearing organs.

With specific reference to the operation of MR scanners, RF hearing has been found to be associated with frequencies ranging from 2.4- to 170-MHz. The gradient magnetic field-induced acoustic noise that occurs during an MR procedure is significantly louder than the sounds associated with RF hearing. Therefore, noises produced by this RF auditory phenomenon are effectively masked and not perceived by patients. Currently, there is no evidence of any detrimental health effect related to the presence of RF hearing.

Noise From Subsidiary Systems. Patient comfort fans and cryogen reclamation systems associated with superconducting magnets of MR systems are the main sources of ambient acoustic noise found in the MR environment. Acoustic noise produced by these subsidiary systems is considerably less than that caused by gradient magnetic fields.

REFERENCES

Alibek S, et al. Acoustic noise reduction in MRI using Silent Scan: An initial experience. Diagn Interv Radiol 2014;20:360-3.

Bandettini PA, et al. Functional MRI of brain activation induced by scanner acoustic noise. Magn Reson Med 1998;39:410-416.

Bongers S, et al. Hearing loss associated with repeated MRI acquisition procedure-related acoustic noise exposure: An occupational cohort study. Occup Environ Med 2017 (In press).

Bowtell RW, Mansfield PM. Quiet transverse gradient coils: Lorentz force balancing designs using geometric similitude. Magn Reson Med 1995;34:494-497.

Brummett RE, Talbot JM, Charuhas P. Potential hearing loss resulting from MR imaging. Radiology 1988;169:539-540.

Chaplain GBB. Anti-noise: The Essex breakthrough. Chart Mech Engin 1983;30:41-47.

Chen CK, Chiueh TD, Chen JH. Active cancellation system of acoustic noise in MR imaging. IEEE Trans Biomed Engin 1999;46:186-190.

Cho ZH, et al. Analysis of acoustic noise in MRI. Magnetic Resonance Imaging 1997;15:815-822.

Costagli M, et al. Assessment of Silent T1-weighted head imaging at 7 T. Eur Radiol 2016;26:1879-88.

Counter SA, Olofsson A, Grahn, Borg E. MRI acoustic noise: Sound pressure and frequency analysis. J Magn Reson Imag 1997;7:606-611.

Elder JA. Special senses. In: United States Environmental Protection Agency, Health Effects Research Laboratory. Biological Effects of Radio frequency Radiation. EPA-600/8-83-026F, Research Triangle Park, 1984, pp. 570-571.

Goldman AM, Gossman WE, Friedlander PC. Reduction of sound levels with anti-noise in MR imaging. Radiology 1989;173:549-550.

Hall DA, et al. Acoustic, psychophysical, and neuroimaging measurements of the effectiveness of active cancellation during auditory functional magnetic resonance imaging. J Acoust Soc Am. 2009;125:347-59.

Hattori Y, Fukatsu H, Ishigaki T. Measurement and evaluation of the acoustic noise of a 3 Tesla MR scanner. Nagoya J Med Sci 2007;69:23-28.

Hedeen RA, Edelstein WA. Characteristics and prediction of gradient acoustic noise in MR imagers. Magn Reson Med 1997;37:7-10.

Heismann B, et al. Sequence-based acoustic noise reduction of clinical MRI scans. Magn Reson Med 2015;73:1104-9

Hutter J, et al. Quiet echo planar imaging for functional and diffusion MRI. Magn Reson Med 2017 (In press).

Hurwitz R, Lane SR, Bell RA, Brant-Zawadzki MN. Acoustic analysis of gradient-coil noise in MR imaging. Radiology 1989;173:545-548.

International Commission on Non-Ionizing Radiation Protection (ICNIRP) statement, medical magnetic resonance procedures: Protection of patients. Health Physics 2004;87:197-216.

Ireland CM, et al. A novel acoustically quiet coil for neonatal MRI system. Concepts Magn Reson Part B Magn Reson Eng 2015;45:107-114.

Jin C, et al. Temporary hearing threshold shift in healthy volunteers with hearing protection caused by acoustic noise exposure during 3-T multisequence MR neuroimaging. Radiology 2017 (In press).

Kaye EA, et al. Adapting MRI acoustic radiation force imaging for *in vivo* human brain focused ultrasound applications. Magn Reson Med 2013;69:724-33.

Lauer AM, et al. MRI acoustic noise can harm experimental and companion animals. J Magn Reson Imag 2012;36:743.

Leithner K, et al. Psychological reactions in women undergoing fetal magnetic resonance imaging. Obstet Gynecol 2008;111(2 Pt 1):396-402.

Lim EY, et al. 3 Tesla magnetic resonance imaging noise in standard head and neck sequence does not cause temporary threshold shift in high frequency. Eur Arch Otorhinolaryngol 2015;272;3109-13.

Lin CY, Chen JH. Real-time active noise control of magnetic resonance imaging acoustic noise. J Acoust Soc Am. 2012;132:1971.

Mansfield PM, Glover PM. Beaumont J Sound generation in gradient coil structures for MRI. Magn Reson Med 1998;39:539-550.

Mansfield PM, et al. Active acoustic screening: Design principles for quiet gradient coils in MRI. Meas Sci Technol 1994;5:1021-1025.

McJury MJ. Acoustic noise levels generated during high field MR imaging. Clinical Radiology 1995;50:331-334.

McJury M. Acoustic Noise and Magnetic Resonance Procedures. In: Magnetic Resonance Procedures: Health Effects and Safety. FG Shellock, Editor, CRC Press, Boca Raton, FL, 2001.

McJury M, Blug A, Joerger C, Condon B, Wyper D. Acoustic noise levels during magnetic resonance imaging scanning at 1.5 T. Brit J Radiol 1994;413-415.

McJury M, Shellock FG. Acoustic noise and MR procedures: A review. J Magn Reson Imag 2000;12:37-45.

McJury M, et al. The use of active noise control (ANC) to reduce acoustic noise generated during MRI scanning: Some initial results. Magnetic Resonance Imaging 1997;15:319-322.

Melnick W. Hearing loss from noise exposure. In: Harris CM, Editor. Handbook of Noise Control. New York: McGraw-Hill, 1979, pp. 2.

Miller LE, Keller AM. Regulation of occupational noise. In: Harris CM, Editor. Handbook of noise control. New York: McGraw-Hill, 1979, pp. 1-16.

Moelker A, et al. Verbal communication in MR environments: Effect of MR system acoustic noise on understanding. Radiology 2004;232:107-113.

Moelker A, Pattynama PM. Acoustic noise concerns in functional magnetic resonance imaging. Human Brain Mapping 2003;20:123-141.

More SR, et al. Acoustic noise characteristics of a 4 Tesla MRI scanner. J Magn Reson Imag 2006;23:388-397.

Ott M, et al. Acoustic noise reduction in T1- and proton-density-weighted turbo spin-echo imaging. MAGMA 2016;29:5-15.

Peelle JE, et al. Evaluating an acoustically quiet EPI sequence for use in fMRI studies of speech and auditory processing. Neuroimage 2010;52:1410-9.

Philbin MK, Taber KH, Hayman LA. Preliminary report: Changes in vital signs of term newborns during MR. Am J Neuroradiol 1996;17:1033-6.

Pierre EY, et al. Parallel imaging-based reduction of acoustic noise for clinical magnetic resonance imaging. Invest Radiol 2014;49:620-6.

Quirk ME, Letendre AJ, Ciottone RA, Lingley JF. Anxiety in patients undergoing MR imaging. Radiology 1989;170:464-466.

Reeves MJ, et al. Neonatal cochlear function: Measurement after exposure to acoustic noise during in utero MR imaging. Radiology 2010;257:802-9.

Robinson DW. Characteristics of occupational noise-induced hearing loss. In: Effects of Noise on Hearing. Henderson D, Hamernik RP, Dosjanjh DS, Mills JH, Editors. Raven Press, New York, 1976, pp. 383-405.

Rondinoni C, et al. Effect of scanner acoustic background noise on strict resting-state fMRI. Braz J Med Biol Res 2013;46:359-67.

Roschmann P. Human auditory system response to pulsed radio frequency energy in RF coils for magnetic resonance at 2.4 to 170 MHz. Magn Reson Med 1991;21:197-215.

Ruckhäberle E, et al. *In vivo* intrauterine sound pressure and temperature measurements during magnetic resonance imaging (1.5 T) in pregnant ewes. Fetal Diagn Ther 2008;24:203-10.

Schmitter S, Bock M. Acoustic noise-optimized verse pulses. Magn Reson Med 2010;64:1446-52.

Segbers M, et al. Shaping and timing gradient pulses to reduce MRI acoustic noise. Magn Reson Med 2010;64:546-53.

Shellock FG, Kanal E. Policies, guidelines, and recommendations for MR imaging safety and patient management. J Magn Reson Imag 1991;1:97-101.

Shellock FG, Morisoli SM, Ziarati M. Measurement of acoustic noise during MR imaging: Evaluation of six "worst-case" pulse sequences. Radiology 1994;191:91-93.

Shellock FG, et al. Determination of gradient magnetic field-induced acoustic noise associated with the use of echo planar and three-dimensional fast spin echo techniques. J Magn Reson Imag 1998;8:1154-1157.

Strainer JC, et al. Functional MR of the primary auditory cortex: An analysis of pure tone activation and tone discrimination. Am J Roentgenol 1997;18:601-610.

Strizek B, et al. Safety of MR imaging at 1.5 T in fetuses: A retrospective case-control study of birth weights and the effects of acoustic noise. Radiology 2015;275:530-7.

Tkach JA, et al. Characterization of acoustic noise in a neonatal intensive care unit MRI system. Pediatr Radiol 2014;44:1011-9

Tomasi DG, Ernst T. Echo planar imaging at 4 Tesla with minimal acoustic noise. J Magn Reson Imag 2003;128-130.

Ulmer JL, et al. Acoustic echo planar scanner noise and pure tone hearing thresholds: The effects of sequence repetition times and acoustic noise rates. J Comp Assist Tomogr 1998;22:480-486.

U.S. Department of Health and Human Services, Food and Drug Administration, Center for Devices and Radiological Health, Criteria for Significant Risk Investigations of Magnetic Resonance Diagnostic Devices, Guidance for Industry and Food and Drug Administration Staff, June 20, 2014.

Zapp J, et al. Sinusoidal echo-planar imaging with parallel acquisition technique for reduced acoustic noise in auditory fMRI. J Magn Reson Imag 2012;36:581-8.

Body Piercing Jewelry

Ritual or decorative body piercing is extremely popular as a form of self-expression. Different types of materials are used to make body piercing jewelry including ferromagnetic and nonferromagnetic metals, as well as nonmetallic materials. The presence of body piercing jewelry that is made from ferromagnetic or conductive material of a certain shape may present a problem for a patient referred for a magnetic resonance (MR) procedure or an individual in the MR environment.

Risks include uncomfortable sensations from movement or displacement that may be mild-to-moderate depending on the site of the body piercing and the ferromagnetic qualities of the jewelry (e.g., mass, degree of magnetic susceptibility, etc.). In extreme cases, serious injuries may occur. In addition, for body piercing jewelry made from electrically conducting material, there is a possibility of MRI-related heating that could cause excessive temperature increases and burns.

Because of potential safety issues, metallic body piercing jewelry should be removed prior to entering the MR environment. However, patients or individuals with body piercings are often reluctant to remove their jewelry. Therefore, if it is not possible to remove metallic body piercing jewelry, the patient or individual should be informed regarding the potential risks. In addition, if the body piercing jewelry is made from ferromagnetic material, some means of stabilization (e.g., application of adhesive tape or bandage) should be used to prevent movement or displacement.

To avoid potential heating of body piercing jewelry made from conductive materials, it is recommended to use gauze, tape, or other similar material to wrap the jewelry in such a manner as to insulate it (i.e. prevent contact) from the underlying skin. The patient should be instructed to immediately inform the MR system operator if heating or other unusual sensation occurs in association with the body piercing jewelry.

According to Muensterer (2004), even temporary or short-term piercing jewelry removal may lead to closure of the subcutaneous tract. Therefore, temporary replacement with a nonmetallic spacer may be indicated. This can be accomplished using the following procedure, as it was applied to umbilical piercing jewelry: (1) Disinfect the piercing and umbilical area with 70% isopropyl alcohol, (2) Open the piercing jewelry by removing the bead from the bar, (3) Place the tip of a tight-fitting intravenous catheter (14 or 16 gauge, without the needle) over the threaded tip of the bar, (4) Advance the intravenous catheter caudally, pushing the piercing out of the skin tract, and (5) Remove the jewelry and leaving the intravenous catheter in the subcutaneous skin tract as a spacer. After the intervention (or MRI examination), reinserted the umbilical piercing jewelry by following the described steps in reverse. Piercing jewelry located in other areas on the body may be replaced for MR examinations in the same way, with minor modifications. Of course, the above procedure should only be performed under the guidance and direction of a physician.

REFERENCES

Armstrong ML, Elkins L. Body art and MRI. Am J Nurs 2005;105:65-6.

Deboer S, Seaver M, Angel E, Armstrong M. Puncturing myths about body piercing and tattooing. Nursing 2008;38:50-54.

Laumann AE, Derick AJ. Tattoos and body piercings in the United States: A national data set. J Am Acad Dermatol 2006;55:413-21.

Muensterer OJ. Temporary removal of navel piercing jewelry for surgery and imaging studies. Pediatrics 2004;114:e384-6.

Shellock FG. MR safety and body piercing jewelry. Signals, No. 45, Issue 2, pp. 7, 2003.

Claustrophobia, Anxiety, and Emotional Distress in the MR Environment

For certain patients that undergo magnetic resonance (MR) examinations, the experience may be associated with emotional distress. Referring physicians, radiologists, and MRI technologists can best manage affected patients by understanding the etiology of the problem and knowing the appropriate maneuver or intervention to implement in order to counter-act the condition.

The experience of "psychological distress" in the MR environment includes all subjectively unpleasant experiences attributable to the procedure. Distress for the patient can range from mild anxiety that can be handled with simple reassurance, to a more serious panic attack that may require psychiatric intervention or medication. Severe psychological reactions to MR examinations are characterized by the rapid onset of at least four of the following: nausea, paresthesias, palpitations, chest pain, faintness, dyspnea, choking sensation, sweating, trembling, vertigo, depersonalization, and fear of losing control or dying.

Many symptoms of a panic attack mimic over-activity of the sympathetic nervous system, prompting concern that catecholamine responses may precipitate cardiac arrhythmias or ischemia in susceptible patients. However, to date, this has not been observed in the clinical MR setting. Nevertheless, for a medically unstable patient, it is advisable to have physiologic monitoring and support readily available.

In the mildest form, distress is the normal amount of anxiety that a person may experience when undergoing a diagnostic procedure. Moderate distress, severe enough to be described as a dysphoric psychological reaction, has been reported by as many as 65% of the patients examined by MR imaging. The most severe forms of psychological distress described by patients include anxiety, claustrophobia, or panic attacks.

Claustrophobia is a disorder characterized by the marked, persistent, and excessive fear of enclosed spaces. In such affected individuals, exposure to an enclosed space such as that found with certain MR systems, almost invariably provokes an immediate anxiety response that, in its most extreme form, is indistinguishable from the panic attack described above.

The actual incidence of distress in the MR environment is highly variable across studies due to differences in outcome measurements used to describe this phenomenon. Some investigations indicated that as many as 20% of the individuals attempting to undergo MR procedures can't complete the exams secondary to serious distress such as claustrophobia or other unwanted sensations. In contrast, other investigations have reported that as few as 0.7% of individuals have incomplete or failed MR procedures due to distress.

THE IMPACT OF EMOTIONAL DISTRESS

Patient distress can contribute to adverse outcomes for the MR procedure. These adverse outcomes include unintentional exacerbation of patient distress, a compromise in the quality and, thus, the diagnostic aspects of the imaging study and decreased efficiency of the MRI facility due to delayed, prematurely terminated, or cancelled studies. Patient compliance during an MR procedure, such as the ability to remain in the MR system and to hold still long enough to complete the study, is of paramount importance to achieve a diagnostically acceptable examination. If a good quality study can't be obtained, the patient may require an invasive procedure in place of the inherently safer MR examination. Thus, for the distressed patient unable to undergo an MR procedure, there may be clinical, medico-legal, and economic related implications.

Increasing pressure to use MR system time efficiently to cover the costs of this expensive diagnostic imaging equipment puts greater stress on both staff and patients. The ability of referring physicians, radiologists, and MRI technologists to detect patient distress at the earliest possible time, to discover the source of the distress, and to provide appropriate intervention can greatly improve patient comfort, the quality of imaging, and efficiency of the facility.

FACTORS THAT CONTRIBUTE TO DISTRESS

Many factors contribute to distress experienced by certain patients undergoing MR procedures. Most commonly cited are concerns about the physical environment of the MR system. Also well documented is the anxiety associated with the underlying medical problem necessitating the MR examination. Certain individuals, such as those with psychiatric illnesses, may be predisposed to suffer greater distress.

The physical environment of the MR system is clearly one important source of distress. Sensations of apprehension, tension, worry, claustrophobia, anxiety, fear, and panic attacks have been directly attributed to the confining dimensions of the MR system. For example, for some scanners, the patient's "line of sight" may be three to ten inches from the inside of the MR system, prompting feelings of uncontrolled confinement and detachment.

Similar distressing sensations have been attributed to other aspects of the MR environment including the prolonged duration of the examination, the acoustic noise, the temperature and humidity within the MR system, and the stress related to restriction of movement. Additionally, being inside of the scanner may produce a feeling of sensory deprivation which is also known to be a precursor of anxiety states.

Adverse psychological reactions are sometimes associated with MR procedures simply because the examination may be perceived by the patient as a "dramatic" medical test with an associated uncertainty of outcome, such that there may be fear of the presence of disease or other condition. In fact, any type of diagnostic procedure can produce anxiety for the patient.

MR systems that have an architecture that utilizes a vertical magnetic field offer a more open design that is presumed to reduce the frequency of distress associated with MR procedures. The latest versions of these "open" MR systems, despite having static magnetic field strengths of 0.3-Tesla or lower, have improved technology (i.e. faster gradient fields, optimized surface coils, etc.) that permit acceptable image quality for most types of standard, diagnostic imaging procedures. The latest generation of high-field-strength (1.5-Tesla and 3-Tesla) MR systems have shorter and wider bore configurations that likely mitigate feelings of being enclosed or being overly confined. In fact, Hunt, et al. (2011) reported that the use of a 1.5-Tesla, wide-short-bore scanner increased the examination success rate in patients with claustrophobia and substantially reduced the need for anesthesia-assisted MRI examinations, even when claustrophobia was severe. However, Enders, et al. (2011) indicated that there was no substantial difference between claustrophobia in patients undergoing MRI using a short-bore versus an open MR system.

In 1993, a specially designed, low-field-strength (0.2-Tesla) MR system (Artoscan, Lunar Corporation/General Electric Medical Systems, Madison, WI and Esaote, Genoa, Italy) became commercially available for MR imaging of extremities. The use of this dedicated extremity MR system provides an accurate, reliable, and relatively inexpensive means (i.e. in comparison to the use of a whole-body MR system) of evaluating musculoskeletal abnormalities.

The architecture of the extremity MR system has no confining features or other aspects that would typically create patient-related problems. This is because only the body part that requires imaging is placed inside the bore of the magnet during the MR examination. One research study reported that 100% of the MR examinations were completed without being interrupted or cancelled for patient-related problems. The unique design of the extremity MR system is believed to have contributed to the successful completion of the MR procedures in the patients of this study.

Patients with pre-existing psychiatric disorders may be at greater risk for experiencing distress in the MR environment. Accordingly, patients with pre-existing conditions should be identified prior to MR examinations to implement anxiety-minimizing efforts (see below). Patients with other psychiatric illnesses such as depression and any illness complicated by thought dysfunction, such as schizophrenia or manic-depressive disorder, may also be at increased risk for distress in the MR environment.

Patients with psychiatric illnesses may, under normal circumstances, be able to tolerate the MR environment without a problem, as is clear from the thousands of subjects who participate in clinical neuroimaging and functional MRI research studies each year. However, the increased stress due to their medical illness or fear of medical illness can exacerbate their psychiatric symptoms to such an extent that they may have difficulty complying with MR procedures.

TECHNIQUES TO MINIMIZE PATIENT DISTRESS

Various procedures exist to minimize distress or anxiety in patients undergoing MR procedures (**Table 1**). Some measures should be employed for all examinations, while others may be required only if the patient experiences distress due to the factors described above.

Table 1. Techniques to manage patients with distress associated with MR procedures.

1) Prepare and educate the patient concerning specific aspects of the MR procedure (e.g., MR system dimensions, gradient noise, intercom system, constant monitoring by the MRI technologist, etc.).
2) Allow an appropriately screened relative or friend to remain with the patient during the MR examination.
3) Maintain verbal, visual, and/or physical contact with the patient during the MR procedure.
4) Use an appropriate stereo system to provide music to the patient.
5) Use an appropriate video monitor or goggles to provide a visual distraction to the patient.

6) Use a virtual reality environment system to provide audio and visual distraction.
7) Place the patient prone for the examination.
8) Position the patient feet-first instead of head-first into the MR system.
9) Use mirrors or prism glasses to redirect the patient's line of sight.
10) Use a blindfold so that the patient is not aware of the surroundings.
11) Use bright lights inside of the MR system.
12) Use a fan inside of the MR system.
13) Use vanilla scented oil or other aroma therapy.
14) Use relaxation techniques such as controlled breathing or mental imagery.
15) Use systematic desensitization.
16) Use medical hypnosis.
17) Use a sedative or other similar medication.

For All Patients Undergoing MR Procedures

Referring clinicians should take time to explain the reason for the MR procedure and what he/she expects to learn from the results with respect to the implications for treatment and prognosis. The single most important step is to educate the patient about the aspects of the MR examination that may be challenging or difficult. This includes conveying, in terms that are understandable to the patient, the internal dimensions of the MR system, the level of gradient magnetic field-induced acoustic noise to expect, and the estimated time duration of the examination.

Studies have documented a decrease in the incidence of premature termination of MR examinations when patients were provided with detailed information about the procedures. Accordingly, patients should be provided with an appropriate brochure or video presentation supplemented by a question and answer session with an MR-trained healthcare professional prior to the examination.

Many details of patient positioning in the MR system can increase comfort and, thus, minimize distress. Taking time to ensure comfortable positioning with sufficient padding and blankets to alleviate undue discomfort or pain is also important. Adequate ear protection should be provided routinely to decrease acoustic noise from the MR system, as needed (i.e. this is typically not required for low-field-strength MR scanners). Demonstration of the two-way intercom system, "squeeze ball", or other monitoring technique to reassure the patient that the MR staff is readily available during the examination is vital for proper patient management.

For Mildly-to-Moderately Distressed Patients

If a patient continues to experience distress after the afore-mentioned measures are implemented, additional interventions are required. Frequently, all that is necessary to successfully complete an MR examination is to allow an appropriately screened relative or friend to remain with the patient. A familiar person in the MR system room will often help an anxious patient develop an increased sense of security. If a supportive companion is not present, a staff member can maintain contact with the patient during the examination to decrease psychological distress.

Placing the patient prone so that the opening of the MR system can be seen will provide a sensation of being in a device that is more spacious. As such, prone positioning can alleviate the "closed-in" feelings frequently associated with being supine. Unfortunately, prone positioning may not be practical or appropriate if the patient has certain underlying medical conditions (e.g., shortness of breath, the presence of chest tubes, wearing a cervical fixation device, etc.). Another method of positioning the patient that may help is to place the individual feet-first instead of head-first into the scanner.

Mirrors or prism glasses can be used to permit the patient to maintain a vertical view of the outside of the MR system in order to minimize phobic responses. Using a blindfold or "eye pillow" (e.g., small pillow containing flax seeds) so that the patient is unaware of the close surroundings has also been suggested to be an effective technique for enabling anxious patients to successfully undergo MR procedures.

The environment of the MR system may be changed to optimize the management of apprehensive patients. For example, the presence of higher lighting levels tends to make most individuals feel less anxious. Therefore, the use of bright lights at either end and inside of the MR system can produce a less imposing environment for the patient. Using a fan inside of the scanner to increase airflow will also help reduce the sensation of confinement. In addition, aroma therapy (e.g., placing a cotton pad moistened with a few drops of lemon, vanilla, or cucumber oil in the MR system) can help reduce distress by providing the patient with a pleasant, olfactory stimulation.

Specialized systems that transmit music or audio communication through headphones have been developed specifically for use with MR systems.

Reports have indicated that these devices successfully reduced symptoms of anxiety in patients during MR procedures. Furthermore, it is possible to provide visual stimulation to the patient via monitors or special goggles. Use of visual stimuli to distract patients tends to reduce distress. Finally, a system may be used to provide a calming virtual reality environment for the patient that may likewise serve as an acceptable means of audio and visual distraction from the MR procedure (this device is frequently used for functional MRI studies).

For Severely Distressed or Claustrophobic Patients

Patients who are at high risk for severe distress in the MR environment and can be identified by their referring clinician or by the scheduling MR staff person should be offered the opportunity to have pre-MR procedure behavioral therapy. MR procedures conducted in patients that previously refused or were unable to tolerate the MR environment have been reported to be successfully managed using relaxation techniques, systematic desensitization, and medical hypnosis.

In the majority of MRI facilities, patients severely affected by claustrophobia, anxiety, or panic attacks in response to MR procedures usually need sedation when attempts to counteract their distress fail. Using a short-acting sedative or an anxiolytic medication may be the only means of managing a patient with a high degree of anxiety.

Importantly, the use of sedation in the MR environment requires special preparation involving several important patient management considerations. For example, the time when the patient is administered the medication for optimal effect prior to the examination must be considered along with the possibility that an adverse reaction may occur. The use of acceptable monitoring equipment operated by appropriately trained and experienced healthcare professionals is required to ensure patient safety. In addition, provisions must be available for an area to permit adequate recovery of the patient after an MR procedure that involves sedation.

REFERENCES

Adamietz B, et al. Tolerance of magnetic resonance imaging in children and adolescents performed in a 1.5 Tesla MR scanner with an open design. Rofo 2007;179:826-831.

Bangard C, et al. MR imaging of claustrophobic patients in an open 1.0T scanner: Motion artifacts and patient acceptability compared with closed bore magnets. Eur J Radiol 2007;64:152-7.

Bigley J, et al. Neurolinguistic programming used to reduce the need for anaesthesia in claustrophobic patients undergoing MRI. 2010;83:113-7.

Dewey M, et al. Claustrophobia during magnetic resonance imaging: Cohort study in over 55,000 patients. J Magn Reson Imag 2007;26:1322-7.

Enders J, et al. Reduction of claustrophobia with short-bore versus open magnetic resonance imaging: A randomized controlled trial. PLoS One 2011;6:e23494

Eshed I, et al. Claustrophobia and premature termination of magnetic resonance imaging examinations. J Magn Reson Imag 2007;26:401-404.

Gollub RL, Shellock FG. Claustrophobia, Anxiety, and Emotional Distress in the Magnetic Resonance Environment. In, Magnetic Resonance Procedures: Health Effects and Safety. FG Shellock, Editor, CRC Press, Boca Raton, FL, 2001.

Harris LM, Cumming SR, Menzies RG. Predicting anxiety in magnetic resonance imaging scans. International Journal of Behavioral Medicine 2004;11:1-7.

Hunt CH, et al. Wide, short bore magnetic resonance at 1.5 T: Reducing the failure rate in claustrophobic patients. Clin Neuroradiol 2011;21;141-4.

Klaming L, et al. The relation between anticipatory anxiety and movement during an MR examination. Acad Radiol 2015 Dec;22(12):1571-8.

McGuinness TP. Hypnosis in the treatment of phobias: A review of the literature. Am J Clin Hypnosis 1984;26:261.

Munn Z, et al. Interventions to reduce anxiety, distress and the need for sedation in adult patients undergoing magnetic resonance imaging: A systematic review. Int J Evid Based Healthcare 2013;11:265-74.

Murphy KJ, Brunberg JA. Adult claustrophobia, anxiety and sedation in MRI. Magnetic Resonance Imaging 1997;15:51.

Parmar R, et al. Foot massage, touch, and presence in decreasing anxiety during a magnetic resonance imaging: A feasibility study. J Altern Complement Med 2017 (In press).

Sarji SA, Abdullah BJ, Kumar G, et al. Failed magnetic resonance imaging examinations due to claustrophobia. Australas Radiol 1998;42:293.

Shellock FG, Stone KR, Resnick D, et al. Subjective perceptions of MRI examinations performed using an extremity MR system. Signals 2000;32:16.

Spouse E, Gedroyc WM. MRI of the claustrophobic patient: Interventionally configured magnets. Br J Radiol 2000;73:146-151.

Szeszak S, et al. Animated educational video to prepare children for MRI without sedation: Evaluation of the appeal and value. Pediatr Radiol 2016;46:1744-1750.

Tazegul G, et al. Can MRI related patient anxiety be prevented? Magn Reson Imaging 2015;33:180-3.

Thorpe S, Salkovskis PM, Dittner A. Claustrophobia in MRI: The role of cognitions. Magnetic Resonance Imaging 2008;26:1081-8.

Viggiano MP, et al. Impact of psychological interventions on reducing anxiety, fear and the need for sedation in children undergoing magnetic resonance imaging. Pediatr Rep 2015;7:5682.

Weinreb J, et al. Magnetic resonance imaging: Improving patient tolerance and safety. Am J Roentgenol 1984;143:1285.

Epicardial Pacing Leads and Intracardiac Pacing Leads

Temporary Epicardial Pacing Leads and Temporary Intracardiac Pacing Leads

Although there is a theoretical risk that MRI examinations in patients with retained temporary *epicardial* leads (which consist of electrically conductive materials) could lead to cardiac excitation or thermal injury, such retained leads which are relatively short in length and do not form large conducting loops have not been found to pose a substantial hazard to patients during MRI procedures.

In 1997, Hartnell, et al. reported findings in 51 patients with retained temporary epicardial pacing wires who underwent clinical MRI procedures. Of those patients examined with electrocardiographic monitoring, no arrhythmias were noted, and for all patients, no symptoms suggestive of arrhythmia or other cardiac dysfunction were identified (although the anatomic region examined and the levels of RF power deposition used in the examinations were not specifically described). While the data in the Hartnell, et al. article may be somewhat flawed and, thus, should be considered mostly anecdotal, to date, there is no report of a complication associated with performing MRI in a patient with retained temporary epicardial leads.

By comparison, an *ex vivo* study of temporary *intracardiac* (i.e., endocardial), pacing leads reported temperature increases of up to 63.1 degrees C. Preliminary results of an investigation confirmed that even unconnected temporary transvenous pacing (as well as permanent pacing leads) leads can undergo high temperature increases at 1.5-Tesla/64-MHz. In a chronic-pacemaker animal model undergoing an MRI examination at 1.5-Tesla, temperature increases of up to 20 degrees C were recorded, although pathological and histological examination did not demonstrate heat-induced damage of the myocardium. The MRI conditions that generated such elevated lead temperatures included the use of the transmit body RF coil to deliver RF energy over the area of the intracardiac pacing lead (e.g., as would be used during an MRI examination of the chest/thorax).

To the best of knowledge of the members of a multi-disciplinary group of experts (i.e. the Consensus Group: Levine GN, Gomes AS, Arai AE, Bluemke DA, Flamm SD, Kanal E, Manning WJ, Martin ET, Smith JM, Wilke N, Shellock FG; Safety of magnetic resonance imaging in patients with cardiovascular devices: an American Heart Association scientific statement from the Committee on Diagnostic and Interventional Cardiac Catheterization, Council on Clinical Cardiology, and the Council on Cardiovascular Radiology and Intervention: endorsed by the American College of Cardiology Foundation, the North American Society for Cardiac Imaging, and the Society for Cardiovascular Magnetic Resonance) there is only limited information pertaining to the MRI safety aspects of temporary cardiac pacemakers (i.e., leads and external pulse generators). For example, a report by Pfeil, et al. (2011) suggested that temporary pacemaker myocardial pacing leads may be "compatible with MR scanning" at 1.5-Tesla, but further in vivo studies and carefully monitored patient investigations are needed before final safety recommendations can be made. Of note is that extra caution must be applied when using the transmit RF body coil over the area where the permanent pacing lead is located. Additionally, the possibility of induced currents must be considered.

Thus, because of the relatively low risk, patients with retained temporary *epicardial* pacing leads may undergo MRI procedures and, importantly, patients do not need to be routinely screened for the presence of such leads before scanning. Because of the possible increased risks involved with the external pulse generators used with temporary epicardial pacing leads, these devices should not be connected when a patient is undergoing MRI.

By comparison, scanning patients with temporary *intracardiac* pacing leads (without the pulse generator) is not recommended, although lead heating might be minimized or avoided by scanning anatomic regions above (e.g., head/brain) or below (e.g., lower extremities) the cardiac pacing leads. Furthermore, because the harsh electromagnetic environment associated with the MR system can alter the operation of an external pulse generator or damage it, it may not be possible to reliably pace the patient during the MRI examination, which makes the issue of scanning a patient with a temporary intracardiac, transvenous lead irrelevant in most cases.

Abandoned Permanent Intracardiac Pacing Leads

Over the lifetime of using a permanent cardiac pacemaker, an intracardiac pacing lead may be "abandoned" and replaced due to lead fracture, insulation breaks, dislodgement, or other failures and abnormalities in pacing or sensing. For an abandoned lead that is not connected to a pulse generator, substantial heating may occur in relation to MRI examinations, as reported by Langman, et al. (2011, 2012).

A study by Higgins, et al. (2014) that involved patients with abandoned pacemaker and implantable cardioverter defibrillator (ICD) leads reported that the use of MRI in patients with abandoned cardiac device leads may be feasible when performed under careful monitoring conditions and with other precautions in place. However, until further studies define safe-scanning conditions for abandoned intracardiac pacing leads, MRI healthcare professionals should be aware of the higher risk of RF-induced lead tip heating and other possible MRI-related issues.

Abandoned Permanent Epicardial Pacing Leads

It should be noted that, retained temporary epicardial cardiac pacing leads (commonly found post cardiac surgery) are not the same as epicardially implanted permanent cardiac pacing leads. Permanent epicardial pacing leads are less commonly found in patients (less than 1% of all permanent pacing leads) than permanent intracardiac pacing leads.

Permanent epicardial pacing leads are implanted by surgeons, usually in the setting of recurring hardware infection to avoid endocardial indwelling (i.e., intracardiac pacing leads) or in congenital heart disease where access to cardiac chambers is a difficulty from an endocardial approach (Personal Communication, Saman Nazarian, M.D., Ph.D., Cardiac Electrophysiology, The University of Pennsylvania Perelman School of Medicine Philadelphia, PA). Because of the inherent qualities (i.e., materials, length of leads, etc.) of these pacing leads, it is advisable to exercise caution for patients with abandoned permanent epicardial cardiac pacing leads similar to how patients with abandoned intracardiac pacing leads are managed with respect to MRI issues.

[Portions of this section are excerpted with permission from Levine GN, Gomes AS, Arai AE, Bluemke DA, Flamm SD, Kanal E, Manning WJ, Martin ET, Smith JM, Wilke N, Shellock FG. Safety of magnetic resonance imaging in patients with cardiovascular devices: An American Heart Association scientific statement from the Committee on Diagnostic and Interventional Cardiac Catheterization. Circulation 2007;116:2878-2891. Reviewed and updated 2018.]

REFERENCES

Achenbach S, et al. Effects of magnetic resonance imaging on cardiac pacemakers and electrodes. Am Heart J 1997;134:467-473.

Bottomley PA, Kumar A, et al. Designing passive MRI-safe implantable conducting leads with electrodes. Med Phys 2010;37:3828-43.

Dempsey MF, Condon B, Hadley DM. Investigation of the factors responsible for burns during MRI. J Magn Reson Imag 2001;13:627–631.

Hartnell GG, et al. Safety of MR imaging in patients who have retained metallic materials after cardiac surgery. Am J Roentgenol 1997;168:1157–1159.

Higgins JV, et al. Safety and outcomes of magnetic resonance imaging in patients with abandoned pacemaker and defibrillator leads. Pacing Clin Electrophysiol 2014;37:1284-90.

Langman DA, et al. Abandoned pacemaker leads are a potential risk for patients undergoing MRI. Pacing Clin Electrophysiol 2011;34:1051-3.

Langman DA, et al. Pacemaker lead tip heating in abandoned and pacemaker-attached leads at 1.5 Tesla MRI. J Magn Reson Imag 2011;33:426-31.

Langman DA, et al. The dependence of radiofrequency induced pacemaker lead tip heating on the electrical conductivity of the medium at the lead tip. Magn Reson Med 2012;68:606-13.

Levine GN, et al. Safety of magnetic resonance imaging in patients with cardiovascular devices: An American Heart Association scientific statement from the Committee on Diagnostic and Interventional Cardiac Catheterization. Circulation 2007;116:2878-2891.

Luechinger R, et al. *In vivo* heating of pacemaker leads during magnetic resonance imaging. Eur Heart J 2005;26:376-383.

Pfeil A, et al. Compatibility of temporary pacemaker myocardial pacing leads with magnetic resonance imaging: An *ex vivo* tissue study. Int J Cardiovasc Imaging 2011;28:317-26.

Shellock FG, Valencerina S, Fischer L. MRI-related heating of pacemaker at 1.5- and 3-Tesla: Evaluation with and without pulse generator attached to leads. Circulation 2005;112;Supplement II:561.

Yu Z, et al. Potential for high-permittivity materials to reduce local SAR at a pacemaker lead tip during MRI of the head with a body transmit coil at 3 T. Magn Reson Med 2017;78:383-386.

Guidelines for the Management of Patients with Coronary Artery Stents Referred for MRI Procedures

In the clinical magnetic resonance imaging (MRI) setting, there is often misunderstanding associated with the management of patients with coronary artery stents, including confusion regarding stents labeled "MRI Safe/MRI Compatible" (i.e. due to labeling applied prior to the change in terminology, 2005) or "MR Conditional", the timing of performing MRI following stent placement, and regarding what MRI limitations may exist (e.g., those related to the acceptable static magnetic field strength, maximum spatial gradient magnetic field, whole body averaged specific absorption rate or SAR, and other conditions)(1-3). This may result in restricted access to MRI for certain patients, particularly those with coronary artery stents for which there is unknown labeling information.

Notably, the previous belief that it may be necessary to wait six weeks or longer after implantation of certain coronary artery stents to allow for endothelialization or other mechanism to prevent migration has been refuted because there are no known coronary artery stents made from ferromagnetic metallic materials (4-22).

MRI labeling information exists for many coronary artery stents (3, 22). By following the pertinent MRI labeling information (i.e. presented in the Instructions for Use, Patient Identification Card, etc.), patients with coronary artery stents have safely undergone MRI examinations, including those performed at 1.5- and 3-Tesla. Importantly, there has never been an adverse event reported in association with performing MRI in patients with these particular implants.

Unfortunately, the standard policy that MRI labeling information is required before allowing MRI in patients with coronary artery stents limits access to this important diagnostic imaging modality for those patients for which labeling is unavailable. However, in consideration of the relevant peer-reviewed literature and other related documents, it is acceptable and safe to perform MRI examinations in all patients with coronary artery stents by following specific guidelines developed by taking into consideration possible safety concerns (i.e. magnetic field interactions and MRI-related heating) for these implants.

By adhering to these admittedly conservative MRI conditions, all patients with coronary artery stents can benefit from the diagnostic imaging information provided by one of the most important noninvasive imaging modalities.

Guidelines. The following guidelines apply to using MRI in all patients with coronary artery stents (including two or more overlapped stents):

1)   Patients with all commercially available coronary artery stents (including drug-eluting and non-drug eluting or bare metal versions) can be scanned at 1.5-Tesla/64-MHz or 3-T/128-MHz, regardless of the value of the spatial gradient magnetic field.

2)   Patients with all commercially available coronary artery stents can undergo MRI immediately after placement of these implants.

3)   The MRI examination must be performed using the following parameters:

  • 1.5-Tesla or 3-Tesla, only
  • Whole body averaged specific absorption rate (SAR) of 2-W/kg, operating in the Normal Operating Mode for the MR system
  • Maximum imaging time, 15 minutes per pulse sequence (multiple sequences per patient are allowed)

Important Note: Any deviation from the above MRI conditions requires prior approval by the Radiologist or supervising physician.

Important Note: These guidelines must be reviewed on an annual basis to confirm that no new coronary artery stent has become available that substantially deviates from the above MRI conditions or that is labeled, MR Unsafe.

Important Note: This information does not apply to other stents such as peripheral vascular stents, abdominal aortic aneurysm (AAA) stent grafts, biliary stents, ureteral stents, or stents used for other applications (e.g., tracheobronchial stents, esophageal stents, etc.).

[The Guidelines for the Management of Patients with Coronary Artery Stents Referred for MRI Procedures should only be implemented for use after careful review by the supervising radiologist or physician responsible for the MRI facility and adoption as a written policy.]

REFERENCES

1. Shellock FG, Crues JV. MR procedures: Biologic effects, safety, and patient care. Radiology 2004;232:635-652.

2. Shellock FG, Woods TO, Crues JV. MRI labeling information for implants and devices: Explanation of terminology. Radiology 2009;253:26-30.

3. Shellock FG. Reference Manual for Magnetic Resonance Safety, Implants, and Devices: 2017 Edition. Biomedical Research Publishing Group, Los Angeles, CA, 2017.

4. Levine GN, et al. Safety of magnetic resonance imaging in patients with cardiovascular devices: An American Heart Association scientific statement from the Committee on Diagnostic and Interventional Cardiac Catheterization. Circulation 2007;116:2878-2891.

5. Ahmed S, Shellock FG. Magnetic resonance imaging safety: Implications for cardiovascular patients. Journal of Cardiovascular Magnetic Resonance 2001;3:171-181

6. Curtis JW, Lesniak DC, Wible JH, Woodard PK. Cardiac magnetic resonance imaging safety following percutaneous coronary intervention. Int J Cardiovasc Imaging.2013;29:1485-90.

7. Gerber TC, et al. Clinical safety of magnetic resonance imaging early after coronary artery stent placement. J Am Coll Cardiol 2003;42:1295-8.

8. Hug J, et al. Coronary arterial stents: Safety and artifacts during MR imaging. Radiology 2000;216:781-787.

9. Jehl J, et al. Clinical safety of cardiac magnetic resonance imaging at 3 T early after stent placement for acute myocardial infarction. Eur Radiol 2009;19:2913-8.

10. Kaya MG, et al. Long-term clinical effects of magnetic resonance imaging in patients with coronary artery stent implantation. Coron Artery Dis 2009; 20:138-42.

11. Patel MR, et al. Acute myocardial infarction: Safety of cardiac MR imaging after percutaneous revascularization with stents. Radiology 2006;240:674-680.

12. Porto I, et al. Safety of magnetic resonance imaging one to three days after bare metal and drug-eluting stent implantation. Am J Cardiol 2005;96:366-8.

13. Shellock FG. MR safety at 3-Tesla: Bare metal and drug eluting coronary artery stents. Signals No. 53, Issue 2, pp. 26-27, 2005.

14. Shellock FG. Biomedical implants and devices: Assessment of magnetic field interactions with a 3.0-Tesla MR system. J Magn Reson Imag 2002;16:721-732.

15. Shellock FG, Morisoli S, Kanal E. MR procedures and biomedical implants, materials, and devices: 1993 update. Radiology 1993;189:587-599.

16. Shellock FG, Shellock VJ. Stents: Evaluation of MRI safety. Am J Roentgenol 1999;173:543-546.

17. Sommer T, et al. High field MR imaging: Magnetic field interactions of aneurysm clips, coronary artery stents and iliac artery stents with a 3.0 Tesla MR system. Rofo 2004;176:731-8.

18. Spuentrup E, et al. Magnetic resonance-guided coronary artery stent placement in a swine model. Circulation 2002;105:874-879.

19. Syed MA, et al. Long-term safety of cardiac magnetic resonance imaging performed in the first few days after bare-metal stent implantation. J Magn Reson Imaging. 2006;24:1056-61.

20. Tejedor-Viñuela P, et al. Safety of early cardiac magnetic resonance imaging in acute myocardial infarction patients with stents. Rev Esp Cardiol 2006;59:1261-7.

21. Wang Y, et al. Magnetic resonance compatibility research for coronary metal stents. Zhongguo Yi Liao Qi Xie Za Zhi. 2015;39:61-3.

Guidelines for the Management of Patients with Heart Valve Prostheses and Annuloplasty Rings Referred for MRI Procedures

In the clinical magnetic resonance imaging (MRI) setting, it is often necessary to manage patients with heart valve prostheses [including transcatheter aortic valve replacements (TAVR), transcatheter aortic valve implantation (TAVI) devices, percutaneous aortic valve replacement (PAVR) implants, transcatheter heart valves (THV), as well as other similar valve implants used in association with minimally invasive procedures] and annuloplasty rings (1-20).

MRI labeling information exists for many heart valve prostheses and annuloplasty rings. By following the pertinent MRI labeling information (i.e. presented in the Instructions for Use, Patient Identification Card, etc.), patients with heart valve prostheses and annuloplasty rings have safely undergone MRI examinations, including those performed at 1.5- and 3-Tesla (15, 20). Notably, there has never been an adverse event reported in association with performing MRI in patients with these particular implants.

Unfortunately, the standard policy that MRI labeling information is required before allowing the use of MRI in a patients with heart valve prostheses and annuloplasty rings limits access to this important diagnostic imaging modality for those patients for which labeling information is unavailable. However, in consideration of the relevant peer-reviewed literature and other related documents (1-21), it is acceptable and safe to perform MRI examinations in all patients with heart valve prostheses and annuloplasty rings by following specific guidelines developed by taking into consideration possible safety concerns (i.e. magnetic field interactions and MRI-related heating) for these implants.

Notably, by adhering to these admittedly conservative MRI conditions, all patients with heart valves and annuloplasty rings can benefit from the diagnostic imaging information provided by one of the most important noninvasive imaging modalities.

Guidelines. The following guidelines apply to using MRI in all patients with heart valve prostheses and annuloplasty rings:

1) Patients with all commercially available heart valve prostheses and annuloplasty rings can be scanned at 1.5-Tesla/64-MHz or 3-T/128-MHz, regardless of the value of the spatial gradient magnetic field.
2) Patients with all commercially available heart valve prostheses and annuloplasty rings can undergo MRI immediately after placement of these implants.
3) The MRI examination must be performed using the following parameters:

   - 1.5-Tesla or 3-Tesla, only
   - Whole body averaged specific absorption rate (SAR) of 2-W/kg, operating in the Normal Operating Mode for the MR system
   - Maximum imaging time, 15 minutes per pulse sequence (multiple sequences per patient are allowed)

Important Note: Any deviation from the above MRI conditions requires prior approval by a radiologist or supervising physician.

Important Note: These guidelines must be reviewed on an annual basis to confirm that no new heart valve prosthesis or annuloplasty ring has become available that substantially deviates from the above MRI conditions or that is labeled, MR Unsafe.

[The Guidelines for the Management of Patients with Heart Valve Prostheses and Annuloplasty Rings Referred for MRI Procedures should only be implemented for use after careful review by the supervising radiologist or physician responsible for the MRI facility and adoption as a written policy.]

REFERENCES

(1) Ahmed S, Shellock FG. Magnetic resonance imaging safety: Implications for cardiovascular patients. Journal of Cardiovascular Magnetic Resonance 2001;3:171-181.
(2) Edwards MB, Taylor KM, Shellock FG. Prosthetic heart valves: Evaluation of magnetic field interactions, heating, and artifacts at 1.5-Tesla. J Magn Reson Imag 2000;12:363-369.
(3) Frank H, Buxbaum P, Huber L, et al. *In vitro* behavior of mechanical heart valves in 1.5-T superconducting magnet. Eur J Radiol 1992;2:555-558.

(4) Hassler M, et al. Effects of magnetic fields used in MRI on 15 prosthetic heart valves. J Radiol 1986;67:661-666.

(5) Levine GN, et al. Safety of magnetic resonance imaging in patients with cardiovascular devices: An American Heart Association scientific statement from the Committee on Diagnostic and Interventional Cardiac Catheterization. Circulation 2007;116:2878-2891.

(6) Maragiannis D, et al. Functional assessment of bioprosthetic aortic valves by CMR. JACC Cardiovasc Imaging 2016;9:785-93.

(7) Myers PO, et al. Safety of magnetic resonance imaging in cardiac surgery patients: Annuloplasty rings, septal occluders, and transcatheter valves. Ann Thorac Surg 2012;93:1019.

(8) Pruefer D, et al. *In vitro* investigation of prosthetic heart valves in magnetic resonance imaging: Evaluation of potential hazards. J Heart Valve Disease 2001;10:410-414.

(9) Randall PA, et al. Magnetic resonance imaging of prosthetic cardiac valves *in vitro* and *in vivo*. Am J Cardiol 1988;62:973-976.

(10) Saeedi M, Thomas A, Shellock FG. Evaluation of MRI issues at 3-Tesla for a transcatheter aortic valve replacement (TAVR) bioprosthesis. Magnetic Resonance Imaging 2015;33:497-501.

(11) Shellock FG. Biomedical implants and devices: Assessment of magnetic field interactions with a 3.0-Tesla MR system. J Magn Reson Imag 2002;16:721-732.

(12) Shellock FG. Prosthetic heart valves and annuloplasty rings: Assessment of magnetic field interactions, heating, and artifacts at 1.5-Tesla. Journal of Cardiovascular Magnetic Resonance 2001;3:159-169.

(13) Shellock FG, Morisoli SM. Ex vivo evaluation of ferromagnetism, heating, and artifacts for heart valve prostheses exposed to a 1.5-Tesla MR system. J Magn Reson Imaging 1994;4:756-758.

(14) Shellock FG, Shellock VJ. MRI Safety of cardiovascular implants: Evaluation of ferromagnetism, heating, and artifacts. Radiology 2000;214:P19H.

(15) Shellock FG. Reference Manual for Magnetic Resonance Safety, Implants, and Devices: 2017 Edition. Biomedical Research Publishing Group, Los Angeles, CA, 2017.

(16) Shellock FG, Shellock VJ. MRI Safety of cardiovascular implants: Evaluation of ferromagnetism, heating, and artifacts. Radiology 2000;214:P19H.

(17) Shellock FG. Biomedical implants and devices: Assessment of magnetic field interactions with a 3.0-Tesla MR system. J Magn Reson Imag 2002;16:721-732.

(18) Soulen RL. Magnetic resonance imaging of prosthetic heart valves [Letter]. Radiology 1986;158:279.

(19) Soulen RL, Budinger TF, Higgins CB. Magnetic resonance imaging of prosthetic heart valves. Radiology 1985;154:705-707.

(20) Shellock FG, Crues JV. MR procedures: Biologic effects, safety, and patient care. Radiology 2004;232:635-652.

(21) Shellock FG, Woods TO, Crues JV. MRI labeling information for implants and devices: Explanation of terminology. Radiology 2009;253:26-30.

Guidelines for the Management of the Post-Operative Patient Referred for a Magnetic Resonance Procedure*

There is often confusion regarding the issue of performing a magnetic resonance (MR) procedure during the post-operative period in a patient with a metallic implant or device. Studies have supported that, if the metallic object is a "passive implant" (i.e. there is no electronically- or magnetically-activated component associated with the operation of the device) and it is made from nonferromagnetic material, the patient may undergo an MR procedure immediately after implantation using an MR system operating at 1.5-Tesla or less (or, the field strength that was used to test the implant/device, including 3-Tesla). In fact, there are several reports that describe placement of vascular stents, coils, filters, and other implants using MR-guided procedures that include the use of high-field-strength (1.5- and 3-Tesla) MR systems. Additionally, a patient or individual with a nonferromagnetic, passive implant is allowed to enter the MR environment associated with a scanner operating at 1.5-Tesla (or, the field strength that was used to test the implant/device, including 3-Tesla) or less immediately after its implantation.

For an implant or device that exhibits magnetic qualities, it may be necessary to wait a period of six weeks after implantation before performing an MR procedure or allowing the individual or patient to enter the MR system room. For example, certain magnetic coils, stents, or filters become firmly incorporated into tissue a minimum of six weeks following placement. In these cases, retentive or counter-forces provided by tissue ingrowth, scarring, granulation, or other mechanisms serve to prevent these objects from presenting risks or hazards to patients or individuals in the MR environment with regard to movement or dislodgement.

However, patients with implants or devices that are magnetic but rigidly fixed in the body (e.g., bone screws, certain orthopedic implants, and other similar devices) may undergo MRI immediately after implantation.

Specific information pertaining to the recommended post-operative waiting period may be found in the labeling or product insert for an implant or device.

Of course, the information above pertains to magnetic field interactions and further consideration must be given to MRI-related heating and possibly other factors for the implant or device under consideration.

Special Note: If there is any concern regarding the integrity of the tissue with respect to its ability to retain the implant or object in place or the implant cannot be properly identified, the patient or individual should not be exposed to the MR environment.

[*The document, Guidelines for the Management of the Post-Operative Patient Referred for a Magnetic Resonance Procedure, was developed by the Institute for Magnetic Resonance Safety, Education, and Research (www.IMRSER.org) and published with permission. Reviewed and updated 2018.]

REFERENCES

Bueker A, et al. Real-time MR fluoroscopy for MR-guided iliac artery stent placement. J Magn Reson Imag 2000;12:616-622.

Manke C, Nitz WR, Djavidani B, et al. MR imaging-guided stent placement in iliac arterial stenoses: A feasibility study. Radiology 2001;219:527-534.

Porto I, et al. Safety of magnetic resonance imaging one to three days after bare metal and drug-eluting stent implantation. Am J Cardiol 2005;96:366-8.

Rutledge JM, et al. Safety of magnetic resonance immediately following Palmaz stent implant: A report of three cases. Catheter Cardiovasc Interv 2001;53:519-523.

Shellock FG. Guidelines for the Management of the Post-Operative Patient Referred for a Magnetic Resonance Procedure. Signals, No. 47, Issue 3, pp. 14, 2003.

Shellock FG. Magnetic Resonance Procedures: Health Effects and Safety. CRC Press, LLC, Boca Raton, FL, 2001.

Shellock FG, Crues JV. MR procedures: Biologic effects, safety, and patient care. Radiology 2004;232:635-652.

Spuentrup E, et al. Magnetic resonance-guided coronary artery stent placement in a swine model. Circulation 2002;105:874-879.

Syed MA, et al. Long-term safety of cardiac magnetic resonance imaging performed in the first few days after bare-metal stent implantation. J Magn Reson Imaging 2006;24:1056-61.

Tsai LL, et al. A practical guide to MR imaging safety: What radiologists need to know. Radiographics 2015;35:1722-37.

Weidman EK, et al. MRI safety: A report of current practice and advancements in patient preparation and screening. Clin Imaging 2015;39:935-7.

Guidelines for Screening Patients for MR Procedures and Individuals for the MR Environment

The establishment of thorough and effective screening procedures for patients and other individuals is one of the most critical components of a program that guards the safety of all those preparing to undergo magnetic resonance (MR) procedures or those needing to enter the MR environment. An important aspect of protecting patients and individuals from MR system-related accidents and injuries involves an understanding of the risks associated with the various implants, devices, accessories, and other objects that may cause problems in this setting. This requires constant attention and diligence to obtain information and documentation about these objects in order to provide the safest MR setting possible.

In addition, because most MR-related incidents have been due to deficiencies in screening methods and/or the lack of properly controlling access to the MR environment (especially with regard to preventing personal items and other potentially problematic objects from entering the MR system room), it is crucial to set up procedures and guidelines to prevent such incidents from occurring.

Magnetic Resonance (MR) Procedure Screening for Patients

Certain aspects of screening patients for MR procedures may take place during the scheduling process. These activities should be conducted by a healthcare worker specially trained in MR safety (i.e. trained to understand the potential hazards and issues associated with the MR environment and MR procedures and to be familiar with the information contained on the screening forms for patients and individuals). While scheduling the patient, it may be ascertained if the patient has an implant or device that may be contraindicated or requires special attention for the MR procedure (e.g., a ferromagnetic aneurysm clip, pacemaker, neurostimulation system, etc.) or if there is a condition that needs careful consideration (e.g., the patient is pregnant, has a disability, history of renal failure, metallic foreign body, etc.). Preliminary screening helps to prevent scheduling patients that may be inappropriate candidates for MR examinations.

After preliminary screening, the patient must undergo comprehensive screening in preparation for the MR examination. Comprehensive screening involves the use of a printed form to document the screening procedure, a careful review of the information on the screening form, and a verbal interview to verify the information and to allow for discussion of concerns that the patient may have. An MR safety trained healthcare professional must conduct this important aspect of patient screening.

The screening form entitled, *Magnetic Resonance (MR) Procedure Screening Form for Patients* was created in conjunction with the Medical, Scientific, and Technology Advisory Board and the Corporate Advisory Board of the Institute for Magnetic Resonance Safety, Education, and Research (IMRSER) **(Figure 1)**. A "downloadable" version of this form may be obtained from the websites, www.IMRSER.org and www.MRIsafety.com. This form is also available in Spanish **(Figure 2**, Translated by Olga Fernandez-Flygare, M.S., Brain Mapping Center, UCLA School of Medicine, Los Angeles, CA and Maelesa Rachele Oriente-Padilla, Loyola-Marymount University, Los Angeles, CA).

Page one of the screening form requests general patient-related information (name, age, sex, height, weight, etc.) as well as information regarding the reason for the MR examination and/or symptoms that may be present. Pertinent information about the patient is required not only to ensure that the medical records are up-to-date, but also in the event that the MRI facility needs to contact the referring physician for additional information regarding the examination or to verify the patient's medical condition.

The form requests information regarding a prior surgical procedure to help determine if there may be an implant or device present that could create a problem. Information is also requested pertaining to prior diagnostic imaging studies that may be helpful to review for assessment of the patient's condition.

Next, questions are posed to determine if there are issues that should be discussed with the patient prior to permitting entry to the MR environment. For example, information is requested regarding any problem with a previous MR examination, an injury to the eye involving a metallic object, or injury from a metallic foreign body. Questions are posed to obtain information about current or recently taken medications as well as the presence of drug allergies. There are also questions asked to assess past and present medical conditions that may affect the MR procedure or the use of an MRI contrast agent.

Important Information: MRI Contrast Agents and Nephrogenic Systemic Fibrosis (NSF). The American College of Radiology (ACR) Contrast Committee and the Subcommittee for MR Safety members recommend pre-screening patients prior to the administration of Gadolinium-Based MR Contrast Agents (GBMCA).

Please review the latest information for the management of patients with underlying health conditions associated with NSF, including information at the following websites:

www.acr.org - Search, "NSF"

www.acr.org/Quality-Safety/Resources/Contrast-Manual

www.fda.gov/Drugs/DrugSafety/ucm223966.htm

In consideration of the above information, questions are posed to the patient to determine if there are conditions that may need to be considered relative to the use of MRI contrast agents and the issue of NSF. For more information on this topic, refer to section, **MRI Contrast Agents and Nephrogenic Systemic Fibrosis (NSF)**.

At the bottom of page one, there is a section for female patients that poses questions that may impact MR procedures. For example, questions regarding the date of the last menstrual period, pregnancy, or late menstrual period are included. A definite or possible pregnancy must be identified prior to permitting the patient into the MR environment so that the risk vs. the benefit of the MR procedure can be considered and discussed with the patient. MR examinations should only be performed in pregnant patients to address important clinical questions. MR facilities should have a clearly defined procedure to follow in the event that the patient has a possible or confirmed pregnancy.

Questions pertaining to the date of the last menstrual period, use of oral contraceptives or hormonal therapy, and fertility medication are necessary for female patients undergoing MRI procedures that are performed to evaluate breast disease or for OB/GYN applications, because these may alter tissue contrast on MR imaging. An inquiry about breastfeeding is included in case the administration of MRI contrast media is being considered for use in nursing mothers.

Page two of the form has the following statement at the top of the page: **"WARNING: Certain implants, devices, or objects may be hazardous to you and/or may interfere with the MR procedure (i.e. MRI, MR**

angiography, functional MRI, MR spectroscopy). Do not enter the MR system room or MR environment if you have any question or concern regarding an implant, device, or object. Consult the MRI Technologist or Radiologist BEFORE entering the MR system room. The MR system magnet is ALWAYS on."

Next, there is a section that lists various implants, devices, and objects to identify anything that could be hazardous to the patient undergoing the MR procedure or that may produce an artifact that could interfere with the interpretation of the MR examination. In general, these items are arranged on the checklist in order of the relative hazard or risk (e.g., aneurysm clip, cardiac pacemaker, implantable cardioverter defibrillator, electronic implant, etc.), followed by items that may produce imaging artifacts that could be problematic for the interpretation of the MR procedure. Additionally, questions are posed to determine if the patient has a breathing problem, movement disorder, or claustrophobia.

Figures of the human body are included on the second page of the form as a means of showing the location of any object inside of or on the body. This information allows the patient to indicate the approximate position of an object that may be hazardous or that could interfere with the interpretation of the MR procedure as a result of producing an artifact.

Page two of the screening form also has an *Important Instructions* section that states: **"Before entering the MR environment or MR system room, you must remove all metallic objects including hearing aids, dentures, partial plates, keys, beeper, cell phone, eyeglasses, hair pins, barrettes, jewelry, body piercing jewelry, watch, safety pins, paperclips, money clip, credit cards, bank cards, magnetic strip cards, coins, pens, pocket knife, nail clipper, tools, clothing with metal fasteners, & clothing with metallic threads. Please consult the MRI Technologist or Radiologist if you have any question or concern BEFORE you enter the MR system room."**

Finally, there is a statement that indicates hearing protection is "advised or required" to prevent possible problems or hazards related to acoustic noise. In general, this should not be an option for a patient undergoing an MR procedure on a high-field-strength MR system. Alternatively, it may be unnecessary for a patient to use hearing protection if undergoing an MR procedure on a low-field-strength MR system because the acoustic noise may not be problematic.

Importantly, undergoing previous MR procedures without incidents does not guarantee a safe subsequent MR examination. Various factors (e.g., the field strength of the MR system, the orientation of the patient, the orientation of a metallic implant or object, etc.) can substantially change the scenario. Thus, a written screening form must be completed each time a patient prepares to undergo an MR examination.

With the use of any type of written questionnaire, limitations exist related to incomplete or incorrect answers provided by the patient. For example, there may be difficulties associated with patients who are impaired with respect to their vision, language fluency, or level of literacy. Therefore, an appropriate accompanying family member or other individual (e.g., referring physician) should be involved in the screening process to verify any information that may impact patient safety. Versions of this form should also be available in other languages, as needed (i.e. specific to the demographics of the MRI facility).

In the event that the patient is comatose or unable to communicate, the written screening form should be completed by the most qualified individual (e.g., physician, family member, etc.) who has knowledge about the patient's medical history and present condition. If the screening information is inadequate, it is advisable to look for surgical scars on the patient and/or to obtain plain films of the skull, chest, and other areas to search for implants that may be hazardous in association with MRI (e.g., aneurysm clips, cardiac pacemakers, neurostimulation systems, etc.).

Following completion of the *Magnetic Resonance (MR) Procedure Screening Form for Patients*, an MR safety trained healthcare professional must review the form's content. Next, a verbal interview must be conducted by the MR safety trained healthcare professional to verify the information on the form and to allow discussion of any question or concern that the patient may have. This provides a mechanism for clarification and confirmation of the answers to the questions posed to the patient so that there is no miscommunication regarding important MR safety issues. In addition, because the patient may not be fully aware of the medical terminology used for a particular implant or device, it is imperative that this particular information on the form be discussed during the verbal interview.

After the comprehensive screening procedure is completed, a patient that is transferred by a stretcher, gurney, or wheelchair to the MR system room should be checked thoroughly for metallic objects such as ferromagnetic oxygen tanks, monitors, unnecessary ECG electrodes, ECG or other leads, sand bags with metal shot, or other objects that could pose a hazard. Obviously, only nonferromagnetic stretchers, gurneys, wheelchairs and accessories should be allowed into the MR system room.

Magnetic Resonance (MR) Environment Screening for Individuals

Before any non-patient individual (e.g., MRI technologist, physician, researcher, relative, visitor, allied healthcare professional, maintenance worker, custodial worker, fire fighter, security officer, etc.) is allowed into the MR environment, he or she must be screened by an MR safety trained healthcare professional. Proper screening for individuals involves the use of a printed form to document the procedure, a review of the information on the form, and a verbal interview to verify the information and to allow discussion of any question or concern that the individual may have before being permitted into the MR environment.

Important Note: If for any reason the individual undergoing screening may need to enter the MR system and, thus, become exposed to the electromagnetic fields used for an MR procedure, this person must be screened using the *Magnetic Resonance (MR) Procedure Screening Form for Patients.*

In general, magnetic resonance (MR) screening forms were developed with patients in mind and, therefore, tend to pose many questions that are inappropriate or confusing to other individuals that may need to enter the MR environment. Therefore, a screening form was created specifically for individuals that need to enter the MR environment and/or MR system room. This form, entitled, *Magnetic Resonance (MR) Environment Screening Form for Individuals* was developed in conjunction with the Medical, Scientific, and Technology Advisory Board and the Corporate Advisory Board of the Institute for Magnetic Resonance Safety, Education, and Research (IMRSER) (**Figure 3**). A "downloadable" version of this form may be obtained from the websites, www.IMRSER.org and www.MRIsafety.com.

At the top of this form, the following statement is displayed: **"The MR system has a very strong magnetic field that may be hazardous to individuals entering the MR environment or MR system room if they have certain metallic, electronic, magnetic, or mechanical implants, devices, or objects. Therefore, <u>all</u> individuals are required to fill out this form BEFORE entering the MR environment or MR system room. Be advised, the MR system magnet is ALWAYS on."**

The screening form for individuals requests general information (name, age, address, etc.) and poses important questions to determine if there are possible problems or issues that should be discussed with the individual prior to permitting entry to the MR environment.

A warning statement is also provided on the form, as follows: **"WARNING: Certain implants, devices, or objects may be hazardous to you in the MR environment or MR system room. <u>Do not enter</u> the MR environment or MR system room if you have any question or concern regarding an implant, device, or object."**

In addition, there is a section that lists implants, devices, and objects to identify the presence of an item that may be hazardous to an individual in the MR environment (e.g., an aneurysm clip, cardiac pacemaker, implantable cardioverter defibrillator, electronic or magnetically activated device, metallic foreign body, etc).

Finally, there is an *Important Instructions* section on the form that states: **"Remove <u>all</u> metallic objects before entering the MR environment or MR system room including hearing aids, beeper, cell phone, keys, eyeglasses, hair pins, barrettes, jewelry (including body piercing jewelry), watch, safety pins, paperclips, money clip, credit cards, bank cards, magnetic strip cards, coins, pens, pocket knife, nail clipper, steel-toed boots/shoes, and tools. Loose metallic objects are especially prohibited in the MR system room and MR environment. Please consult the MRI Technologist or Radiologist if you have any question or concern BEFORE you enter the MR system room."**

The proper use of this written form along with thorough verbal screening of the individual by an MR safety trained healthcare worker will prevent accidents and injuries in the MR environment.

[*The screening forms, *Magnetic Resonance (MR) Procedure Screening Form For Patients* and *Magnetic Resonance (MR) Environment Screening Form for Individuals* were developed in conjunction with the Institute for Magnetic Resonance Safety, Education, and Research (IMRSER) and published with permission. Reviewed and updated 2018.]

REFERENCES

Calamante F, et al. Recommended responsibilities for management of MR safety. J Magn Reson Imaging 2016;44:1067-1069.

Expert Panel on MR Safety, Kanal E, Barkovich AJ, Bell C, et al. ACR guidance document on MR safe practices: 2013. J Magn Reson Imag 2013;37:501-30.

Sawyer-Glover A, Shellock FG. Pre-Magnetic Resonance Procedure Screening, In: Magnetic Resonance Procedures: Health Effects and Safety, FG Shellock, Editor, CRC Press, LLC, Boca Raton, FL, 2001.

Sawyer-Glover A, Shellock FG. Pre-MRI procedure screening: recommendations and safety considerations for biomedical implants and devices. J Magn Reson Imag 2000;12:92-106.

Shellock FG. Biomedical implants and devices: Assessment of magnetic field interactions with a 3.0-Tesla MR system. J Magn Reson Imag 2002;16:721-732.

Shellock FG. MR safety update 2002: Implants and devices. J Magn Reson Imag 2002;16:485-496.

Shellock FG, Crues JV. Commentary. MR safety and the American College of Radiology White Paper. Am J Roentgenol 2002;178:1349-1352.

Shellock FG, Crues JV. MR procedures: Biologic effects, safety, and patient care. Radiology 2004;232:635-652.

Shellock FG, Kanal E. Policies, guidelines, and recommendations for MR imaging safety and patient management. J Magn Reson Imag 1991;1:97-101.

Shellock FG, Kanal E. SMRI Report. Policies, guidelines and recommendations for MR imaging safety and patient management. Questionnaire for screening patients before MR procedures. J Magn Reson Imag 1994;4:749-751, 1994.

Shellock FG, Spinazzi A. MRI safety update: 2008, Part 2, Screening patients for MRI. Am J Roentgenol 2008;191:12-21.

Tsai LL, et al. A practical guide to MR imaging safety: What radiologists need to know. Radiographics 2015;35:1722-37.

Weidman EK, et al. MRI safety: A report of current practice and advancements in patient preparation and screening. Clin Imaging 2015;39:935-7.

www.ACR.org; the website for the American College of Radiology

www.IMRSER.org; website for the Institute for Magnetic Resonance Safety, Education, and Research

Figure 1. Magnetic Resonance (MR) Procedure Screening Form For Patients (Developed in conjunction with the Institute for Magnetic Resonance Safety, Education, and Research, www.IMRSER.org).

MAGNETIC RESONANCE (MR) PROCEDURE SCREENING FORM FOR PATIENTS

Date ___/___/___   Patient Number _____

Name _____   Age _____ Height _____ Weight _____
       Last name   First name   Middle Initial

Date of Birth ___/___/___   Male ☐ Female ☐   Body Part to be Examined _____

        month day   year
Address _____   Telephone (home) (____) ____-____

City _____   Telephone (work) (____) ____-____

State _____ Zip Code _____

Reason for MRI and/or Symptoms _____

Referring Physician _____   Telephone (____) ____-____

1. Have you had prior surgery or an operation (e.g., arthroscopy, endoscopy, etc.) of any kind?   ☐ No   ☐ Yes
   If yes, please indicate the date and type of surgery:
   Date ___/___/___   Type of surgery _____
   Date ___/___/___   Type of surgery _____
2. Have you had a prior diagnostic imaging study or examination (MRI, CT, Ultrasound, X-ray, etc.)?   ☐ No   ☐ Yes
   If yes, please list: Body part   Date   Facility
   MRI   _____   ___/___/___   _____
   CT/CAT Scan   _____   ___/___/___   _____
   X-Ray   _____   ___/___/___   _____
   Ultrasound   _____   ___/___/___   _____
   Nuclear Medicine   _____   ___/___/___   _____
   Other_____ _____   ___/___/___   _____

3. Have you experienced any problem related to a previous MRI examination or MR procedure?   ☐ No   ☐ Yes
   If yes, please describe: _____
4. Have you had an injury to the eye involving a metallic object or fragment (e.g., metallic slivers,
   shavings, foreign body, etc.)?   ☐ No   ☐ Yes
   If yes, please describe: _____
5. Have you ever been injured by a metallic object or foreign body (e.g., BB, bullet, shrapnel, etc.)?   ☐ No   ☐ Yes
   If yes, please describe: _____
6. Are you currently taking or have you recently taken any medication or drug?   ☐ No   ☐ Yes
   If yes, please list: _____
7. Are you allergic to any medication?   ☐ No   ☐ Yes
   If yes, please list: _____
8. Do you have a history of asthma, allergic reaction, respiratory disease, or reaction to a contrast
   medium or dye used for an MRI, CT, or X-ray examination?   ☐ No   ☐ Yes
9. Do you have anemia or any disease(s) that affects your blood, a history of renal (kidney)
   disease, renal (kidney) failure, renal (kidney) transplant, high blood pressure (hypertension),
   liver (hepatic) disease, a history of diabetes, or seizures?   ☐ No   ☐ Yes
   If yes, please describe: _____

For female patients:
10. Date of last menstrual period: ___/___/___   Post menopausal?   ☐ No   ☐ Yes
11. Are you pregnant or experiencing a late menstrual period?   ☐ No   ☐ Yes
12. Are you taking oral contraceptives or receiving hormonal treatment?   ☐ No   ☐ Yes
13. Are you taking any type of fertility medication or having fertility treatments?   ☐ No   ☐ Yes
    If yes, please describe: _____
14. Are you currently breastfeeding?   ☐ No   ☐ Yes

WARNING: Certain implants, devices, or objects may be hazardous to you and/or may interfere with the MR procedure (i.e., MRI, MR angiography, functional MRI, MR spectroscopy). <u>Do not enter</u> the MR system room or MR environment if you have any question or concern regarding an implant, device, or object. Consult the MRI Technologist or Radiologist BEFORE entering the MR system room. The MR system magnet is ALWAYS on.

Please indicate if you have any of the following:

☐ Yes ☐ No Aneurysm clip(s)
☐ Yes ☐ No Cardiac pacemaker
☐ Yes ☐ No Implanted cardioverter defibrillator (ICD)
☐ Yes ☐ No Electronic implant or device
☐ Yes ☐ No Magnetically-activated implant or device
☐ Yes ☐ No Neurostimulation system
☐ Yes ☐ No Spinal cord stimulator
☐ Yes ☐ No Internal electrodes or wires
☐ Yes ☐ No Bone growth/bone fusion stimulator
☐ Yes ☐ No Cochlear, otologic, or other ear implant
☐ Yes ☐ No Insulin or other infusion pump
☐ Yes ☐ No Implanted drug infusion device
☐ Yes ☐ No Any type of prosthesis (eye, penile, etc.)
☐ Yes ☐ No Heart valve prosthesis
☐ Yes ☐ No Eyelid spring or wire
☐ Yes ☐ No Artificial or prosthetic limb
☐ Yes ☐ No Metallic stent, filter, or coil
☐ Yes ☐ No Shunt (spinal or intraventricular)
☐ Yes ☐ No Vascular access port and/or catheter
☐ Yes ☐ No Radiation seeds or implants
☐ Yes ☐ No Swan-Ganz or thermodilution catheter
☐ Yes ☐ No Medication patch (Nicotine, Nitroglycerine)
☐ Yes ☐ No Any metallic fragment or foreign body
☐ Yes ☐ No Wire mesh implant
☐ Yes ☐ No Tissue expander (e.g., breast)
☐ Yes ☐ No Surgical staples, clips, or metallic sutures
☐ Yes ☐ No Joint replacement (hip, knee, etc.)
☐ Yes ☐ No Bone/joint pin, screw, nail, wire, plate, etc.
☐ Yes ☐ No IUD, diaphragm, or pessary
☐ Yes ☐ No Dentures or partial plates
☐ Yes ☐ No Tattoo or permanent makeup
☐ Yes ☐ No Body piercing jewelry
☐ Yes ☐ No Hearing aid
               (Remove before entering MR system room)
☐ Yes ☐ No Other implant _____
☐ Yes ☐ No Breathing problem or motion disorder
☐ Yes ☐ No Claustrophobia

> **Please mark on the figure(s) below the location of any implant or metal inside of or on your body.**

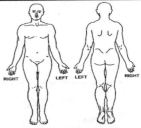

RIGHT   LEFT   LEFT   RIGHT

 IMPORTANT INSTRUCTIONS

Before entering the MR environment or MR system room, you must remove all metallic objects including hearing aids, dentures, partial plates, keys, beeper, cell phone, eyeglasses, hair pins, barrettes, jewelry, body piercing jewelry, watch, safety pins, paperclips, money clip, credit cards, bank cards, magnetic strip cards, coins, pens, pocket knife, nail clipper, tools, clothing with metal fasteners, & clothing with metallic threads.

Please consult the MRI Technologist or Radiologist if you have any question or concern BEFORE you enter the MR system room.

NOTE: You may be advised or required to wear earplugs or other hearing protection during the MR procedure to prevent possible problems or hazards related to acoustic noise.

I attest that the above information is correct to the best of my knowledge. I read and understand the contents of this form and had the opportunity to ask questions regarding the information on this form and regarding the MR procedure that I am about to undergo.

Signature of Person Completing Form: _____   Date ____ / ____ / ____
                                              Signature

Form Completed By: ☐ Patient ☐ Relative ☐ Nurse _____   _____
                                                       Print name   Relationship to patient

Form Information Reviewed By: _____   _____
                                       Print name   Signature

☐ MRI Technologist   ☐ Nurse   ☐ Radiologist   ☐ Other _____

Figure 2. Magnetic Resonance (MR) Procedure Screening Form For Patients: Spanish Version

CUESTIONARIO PREVIO A ESTUDIO CON RESONANCIA MAGNÉTICA (MR)
PARA PACIENTES

Fecha ___/___/___   Número de paciente_____

Nombre_____   Edad_____ Altura_____ Peso_____
Apellido   Primer Nombre   Segundo Nombre

Fecha de nacimiento___/___/___ Varón☐ Hembra☐   Parte del cuerpo a ser examinada_____
Mes Dia Año
Dirección_____   Teléfono (domicilio) (____) ____-_____

Ciudad_____   Teléfono (trabajo) (____) ____-_____

Provincia_____   Código Postal_____

Motivo para el estudio de MRI y/o síntomas_____

Médico que le refirió_____   Teléfono (____) - _____

1. Anteriormente, ¿le han hecho alguna cirugía u operación (e.g., artroscopía, endoscopía, etc.) de cualquier tipo? ☐ No ☐ Sí
Si respondió afirmativamente, indique la fecha y que tipo de cirugía:
Fecha ___/___/___ Tipo de cirugía _____
Fecha ___/___/___ Tipo de cirugía _____
2. Anteriormente, ¿le han hecho algún estudio o exámen de diagnóstico (MRI, CT, Ultrasonido, Rayos-X, etc.)? ☐ No ☐ Sí
Si respondió afirmativamente, descríbalos a continuación:
Parte del Cuerpo   Fecha   Lugar/Institución
MRI _____   ___/___/___   _____
CT/CAT _____   ___/___/___   _____
Rayos-X _____   ___/___/___   _____
Ultrasonido _____   ___/___/___   _____
Medicina Nuclear _____   ___/___/___   _____
Otro_____
3. ¿Ha tenido algún problema relacionado con estudios ó procedimientos anteriores con MR? ☐ No ☐ Sí
Si respondió afirmativamente, descríbalos: _____
4. ¿Se ha golpeado el ojo con un objeto ó fragmento metálico (e.g., astillas metálicas, virutas, objeto extraño, etc.)? ☐ No ☐ Sí
Si respondió afirmativamente, describa el incidente: _____
5. ¿Ha sido alcanzado alguna vez por un objeto metálico u objeto extraño (e.g. perdigones, bala, metralla, etc.)? ☐ No ☐ Sí
Si respondió afirmativamente, describa el incidente: _____
6. ¿Esta actualmente tomando ó ha recientemente tomado algún medicamento o droga? ☐ No ☐ Sí
Si respondió afirmativamente, indique el nombre del medicamento:_____
7. ¿Es Ud. alérgico/a á algún medicamento? ☐ No ☐ Sí
Si respondió afirmativamente, indique el nombre del medicamento:_____
8. ¿Tiene historia de asma, reacción alérgica, enfermedad respiratoria, ó reacción a contrastes ó tinturas usados en MRI, CT, ó
Rayos-X? ☐ No ☐ Sí
9. ¿Tiene anemia u otra enfermedad que afecte su sangre, algún episodio de enfermedad de riñón, fracaso de riñón,
un transplante de riñón, hipertensión, la historia de la diabetes, relativo al higado ó de ataques epilépticos?
Si respondió afirmativamente, descríbalos: _____ ☐ No ☐ Sí

Para los pacientes femeninos:
10. Fecha de su último periodo menstrual: ___/___/___   En la menopausia? ☐ No ☐ Sí
11. ¿Está embarazada ó tiene retraso con su periodo menstrual? ☐ No ☐ Sí
12. ¿Está tomando contraceptivos orales ó recibiendo tratamiento hormonal? ☐ No ☐ Sí
13. ¿Está tomando algún tipo de medicamento para la fertilidad ó recibiendo tratamientos de fertilidad? ☐ No ☐ Sí
Si responde afirmativamente, descríbalos a continuación: _____
14. ¿Está amamantado a su bebé? ☐ No ☐ Sí

Translated with permission 5/05 Olga Fernandez-Flygare, M.S., Brain
Mapping Center, UCLA School of Medicine, Los Angeles, CA

ADVERTENCIA: Ciertos implantes, dispositivos, u objetos pueden ser peligrosos y/o pueden interferir con el procedimiento de resonancia magnética (es decir, MRI, MR angiografía, MRI funcional, MR espectroscopía). <u>No entre</u> a la sala del escáner de MR o a la zona del laboratorio de MR si tiene alguna pregunta o duda relacionadas con un implante, dispositivo, u objeto. Consulte con el técnico o radiólogo de MRI ANTES de entrar a la sala del escáner de MR. **Recuerde que el imán del sistema MR está SIEMPRE encendido.**

Por favor indique si tiene alguno de los siguientes:

- ☐ Sí ☐ No Pinza(s) de aneurisma
- ☐ Sí ☐ No Marcapasos cardíaco
- ☐ Sí ☐ No Implante con desfibrilador para conversión cardíaca (ICD)
- ☐ Sí ☐ No Implante electrónico ó dispositivo electrónico
- ☐ Sí ☐ No Implante ó dispositivo activado magnéticamente
- ☐ Sí ☐ No Sistema de neuroestimulación
- ☐ Sí ☐ No Estimulador de la médula espinal
- ☐ Sí ☐ No Electrodos ó alambres internos
- ☐ Sí ☐ No Estimulador de crecimiento/fusión del hueso
- ☐ Sí ☐ No Implante coclear, otológico, u otro implante del oído
- ☐ Sí ☐ No Bomba de infusión de insulina ó similar
- ☐ Sí ☐ No Dispositivo implantado para infusión de medicamento
- ☐ Sí ☐ No Cualquier tipo de prótesis (ojo, peneal, etc.)
- ☐ Sí ☐ No Prótesis de válvula cardiaca
- ☐ Sí ☐ No Muelle ó alambre del párpado
- ☐ Sí ☐ No Extremidad artificial ó prostética
- ☐ Sí ☐ No Malla metálica (stent), filtro, ó anillo metálico
- ☐ Sí ☐ No Shunt (espinal ó intraventricular)
- ☐ Sí ☐ No Catéter y/u orificio de acceso vascular
- ☐ Sí ☐ No Semillas ó implantes de radiación
- ☐ Sí ☐ No Catéter de Swan-Ganz ó de termodilución

- ☐ Sí ☐ No Parche de medicamentos (Nicotina, Nitroglicerina)
- ☐ Sí ☐ No Cualquier fragmento metálico ó cuerpo extraño
- ☐ Sí ☐ No Implante tipo malla
- ☐ Sí ☐ No Aumentador de tejidos (e.g. pecho)
- ☐ Sí ☐ No Grapas quirúrgicas, clips, ó suturas metálicas
- ☐ Sí ☐ No Articulaciones artificiales (cadera, rodilla, etc.)
- ☐ Sí ☐ No Varilla de hueso/coyuntura, tornillo, clavo, alambre, chapas, etc.
- ☐ Sí ☐ No Dispositivo intrauterino (IUD), diafragma, ó pesario
- ☐ Sí ☐ No Dentaduras ó placas parciales
- ☐ Sí ☐ No Tatuaje ó maquillaje permanente
- ☐ Sí ☐ No Perforación (piercing) del cuerpo
- ☐ Sí ☐ No Audífono *(Quíteselo antes de entrar a la sala del escáner de MR)*
- ☐ Sí ☐ No Otro implante
- ☐ Sí ☐ No Problema respiratorio ó desorden del movimiento
- ☐ Sí ☐ No Claustrofobia

> Por favor marque en la imagen de abajo la localización de cualquier implante o metal en su cuerpo.

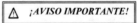

DERECHA   IZQUIERDA   DERECHA

⚠ **¡AVISO IMPORTANTE!**

Antes de entrar a la zona de MR ó a la sala del escáner de MR, tendrá que quitarse todo objeto metálico incluyendo audífono, dentaduras, placas parciales, llaves, beeper, teléfono celular, lentes, horquillas de pelo, pasadores, todas las joyas (incluyendo "body piercing"), reloj, alfileres, sujetapapeles, clip de billetes, tarjetas de crédito ó de banco, toda tarjeta con banda magnética, monedas, plumas, cuchillos, corta uñas, herramientas, ropa con enganches de metal, y ropa con hilos metálicos.

Por favor consulte con el Técnico de MRI ó Radiólogo si tiene alguna pregunta ó duda ANTES de entrar a la sala de escáner de MR.

NOTA: Es posible se le pida usar auriculares u otra protección de sus oídos durante el procedimiento de MR para prevenir problemas ó riesgos asociados al nivel de ruido en la sala del escáner de MR.

Atestiguo que la información anterior es correcta según mi mejor entender. Leo y entiendo el contenido de este cuestionario y he tenido la oportunidad de hacer preguntas en relación a la información en el cuestionario y en relación al estudio de MR al que me voy a someter a continuación.

Firma de la persona llenando este cuestionario: _____ Fecha ___/___/___

                                    Firma

Cuestionario lleno por: ☐Paciente ☐Pariente ☐Enfermera _____ _____

                                     Nombre en letra de texto   Relación con el paciente

Información revisada por: _____

                          Nombre en letra de texto   Firma

☐ Técnico de MRI   ☐Enfermera   ☐ Radiólogo   ☐ Otro

Figure 3. Magnetic Resonance (MR) Environment Screening Form for Individuals (Developed in conjunction with the Institute for Magnetic Resonance Safety, Education, and Research, www.IMRSER.org).

MAGNETIC RESONANCE (MR) ENVIRONMENT SCREENING FORM FOR INDIVIDUALS*

The MR system has a very strong magnetic field that may be hazardous to individuals entering the MR environment or MR system room if they have certain metallic, electronic, magnetic, or mechanical implants, devices, or objects. Therefore, all individuals are required to fill out this form BEFORE entering the MR environment or MR system room. Be advised, the MR system magnet is ALWAYS on.

*NOTE: If you are a patient preparing to undergo an MR examination, you are required to fill out a different form.

Date ___ / ___ / ___   Name _____   Age _____
     month   day   year   Last Name   First Name   Middle Initial

Address _____   Telephone (home) (____) ____ - _____

City _____   Telephone (work) (____) ____ - _____

State _____   Zip Code _____

1. Have you had prior surgery or an operation (e.g., arthroscopy, endoscopy, etc.) of any kind?   ☐ No ☐ Yes
   If yes, please indicate date and type of surgery: Date ___ / ___ / ___   Type of surgery _____
2. Have you had an injury to the eye involving a metallic object (e.g., metallic slivers, foreign body)?   ☐ No ☐ Yes
   If yes, please describe: _____
3. Have you ever been injured by a metallic object or foreign body (e.g., BB, bullet, shrapnel, etc.)?   ☐ No ☐ Yes
   If yes, please describe: _____
4. Are you pregnant or suspect that you are pregnant?   ☐ No ☐ Yes

WARNING: Certain implants, devices, or objects may be hazardous to you in the MR environment or MR system room. Do not enter the MR environment or MR system room if you have any question or concern regarding an implant, device, or object.

Please indicate if you have any of the following:
☐ Yes ☐ No Aneurysm clip(s)
☐ Yes ☐ No Cardiac pacemaker
☐ Yes ☐ No Implanted cardioverter defibrillator (ICD)
☐ Yes ☐ No Electronic implant or device
☐ Yes ☐ No Magnetically-activated implant or device
☐ Yes ☐ No Neurostimulation system
☐ Yes ☐ No Spinal cord stimulator
☐ Yes ☐ No Cochlear implant or implanted hearing aid
☐ Yes ☐ No Insulin or infusion pump
☐ Yes ☐ No Implanted drug infusion device
☐ Yes ☐ No Any type of prosthesis or implant
☐ Yes ☐ No Artificial or prosthetic limb
☐ Yes ☐ No Any metallic fragment or foreign body
☐ Yes ☐ No Any external or internal metallic object
☐ Yes ☐ No Hearing aid
          (Remove before entering the MR system room)
☐ Yes ☐ No Other implant _____

⚠ IMPORTANT INSTRUCTIONS

Remove all metallic objects before entering the MR environment or MR system room including hearing aids, beeper, cell phone, keys, eyeglasses, hair pins, barrettes, jewelry (including body piercing jewelry), watch, safety pins, paperclips, money clip, credit cards, bank cards, magnetic strip cards, coins, pens, pocket knife, nail clipper, steel-toed boots/shoes, and tools. Loose metallic objects are especially prohibited in the MR system room and MR environment.

Please consult the MRI Technologist or Radiologist if you have any question or concern BEFORE you enter the MR system room.

I attest that the above information is correct to the best of my knowledge. I have read and understand the entire contents of this form and have had the opportunity to ask questions regarding the information on this form.

Signature of Person Completing Form: _____   Date ___ / ___ / ___
                                                              Signature

Form Information Reviewed By: _____   _____
                                          Print name   Signature

☐ MRI Technologist   ☐ Radiologist   ☐ Other _____

Guidelines to Prevent Excessive Heating and Burns Associated with Magnetic Resonance Procedures*

Magnetic resonance (MR) imaging is a relatively safe diagnostic modality. However, damaged radiofrequency coils, physiologic monitors, electronically-activated devices, and external accessories or objects made from conductive materials have caused excessive heating, resulting in burn injuries to patients undergoing MR procedures. Heating of implants and similar devices may also occur, but this tends to be problematic primarily for objects made from conductive materials that have elongated shapes or that form loops of a certain diameter. For example, excessive MRI-related heating has been reported for leads, guidewires, catheters (e.g., catheters with thermistors or other conducting components), and external fixation systems, and cervical fixation systems.

In the United States, many incidents of excessive heating have been reported in patients undergoing MR procedures that were unrelated to equipment problems or the presence of conductive external or internal implants or materials [review of data files from U.S. Food and Drug Administration, Center for Devices and Radiological Health, Manufacturer and User Facility Device Experience Database, MAUDE]. In a review of the MAUDE database over a 10 year period, Hardy and Weil (2010) indicated that 419 thermal injuries were associated with MRI.

These incidents included first, second, and third degree burns that were experienced by patients. In many of these cases, the reports indicated that the limbs or other body parts of the patients were in direct contact with transmit body radiofrequency (RF) coils or other transmit RF coils of the MR systems. In other cases, skin-to-skin contact points were suspected to be responsible for these injuries, however, the exact mechanism responsible for these incidents is unknown.

MR systems require the use of RF pulses to create the MR signal. This RF energy is transmitted through free space from the transmit RF coil to the patient. When conducting materials are placed within the RF field, a concentration of electrical currents sufficient to cause excessive heating and tissue damage may occur. Therefore, only devices with carefully designed current paths can be made safe for use during MR procedures. Simply insulating conductive material (e.g., wire or lead) or separating it from the patient may not be sufficient to prevent excessive heating or burns from occurring for some devices.

Furthermore, certain elongated shapes (i.e. depending on the length and the transmit RF frequency) exhibit the phenomenon of "resonance" that increases their propensity to concentrate RF currents. At the operating frequencies of present day MR systems, conducting loops of tens of centimeters in size can create problems and must be avoided, unless high impedance techniques are used to limit the RF current. Importantly, even loops that include small gaps separated by insulation may still conduct currents.

Pietryga, et al. (2013) reported a case of a thermal burn that occurred during MRI that was likely caused by invisible silver embedded microfibers in the fabric of an undershirt. As the prevalence of fabrics containing nondetectable metallic microfibers increases for use in athletic clothing or other garments, the importance of having patients change into gowns or other appropriate attire that do not contain metallic materials is advised as another means of preventing MRI-related burns. A recent case report by Bertrand, et al. (2017) presented information pertaining to a blanket that combusted in an MR system, likely due the presence of copper fibers used for the fabrication of the blanket's material.

To prevent excessive heating and possible burns in association with MR procedures, the following guidelines are recommended:

1) The patient should change into a gown or other appropriate attire that does not contain metallic material.
2) Prepare the patient for the MR procedure by ensuring that there are no unnecessary metallic objects contacting the patient's skin (e.g., drug delivery patches with metallic components, jewelry, necklaces, bracelets, key chains, etc.).
3) Prepare the patient for the MR procedure by using insulation material (i.e. appropriate padding) to prevent skin-to-skin contact points and the formation of "closed-loops" from touching body parts.
4) Insulating material (minimum recommended thickness, 1-cm) should be placed between the patient's skin and transmit RF coil that is used for the MR procedure (alternatively, the transmit RF coil itself should be padded). There should be no direct contact between the patient's skin and the transmit RF body coil of the MR system. This

may be accomplished by having the patient place his/her arms over his/her head or by using elbow pads or foam padding between the patient's tissue and the transmit RF body coil of the MR system. This is especially important for MR examinations that use the transmit RF body coil or other large RF coils for transmission of RF energy.

5) Use only electrically conductive devices, equipment, accessories (e.g., ECG leads, electrodes, etc.), and materials that have been thoroughly tested and determined to be safe or otherwise acceptable for MR procedures.

6) Carefully follow the MR Safe or MR Conditional criteria and recommendations for implants and devices made from electrically-conductive materials (e.g., bone fusion stimulators, neurostimulation systems, cardiac devices, cochlear implants, etc.).

7) Before using electrical equipment, check the integrity of the insulation and/or housing of all components including surface RF coils, monitoring leads, cables, and wires. Preventive maintenance should be practiced routinely for such equipment.

8) Remove all non-essential electrically conductive materials from the MR system prior to the MR procedure (i.e. unused surface RF coils, ECG leads, EEG leads, cables, wires, etc.).

9) Keep electrically conductive materials that must remain in the MR system from directly contacting the patient by placing thermal and/or electrical insulation between the conductive material and the patient.

10) Keep electrically conductive materials that must remain within the transmit body RF coil or other transmit RF coil from forming conductive loops. Note: The patient's tissue is conductive and, therefore, may be involved in the formation of a conductive loop, which can be circular, U-shaped, or S-shaped.

11) Position electrically conductive materials to prevent "cross points". A cross point is the point where a cable crosses another cable, where a cable loops across itself, or where a cable touches either the patient or sides of the transmit RF coil more than once. Even the close proximity of conductive materials with each other should be avoided because cables and RF coils can capacitively-couple (without any contact or crossover) when placed close together.

12) Position electrically conductive materials (e.g., cables, wires, etc.) to exit down the center of the MR system, *not* along the side of the MR system or close to the transmit RF body coil or other transmit RF coil.

13) Do not position electrically conductive materials across an external metallic prosthesis (e.g., external fixation device, cervical fixation device, etc.) or similar device that is in direct contact with the patient.

14) Allow only properly trained individuals to operate devices (e.g., monitoring equipment) in the MR environment.
15) Follow all manufacturer instructions for the proper operation and maintenance of physiologic monitoring or other similar electronic equipment intended for use during MR procedures.
16) Electrical devices that do not appear to be operating properly during the MR procedure should be removed from the patient immediately.
17) RF surface coil decoupling failures can cause localized RF power deposition levels to reach excessive levels. The MR system operator will recognize such a failure as a set of concentric semicircles in the tissue on the associated MR image or as an unusual amount of image non-uniformity related to the position of the transmit RF coil.
18) Do not permit patients to wear clothing items (e.g., sportswear, underwear, yoga pants, etc.) that have metal-based fibers.
19) Closely monitor the patient during the MR procedure. If the patient reports sensations of heating or other unusual sensation, discontinue the MR procedure immediately and perform a thorough assessment of the situation.

The adoption and regular practice of these guidelines will ensure that patient safety is maintained, especially as more conductive materials and electronically-activated devices are used in association with MR procedures.

[*The document, Guidelines to Prevent Excessive Heating and Burns Associated with Magnetic Resonance Procedures, was developed by the Institute for Magnetic Resonance Safety, Education, and Research (IMRSER) and published with permission. Reviewed and updated 2018.]

REFERENCES

Abdel-Rehim S, et al. Burns from ECG leads in an MRI scanner: Case series and discussion of mechanisms. Ann Burns Fire Disasters 2014;27:215-8.

Bashein G, Syrory G. Burns associated with pulse oximetry during magnetic resonance imaging. Anesthesiology 1991;75:382-3.

Bennett MC, et al. Mechanisms and prevention of thermal injury from gamma radiosurgery headframes during 3T MR imaging. J Appl Clin Med Phys 2012;13:3613.

Bertrand A, et al. A new fire hazard for MR imaging systems: Blankets-case report. Radiology 2017 (In press).

Brown TR, Goldstein B, Little J. Severe burns resulting from magnetic resonance imaging with cardiopulmonary monitoring. Risks and relevant safety precautions. Am J Phys Med Rehabil 1993;72:166-7.

Chou C-K, et al. Absence of radiofrequency heating from auditory implants during magnetic resonance imaging. Bioelectromagnetics 1997;44:367-372.

Dempsey MF, Condon B. Thermal injuries associated with MRI. Clin Radiol 2001;56:457-65.

Dempsey MF, Condon B, Hadley DM. Investigation of the factors responsible for burns during MRI. J Magn Reson Imag 2001;13:627-631.

Diaz F, Tweardy L, Shellock FG. Cervical fixation devices: MRI issues at 3-Tesla. Spine 2010;35:411-5.

ECRI Institute. Health Devices Alert. A new MRI complication? Health Devices Alert May 27, pp. 1, 1988.

ECRI Institute. Thermal injuries and patient monitoring during MRI studies. Health Devices Alert 1991;20:362-363.

ECRI Institute. Hazard Report. Patients can be burned by damaged MRI AV entertainment systems. Health Devices 2008;37:379-80

Friedstat JS, et al. An unusual burn during routine magnetic resonance imaging. J Burn Care Res 2013;34:e110-1.

Haik J, Daniel S, et al. MRI induced fourth-degree burn in an extremity, leading to amputation. Burns 2009;35:294-6.

Hall SC, Stevenson GW, Suresh S. Burn associated with temperature monitoring during magnetic resonance imaging. Anesthesiology 1992;76:152.

Hardy PT, Weil KM. A review of thermal MR injuries. Radiol Technol 2010;81:606-9.

Heinz W, Frohlich E, Stork T. Burns following magnetic resonance tomography study. Z Gastroenterol 1999;37:31-2.

International Commission on Non-Ionizing Radiation Protection (ICNIRP) statement, medical magnetic resonance procedures: Protection of patients. Health Physics 2004;87:197-216.

Jacob ZC, et al. MR imaging-related electrical thermal injury complicated by acute carpal tunnel and compartment syndrome: Case report. Radiology 2010;254:846-50.

Jones S, Jaffe W, Alvi R. Burns associated with electrocardiographic monitoring during magnetic resonance imaging. Burns 1996;22:420-421.

Kainz W. MR heating tests of MR critical implants. J Magn Reson Imag 2007;26:450-1.

Expert Panel on MR Safety, Kanal E, Barkovich AJ, et al. ACR guidance document on MR safe practices: 2013. J Magn Reson Imag 2013;37:501-30.

Kanal E, Shellock FG. Burns associated with clinical MR examinations. Radiology 1990;175:585.

Kanal E, Shellock FG. Policies, guidelines, and recommendations for MR imaging safety and patient management. J Magn Reson Imag 1992;2:247-248.

Karoo RO, et al. Full-thickness burns following magnetic resonance imaging: A discussion of the dangers and safety suggestions. Plast Reconstr Surg 2004;114:1344-1345.

Keens SJ, Laurence AS. Burns caused by ECG monitoring during MR imaging. Anaesthesia 1996;51:1188-9.

Kim LJ, et al. Scalp burns from halo pins following magnetic resonance imaging. Case Report. Journal of Neurosurgery 2003:99:186.

Knopp MV, et al. Unusual burns of the lower extremities caused by a closed conducting loop in a patient at MR imaging. Radiology 1996;200:572-5.

Kugel H, et al. Hazardous situation in the MR bore: Induction in ECG leads causes fire. Eur Radiol 2003;13:690-694.

Lange S, Nguyen QN. Cables and electrodes can burn patients during MRI. Nursing 2006;36:18.

Nakamura T, et al. Mechanism of burn injury during magnetic resonance imaging (MRI)-simple loops can induce heat injury. Front Med Biol Eng 2001;11:117-29.

Newcombe VF, et al. Potential heating caused by intraparenchymal intracranial pressure transducers in a 3-Tesla magnetic resonance imaging system using a body radiofrequency resonator: Assessment of the Codman MicroSensor Transducer. J Neurosurg 2008;109:159-64.

Nyenhuis JA, et al. Heating near implanted medical devices by the MRI RF-magnetic field. IEEE Trans Magn 1999;35:4133-4135.

Pietryga JA, et al. Invisible metallic microfiber in clothing presents unrecognized MRI risks for cutaneous burns. Am J Neuroradiol 2013;34:E47-50.

Ruschulte H, Piepenbrock S, Munte S, Lotz J. Severe burns during magnetic resonance examination. Eur J Anaesthesiol 2005;22:319-320.

Scheel M, et al. Evaluation of intracranial electrocorticography recording strips and tissue partial pressure of oxygen and temperature probes for radio-frequency-induced heating. Acta Neurochir Suppl. 2013;115:149-52.

Shellock FG. Radiofrequency-induced heating during MR procedures: A review. J Magn Reson Imag 2000;12: 30-36.

Shellock FG, Crues JV. MR procedures: Biologic effects, safety, and patient care. Radiology 2004;232:635-652.

Shellock FG, Slimp G. Severe burn of the finger caused by using a pulse oximeter during MRI. Am J Roentgenol 1989;153:1105.

Tanaka R, et al. Overheated and melted intracranial pressure transducer as cause of thermal brain injury during magnetic resonance imaging. J Neurosurg 2012;117:1100-9.

Takahashi T, et al. MRI-related thermal injury due to skin-to-skin contact. Eur J Dermatol 2016;26:296-8.

Tjalma WA. Burning of an ulcerated breast cancer during MRI: A lesson to be learned. JBR-BTR 2014;97:125.

Tsai LL, et al. A practical guide to MR imaging safety: What radiologists need to know. Radiographics 2015;35:1722-37.

Wright BB, et al. A neck burn of unexpected etiology during magnetic resonance imaging of a one year old boy. J Clin Anesth 2014;26:86-7.

Yamazaki M, et al. Investigation of local heating caused by closed conducting loop at clinical MR imaging: Phantom study. Nippon Hoshasen Gijutsu Gakkai Zasshi 2008;20;64:883-5.

Infection Control in the MRI Environment

The magnetic resonance (MR) imaging environment is a complex and potentially dangerous setting with respect to issues involving infection control, particularly because custodial personnel and routine cleaning equipment are not permitted to enter this area without adhering to strict policies and procedures. Importantly, cleaning the MR system room is often the responsibility of the MR system operator, who is rarely trained or certified in infection control. Therefore, it is unreasonable to believe that the MRI environment, especially the MR system and associated accessories (e.g., inside the bore of the scanner, surface coils, the positioning pads/sponges, patient management devices, etc.), can be cleaned safely and effectively by untrained personnel. This important task requires specialized written procedures and proper training.

Patients with serious infections may undergo diagnostic imaging during the course of their treatment. There is frequently a lack of special procedures for managing highly contagious patients, particularly at outpatient imaging centers and mobile MR scanners. Contagious patients may simply be placed on the MR system table and scanned, while the next patient, possibly an immunosuppressed child with a sprained knee, is put on the table directly after this infected patient without properly cleaning the table, pads, and sponges. Obviously, this is a serious situation that deserves attention. Therefore, all MRI facilities must take appropriate action to ensure that the MR environment is not a site for exposing patients and healthcare workers to microorganisms that are capable of causing infectious diseases.

At many MRI centers, there is a misconception that merely placing a clean sheet over the scanner table, without actually cleaning the mattress between patients, will prevent the spread of infectious agents. Of note is that placing clean sheets on a contaminated surface may contaminate the sheets and pose further infectious risk when the sheets are handled. Of further concern is that very few MRI facilities clean inside of the bore of the MR system on a regular basis. Positioning pads and sponges may only be cleaned once a day.

There is also the issue of potentially spreading infectious agents by direct or indirect contact among the imaging staff and patients within the imaging facility. For MR systems in mobile facilities, ensuring proper hygiene is often more difficult, since these sites may not have a sink or running water. Therefore, hand-washing between patients as well as using hand sanitizer regularly is of crucial importance.

Another overlooked area is the presence of torn or frayed positioning pads, sponges, and scanner table mattresses used in association with MRI examinations. Once the covering material has been breached, the surfaces of these items cannot be properly cleaned and should be immediately removed and replaced. It is well known that, if disinfected, a smooth surface can be repeatedly used without problems. However, for items with a porous surface (e.g., those made from "spongy" materials), the presence of infectious agents, including Methicillin-resistant Staphylococcus aureus, MRSA, can be detected even after performing disinfection. Thus, porous surfaces made of such materials cannot be adequately cleaned and disinfected.

Protecting patients and staff takes a concerted effort by all parties involved in the MRI facility. There is no question that infection control has not received the attention that it deserves and there is a growing concern that at least some of the spread of infectious agents could be coming from outpatient imaging centers and radiology departments in hospitals.

The following recommendations are provided for MRI facilities to address infection control standards that are used throughout the healthcare industry:

Recommendations for Infection Control in the MRI Environment

1) Create a written infectious control policy to include cleaning procedures for the MRI environment, as well as a cleaning schedule, and have it posted throughout the center.
2) Implement a mandatory hand-washing / hand-sanitizing procedure between each patient not only for MRI healthcare workers, but also for others who come into contact with patients.
3) Clean the MR scanner table, the area inside the bore of the MR system, and all items that come into contact with the patient. Infection control experts recommend that the cleaning procedure should be performed between patients.
4) Clean all positioning pads and sponges with an approved disinfectant. Infection control experts recommend cleaning after each patient.

5) Periodically inspect the pads with a magnifying glass, particularly at the seams, to identify fraying or tearing. Replace the pads, as needed.

6) Use pillows with a waterproof covering that is designed to be surface wiped. Replace pillows when this barrier is compromised.

7) Promptly remove body fluids and then disinfect all contaminated areas.

8) If the patient has an open wound or history of infection, especially related to MRSA, gloves and gowns must be worn by all staff members coming into contact with the patient. These barriers must be removed before touching other areas that do not come in contact with the patient (e.g., door knobs, scanner console, computer keyboards, etc.).

9) The scanner table, positioning sponges, and pads should be completely cleaned with disinfectant before the next patient is scanned, if this procedure is not already being performed between each patient. For patients with any known infectious process, add 10-15 minutes to the scheduled scan time to ensure that there is enough time to thoroughly clean the room and patient-related surfaces.

10) All furniture should be periodically cleaned. Ideal surfaces are those that are waterproof, nonporous, and easy to clean. Infection control experts recommend that such cleaning be performed between patients.

[Content excerpted with permission provided by Peter Rothschild, M.D. Louisville, KY. Reviewed and updated 2018.]

REFERENCES

Brennan PJ, Abrutyn E. Developing policies and guidelines. Infec Control Hosp Epidemiol 1995;16:512-517.

CNA. MRSA Alert: MRI infection creates new "superbug" concerns. AlertBulletin. Issue 4, 09, www.CNA.com/healthpro

Datta R, Huang SS. Risk of infection and death due to methicillin-resistant Staphylococcus aureus in long-term carriers. Clin Infect Dis 2008;47:176-81.

Guidelines for Environmental Infection Control and Healthcare Facilities Recommendations of CDC and Healthcare Infection Control Practices Advisory Committee (HICPAC) 2003. Available from the Center for Disease Control and Prevention, www.cdc.gov

Haley RW, et al. The efficacy of infection surveilliance and control programs in preventing nosocomial infections in US hospitals. Am J Epidemiology 1985;121:182-205.

Huang SS, Datta R, Platt R. Risk of acquiring antibiotic-resistant bacteria from prior room occupants. Arch Intern Med 2006;166:1945-51.

Huang SS, et al. Impact of routine intensive care unit surveillance cultures and resultant barrier precautions on hospital-wide methicillin-resistant Staphylococcus aureus bacteremia. Clin Infect Dis 2006;43:971-8.

Lawton, RM, et al. Prepackaged hand hygiene educational tools facilitate implementation. Am J Infection Control 2006;34:152-154.

Oie S, et al. Contamination of environmental surfaces by Staphylococcus aureus in a dermatological ward and its preventive measures. J Hosp Infect 1998;40:135-40.

Pulgliese G, et al. Development and implementation of infection control policies and procedures. In: Mayhill CG. Hospital Epidemiology and Infection Control. Philadelphia: Lippincott, Williams and Wilkins, 1999, pp.1357-1366.

Shiomori T, et al. Evaluation of bedmaking-related airborne and surface methicillin-resistant Staphylococcus aureus contamination. J Hosp Infect 2002;50:30-5.

Tsai LL, et al. A practical guide to MR imaging safety: What radiologists need to know. Radiographics 2015;35:1722-37.

Yokoe DS, Classen, D. Improving patient safety through infection control: A new healthcare imperative. Infect Control Hosp Epidemiol 2008;29:S3-S11.

Magnetic Resonance Imaging: Information for Patients*

Message to MR Users: This information is provided as a template for use by MRI facilities. Therefore, an MRI facility is free to utilize this information, as needed, and to modify, adapt, or otherwise change the content relative to the specific facility and conditions.

What is magnetic resonance imaging (MRI)?

MRI, or magnetic resonance imaging, is a means of "seeing" inside of the body in order for doctors to find certain diseases or abnormal conditions. MRI does not rely on the type of radiation (i.e. ionizing radiation) used for an X-ray or computed tomography (CT). The MRI examination requires specialized equipment that uses a powerful, constant magnetic field, rapidly changing local magnetic fields, radiofrequency energy, and dedicated equipment including a powerful computer to create very clear pictures of internal body structures.

During the MRI examination, the patient is placed within the MR system or "scanner". The powerful, constant magnetic field aligns a tiny fraction of subatomic particles called protons that are present in most of the body's tissues. Radiofrequency energy is applied to cause these protons to produce signals that are picked up by a receiver within the scanner. The signals are specially characterized using the rapidly changing, local magnetic field and computer-processed to produce images of the body part of interest.

What is MRI used for?

MRI has become the preferred procedure for diagnosing a large number of potential problems in many different parts of the body. In general, MRI creates pictures that can show differences between healthy and unhealthy tissue. Doctors use MRI to examine the brain, spine, joints (e.g., knee, shoulder, wrist, and ankle), abdomen, pelvic region, breast, blood vessels, heart and other body parts.

Is MRI safe?

To date, over 500 million patients have had MRI examinations. MRI has been shown to be extremely safe as long as proper safety precautions are taken. In general, the MRI procedure produces no pain and causes no known short-term or long-term tissue damage of any kind.

The powerful magnetic field of the scanner can attract certain metallic objects that are "ferromagnetic", causing them to move suddenly and with great force towards the center of the MR system. This may pose a risk to the patient or anyone in the path of the object. Therefore, great care is taken to prevent ferromagnetic objects from entering the MR system room. It is vital that you remove metallic objects in advance of an MRI examination, including watches, jewelry, and items of clothing that have metallic threads or fasteners.

The MRI facility has a screening procedure that, when carefully followed, will ensure that the MRI technologist and radiologist knows about the presence of metallic implants and materials so that special precautions can be taken (see below). In some unusual cases, the examination may be cancelled because of concern related to a particular implant or device. For example, if an MRI is ordered, it may be cancelled if the patient has a ferromagnetic aneurysm clip because of the risk of dislodging the clip from the blood vessel. Also, the magnetic field of the scanner can damage an external hearing aid or cause a heart pacemaker to malfunction. If you have a bullet, shrapnel, or similar metallic fragment in your body there is a potential risk that it could change position, possibly causing injury.

How to prepare for the MRI examination.

There's no special preparation necessary for the MRI examination. Unless your doctor specifically requests that you not eat or drink anything before the exam, there are no food or drink restrictions. Continue to take any medication prescribed by your doctor unless otherwise directed.

You won't be allowed to wear anything metallic during the MRI examination, so it would be best to leave watches, jewelry or anything made from metal at home. Even some cosmetics contain small amounts of metals, so it is best to not wear make-up.

In order to prevent metallic objects from being attracted by the powerful magnet of the MR system, you may receive a gown (which is advisable) to wear during your examination. Items that need to be removed before entering the MR system room include:

- Purse, wallet, money clip, credit cards, other cards with magnetic strips
- Electronic devices such as beepers or cellular phones
- Hearing aids
- Metallic jewelry, watches
- Pens, paper clips, keys, nail clippers, coins
- Hair barrettes, hairpins
- Any article of clothing that has a metallic zipper, buttons, snaps, hooks, under-wires, or metallic threads
- Shoes, belt buckles, safety pins

Before the MRI procedure, you will be asked to fill out a screening form asking about anything that might create a health risk or interfere with the examination. You will also undergo an interview by a member of the MRI facility to ensure that you understand the questions on the form. Even if you have undergone an MRI procedure before at this or another facility, you will still be asked to complete an MRI screening form.

Examples of items or things that may create a health hazard or other problem during an MRI exam include:

- Pacemaker
- Implantable cardioverter defibrillator (ICD)
- Neurostimulation system
- Aneurysm clip
- Metallic implant
- Implanted drug infusion device
- Foreign metal objects, especially if in or near the eye
- Shrapnel or bullet
- Permanent cosmetics or tattoos
- Dentures/teeth with magnetic keepers
- Other implants that involve magnets
- Medication patch (i.e. transdermal patch) that contains metallic foil

Check with the MRI technologist or radiologist at the MRI facility if you have questions or concerns about any implanted object or health condition that could impact the MRI procedure. This is particularly important if you have undergone surgery involving the brain, ear, eye, heart, or blood vessels.

Important Note: If you are pregnant or think that you could be pregnant, you must notify your physician and the radiologist, or the MRI technologist at the MRI facility prior to the MRI procedure.

Before entering the MR system room, any friend or relative that might be allowed to accompany you will be asked questions to ensure that he or she may safely enter the room and will likewise be instructed to remove all metallic objects. Additionally, this individual will need to fill out a screening form.

What is the MRI examination like?

The MRI examination is performed in a special room that houses the MR system or "scanner". You will be escorted into the room by a staff member of the MRI facility and asked to lie down on a comfortably padded table that gently glides you into the scanner.

In order to prepare for the MRI examination, you may be required to wear earplugs or headphones to protect your hearing because, when certain scanners operate, they may produce loud noises. These loud noises are normal and should not worry you.

For some MRI studies, a contrast agent called "gadolinium" may be injected into a vein to help obtain a clearer picture of the body part that is undergoing examination. At some point during the procedure, a nurse or MRI technologist will slide the table out of the scanner to inject the contrast agent. This is typically done through a small needle connected to an intravenous line that is placed in an arm or hand vein. A saline solution will drip through the intravenous line to prevent clotting until the contrast agent is injected at some point during the exam. Unlike contrast agents used in X-ray studies, MRI contrast agents do not contain iodine and, therefore, rarely cause allergic reactions or other problems.

The most important thing for you to do is to relax and remain still. Most MRI exams take between 15 to 45 minutes to complete depending on the body part imaged and how many images are needed, although some may take 60 minutes or longer. You'll be told ahead of time how long your scan is expected to take.

You will be asked to remain perfectly still during the time the imaging takes place, but between sequences some minor movement may be allowed. The MRI technologist will advise you, accordingly.

When the MRI procedure begins, you may breathe normally, however, for certain examinations it may be necessary for you to hold your breath for a short period of time.

During your MRI examination, the MR system operator will be able to speak to you, hear you, and observe you at all times. Consult the MR system operator if you have any question or feel anything unusual.

When the MRI procedure is over, you may be asked to wait until the images are examined to determine if more images are needed. After the scan, you have no restrictions and can go about your normal activities.

Once the entire MRI examination is completed, the pictures will be reviewed by a radiologist, a specially-trained physician who is able to interpret the images for your doctor. The radiologist will send your doctor a report. You should contact your doctor to go over your results and discuss your next step.

DISCLAIMER

This information is provided for the sole purpose of educating you as to the basics of the MRI examination. You should rely on your physician, a radiologist, or an MRI technologist for specific information about your own examination.

[*Developed in conjunction with the Safety Committee of the International Society for Magnetic Resonance in Medicine, www.ISMRM.org. Reviewed and updated 2018.]

Metallic Foreign Bodies
and Screening

A patient or individual with a history of being injured by a metallic foreign body such as a bullet, shrapnel, or other metallic object should be thoroughly screened and evaluated prior to admission to the area of the MR system. This is particularly important because serious injury may occur as a result of movement or dislodgment of the metallic foreign body as it is attracted by the powerful static magnetic field. In addition, excessive heating may occur, although this tends to happen only if the object is made from conductive material and has an elongated shape or forms a loop of a certain diameter.

The relative risk of injury is dependent on the ferromagnetic properties of the foreign body, the geometry and dimensions of the object, the strength of the static magnetic field, and the strength of the spatial gradient magnetic field of the MR system. Additionally, the potential for injury is related to the amount of force with which the object is "fixed" or retained within the tissue (i.e. counter-force or retention force from scarring or encapsulation may prevent migration of the metal) and whether or not it is positioned in or adjacent to a sensitive site of the body such as vital neural, vascular, or soft tissue structure.

The use of plain film radiography or computed tomography (CT) is recommended to detect metallic foreign bodies for individuals and patients prior to admission to the MR environment. This includes screening for the presence of metallic orbital foreign bodies (see **Metallic Orbital Foreign Bodies and Screening**). The sensitivity of plain film radiography is considered to be sufficient to identify any metal object with a mass large enough to present a hazard to an individual or patient in the MR environment.

In 2013, Karacozoff and Shellock (2013) reported that a particular ferromagnetic detection system (Ferroguard Screener, Metrasens) may provide an additional means of guiding the decision regarding management of patients with metallic foreign bodies insofar as this device was successfully utilized to identify a ferromagnetic, armor-piercing bullet.

REFERENCES

Boutin RD, et al. Injuries associated with MR imaging: Survey of safety records and methods used to screen patients for metallic foreign bodies before imaging. Am J Roentgenol 1994;162:189.

Elster AD, et al. Patient screening prior to MR imaging: A practical approach synthesized from protocols at 15 U.S. medical centers. Am J Roentgenol 1994;162:195.

Eshed I, et al. Is magnetic resonance imaging safe for patients with retained metal fragments from combat and terrorist attacks? Acta Radiol 2010;51:170-4.

Karacozoff AM, Shellock FG. Armor-piercing bullet: 3-Tesla MRI findings and identification by a ferromagnetic detection system. Military Medicine 2013;178:e380-5.

International Commission on Non-Ionizing Radiation Protection (ICNIRP) statement, medical magnetic resonance procedures: Protection of patients. Health Physics 2004;87:197-216.

Jarvik JG, Ramsey JG. Radiographic screening for orbital foreign bodies prior to MR imaging: Is it worth it? Am J Neuroradiol 2000;1:245.

Mani, RL. In search of an effective screening system for intraocular metallic foreign bodies prior to MR - An important issue of patient safety. Am J Neuroradiol 1988;9:1032.

Murphy KJ, Burnberg JA. Orbital plain film as a prerequisite for MR imaging: Is a known history of injury sufficient screening criteria? Am J Roentgenol 1996;167:1053.

Otto PM, et al. Screening test for detection of metallic foreign objects in the orbit before magnetic resonance imaging. Invest Radiol 1992;27:308-311.

Seidenwurm DJ, et al. Cost utility analysis of radiographic screening for an orbital foreign body before MR imaging. Am J Neuroradiol 2000;21:426.

Shellock FG, Crues JV. MR procedures: Biologic effects, safety, and patient care. Radiology 2004;232:635-652.

Shellock FG, Crues JV, Editors. MRI Bioeffects, Safety, and Patient Management. Biomedical Research Publishing Group, Los Angeles, CA, 2014.

Shellock FG, Kanal E. SMRI Safety Committee. Policies, guidelines, and recommendations for MR imaging safety and patient management. J Magn Reson Imag 1991;1:97-101.

Williams S, et al. Ferrous intraocular foreign bodies and magnetic resonance imaging. Am J Ophthalmology 1998;105:398.

Zhang Y, et al. Tiny ferromagnetic intraocular foreign bodies detected by magnetic resonance imaging: A report of two cases. J Magn Reson Imag 2009;29:704-7.

Metallic Orbital Foreign Bodies and Screening

The case report in 1986 by Kelly, et al. regarding a patient that sustained an orbital injury from a metallic foreign body led to substantial controversy regarding the procedure required to screen patients prior to MR procedures. Notably, this incident is one of the few serious eye injuries that has occurred in the MR environment. Accordingly, the policy of performing radiographic screening for orbital foreign bodies in patients or individuals simply because of a history of occupational exposure to metallic fragments must be reconsidered.

A study by Seidenwurm, et al. (2000) evaluated the practical aspects and cost-effectiveness of using a clinical versus radiographic technique to initially screen patients for orbital foreign bodies before MR procedures. The cost of screening was determined on the basis of published reports, disability rating guides, and a practice survey. A sensitivity analysis was performed for each variable. For this analysis, the benefits of screening were avoidance of immediate, permanent, nonameliorable, or unilateral blindness.

The findings of Seidenwurm, et al. support the fact that the use of clinical screening before radiography increases the cost-effectiveness of foreign body screening by an order of magnitude (i.e. assuming base case ocular foreign body removal rates). From a clinical screening standpoint for a metallic foreign body located in the orbit, asking the patient "Did a doctor get it all out?" serves this purpose.

Seidenwurm, et al. implemented the following policy with regard to screening patients with suspected metallic foreign bodies, "If a patient reports injury from an ocular foreign body that was subsequently removed by a doctor or that resulted in negative findings on any examination, we perform MR imaging. Those persons with a history of injury and no subsequent negative eye examination are screened radiographically." Of note is that Seidenwurm, et al. performed more than 100,000 MRI procedures under this protocol without incident.

Thus, an occupational history of exposure to metallic fragments, by itself, is insufficient to mandate radiographic orbital screening. Therefore, guidelines for foreign body screening should be based on this information and because radiographic screening before MR procedures on the basis of occupational exposure alone is neither clinically necessary nor cost-effective.

Clinical Screening Protocol. The procedure to follow with regard to patients with suspected metallic orbital foreign bodies involves asking them if they had an ocular injury. If they sustained an ocular injury, they are asked whether they had a medical examination at the time of the injury and whether they were told by the examining doctor, "It's all out." If they did not have an injury, if they were told their ophthalmologic examination was normal, and/or if the foreign body was removed entirely at the time of the injury, then they can proceed to MR imaging.

Radiographic Screening Protocol. Based on the results of the clinical screening protocol, patients are screened radiographically if they sustained an ocular injury related to a metallic foreign object and they were told that the eye examination revealed that the foreign body was not removed. In such a case, the MRI examination is postponed and the patient is scheduled for screening radiography.

In the event that the removal of the entire metallic foreign body cannot be verified or if there is insufficient information to confirm that there is no metallic foreign body present, screening radiography should be used prior to MRI.

SCREENING ADOLESCENTS FOR METALLIC ORBITAL FOREIGN BODIES

A case report by Elmquist and Shellock (1996) illustrates that special precautions are needed for screening adolescent patients prior to MR procedures. This article described an incident in which a 12-year-old patient accompanied by his parent completed all routine screening procedures prior to MR imaging of the lumbar spine. The patient and parent provided negative answers to all questions regarding prior injuries by metallic objects and the presence of metallic foreign bodies.

While entering the MR system room, the adolescent patient appeared to be anxious about the examination. He was placed in a feet-first, supine position on the MR system table and prepared for the procedure. As the patient was moved slowly toward the opening of a 1.5-Tesla MR system, he complained of a pressure sensation in his left eye. The MRI technologist immediately removed the patient from the MR environment.

Once again, the patient was questioned regarding a previous eye injury. The patient denied sustaining such an injury. Despite that patient's response, a metallic foreign body in the orbit was suspected. Therefore, plain film radiographs of the orbits were obtained and revealed a metallic foreign body in the left orbit. The patient and parent were counseled regarding the implications of future MR procedures with respect to the possibility of significant eye injury related to movement or dislodgment of the metallic object. This case demonstrates that routine safety protocols may be insufficient for adolescents referred for MR procedures. Accordingly, it is recommended to provide adolescents with additional screening that includes private counseling about the hazards associated with the MR environment.

REFERENCES

Boutin RD, et al. Injuries associated with MR imaging: Survey of safety records and methods used to screen patients for metallic foreign bodies before imaging. Am J Roentgenol 1994;162:189.

Elmquist C, Shellock FG, Stoller D. Screening adolescents for metallic foreign bodies before MR procedures. J Magn Reson Imag 1996;5:784.

Elster AD, et al. Patient screening prior to MR imaging: A practical approach synthesized from protocols at 15 U.S. medical center. Am J Roentgenol 1994;162:195.

Expert Panel on MR Safety, Kanal E, Barkovich AJ, Bell C, et al. ACR guidance document on MR safe practices: 2013. J Magn Reson Imag 2013;37:501-30.

Jarvik JG, Ramsey JG. Radiographic screening for orbital foreign bodies prior to MR imaging: Is it worth it? Am J Neuroradiol 2000;21:245.

Kelly WM, et al. Ferromagnetism of intraocular foreign body causes unilateral blindness after MR study. Am J Neuroradiol 1986;7:243.

Lawrence DA, et al. Undetected intraocular metallic foreign body causing hyphema in a patient undergoing MRI: A rare occurrence demonstrating the limitations of pre-MRI safety screening. Magn Reson Imaging 2015;33:358-61.

Mani RL. In search of an effective screening system for intraocular metallic foreign bodies prior to MR - An important issue of patient safety. Am J Neuroradiol 1988;9:1032.

Murphy KJ, Brunberg JA. Orbital plain film as a prerequisite for MR imaging: Is a known history of injury sufficient screening criteria? Am J Roentgenol 1996;167:1053-5.

Seidenwurm DJ, et al. Cost utility analysis of radiographic screening for an orbital foreign body before MR imaging. AJNR 2000;21:426-233.

Shellock FG. New recommendations for screening patients for suspected orbital foreign bodies. Signals, No. 36, Issue 4, pp. 8-9, 2001.

Shellock FG, Kanal E. SMRI Safety Committee. Policies, guidelines, and recommendations for MR imaging safety and patient management. J Magn Reson Imag 1991;1:97-101.

Williams S, et al. Ferrous intraocular foreign bodies and magnetic resonance imaging. Am J Opthalmol 1998;05:398.

Zhang Y, et al. Tiny ferromagnetic intraocular foreign bodies detected by magnetic resonance imaging: A report of two cases. J Magn Reson Imag 2009;29:704-7.

Monitoring Patients in the MR Environment

Conventional monitoring equipment and accessories were not designed to operate in the harsh magnetic resonance (MR) environment that utilizes electromagnetic fields that can adversely affect or alter the operation of these devices. Fortunately, physiologic monitors and other patient support devices have been developed or specially-modified to perform properly in this setting.

MR healthcare professionals must consider the ethical and medico-legal ramifications of providing proper patient care that includes identifying patients that require monitoring in the MR setting and following a proper protocol to ensure their safety by using appropriate equipment, devices, and accessories. The early detection and treatment of complications that may occur in high-risk, critically-ill, sedated, or anesthetized patients undergoing MR procedures can prevent relatively minor problems from becoming life-threatening situations.

GENERAL POLICIES AND PROCEDURES

Monitoring during an MR examination is indicated whenever a patient requires observations of vital physiologic parameters due to an underlying health problem or is unable to respond or alert the MRI technologist or other healthcare professional regarding pain, respiratory problem, cardiac distress, or difficulty that might arise during the procedure. In addition, a patient should be monitored if there is a greater potential for a change in physiologic status during the MR exam. **Table 1** summarizes the patients that may require monitoring during MR procedures. Besides patient monitoring, various support devices and accessories may be needed for use in high-risk patients to ensure safety.

Because of the widespread use of MRI contrast agents and the potential for adverse effects or idiosyncratic reactions to occur, it is prudent to have monitoring equipment and accessories readily available for the proper management and support of patients who may experience side-effects. This is emphasized because adverse events, while extremely rare, may be serious or life threatening.

In 1992, the Safety Committee of the Society for Magnetic Resonance Imaging first published guidelines and recommendations concerning the monitoring of patients during MR procedures. This information indicates that all patients undergoing MR examinations should be visually and/or verbally (e.g., intercom system) monitored, and that patients who are sedated, anesthetized, or are unable to communicate must be physiologically monitored and supported by the appropriate means.

Importantly, guidelines issued by the Joint Commission indicate that patients receiving sedatives or anesthetics require monitoring during administration and recovery from these medications. Other professional organizations, including the American College of Radiology (ACR), and the American Society of Anesthesiologists (ASA), similarly recommend the need to monitor certain patients using proper equipment and techniques.

Table 1. Patients that require monitoring and support during MR procedures.

- Physically or mentally unstable patients.
- Patients with compromised physiologic functions.
- Patients who are unable to communicate.
- Neonatal and pediatric patients.
- Sedated or anesthetized patients.
- Patients undergoing MR-guided interventional or intraoperative procedures.
- Critically-ill or high-risk patients.
- Patients who may have a reaction to an MRI contrast agent or medications.

SELECTION OF PARAMETERS TO MONITOR

The proper selection of the specific physiologic parameters that should be monitored during the MR procedure is crucial for patient safety. Various factors must be considered including the patient's medical history, present condition, the use of medication and possible side effects, as well as aspects of the MR procedure to be performed. For example, if the patient requires general anesthesia during the MR procedure, monitoring multiple physiologic parameters is required. Policies and procedures for the management of the patient in the MR environment should be comparable to those used in the operating room or critical care setting, especially with respect to monitoring and support requirements. Specific recommendations for physiologic monitoring of patients during MR examinations should be developed in consideration of "standard of care" issues as well as in consultation with anesthesiologists and other similar healthcare specialists. Notably, the Society of Anesthesiologists Task Force on Anesthetic Care for Magnetic Resonance Imaging recently presented a practice advisory on anesthetic care for patients undergoing MRI (2015).

PERSONNEL INVOLVED IN PATIENT MONITORING

Only healthcare professionals with appropriate training and experience should be permitted to monitor and manage patients during MR procedures. The healthcare professional must be experienced with the operation of the monitoring equipment and accessories used in the MR environment and should be able to recognize equipment malfunctions, device problems, and recording artifacts. Furthermore, this individual should be well-versed in screening patients for conditions that may complicate the procedure. For example, patients with asthma, congestive heart failure, obesity, obstructive sleep apnea, and other conditions are at increased risk for having problems during sedation or anesthesia. Also, the healthcare professional must be able to identify and manage adverse events using appropriate equipment and procedures.

Policies and procedures must be implemented to continue physiologic monitoring and management of the patient by trained personnel after the MR procedure is performed. This is especially needed for a patient recovering from the effects of a sedative or general anesthesia.

The monitoring of physiologic parameters and management of the patient during an MR procedure is typically the responsibility of several individuals depending on the level of training for the healthcare professional and in consideration of the condition, medical history, and procedure that is to be performed for the patient. These individuals include anesthesiologists, nurses, MRI technologists, or radiologists.

EMERGENCY PLAN

The development, implementation, and regular practice of an emergency plan that addresses and defines the activities, use of equipment, and other pertinent issues related to a medical emergency are important for patient safety. For example, a plan needs to be developed for handling patients if there is the need to remove them from the MR system room to perform cardiopulmonary resuscitation. Obviously, taking necessary equipment such as a cardiac defibrillator, intubation instruments, or other similar devices near the MR system could pose a substantial hazard to the patients and healthcare workers if these are not safe for use in the MR environment. Healthcare professionals who are members of the cardiopulmonary resuscitation (i.e. "Code Blue") team must be specially trained to conduct their activities in the MR setting.

For out-patient or mobile MRI facilities, it is necessary to educate outside emergency personnel (e.g., paramedics, firefighters, etc.) regarding the potential hazards associated with the MR environment. Typically, MRI facilities not affiliated with or in close proximity to a hospital must contact paramedics to handle medical emergencies and to transport patients to the hospital for additional care. Therefore, personnel responsible for summoning the paramedics, notifying the hospital, and performing other integral activities must be designated beforehand to avoid problems and confusion during an actual emergent event. To ensure proficiency with the various afore-mentioned tasks, it is advisable to regularly conduct a "mock" emergency.

TECHNIQUES AND EQUIPMENT USED TO MONITOR AND SUPPORT PATIENTS

Physiologic monitoring and support of patients is not a trivial task in the MR environment. The types of equipment for patient monitoring and support must be considered carefully and utilized properly to ensure the safety of both patients and MR healthcare professionals.

Several potential problems and hazards are associated with the performance of patient monitoring and support in the MR environment. Physiologic monitors and accessories that contain ferromagnetic components (e.g., transformers, outer casings, etc.) can be strongly attracted by the static magnetic field used of the MR system, posing a serious "missile" or projectile hazard to patients and healthcare workers.

Necessary or critical devices that have ferromagnetic components should be permanently fixed to the floor or tethered to the wall and properly labeled with warning information to prevent them from being moved too close to the MR system. All personnel involved with MR procedures should be aware of the importance of the placement and use of the equipment, especially with regard to the hazards of moving portable equipment too close to the MR system to prevent serious missile-related and other accidents.

Electromagnetic fields associated with the MR system can significantly effect the operation of conventional monitoring equipment. In addition, the monitoring equipment, itself, may emit spurious electromagnetic noise that, in turn, produces artifacts on the MR images.

Physiologic monitors that contain microprocessors or other similar components may "leak" and produce electromagnetic interference that can substantially alter MR images. To prevent adverse interactions between the MR system and physiologic monitors, RF-shielded cables, RF filters, special outer RF-shielded enclosures, or fiber-optic techniques can be utilized to prevent image-related or other problems in the MR environment.

During the operation of MR systems, electrical currents may be generated in the conductive materials of monitoring equipment that are used as part of the interface to the patient. These currents can be of sufficient magnitude to cause excessive heating and thermal injury to the patient. Serious burns have occurred in association with MR procedures that were directly attributed to the utilization of monitoring devices. These injuries were related to the use of electrocardiographic lead wires, plethysmographic gating systems, pulse oximeters, and other types of monitoring equipment comprised of wires, cables, or similar components made from conductive materials. Therefore, it is important to follow the instructions and recommendations from the manufacturers with regard to the use of the devices in the MR environment. Fortunately, modern-day physiologic monitoring devices utilize fiber-optic techniques to prevent many of the afore-mentioned issues that exist with "hard-wire" cables, wires, and patient-monitor interfaces.

MONITORING EQUIPMENT AND SUPPORT DEVICES

This section describes the physiologic parameters that may be assessed in patients during MR examinations using appropriate monitoring equipment for the MR environment. In addition, various devices and accessories that are useful for the support and management of patients are presented.

Electrocardiogram and Heart Rate

Monitoring the patient's electrocardiogram (ECG) in the MR environment is particularly challenging because of the inherent distortion of the ECG waveform that occurs using MR systems operating at high field strengths. This effect is observed as blood, a conductive fluid, flows through the large vascular structures in the presence of the static magnetic field of the MR system. The resulting induced biopotential is seen primarily as an augmented T-wave amplitude, although other non-specific waveform-changes are also apparent on the ECG. Since altered T-waves or ST segments may be associated with cardiac disorders, static magnetic field-induced ECG-distortions may be problematic for certain patients. For this reason, it may be necessary to obtain a baseline recording of the ECG prior to placing the patient inside the MR system along with a recording obtained immediately after the MR procedure to determine the cardiac status of the patient.

Additional artifacts caused by the static, gradient, and RF fields of the MR system can severely distort the ECG, making observation of morphologic changes and detection of arrhythmias difficult. ECG artifacts that occur in the MR environment may be decreased substantially by implementing several simple techniques that include, the following:

- Use ECG electrodes that have minimal metal or those recommended by the manufacturer
- Select electrodes and cables that contain nonferromagnetic metals
- Place the limb electrodes in close proximity to one another
- Position the line between the limb electrodes and leg electrodes parallel to the magnetic field flux lines
- Maintain a small area between the limb and leg electrode
- Twist or braid the ECG leads
- Position the area of the electrodes near or in the center of the MR system

The use of proper ECG electrodes (i.e. those tested and deemed to be acceptable for patients by the monitoring equipment manufacturer) is required to ensure patient safety and proper recording of the ECG in the MR environment. Accordingly, ECG electrodes have been specially developed for use during MR procedures to protect the patient from potentially hazardous conditions. These ECG electrodes were also designed to reduce imaging artifacts.

Fiber-optic ECG recording techniques may be used to prevent burns during MR examinations. For example, one such fiber-optic system acquires the ECG waveform using a special transceiver that resides in the MR system bore along with the patient and is located near the ECG electrodes. A module digitizes and optically encodes the ECG waveform and transmits it to the monitor using a fiber-optic cable. The use of this fiber-optic ECG technique eliminates the potential for burns associated with hard-wired ECG systems by removing the conductive patient cable and the "antenna effect" that are typically responsible for excessive heating.

Besides using an ECG monitor, the patient's heart rate may be determined continuously during the MR procedure using other acceptable devices including a photoplethysmograph and a pulse oximeter. A noninvasive, heart rate and blood pressure monitor (see section below) can also be utilized to obtain intermittent or semi-continuous recordings of heart rate during the MR examination.

Blood Pressure

Conventional, manual sphygmomanometers may be adapted for use during MR procedures. This is typically accomplished by lengthening the tubing from the cuff to the device so that the mercury column and other primary components may be positioned an acceptable distance (e.g., at 200-gauss or higher fringe field level) from the MR system. Blood pressure measuring devices that incorporate a spring-gauge may be adversely affected by magnetic fields, causing them to work erroneously in the MR setting. Therefore, spring-gauge blood pressure devices should undergo pre-clinical testing before being used to monitor patients.

A blood pressure monitor that uses the oscillometric method may be utilized to obtain semi-continuous recordings of systolic, diastolic, and mean blood pressures as well as pulse rate. These devices can record systemic blood pressure in adult, pediatric, and neonate patients, selecting the appropriate blood pressure cuff size for the subject. However, the intermittent inflation of the blood pressure cuff by an automated, noninvasive blood pressure monitor may disturb lightly sedated patients, especially infants or neonates, causing them to move and disrupt the MR procedure. For this reason, the use of a noninvasive blood pressure monitor may not be the best instrument to conduct physiologic monitoring in every patient.

Respiratory Rate and Apnea

Because respiratory depression and upper airway obstruction are frequent complications associated with the use of sedatives and anesthetics, monitoring techniques that detect a decrease in respiratory rate, hypoxemia, or airway obstruction should be used during the administration of these drugs. This is particularly important in the MR environment because visual observation of the patient's respiratory efforts is often difficult.

Respiratory rate monitoring can be performed during MR procedures by various techniques. The impedance method that utilizes chest leads and electrodes (similar to those used to record the ECG) may be used to monitor respiratory rate. This technique of recording respiratory rate measures a difference in electrical impedance induced between the leads that correspond to changes in respiratory movements. Unfortunately, the electrical impedance method of assessing respiratory rate tends to be inaccurate in pediatric patients because of the small volumes and associated motions of the relatively small thorax.

Respiratory rate may also be monitored using a rubber bellows placed around the patient's thorax or abdomen (i.e. for "chest" or "belly" breathers). The bellows is attached to a pressure transducer that records body movements associated with inspiration and expiration. However, the bellows monitoring technique, like the electrical impedance method, is only capable of recording body movements associated with respiratory efforts. Therefore, these respiratory rate monitoring techniques do not detect apneic episodes related to upper airway obstruction (i.e. absent airflow despite respiratory effort) and may not provide sufficient sensitivity for assessing patients during MR procedures. For this reason, assessment of respiratory rate and identification of apnea should be accomplished using more appropriate monitoring devices.

Respiratory rate and apnea may be monitored during MR procedures using an end-tidal carbon dioxide monitor or a capnometer. These devices measure the level of carbon dioxide during the end of the respiratory cycle (i.e. end-tidal carbon dioxide). Additionally, capnometers provide quantitative data with respect to end-tidal carbon dioxide that is important for determining certain aspects of gas exchange in patients. The waveform provided on the end-tidal carbon dioxide monitors is also useful for assessing whether the patient is having difficulties breathing. The interface between the patient for the end-tidal carbon dioxide monitor and capnometer is a nasal or oro-nasal cannula that is made from plastic. This interface prevents potential adverse interactions between the monitor and the patient during an MR examination.

Oxygen Saturation

Oxygen saturation is a crucial variable to measure in sedated and anesthetized patients. This physiologic parameter is measured using pulse oximetry, a monitoring technique that assesses the oxygenation of tissue. Additionally, the patient's heart rate may be calculated by measuring the frequency that pulsations occur as the blood moves through the vascular bed. Thus, a pulse oximeter can be used to determine oxygen saturation and pulse rate on a continuous basis by measuring the transmission of light through a vascular site such as the ear lobe, finger-tip, or toe. Notably, anesthesiologists consider the use of pulse oximetry to be the standard practice for monitoring sedated or anesthetized patients.

Commercially-available, specially-modified pulse oximeters that have hard-wire cables have been used to monitor sedated patients during MR procedures with moderate success. Unfortunately, these pulse oximeters tend to work intermittently during the operation of the MR system, primarily due to interference from the gradient and/or radio frequency electromagnetic fields. Of greater concern is the fact that pulse oximeters with hard-wire cables have been responsible for many patient burn injuries during MRI examinations, presumably as a result of excessive current being induced in the conductive cables.

Pulse oximeters have been developed that use fiber-optic technology to obtain and transmit the physiologic signals from the patient. These devices operate without interference by the electromagnetic fields used for MR procedures. Several different fiber-optic pulse oximeters are commercially available for use in the MR environment.

Temperature

There are several reasons to monitor body and/or skin temperatures during MR procedures. These reasons include recording temperatures in neonates with inherent problems retaining body heat (a tendency that is augmented during sedation or anesthesia), in patients during MR procedures that use high levels of RF power, and in patients with underlying conditions that impair their ability to dissipate heat.

Skin and body temperatures may be monitored during MR procedures using a variety of techniques. However, it should be noted that the use of hard-wire, thermistor or thermocouple-based techniques to record temperatures in the MR environment typically cause artifacts or erroneous measurements due to direct heating of the temperature probes. A more appropriate, effective and easier technique of recording temperatures during MR examinations is with the use of a fluoroptic thermometry system. Notably, monitoring skin temperature, only, is insufficient to ensure patient safety as this parameter does not provide proper information relative to "deep" body or core temperature. (See section, "**Monitoring Body Temperature During MRI**").

The fluoroptic monitoring system has several important features that make it particularly useful for temperature monitoring during MR procedures. For example, this device incorporates fiber-optic probes that are small but efficient in carrying optical signals over long paths, it provides noise-free applications in electromagnetically hostile environments, and it has fiber-optic components that will not pose a risk to patients.

Multi-Parameter Physiologic Monitoring Systems

In certain cases, it is necessary to monitor several different physiologic parameters simultaneously in patients undergoing MR examinations. While several different stand-alone units may be used to accomplish this task, the most efficient means of recording multiple parameters is by utilizing a monitoring system that permits the measurement of different physiologic functions such as heart rate, respiratory rate, blood pressure, and oxygen saturation.

Currently, there are a number of multi-parameter patient monitoring systems that are acceptable for use in the MRI environment, even in the 3-Tesla setting. Typically, these devices are designed with components positioned within the MR system room and incorporate special circuitry to substantially reduce the artifacts that effect the recording of ECG and other physiologic variables.

Ventilators

Devices used for mechanical ventilation of patients typically contain mechanical switches, microprocessors, and ferromagnetic components that may be adversely effected by the electromagnetic fields used by MR systems. Ventilators that are activated by high pressure oxygen and controlled by the use of fluidics (i.e. no requirements for electricity) may still have ferromagnetic parts that can malfunction as a result of interference from MR systems.

Ventilators have been modified or specially-designed for use during MR procedures performed in adult as well as neonatal patients. These devices tend to be constructed from non-ferromagnetic materials and have undergone pre-clinical evaluations to ensure that they operate properly in the MR environment, without producing artifacts on MR images.

Some ventilators only operate properly and are approved at a "safe" distance from the MR system due to the presence of ferromagnetic parts, including batteries. Thus, these devices are labeled "MR Conditional' and the conditions for use must be followed carefully. Therefore, it is advisable to permanently fix these ventilators to the floor or tether them to prevent missile-related accidents. Furthermore, these devices must be properly labeled with warning information to prevent them from being moved too close to the MR system. Healthcare professionals should be trained regarding the specific MR Conditional aspects of these ventilators.

Additional Devices and Accessories

A variety of devices and accessories are often necessary for support and management of high-risk or sedated patients in the MR setting. Gurneys, oxygen tanks, gas regulators, stethoscopes, suction devices, infusion pumps, power injectors, and other similar devices and accessories shown to be acceptable for the MR environment may be obtained from various manufacturers and distributors. Additionally, there are gas anesthesia systems available that were designed for use in patients undergoing MR procedures.

SEDATION

Whenever sedatives are used, it is imperative to perform physiologic monitoring to ensure patient safety. In addition, it is important to have the necessary equipment readily available in the event of an emergency. These requirements should also be followed for patients undergoing sedation in the MR environment.

There is controversy regarding who should be responsible for performing sedation of patients in the MR setting. (For the sake of discussion, the terms "sedation" and "anesthesia" are used interchangeably since they are actually part of the same continuum.) Obviously, there are medical, regulatory, administrative, and financial issues to be considered.

In general, for patients with conditions that complicate sedation procedures, a nurse under the direction of an anesthesiologist or a specially trained radiologist may be responsible for preparing, sedating, monitoring, and recovering these cases. However, for patients with serious medical or other unusual problems, it is advisable to utilize anesthesia consultation to properly manage these individuals before, during, and after MR procedures.

In addition, the MRI facility should establish policies and guidelines for patient preparation, monitoring, sedation, and management during the post-sedation recovery period. These policies and guidelines should be based on standards established by the American Society of Anesthesiologists (ASA), the American College of Radiology (ACR), the American Academy of Pediatrics Committee on Drugs (AAP-COD), and the Joint Commission on Accreditation of Healthcare Organizations (JCAHO).

Practice Guidelines for Sedation and Anesthesia from the American Society of Anesthesiologists indicate that a trained healthcare professional must be present that is responsible for monitoring the patient if a sedative or anesthetic agent is used. Furthermore, the following aspects of patient monitoring must be performed:

1) Visual monitoring
2) Assessment of the level of consciousness
3) Evaluation of ventilatory status
4) Evaluation of oxygen status assessed via the use of pulse oximetry
5) Determination of hemodynamic status via the use of blood pressure monitoring and electrocardiography if significant cardiovascular disease is present in the patient

Healthcare professionals must be able to recognize complications of sedation, such as hypoventilation and airway obstruction, as well as be able to establish a patent airway for positive-pressure ventilation.

Patient Preparation

Special patient screening must be conducted to identify conditions that may complicate sedation in order to properly prepare the patient for the administration of a sedative. This screening procedure should request important information from the patient that includes the following: major organ system disease (e.g., diabetes, pulmonary, cardiac, or hepatic disease), prior experience or adverse reactions to sedatives or anesthetics, current medications, allergies to drugs, and a history of alcohol, substance, or tobacco abuse.

In addition, the "nothing by mouth" (NPO) interval for the patient must be determined to reduce the risk of aspiration during the procedure. The ASA "Practice Guidelines Regarding Preoperative Fasting" recommend a minimum NPO periods of two hours for clear liquids, four hours for breast milk, six hours for infant formula, and six hours for a "light meal". The NPO period is extremely important because sedatives may depress the patient's gag reflex.

Administration of Sedation

A thorough discussion of sedation techniques, especially with regard to the use of various pharmacologic agents, is outside the scope of this monograph. Therefore, a review of more recent peer-reviewed papers on this topic is recommended.

Documentation

During the use of sedation, written records must be maintained that indicate the patient's vital signs as well as the name, dosage, and time of administration for all drugs that are given to the patient. The use of a time-based anesthesia-type record is the best means of maintaining written documentation for sedation of patients in the MR environment.

Post-Sedation Recovery

After sedation, the medical care of the patient must continue. This is especially important for pediatric patients because certain medications have relatively long half-lives (e.g., chloral hydrate, pentobarbitol, etc.). Therefore, an appropriate room with monitoring and emergency equipment must be available to properly manage these patients.

Prior to allowing the patient to leave the MRI facility, the patient should be alert, oriented, and have stable vital signs. In addition, a responsible adult should accompany the patient home. Written instructions that include an emergency telephone number should be provided to the patient.

REFERENCES

ACR–SIR Practice Guideline for Sedation/Analgesia, Amended 2014. American College of Radiology (acr.org), Reston, VA.

American Academy of Pediatrics; American Academy of Pediatric Dentistry, Guidelines for monitoring and management of pediatric patients during and after sedation for diagnostic and therapeutic procedures: An update. Pediatrics 2006;118:2587-602.

Dalal PG, et al. Sedation and anesthesia protocols used for magnetic resonance imaging studies in infants: Provider and pharmacologic considerations. Anesth Analg 2006;103:863-8.

De Sanctis Briggs V. Magnetic resonance imaging under sedation in newborns and infants: A study of 640 cases using sevoflurane. Paediatr Anaesth 2005;15:9-15.

Gooden CK. Anesthesia for magnetic resonance imaging. Curr Opin Anaesthesiol 2004;17:339-42.

Greenberg KL, Weinreb J, Shellock FG. "MR conditional" respiratory ventilator system incident in a 3-T MRI environment. Magnetic Resonance Imaging 2011;29:1150-4.

Henrichs B, Walsh RP. Intraoperative magnetic resonance imaging for neurosurgical procedures: Anesthetic implications. AANA J 2011;79:71-7.

Holshouser B, Hinshaw DB, Shellock FG. Sedation, anesthesia, and physiologic monitoring during MRI. J Magn Reson Imag 1993;3:553-558.

Johnston T, et al. Intraoperative MRI: Safety. Neurosurg Clin N Am 2009;20:147-53.

Kanal E, Shellock FG. Policies, guidelines, and recommendations for MR imaging safety and patient management. Patient monitoring during MR examinations. J Magn Reson Imag 1992;2:247.

Kanal E, Shellock FG. Patient monitoring during clinical MR imaging. Radiology 1992;185:623.

Lo C, et al. Effect of magnetic resonance imaging on core body temperature in anaesthetised children. Anaesth Intensive Care 2014;42:333-9.

Expert Panel on MR Safety, Kanal E, Barkovich AJ, et al. ACR guidance document on MR safe practices: 2013. J Magn Reson Imag 2013;37:501-30.

Machata AM, et al. Effect of brain magnetic resonance imaging on body core temperature in sedated infants and children. Br J Anaesth 2009;102:385-9.

McArdle C, et al. Monitoring of the neonate undergoing MR imaging: Technical considerations. Radiology 1986;159:223.

McClain CD, et al. Anesthetic concerns for pediatric patients in an intraoperative MRI suite. Curr Opin Anaesthesiology 2011;24:480-6.

Nasr VG, et al. Performance validation of a modified magnetic resonance imaging-compatible temperature probe in children. Anesth Analg 2012;114:1230-4.

Reinking Rothschild D. Chapter 5, Sedation for open magnetic resonance imaging. In, Open MRI, P. A. Rothschild and D. Reinking Rothschild, Editors, Lippincott, Williams and Wilkins, Philadelphia, 2000, pp. 39.

Practice advisory on anesthetic care for magnetic resonance imaging: an updated report by the American Society of Anesthesiologists Task Force on Anesthetic Care for Magnetic Resonance Imaging. Anesthesiology 2015;122:495-520.

Practice advisory on anesthetic care for magnetic resonance imaging: A report by the Society of Anesthesiologists Task Force on Anesthetic Care for Magnetic Resonance Imaging. Anesthesiology 2009;110:459-79.

Practice Guidelines for Sedation and Analgesia by Non-Anesthesiologists. An updated report by the American Society of Anesthesiologists Task Force on Sedation and Analgesia by Non-Anesthesiologists. Anesthesiology 2002; 96:1004–17.

Schulte-Uentrop L, Goepfert MS. Anaesthesia or sedation for MRI in children. Curr Opin Anaesthesiol 2010;23:513-7.

Serafini G, Zadra N. Anaesthesia for MRI in the paediatric patient. Curr Opin Anaesthesiology 2008;21:499-503.

Shellock FG. Chapter 11, Patient monitoring in the MR environment. In: Magnetic Resonance Procedures: Health Effects and Safety. CRC Press, Boca Raton, FL, 2001, pp. 217-241.

Tsai LL, et al. A practical guide to MR imaging safety: What radiologists need to know. Radiographics 2015;35:1722-37.

Monitoring Body Temperature During MRI

Introduction

Magnetic resonance imaging (MRI) has been an important diagnostic imaging modality for more than 30 years. Advancements in technology and imaging protocols have contributed to the growth of MRI applications and expanded the demographic of patient populations from neonates to high-risk patients. The use of sedation or anesthesia is necessary for certain MRI examinations, especially for pediatric or critically-ill patients (1). Importantly, the volume of pediatric patients undergoing MRI or computed tomography (CT) procedures under sedation or anesthesia has grown at an annual rate of 8% to 9% (2). This monograph focuses on the need to monitor body temperature in patients during MRI and discusses the sites to record temperature based on efficacy and stability of the measurement, as well as the response time (i.e. the temporal resolution) during temperature fluctuations.

Monitoring Patients in the MRI Environment

Conventional monitoring equipment and accessories were not designed to operate in the harsh MRI environment that utilizes electromagnetic fields that can adversely affect or alter the operation of these devices (3). Fortunately, various monitors and other patient support devices have been developed to perform properly during MRI procedures.

MRI healthcare professionals must consider the ethical and medico-legal ramifications of providing proper patient care that includes identifying patients that require monitoring in the MRI setting and following a proper protocol to ensure their safety by using appropriate equipment, devices, and accessories (3). The early detection and treatment of complications that may occur in high-risk, critically-ill, sedated, or anesthetized patients undergoing MRI examinations can prevent relatively minor issues from becoming life-threatening situations.

General Policies and Procedures

Patients undergoing MRI examinations while under sedation or general anesthesia require the same standard of care that is provided in operating rooms and intensive care units (ICU) (4, 5). This involves monitoring vital physiological parameters including the electrocardiogram (ECG), oxygen saturation, blood pressure, end tidal carbon dioxide (CO_2), and body temperature (6, 7). The use of sedation or anesthesia is necessary for certain MRI examinations, especially for pediatric or critically-ill patients (3, 8). Importantly, children represent the largest group requiring sedation for MRI exams (3, 8). Sedation is used on children to minimize discomfort, motion and anxiety during the procedure (8, 9). The American Academy of Pediatrics and the American College of Radiology have published guidelines for monitoring children and adults during sedation (8, 10). The vital signs that must be monitored include the heart rate, blood pressure, respiratory rate, oxygen saturation, blood oxygenation, and body temperature (8).

Because of the widespread use of MRI contrast agents and the potential for adverse effects or idiosyncratic reactions to occur, it is prudent to have appropriate monitoring equipment and accessories readily available for the proper management and support of patients who may experience side-effects. This is emphasized because adverse events, while extremely rare, may be serious or life threatening. In addition, patients may have adverse reactions to other medications while undergoing MRI procedures.

In 1992, the Safety Committee of the Society for Magnetic Resonance Imaging published guidelines and recommendations concerning the monitoring of patients during MRI procedures (11). This information indicates that all patients undergoing MRI examinations should be visually (e.g., using a camera system) and/or verbally (e.g., intercom system) monitored, and that patients who are sedated, anesthetized, or are unable to communicate should be physiologically monitored and supported by the appropriate means.

Injuries and fatalities have occurred in association with MRI examinations. These may have been prevented with the proper use of monitoring equipment and devices (3, 4, 11). Notably, guidelines issued by the Joint Commission on Accreditation of Healthcare Organizations (JCAHO) indicate that patients receiving sedatives or anesthetics require monitoring during administration and recovery from these medications (12). Other professional organizations similarly recommend the need to monitor certain patients using proper equipment and techniques (5, 6, 8, 9, 13).

Why Monitor Body Temperature?

In human subjects, "deep" body or core temperature is regulated between 36 and 38 degrees C by the hypothalamus and continuously fluctuates due to diurnal, internal, and external factors (14). Importantly, the regulation of body temperature is suppressed by anesthesia and generally results in patients becoming hypothermic (15, 16). Side-effects of a decrease in body temperature can range from hypovolemia, myocardial ischemia, cardiac arrhythmia, pulmonary edema, decreased cerebral blood flow in cases of mild hypothermia, to mortality related to extreme hypothermia (17).

Additionally, some patients may experience malignant hyperthermia, which is a rare life-threatening condition that is usually triggered by exposure to certain drugs used for general anesthesia. In susceptible individuals, these drugs can induce a drastic and uncontrolled increase in skeletal muscle oxidative metabolism, which overwhelms the body's capacity to supply oxygen, remove carbon dioxide, and regulate body temperature. Malignant hyperthermia can eventually lead to circulatory collapse and death if not quickly identified and treated.

The anesthesiologist or nurse anesthetist may not be able to clearly visualize or have close access to the patient during the MRI procedure due to the design of the MR system. The anesthesiologist or nurse anesthetist may not be in the immediate proximity of the patient during the MRI procedure due to the design of the MR system. Therefore, it is imperative to continuously monitor the body temperature and provide real time information to the anesthesia healthcare professional. It is also important that the measurement site has clinical relevance and a relatively "fast" response time to any fluctuation in body temperature because the anesthesiologist or nurse anesthetist is unable to visualize the discoloration of the patient's skin in cases of sudden temperature changes.

Measuring Body Temperature During an MRI

The accuracy and efficacy of the measurement of body temperature has been a topic of discussion for many years (14, 18-20). The measurement of temperature in a human subject is affected by the following factors (14, 21):

- The site of measurement (e.g., skin, oral, esophagus, rectal, pulmonary artery, hypothalamus, bladder, tympanic membrane, axillary area).
- Environmental conditions (temperature and humidity).
- The measurement technique (e.g., mercury thermometer, electronic thermometer, thermistor probe or catheter, thermocouple-based probe, infrared radiation readers, fiber-optic method).

The most accurate body temperature is measured at the hypothalamus, but this site is not accessible by any practical means. However, a "deep" body site that directly reflects the temperature "sensed" by the hypothalamus will provide clinically relevant information (14). For example, sites that provide correlation to deep body temperature are pulmonary artery blood, urinary bladder, the esophagus, and the rectum (18, 19, 22). Notably, the temporal resolution for each site varies, which can dramatically impact the ability to recognize clinically important changes that may require prompt patient management (14, 18).

When monitoring temperature during MRI, the decision on which body site to use should be based on accuracy as well as accessibility. There may be limitations on the type of equipment available for temperature measurements in the MR system room (3, 8, 23). For example, hard wire thermistor or thermocouple-based sensors are prone to measurement errors due to electromagnetic interference (EMI) and may introduce artifacts in the MR images (3). Fiber-optic sensors (i.e. fluoroptic thermometry) are optimally used to record temperatures in the MRI environment because they safe and unaffected by EMI (3).

In the MRI setting, anesthesiologists, nurse anesthetists, and clinicians may be feel that they are limited to measure "surface" temperatures, such as those in on the skin surface, axilla, and groin. However, these temperature measurement sites are very problematic insofar as they do not properly reflect "deep" body temperature and exhibit considerable temporal differences when changes occur. Another option is to use a minimally invasive measurement technique to record temperature in the rectum or esophagus.

While a so-called "surface" temperature site (i.e. skin, axilla, and groin) may be used for temperature recordings during MRI mainly because of the ease of obtaining the measurement with currently available equipment, this method does not provide an accurate representation of body temperature and is susceptible to substantial variations and erroneous information relative to the "deep" body temperature due to the specific site selected for temperature probe placement, patient movement, and environmental conditions (14, 19, 20).

Importantly, recording skin or other surface temperature during MRI can be influenced by the level of the patient's perspiration due to RF heating and the use of blankets or air circulation from the fan in the bore of the MR system. Additionally, investigations have demonstrated that peripheral vasoconstriction resulting from skin surface cooling decreases the surface temperature without influencing the core or deep body temperature (24).

While the measurement of "deep" body temperature requires additional set up time and is minimally invasive, it provides a more accurate representation of body temperature (14). The two most prevalent core temperature measurement sites used in the MRI setting are the rectum and esophagus.

Rectal temperature measurements are highly accurate and usually within 0.6 degrees C of the deep body temperature (14). The main drawback to this temperature measurement site is associated with a lag or delay in the temporal response to changing body temperature due to the presence of thermal inertia from the intervening tissues (i.e. between the rectum and hypothalamus). This temporal delay may also be caused by the presence of feces and poor blood supply in the rectum (14, 25). A clinical investigation reported that the rectal temperature substantially lagged in response to changes in body temperature (25). The lack of temporal resolution can expose the patient to a hypothermic or hyperthermic condition for an extended period without it being recognized by the clinician. Also, special care must be taken when placing a rectal temperature probe in neonatal or pediatric patients to prevent perforation and infection (14, 25).

Esophageal temperature measurements provide a high level of accuracy and good temporal correlation to deep body temperature due to the close proximity to the aorta, a deep body site (20). In addition to the accuracy, the temperature recorded in the esophagus is responsive to fluctuations in body temperature and readily tracks changes compared to rectal or surface temperature measurement sites (14, 25). The only caveat is that the accuracy of measuring temperature in the esophagus is directly related to the proper positioning of the temperature sensor (14, 19). Airflow in the trachea can impact the measured temperature if the probe is not inserted deep enough into the esophagus. The recommended position for the temperature sensor is in the lower one-third of the esophagus for an accurate core temperature measurement (14).

Monitoring Body Temperature During MRI: Recommendations

In consideration of the available temperature measurement sites that may be monitored during MRI, especially with regard to which site provides the most accurate information along with the best temporal resolution, the temperature of the esophagus will provide the most acceptable and clinically relevant information. Furthermore, esophageal temperature is insensitive to ambient air circulation and patient perspiration during the MRI examination and has the added benefit of fast response time to temperature fluctuations in the deep body compared to the measurement of temperature in the rectum. The current availability of temperature probes and recording equipment properly designed for use in the MRI setting, permits the monitoring of body temperature in the esophagus, which provides physiologic information that is vital to patient care.

[Excerpted with permission from Thacker V, Shellock FG. Monitoring Body Temperature During MRI.]

REFERENCES

1. Schulte-Uentrop L, Goepfert MS. Anaesthesia or sedation for MRI in children. Curr Opin Anaesthesiol 2010;23:513-7.
2. Watchel RE, Dexter F, Dow AJ. Growth rates in pediatric diagnostic imaging and sedation. Anesthesia and Analgesia 2009;108:1616-1621.
3. Shellock FG. Chapter 11, Patient Monitoring in the MRI Environment. In: Magnetic Resonance Procedures: Health Effects and Safety. CRC Press, Boca Raton, FL, 2001, pp. 217-241.
4. Kanal E, Shellock, FG. Patient monitoring during clinical MR imaging. Radiology 1992;185:623.
5. Practice Advisory on Anesthetic Care for Magnetic Resonance Imaging, Anesthesiology 2009;110:459–79
6. Standards For Basic Anesthetic Monitoring (Approved By The ASA House of Delegates on October 21, 1986, And Last Amended On October 25, 2005)
7. Holshouser, B., Hinshaw, D. B., and Shellock, F. G. Sedation, anesthesia, and physiologic monitoring during MRI. J Magn Reson Imag 1993;3:553-558.
8. American Academy of Pediatrics, American Academy of Pediatric Dentistry, Cote CJ, Wilson S.Work Group on Sedation. Guidelines for monitoring and management of pediatric patients during and after sedation for diagnostic and therapeutic procedures: An update. Pediatrics 2006;118:2587-602.
9. Kanal E, Barkovich AJ, et al. ACR guidance document for safe MR practices: 2007. Am J Roentgenol 2007;188:1447-1474.
10. American College of Radiology, ACR standard for the use of intravenous conscious sedation, and ACR standard for pediatric sedation/analgesia. In, 1998 ACR Standards, Reston, VA, American College of Radiology, 1998.
11. Kanal E, Shellock, FG. Policies, guidelines, and recommendations for MR imaging safety and patient management. Patient monitoring during MR examinations. J Magn Reson Imag 1992;2:247.
12. Joint Commission on Accreditation of Healthcare Organizations. Sedation and anesthesia care standards. Oakbrook Terrace, IL:2003.
13. Dalal PG, et al. Sedation and anesthesia protocols used for magnetic resonance imaging studies in infants: Provider and pharmacologic considerations. Anesth Analg 2006;103:863-8.

14. Knies RC. Temperature Measurement in Acute Care: The Who, What, Where, When, Why, and How? Web Article http://enw.org/Research-Thermometry.htm (Accessed June 24, 2014).

15. Michiaki Y. Anesthesia and body temperature: Temperature regulation under general anesthesia combined with epidural anesthesia. Journal of Clinical Anesthesia 2000;24:1416-1424.

16. Takashi M. Anesthesia and body temperature: General anesthesia and thermoregulation. Journal of Clinical Anesthesia 2000;24:1408-1415.

17. Schubert A. Side effects of mild hypothermia. Journal of Neurological Anesthesiology 1995;7:139-147

18. Lilly JK, Boland JP, Zekan S. Urinary bladder temperature monitoring: A new index of body core temperatures. Critical Care Medicine 1980;8:742-744.

19. Lefrant J–Y, et al. Temperature Measurement in intensive care patients: Comparison of urinary bladder, esophageal, rectal, axillary, and inguinal methods versus pulmonary artery core method. Intensive Care Med 2003;29:414-418.

20. Robinson J, Charlton J, Seal R, Spady D, Joffres MR. Esophageal, rectal, axillary, tympanic, and pulmonary artery temperatures during cardiac surgery. Canadian Journal of Anesthesiology 1998;45:317-323.

21. Takashi A. Anesthesia and body temperature: Interoperative monitoring of body temperature and its significance. Journal of Clinical Anesthesia 2000;24:1432-1443.

22. Shellock FG, Rubin SA. Simplified and highly accurate core temperature measurements. Med Prog Technol 1982;8:187-8.

23. Gooden CK. Anesthesia for magnetic resonance imaging. Curr Opin Anaesthesiol 2004;17:339-42.

24. Wilson TE, et al. Skin surface cooling elicits peripheral and visceral vasoconstriction in humans. Journal of Applied Physiology 2007;103:1257-1262.

25. Newsham KR, et al. Comparison of rectal and tympanic thermometry: Discussion. Southern Medical Journal 2002;95;804-810.

MRI Contrast Agents: ACR–ASNR Position Statement on the Use of Gadolinium Contrast Agents

Following U.S. Food and Drug Administration (FDA) approval in 1988, gadolinium-based contrast agents (GBCAs) have been used for diagnosis and treatment guidance in more than 300 million patients worldwide. GBCAs increase the conspicuity of diseased tissues. All GBCAs share a common structure of an organic ligand that tightly binds to and improves the stability, solubility, and safety of the central gadolinium heavy metal ion. In typical patients, the chelate is mostly eliminated via the kidneys, with some amount of liver excretion demonstrated for a few of the agents.

Since 2006, radiologists have withheld some GBCAs from patients with acute kidney injury and/or severe chronic kidney disease, if the estimated glomerular filtration rate (GFR) is <30 mL/min/1.73 m2, because of the increased risk of nephrogenic systemic fibrosis (NSF). NSF is a rare but serious systemic disease characterized by fibrosis of the skin and other tissues throughout the body in renally impaired individuals. As a result of judicious use of GBCAs among patients with compromised renal function and a decrease in utilization of those GBCAs that are more highly associated with NSF, there has been a drastic reduction in the number of cases encountered since restrictive guidelines were put into place after the association of NSF with GBCAs was identified in 2006.

Recently, residual gadolinium has been found within the brain tissue of patients who received multiple doses of GBCAs over their lifetimes. For reasons that remain unclear, gadolinium deposition appears to occur preferentially in certain specific areas of the brain, even in the absence of clinically evident disease and in the setting of an intact blood brain barrier. Such deposition is not expected, and led the FDA to publish a Safety Alert in July of 2015 indicating that they were actively investigating the risk and clinical significance of these gadolinium deposits. To date, no adverse health effects have been uncovered, but the radiology community has initiated a rigorous investigation.

Gadolinium deposition in the brain may be dose dependent and can occur in patients with no clinical evidence of kidney or liver disease. Fortunately, there have been no reports to date to suggest these deposits are associated with histologic changes that would suggest neurotoxicity, even among GBCAs with the highest rates of deposition. Although there are no known adverse clinical consequences associated with gadolinium deposition in the brain, additional research is warranted to elucidate the mechanisms of deposition, the chelation state of these deposits, the relationship to GBCA stability and binding affinity, and theoretical toxic potential, which may be different for different GBCAs. Until we fully understand the mechanisms involved and their clinical consequences, the safety and tissue deposition potential of all GBCAs must be carefully evaluated.

GBCAs provide crucial, life-saving medical information. Each time a gadolinium-enhanced MRI study is considered, it would be prudent to consider the clinical benefit of the diagnostic information or treatment result that MRI or MRA may provide against the unknown potential risk of gadolinium deposition in the brain for each individual patient. Particular attention should be paid to pediatric and other patients who may receive many GBCA-enhanced MRI studies over the course of their lifetimes. If the decision for an individual patient is made to use a GBCA for an MRI study, multiple factors need to be considered when selecting a GBCA, including diagnostic efficacy, relaxivity, rate of adverse reactions, dosing/concentration, and propensity to deposit in more sensitive organs such as the brain. As this gadolinium deposition phenomenon remains a relatively undefined clinical phenomenon, and accurate and complete data may be useful as investigations proceed, the identity and dose of GBCA used should be recorded after each intravenous administration.

The radiology community will continue to assess the safety of GBCAs and modify clinical practice recommendations accordingly as new data becomes available.

Date: May 2016

MRI Contrast Agents and Adverse Reactions

Gadolinium-based contrast media (GBCM) have been approved for parenteral use since the late 1980s. These agents can be differentiated on the basis of chelate chemistry, stability, viscosity, osmolality, and, in some cases, effectiveness for specific applications. GBCM are extremely well tolerated by the vast majority of patients in whom they are injected. Acute adverse reactions are encountered with a lower frequency than is observed after administration of iodinated contrast media.

Adverse Reactions

The adverse event rate for GBCM administered at clinical doses (0.1–0.2 mmol/kg for most GBCM) ranges from 0.07% to 2.4%. Most reactions are mild and physiologic, including coldness, warmth, or pain at the injection site; nausea with or without vomiting; headache; paresthesias; and dizziness. Allergic-like reactions are uncommon and vary in frequency from 0.004% to –0.7%. The manifestations of an allergic-like reaction to a GBCM are similar to those of an allergic-like reaction to an iodinated contrast medium. Severe life-threatening anaphylactic reactions occur (1-6) but are exceedingly rare (0.001% to 0.01%) (7-9). In an accumulated series of 687,000 doses there were only five severe reactions (10). In a survey of 20 million administered doses, there were 55 severe reactions. A large single-institution study that included more than 100,000 GBCM injections demonstrated an allergic-like reaction frequency of 0.15%, with 0.13% mild reactions and 0.006% severe reactions (six reactions) (11). Fatal reactions to gadolinium chelate agents occur but are extremely rare (12).

GBCM administered to patients with acute kidney injury or severe chronic kidney disease can result in a syndrome of nephrogenic systemic fibrosis (NSF) (13, 14). For more information, see the section on Nephrogenic Systemic Fibrosis (ACR Manual on Contrast Media – Version 10.2, 2016, www.ACR.org). GBCM are not considered nephrotoxic at dosages approved for MR imaging.

Risk Factors
The frequency of acute adverse reactions to GBCM is about eight times higher in patients with a previous reaction to GBCM. At many

institutions, a prior allergic-like reaction to GBCM is often an indication for corticosteroid prophylaxis prior to subsequent exposures. One GBCM, gadobenate dimeglumine, has FDA labeling contraindicating use in patients who have a history of an allergic-like reaction to GBCM. Some reports have suggested that GBCM that have been most commonly associated with NSF are less likely to be associated with allergic-like reactions and vice versa (15).

Patients with asthma and various other allergies may have a mild increased risk for an allergic-like reaction to GBCM compared to the general population, but many institutions do not have special procedures for these patients given the extremely low overall reaction rate for GBCM. There is no cross-reactivity between GBCM and iodinated contrast media.

In a patient with previous moderate or severe allergic-like reactions to a specific GBCM, it may be prudent to use a different GBCM and premedicate for subsequent MR examinations, although there are no published studies to confirm that this approach is efficacious in reducing the likelihood of a repeat contrast reaction.

The Safety of Gadolinium-Based Contrast Media in Patients with Sickle Cell Disease

Early in vitro research investigating the effects of a strong external magnetic field (e.g., MR magnet) on red blood cells (erythrocytes) suggested that fully deoxygenated sickle erythrocytes align perpendicularly to a magnetic field. It was hypothesized that this alignment could further restrict sickle erythrocyte flow through small vessels and promote vaso-occlusive complications in sickle cell patients (16). Based on this supposition, FDA package inserts suggested caution in patients with sickle cell disease for two GBCM approved for use in the United States (gadoversetamide [OptiMARK, Mallinckrodt] and gadoteridol [Prohance, Bracco Diagnostics]).

To the best of our knowledge and noted in a review of the literature (17), there has been no documented *in vivo* vaso-occlusive or hemolytic complication directly related to the IV administration of GBCM in a sickle cell disease patient. A small retrospective study with a control group showed no significantly increased risk of vaso-occlusive or hemolytic adverse events when administering GBCM to sickle cell disease patients (18). Additionally, several small scientific studies (19-21) of patients with sickle cell disease have employed MR imaging with GBCM without reported adverse effects.

Therefore, the risk to patients with sickle cell disease from IV-administered GBCM at approved dosages is very low or nonexistent, and there is no reason to withhold these agents from these patients when their use is otherwise indicated.

Breath-holding Difficulty with Gadoxetate Disodium

Several studies have noted that gadoxetate disodium may be associated with transient severe respiratory motion-related artifact that manifests in the arterial phase of dynamic T1-weighted gradient echo imaging and resolves shortly thereafter (22-26). This manifestation has been described as "transient dyspnea". At one institution, patient surveys showed that significantly more patients complained of subjective shortness of breath following gadoxetate disodium compared to gadobenate dimeglumine exposure (22). The reported rate of occurrence of "transient dyspnea" has varied by site, imaging acquisition parameters, and administered volume, ranging from 4% to 14% (22-26).

Based on the volume-effect relationship and the lack of identifiable atopic covariates, this appears to be a physiologic reaction, manifesting as dyspnea or breath-holding difficulty that is unique to this agent (25). The event is self-limited and does not appear to relate to allergic-like bronchospasm (22, 24, 25). Therefore, corticosteroid prophylaxis is unlikely to be beneficial and is not felt to be indicated. Strong risk factors include a larger administered volume irrespective of patient weight (20 mL doses are twice as likely to cause the artifact as 10 mL doses) (25), chronic obstructive pulmonary disease (patients with COPD have a 35–40% event rate) (25), and readministering the agent to patients who have previously had a similar reaction (previously affected patients have a 60% event rate on subsequent studies compared to a 5% event rate in the unaffected population) (26). Imaging strategies to avoid the artifact include minimizing the injected volume (≤ 10 mL), avoiding the agent in patients who have experienced it before, and acquiring more than one arterial phase with a short temporal footprint (22-26).

Treatment of Acute Adverse Reactions

Treatment of acute adverse reactions to GBCM is similar to that for acute reactions to iodinated contrast media (see Tables 2 and 3, ACR Manual on Contrast Media – Version 10.2, 2016, www.ACR.org). In any facility where contrast media are injected, it is imperative that personnel trained in recognizing and handling reactions and the equipment and medications to do so be on site or immediately available. Most MR facilities take the position that patients requiring treatment should be taken out of the imaging room immediately and away from the magnet so that none of the resuscitative equipment becomes a magnetic hazard.

Extravasation

Extravasation events to GBCM are rare, with one series demonstrating a rate of 0.05% (28,000 doses). Laboratory studies in animals have demonstrated that both gadopentetate dimeglumine and gadoteridol are less toxic to the skin and subcutaneous tissues than are equal volumes of iodinated contrast media (27, 28). The small volumes typically injected for MR studies limit the chances of developing compartment syndrome. For these reasons the likelihood of a significant injury resulting from extravasated MR contrast media is extremely low.

Serum Calcium Determinations

Some linear nonionic GBCM (e.g., gadoversetamide, gadodiamide) may interfere with total serum calcium values as determined with some calcium assay methods (29, 30). These GBCM do not cause actual reductions in serum calcium. Rather, they interfere with the test, leading to falsely low serum calcium laboratory values. In one report by Brown, et al. (30), calcium levels measured by only one of three different assays (the orthocresolphthalein assay) showed a temporary decrease for just two of four studied GBCM (gadopentetate and gadoteridol had no effect), the length and severity of which closely mirrored the concentration of the measured GBCM in blood.

Off-Label Use of MRI Contrast Agents

In the past, radiologists often used GBCM in an off-label fashion (e.g., off-label higher doses or off-label indications). By definition, such usage is not approved by the FDA. However, physicians have some latitude in off-label GBCM use as guided by clinical circumstances as long as they can justify such usage in individual cases. Examples include MR angiography, cardiac applications, and pediatric applications in patients younger than two years of age. In addition, no GBCM is approved in the United States for use in a power injector. Off-label dosing of GBCM is now used much less commonly. Extremely high doses of GBCM much greater than FDA labeling (which were used frequently in the past) have largely been abandoned, especially in patients with severe chronic kidney disease and acute kidney injury due to concerns regarding nephrogenic systemic fibrosis.

REFERENCES

1. Weiss KL. Severe anaphylactoid reaction after i.v. Gd-DTPA. Magn Reson Imaging. 1990;8:817-818.

2. Omohundro JE, et al. Laryngospasm after administration of gadopentetate dimeglumine. J Magn Reson Imaging. 1992;2:729-730.

3. Tardy B, et al. Anaphylactic shock induced by intravenous gadopentetate dimeglumine. Lancet. 1992;339:494.

4. Takebayashi S, et al. Severe adverse reaction to iv gadopentetate dimeglumine. AJR Am J Roentgenol. 1993;160:659.

5. Witte RJ. Life-threatening anaphylactoid reaction after intravenous gadoteridol administration in a patient who had previously received gadopentetate dimeglumine. AJNR Am J Neuroradiol. 1994;15:523-524.

6. Murphy KJ, et al. Adverse reactions to gadolinium contrast media: a review of 36 cases. AJR Am J Roentgenol. 1996;167:847-849.

7. Murphy KJ, Cohan RH. Adverse reactions to gadolinium contrast media: a review of 36 cases. 1996;167:847-849.

8. Runge VM. Safety of approved MR contrast media for intravenous injection. J Magn Reson Imaging. 2000;12(2):205-213.

9. Runge VM. Safety of magnetic resonance contrast media. Top Magn Reson Imaging. 2001;12(4):309-314.

10. Murphy KP. Occurrence of adverse reactions to gadolinium-based contrast material and management of patients at increased risk: a survey of the American Society of Neuroradiology Fellowship Directors. Acad Radiol. 1999;6:656-664.

11. Davenport MS, et al. Effect of abrupt substitution of gadobenate dimeglumine for gadopentetate dimeglumine on rate of allergic-like reactions. Radiology. 2013;266:773-782.

12. Jordan RM, Mintz RD. Fatal reaction to gadopentetate dimeglumine. AJR Am J Roentgenol 1995;164:743-744.

13. Kanal E, et al. ACR guidance document for safe MR practices: 2007. AJ Am J Roentgenol 2007;188:1447-1474.

14. Kuo PH, et al. Gadolinium-based MR contrast agents and nephrogenic systemic fibrosis. Radiology 2007;242:647-649.

15. Jung JW, et al. Immediate hypersensitivity reaction to gadolinium-based MR contrast media. Radiology 2012;264:414-422.

16. Brody AS, et al. AUR memorial Award. Induced alignment of flowing sickle erythrocytes in a magnetic field. A preliminary report. Invest Radiol. 1985;20:560-566.

17. Kanal E, Shellock FG, Talagala L. Safety considerations in MR imaging. Radiology. 1990;176:593-606.

18. Dillman JR, et al. Safety of gadolinium-based contrast material in sickle cell disease. J Magn Reson Imaging 2011;34:917-920.

19. Umans H, et al. The diagnostic role of gadolinium enhanced MRI in distinguishing between acute medullary bone infarct and osteomyelitis. Magn Reson Imaging 2000;18:255-262.

20. Westwood MA, et al. Myocardial tissue characterization and the role of chronic anemia in sickle cell cardiomyopathy. J Magn Reson Imaging. 2007;26:564-568.

21. Zimmerman RA. MRI/MRA evaluation of sickle cell disease of the brain. Pediatr Radiol 2005;35:249-257.

22. Davenport M, et al. Comparison of acute transient dyspnea after intravenous administration of gadoxetate disodium and gadobenate dimeglumine: effect on arterial phase image quality. Radiology 2013;266:452-461.

23. Pietryga JA, t al. Respiratory motion artifact affecting hepatic arterial phase imaging with gadoxetate disodium: examination recovery with a multiple arterial phase acquisition. Radiology 2014;271:426-434.

24. Davenport MS, et al. Matched within-patient cohort study of transient arterial-phase respiratory motion related artifact in MRI of the liver: Gd-EOB-DTPA vs. Gd-BOPTA. Radiology 2014;272:123-131.

25. Davenport MS, et al. Dose-toxicity relationship of gadoxetate disodium and transient post-injection dyspnea. AJR Am J Roentgenol 2014;203:796-802.

26. Bashir MR, et al. Respiratory motion artifact affecting hepatic arterial phase imaging with gadoxetate disodium is more common in patients with a prior episode of arterial phase motion associated with gadoxetate disodium. Radiology 2015;274:141-148.

27. McAlister WH, et al. The effect of Gd-dimeglumine on subcutaneous tissues: a study with rats. AJNR 1990;11:325-327.

28. Cohan RH, et al. Extravascular toxicity of two magnetic resonance contrast agents. Preliminary experience in the rat. Invest Radiol. 1991;26:224-226.

29. Lin J IJ, et al. Interference of magnetic resonance imaging contrast agents with the serum calcium measurement technique using colorimetric reagents. J Pharm Biomed Anal. 1999;21:931-943.

30. Brown JJ, et al. Measurement of serum calcium concentration after administration of four gadoliniumbased contrast agents to human volunteers. AJR Am J Roentgenol. 2007;189:1539-1544.

MRI Contrast Agents and Breast Feeding Mothers

Administration Of Contrast Media To Women Who Are Breast Feeding

Imaging studies requiring either iodinated or gadolinium-based contrast media are occasionally required in patients who are breast feeding. Both the patient and the patient's physician may have concerns regarding potential toxicity to the infant from contrast media that is excreted into the breast milk.

The literature on the excretion into breast milk of iodinated and gadolinium-based contrast media and the gastrointestinal absorption of these agents from breast milk is very limited; however, several studies have shown that the expected dose of contrast medium absorbed by an infant from ingested breast milk is extremely low.

Iodinated X-ray Contrast Media (Ionic and Nonionic)
Background
The plasma half-life of intravenously administered iodinated contrast medium is approximately 2 hours, with nearly 100% of the media cleared from the bloodstream in patients with normal renal function within 24 hours. Because of its low lipid solubility, less than 1% of the administered maternal dose of iodinated contrast medium is excreted into the breast milk in the first 24 hours (1, 2). In addition, less than 1% of the contrast medium ingested by the infant is absorbed from its gastrointestinal tract (3). Therefore, the expected systemic dose absorbed by the infant from the breast milk is less than 0.01% of the intravascular dose given to the mother. This amount represents less than 1% of the recommended dose for an infant being prescribed iodinated contrast material related to an imaging study (usually 1.5 to 2 mL/kg). The potential risks to the infant include direct toxicity and allergic sensitization or reaction, which are theoretical concerns but have not been reported.

The likelihood of either direct toxic or allergic-like manifestations resulting from ingested iodinated contrast material in the infant is extremely low. As with other medications in milk, the taste of the milk may be altered if it contains contrast medium (1-4).

Recommendation
Because of the very small percentage of iodinated contrast medium that is excreted into the breast milk and absorbed by the infant's gut, we believe that the available data suggest that it is safe for the mother and infant to continue breast-feeding after receiving such an agent.

Ultimately, an informed decision to temporarily stop breast-feeding should be left up to the mother after these facts are communicated. If the mother remains concerned about any potential ill effects to the infant, she may abstain from breast-feeding from the time of contrast administration for a period of 12 to 24 hours.

There is no value to stop breast feeding beyond 24 hours. The mother should be told to express and discard breast milk from both breasts during that period. In anticipation of this, she may wish to use a breast pump to obtain milk before the contrast-enhanced study to feed the infant during the 24-hour period following the examination.

Gadolinium-Based Contrast Agents
Background
Like iodinated contrast media, gadolinium-based contrast media have a plasma half-life of approximately 2 hours and are nearly completely cleared from the bloodstream in patients with normal renal function within 24 hours. Also similar to iodinated contrast media, gadolinium-based contrast media are excreted into the breast milk. It is likely that the overwhelming bulk of gadolinium excreted in the breast milk is in a stable and chelated form (6).

Less than 0.04% of the intravascular dose given to the mother is excreted into the breast milk in the first 24 hours (4-6). Because less than 1% of the contrast medium ingested by the infant is absorbed from its gastrointestinal tract (6, 7), the expected systemic dose absorbed by the infant from the breast milk is less than 0.0004% of the intravascular dose given to the mother. This ingested amount is far less than the permissible dose for intravenous use in neonates. The likelihood of an adverse effect from such a minute fraction of gadolinium chelate absorbed from breast milk is remote (2). However, the potential risks to the infant include direct toxicity (including toxicity from free gadolinium, because it is unknown how much, if any, of the gadolinium in breast milk is in the unchelated form) and allergic sensitization or reaction. These are theoretical concerns but none of these complications have been reported

(5). As in the case with iodinated contrast medium, the taste of the milk may be altered if it contains a gadolinium-based contrast medium (2).

Recommendation

Because of the very small percentage of gadolinium-based contrast medium that is excreted into the breast milk and absorbed by the infant's gut, we believe that the available data suggest that it is safe for the mother and infant to continue breast-feeding after receiving such an agent (6).

Ultimately, an informed decision to temporarily stop breast-feeding should be left up to the mother after these facts are communicated. If the mother remains concerned about any potential ill effects to the infant, she may abstain from breast-feeding from the time of contrast administration for a period of 12 to 24 hours. There is no value to stop breast feeding beyond 24 hours. The mother should be told to express and discard breast milk from both breasts after contrast administration until breast feeding resumes. In anticipation of this, she may wish to use a breast pump to obtain milk before the contrast-enhanced study to feed the infant during the 24-hour period following the examination.

REFERENCES

1. Bettman MA. Frequently asked questions: Iodinated contrast agents. Radiographics 2004; 24:S3-S10

2. Webb JAW, et al. The use of iodinated and gadolinium contrast media during pregnancy and lactation. Eur Radiol 2005; 15: 1234-1240.

3. Trembley E, Therasse E, Thomassin N, et al. Quality Initiatives Guidelines for use of medical imaging during pregnancy and lactation. Radiographics 2012; 32: 897-911.

4. Wang PI, et al. Imaging of pregnant and lactating patients: Part 1. evidence-based review and recommendations. AJR 2012; 198:778-784.

5. Rofsky NM, et al. Quantitative analysis of gadopentate diglumine excreted in breast milk. JMRI 1993;3:131-132.

6. Kubik-Huch RA, et al. Gadopentetate diglumine excretion into human breast milk during lactation. Radiology 2000; 216:555-558.

MRI Contrast Agents: Intracranial Gadolinium Retention

Intracranial Gadolinium Retention and High Signal Intensity in Globus Pallidus and Dentate Nucleus on Unenhanced T1-weighted MR Images: A Review of the Literature*

[*Special thanks to Alberto Spinazzi, M.D., Global Medical and Regulatory Affairs, Bracco Diagnostics, Inc.]

Introduction

Some patients exposed to multiple administrations of certain gadolinium-based contrast agents (GBCAs) may exhibit progressively increased signal intensity (SI) in the globus pallidus (GP) and the dentate nucleus (DN) on unenhanced T1-weighted brain images (1-10). This monograph provides a cumulative review of relevant literature relating to this abnormal imaging finding and to the potential deposition of gadolinium in brain tissues.

Studies described in this document were published in the peer-reviewed literature. The first report on abnormal T1 shortening seen in the GP and DN was available online in December 2013 and published in March 2014 (1). A systematic and comprehensive online search was performed using the following databanks: Embase, Biosis, Medline, and Derwent Drug File for publications printed from December 2013 through September 2015. The search was conducted using the search terms: "gadolinium" or "gadolinium-based contrast agent" or "gadolinium deposition" or "gadolinium retention" or "dentate nucleus" or "globus pallidus" or "brain". The results were limited to human data and excluded duplicates, review articles, case reports, editorials, conference abstracts or papers, news, and commentaries. Due to the limited precision of the index terms used by the online databases, a screening was performed by experienced medical reviewers to include citations that were pertinent.

Imaging Findings

Certain patients exposed to multiple administrations of GBCAs may exhibit progressively increased SI in the GP and the DN on unenhanced T1-weighted brain images (1-10). Abnormal T1 shortening has been observed after serial application of certain GBCAs and not others. Kanda, et al. (3) reported that, while a significant increase in SI in the DN and GP occurred after multiple doses of the linear GBCA Magnevist (active ingredient: gadopentetate dimeglumine), this abnormal finding did not occur after multiple doses of the macrocyclic GBCA ProHance (active ingredient: gadoteridol). Radbruch, et al. (6) showed that SI increase in the DN and GP on T1-weighted images is caused by serial application of Magnevist but not by the macrocyclic GBCA Dotarem (active ingredient: gadoterate meglumine). Ramalho, et al. (7) reported that patients who received the linear GBCA Omniscan (active ingredient: gadodiamide) showed a significant increase in signal intensity in the DN and GP compared to other brain areas (thalamus, TH, and middle cerebral peduncles, MCP). Conversely, those who received the linear GBCA MultiHance did not show a significant increase in SI in the DN or GP. These results were not confirmed by Weberling, et al. (10) who instead reported an increase in SI in the DN after serial injections of MultiHance (active ingredient: gadobenate dimeglumine). Differences in patient population and study methodology may explain the different results from these two studies, especially less rigorous control of previous exposure to other GBCAs in the study by Weberling, et al. (10). T1 hyperintensity in the GP and DN following repeated administrations of Omniscan were observed by Errante, et al. (2), Quattrocchi, et al. (4) and McDonald, et al. (5), while Stojanov, et al. (8) reported a significant increase in SI in the DN and GP in patients with multiple sclerosis following multiple exposure to the macrocyclic GBCA Gadavist (active ingredient: gadobutrol).

In summary, abnormal T1 shortening was observed following repeated prior administration of the linear agents Omniscan and Magnevist, and of an agent with a macrocyclic ligand, Gadavist. Inconsistent results were reported for the linear GBCA MultiHance. Increased SI in the GP or DN has not been reported following serial exposure to the macrocyclic GBCAs ProHance and Dotarem, or the linear agents OptiMARK (active ingredient: gadoversetamide), Eovist (active ingredient: gadoxetate disodium), and Ablavar (active ingredient: gadofoveset trisodium).

Importantly, none of the authors of the clinical investigations published so far has ever reported any symptoms in their patients that would relate to damage to the GP, the DN, or other brain structures (1-10).

Evidence of Gadolinium Deposition in Brain Tissues

Two investigations have associated abnormal T1 shortening in the GP and DN with deposition of gadolinium in brain autopsy specimens. Kanda, et al. (11) conducted an investigation using brain tissues obtained at autopsy in five subjects who were exposed to multiple administrations of GBCAs (GBCA group) and five subjects with no history of GBCA administration (non-GBCA group). The GBCAs involved were Magnevist, Omniscan, and ProHance. By using inductively coupled plasma mass spectroscopy to determine the presence and concentration of gadolinium in the brain tissues, Kanda, et al. (11) showed that, following repeated GBCA administration, gadolinium accumulates in the brain, and that the concentration of gadolinium was higher in the DN and GP than in other regions. Gadolinium was detected in all specimens in the GBCA group. Of note, gadolinium was also present in some specimens in the non-GBCA group. However, the gadolinium concentration was significantly higher in the GBCA group.

A study by McDonald, et al. (5) reported that, in patients with hyperintensity in the DN and GP on unenhanced T1-weighted MR images following exposure to multiple doses of Omniscan, the majority of gadolinium deposits were in the endothelial walls, with a smaller fraction in the brain interstitium. Importantly, no signs of neuronal damage were observed at microscopy of the involved brain tissues.

The findings of McDonald, et al. (5) are consistent with those previously reported by Sanyal, et al. (12) who performed an analysis of tissues obtained during autopsy of a patient with verified advanced nephrogenic systemic fibrosis (NSF). Using light microscopy and scanning electron microscopy/energy-dispersive X-ray spectroscopy, Sanyal, et al. (12) found gadolinium deposits in the perivascular glial cells in the cerebellum but not in the pons, thalamus or corpus striatum.

Gadolinium Form in Brain Tissues

Free gadolinium ions are not expected to survive in a physiological environment. Studies performed in human plasma have shown that the gadolinium ions released in transmetallation reactions distribute into a number of species, mostly phosphates, or complexes with small (e.g. citrate) and large (e.g., albumin) biomolecules (13, 14). Neither Kanda, et al. (11) nor McDonald, et al. (5) determined the form in which gadolinium is retained in brain tissues, while Sanyal, et al. (12) could only find insoluble gadolinium phosphates. Gadolinium phosphates have very low solubility and precipitate into particles that have little or no effect on water proton relaxation rate, that is, on SI on T1-weighted images (13,

14). Therefore, the enhanced SI observed in the DN and GP on T1-weighted images is not expected to be dependent on gadolinium phosphate complexes but is likely due either to intact molecules of the administered GBCA or to the formation of soluble gadolinium complexes. Other metals (e.g., manganese) could also contribute to the overall effect on SI. In none of the three studies aimed at determining the presence of gadolinium in the brain was investigation made of the presence and concentration of other metals or factors that could contribute to SI increase in the DN and GP on T1-weighted images (5, 11, 12).

Factors That May Influence the Deposition of Gadolinium in Brain Tissues

The central nervous system (CNS) is sealed from the blood milieu by the blood-brain barrier (BBB), localized at the level of the endothelial cells within CNS microvessels, and the blood-cerebrospinal fluid (CSF) barrier (BCSFB), established by choroid plexus epithelial cells (15). The lack of permeability of the BBB and the absence of intra-parenchymal enhancement on post-contrast scans suggest that it is an unlikely pathway for gadolinium penetration under normal conditions (16, 17). There is a list of pathologies affecting the CNS that involve an element of BBB dysfunction, including multiple sclerosis, hypoxia and ischemia, edema, Parkinson's disease, dementia or Alzheimer's disease, epilepsy, primary or secondary tumors, acute brain injuries, lysosomal storage diseases, and diabetes (15, 17). If there is BBB disruption, for example in patients with diabetes or focal lesions, SI increases following administration of GBCAs are usually observed in several areas of the brain. A study by Starr, et al. (18) in patients with type II diabetes revealed SI increases in several brain areas after injection of a GBCA with the greatest increase observed in the basal ganglia. The SI increase seen in diabetic subjects was consistent with previous theoretical models and similar to that observed in single lesions in multiple sclerosis. Importantly, there were no signs of gadolinium retention or accumulation, at least after a single exposure to a GBCA: after 30 minutes, the SI time profile for diabetic subjects was similar to that of the healthy controls in all brain areas, with statistical linear decline closer to a real time exponential decline and consistent with first order kinetics (18). Whether and how gadolinium, in any form (intact GBCA molecule or other compounds), may progressively accumulate in the DN and GP in patients who have, or have had, BBB disruption is unknown. Sanyal, et al. (12) found gadolinium in the perivascular glial cells in the cerebellum of a patient who had developed NSF but no gadolinium deposits were found in the brain interstitium, that is, there was no evidence that gadolinium, in any form, had crossed the BBB. Only

McDonald, et al. (5) found gadolinium deposits in the brain interstitium, even if a much larger fraction was observed in the endothelial walls.

The BCSFB is the morphological correlate of the BBB and is found at the level of unique apical tight junctions between the choroid plexus epithelial cells. These tight junctions inhibit paracellular diffusion of water-soluble molecules across this barrier (15). In addition to its barrier function, choroid plexus epithelial cells have a secretory function and produce the CSF. The barrier and secretory function of the choroid plexus epithelial cells are maintained by the expression of numerous transport systems that allow the directed transport of ions and nutrients into the CSF and the removal of toxic agents from the CSF. Unlike the BBB, the BCSFB is selectively permeable and it has been hypothesized that the BCSFB could allow the passage of GBCAs, or other gadolinium compounds, under certain conditions (17). CSF SI changes following administration of GBCAs have been observed with major disruptions of the BBB in studies involving neurologic disorders such as ischemic stroke, epilepsy, tumors, and acute brain injuries (17, 19, 20). Significantly reduced renal function has been described as a predisposing condition leading to elevated gadolinium compounds (a form never determined) in the CSF (21). However, the increased SI in the DN and GP on unenhanced T1-weighted MR images was shown to be independent of renal function status (1, 8). Thus, apart from repeated exposure to some, though not all, GBCAs, no other predisposing factors have been identified and it is not clear how gadolinium can get to and be retained in the brain interstitium.

Conclusions

Abnormal T1 shortening in the DN and GP on unenhanced images was observed in some patients exposed to repeated prior administration of some linear GBCAs and a macrocyclic GBCA. This imaging finding was associated with the presence and higher concentrations of gadolinium in these deep brain areas. The majority of gadolinium deposits have been observed in the endothelial walls, with a smaller fraction in the brain interstitium. No signs of neuronal damage could be observed at microscopy of the involved brain tissues. It is not clear in which form gadolinium is retained in brain tissues and which form may contribute to the effect on SI. Differently from NSF, which is observed exclusively in patients with severely reduced renal function, no groups of patients likely to be at increased risk of gadolinium accumulation in the brain have been identified. No clinical conditions have been associated with progressively increased SI in the GP and DN on unenhanced T1-weighted brain images. So far, no specific clinical guidelines on how to manage patients requiring multiple exposures to GBCAs have been released by any scientific society or regulatory authority.

REFERENCES

1. Kanda T, et al. High signal intensity in the dentate nucleus and globus pallidus on unenhanced T1-weighted MR images: relationship with increasing cumulative dose of a gadolinium-based contrast material. Radiology 2014;270:834-841.

2. Errante Y, et al. Progressive increase of T1 signal intensity of the dentate nucleus on unenhanced magnetic resonance images is associated with cumulative doses of intravenously administered gadodiamide in patients with normal renal function, suggesting dechelation. Invest Radiol 2014;49:685-690.

3. Kanda T, et al. High signal intensity in dentate nucleus on unenhanced T1-weighted MR images: Association with linear versus macrocyclic gadolinium chelate administration. Radiology 2015;275:803-809.

4. Quattrocchi CC, et al. Gadodiamide and dentate nucleus T1 hyperintensity in patients with meningioma evaluated by multiple follow-up contrast-enhanced magnetic resonance examinations with no systemic interval therapy. Invest Radiol 2015;50:470-472.

5. McDonald RJ, et al. Intracranial gadolinium deposition after contrast-enhanced MR imaging. Radiology 2015;275:772-782.

6. Radbruch A, et al. Gadolinium retention in the dentate nucleus and globus pallidus is dependent on the class of contrast agent. Radiology 2015;275:783-791.

7. Ramalho J, et al. High signal intensity in globus pallidus and dentate nucleus on unenhanced T1-weighted MR images: Evaluation of two linear gadolinium-based contrast agents. Radiology 2015;276:836-844.

8. Stojanov DA, et al. Increasing signal intensity within the dentate nucleus and globus pallidus on unenhanced T1W magnetic resonance images in patients with relapsing-remitting multiple sclerosis: Correlation with cumulative dose of a macrocyclic gadolinium-based contrast agent, gadobutrol. Eur Radiol 2016;26:807-15.

9. Adin ME, et al. Hyperintense dentate nuclei on T1-weighted MRI: Relation to repeat gadolinium administration. AJNR Am J Neuroradiol 2015;36:1859-65.

10. Weberling LD, et al. Increased signal intensity in the dentate nucleus on unenhanced T1-weighted images after gadobenate dimeglumine administration. Invest Radiol 2015;50:743-748.

11. Kanda T, et al. Gadolinium-based contrast agent accumulates in the brain even in subjects without severe renal dysfunction: Evaluation of autopsy brain specimens with inductively coupled plasma mass spectroscopy. Radiology 2015;276:228-232.

12. Sanyal S, et al. Multiorgan gadolinium (Gd) deposition and fibrosis in a patient with nephrogenic systemic fibrosis. An autopsy-based review. Nephrol Dial Transplant 2011;26:3616-3626.

13. Baranyai Z, et al. The role of equilibrium and kinetic properties in the association of Gd[DTPA-bis (methylamide)] (Omniscan) at near to physiological conditions. Chem Eur Journal 2015;21:4789-4799.

14. Aime S. and Caravan P. Biodistribution of gadolinium-based contrast agents, including gadolinium deposition. J Mag Res Imag 2009;30:1259-1267.

15. Engelhardt B, Sorokin L. The blood-brain and the blood-cerebrospinal fluid barriers: Function and dysfunction. Semin Immunopathol 2009;31:497-511.

16. Abbott NJ, et al. Structure and function of the blood brain barrier. Neurobiol Dis 2010;37:13-25.

17. Levy LM. Exceeding the limits of the normal blood brain barrier: Quo vadis gadolinium? Am J Neuroradiol 2007;28:1835-1836.

18. Starr JM, et al. Increased blood brain barrier permeability in type II diabetes demonstrated by gadolinium magnetic resonance imaging. J Neurol Neurosurg Psychiatry 2003;74:70-76.

19. Morris JM, Miller GM. Increased signal in the subarachnoid space on fluid-attenuated inversion recovery imaging associated with the clearance dynamics of gadolinium chelate: A potential diagnostic pitfall. AJNR Am J Neuroradiol 2007;28:1964-1967

20. Bozzao A, et al. Cerebrospinal fluid changes after intravenous injection of gadolinium chelate: Assessment by FLAIR MR imaging. Eur Radiol 2003;13:592–597

21. Rai AT, Hogg JP. Persistence of gadolinium in CSF: A diagnostic pitfall in patients with end-stage renal disease. AJNR Am J Neuroradiol 2001;22:1357–1361.

MRI Contrast Agents and Pregnant Patients

Gadolinium-Based Contrast Agents (GBCAs)

Mutagenic effect of gadolinium-based contrast agents

To date, there have been no known adverse effects to human fetuses reported when clinically recommended dosages of gadolinium-based contrast agents (GBCAs) have been given to pregnant women. A single cohort study of 26 women exposed to gadolinium chelates during the first trimester of pregnancy showed no evidence of teratogenesis or mutagenesis in their progeny (10). However, no well-controlled studies of the teratogenic effects of these media in pregnant women have been performed.

Risk of nephrogenic systemic fibrosis

There are no known cases of nephrogenic systemic fibrosis (NSF) linked to the use of GBCAs in pregnant patients. However, gadolinium chelates may accumulate in the amniotic fluid. Therefore, there is the potential for the dissociation of the toxic free gadolinium ion, conferring a potential risk for the development of NSF in the child or mother.

Recommendations for the use of GBCA-enhanced MRI examinations in pregnant patients

Because it is unclear how GBCAs will affect the fetus, these agents should be administered with caution to pregnant or potentially pregnant patients. GBCAs should only be used if their usage is considered critical and the potential benefits justify the potential unknown risk to the fetus. If a GBCA is to be used in a pregnant patient, one of the agents believed to be at low risk for the development of NSF (11) should be used at the lowest possible dose to achieve diagnostic results. In pregnant patients with severely impaired renal function, the same precautions should be observed as in non-pregnant patients.

The ACR Committee on Drugs and Contrast Media recommends the following concerning the performance of contrast-enhanced MRI examinations in pregnant patients:

Each case should be reviewed carefully by members of the clinical and radiology service groups, and a GBCA should be administered only when there is a potential significant benefit to the patient or fetus that outweighs the possible but unknown risk of fetal exposure to free gadolinium ions.

A. The radiologist should confer with the referring physician and document the following in the radiology report or the patient's medical record:

   1. That information requested from the MRI study cannot be acquired without the use of IV contrast or by using other imaging modalities.

   2. That the information needed affects the care of the patient and/or fetus during the pregnancy.

   3. That the referring physician is of the opinion that it is not prudent to wait to obtain this information until after the patient is no longer pregnant.

B. It is recommended that informed consent be obtained from the patient after discussion with the referring physician.

Premedication of pregnant patients (with prior allergic-like reactions to iodinated or gadolinium-based contrast media)

Diphenhydramine and corticosteroids (most commonly prednisone and methylprednisolone) are commonly used for prophylaxis in patients at risk for allergic-like contrast reactions to contrast media. Diphenhydramine is classified as FDA category B. (FDA category B: Animal reproductive studies have failed to demonstrate a risk to the fetus, and there are no adequate well-controlled studies in pregnant women.) Prednisone (FDA category C) and dexamethasone (FDA category C) traverse the placenta; however, most of these agents are metabolized within the placenta before reaching the fetus, and therefore are not associated with teratogenicity in humans. (FDA category C: Animal reproduction studies have shown an adverse effect on fetus, and there are no adequate and well-controlled studies in humans, but potential benefits may warrant use of the drug in pregnant women despite potential risks.) However, sporadic cases of fetal adrenal suppression have been reported. Methylprednisolone is also classified as a category C drug and carries a small risk to the fetus for the development of a cleft lip if used before 10 weeks of gestation (12, 13).

Recommendations for the use of corticosteroid premedication in pregnant patients

Expert opinion indicates that the use of steroids in pregnancy is generally safe (14,15), although common specific regimens for premedication prior to contrast media administration have not been tested. Severe anaphylaxis in a pregnant female represents an even greater risk to the fetus than to the mother herself (16). Given this information, we recommend that otherwise-indicated premedication to reduce the risk of contrast media reaction not be withheld because the patient is pregnant and a standard PO or IV regimen be employed (see Chapter on Patient Selection and Premedication Strategies, ACR Manual on Contrast Media – Version 10.2, 2016, www.ACR.org). Both referring clinician and their pregnant patients receiving premedication prior to contrast media administration should indicat that they understand the potential risks and benefits of the medications being used, as well as alternative diagnostic options.

REFERENCES

1. Dean PB. Fetal uptake of an intravascular radiologic contrast medium. Rofo. 1977;127:267-270.
2. Moon AJ, Katzberg RW, Sherman MP. Transplacental passage of iohexol. J Pediatr. 2000;136:548-549.
3. Panigel M, Wolf G, Zeleznick A. Magnetic resonance imaging of the placenta in rhesus monkeys, Macaca mulatta. J Med Primatol. 1988;17(1):3-18.
4. Kanal E, Barkovich AJ, Bell C, et al. ACR guidance document for safe MR practices: 2007. AJR Am J Roentgenol. 2007;188(6):1447-1474.
5. Atwell TD, et al. Neonatal thyroid function after administration of IV iodinated contrast agent to 21 pregnant patients. AJR Am J Roentgenol. 2008;191:268-271.
6. Bourjeily G, et al. Neonatal thyroid function: effect of a single exposure to iodinated contrast medium in utero. Radiology. 2010;256:744-750.
7. Kochi MH, et al. Effect of in utero exposure of iodinated intravenous contrast on neonatal thyroid function. J Comput Assist Tomogr. 2012;36:165-169.
8. McKay DB, Josephson MA. Pregnancy in recipients of solid organs--effects on mother and child. N Engl J Med. 2006;354:1281-1293.
9. Rajaram S, et al. Effect of antenatal iodinated contrast agent on neonatal thyroid function. Br J Radiol. 2012;85:e238-242.
10. De Santis M, et al. Gadolinium periconceptional exposure: pregnancy and neonatal outcome. Acta Obstet Gynecol Scand. 2007;86:99-101.
11. Thomsen HS, et al. Nephrogenic systemic fibrosis and gadolinium-based contrast media: updated ESUR Contrast Medium Safety Committee guidelines. Eur Radiol. 2013;23:307-318.

12. Niebyl JR. Clinical practice. Nausea and vomiting in pregnancy. N Engl J Med. 2010;363:1544-1550.

13. Wang PI, et al. Imaging of pregnant and lactating patients: part 1, evidence-based review and recommendations. AJR Am J Roentgenol. 2012;198:778-784.

14. Bonanno C, Wapner RJ. Antenatal corticosteroids in the management of preterm birth: are we back where we started? Obstet Gynecol Clin North Am. 2012;39:47-63.

15. Gerosa M, et al. Safety considerations when prescribing immunosuppression medication to pregnant women. Expert Opin Drug Saf. 2014;13:1591-1599.

16. Simons FE, Schatz M. Anaphylaxis during pregnancy. J Allergy Clin Immunol. 2012;130(3):597-606.

MRI Contrast Agents and Nephrogenic Systemic Fibrosis (NSF)

[Special thanks to Alberto Spinazzi, M.D., Global Medical and Regulatory Affairs, Bracco Diagnostics, Inc.]

Definition

Even though the first cases of nephrogenic systemic fibrosis (NSF) were identified in 1997, and the first published report of 14 cases appeared in 2000 (1), NSF has only recently received great attention, especially because of its possible association with exposure to gadolinium-based contrast agents (GBCAs). "Nephrogenic" does not mean that the disease is caused by factors originating in the kidney, but that NSF has been observed only in patients with chronic kidney disease, while "systemic" emphasizes the systemic nature of this fibrosing disorder (2). It was previously known as "Nephrogenic Fibrosing Dermopathy", since its most prominent and visible effects are observed in the skin, where the histopathologic findings closely parallel those observed in wound healing reactions (1, 3, 4, 5). The nomenclature of the disease has been changed to NSF based on autopsy case reports of individual NSF patients that have reported variable degrees of myocardial, pericardial, and pleural fibrosis, along with the involvement of nerves and skeletal muscles (6, 7, 8). The disease is progressive and can be associated with a fatal outcome. There is still no definitive cure.

Diagnosis

NSF cannot be detected using a single diagnostic test. A confident diagnosis can usually be reached through the combination of a good clinical history, a good physical exam and the histopathologic examination of a biopsy specimen of involved skin. The main elements that should guide physicians in the diagnostic process are the clinical presentation in the setting of severe renal insufficiency and, more important, confirmatory cutaneous histopathologic findings (9).

So far, NSF has been observed only in patients with acute or chronic severe renal insufficiency (glomerular filtration rate, GFR, <30 mL/min/1.73m^2), or acute renal insufficiency of any severity due to the hepato-renal syndrome or in the perioperative liver transplantation period (9). The majority of patients with NSF have a GFR <15 mL/min and are receiving (or have received) either hemodialysis, peritoneal dialysis, or both (9).

The skin changes can mimic progressive systemic sclerosis with a predilection for the extremity involvement that can extend to the torso. It has not been reported to occur on the face, palms, or soles. Unlike scleroderma, NSF usually spares the face. Skin lesions usually begin with swelling, progressing to erythematous papules and coalescing hyperpigmented, browny plaques with *peau d'orange* surface. Peripheral irregular fingerlike or ameboid projections may be present along with islands of sparing. Bullae and nodules have also been reported. The skin involvement is often symmetrical and bilateral. Upon eye examination, new onset of white-yellow scleral plaques with dilated capillary loops may be seen in patients less than 45 years of age (1, 4, 9, 10).

The involved skin and subcutis usually becomes markedly thickened and hardened, with a wooden consistency to palpation. The induration characteristically involves the distal extremities first, gradually proceeding to involve the proximal extremities to the level of the mid-thigh and mid-upper arms (1, 9, 10). The involvement of the skin and subcutis overlying joints often causes a decrease in function of the hands and feet first, and then of more proximal joints in affected extremities, with elbows angled inwards and downwards and the body stooped over. Pedal plantar flexion may be sufficiently severe, making walking difficult or impossible. Joint contractures may develop very rapidly, with patients becoming wheelchair bound days to weeks after NSF starts, so that patients may become wheelchair dependent (9, 10).

If renal function is restored, the skin lesions may stabilize or even regress (9). Occasional patients (estimated at less than 5%) have rapidly progressive, fulminant NSF, associated with an accelerated loss of mobility, and often severe pain (9, 10).

Patients with NSF may complain of itching and sharp pain. Itching and pain may be localized in the affected areas, in the rib cage or hips. Loss of appetite and muscle weakness are commonly described (9, 10).

When the above noted signs and symptoms are observed in patients with severe renal insufficiency, a biopsy should be performed to obtain specimens of involved skin.

Histologically, NSF is characterized by dermal fibrosis (11). There is always an increased number of fibrocytes, that are CD34 and procollagen I positive when stained immunohistochemically (11). This dual positivity is characteristic of so-called "circulating fibrocytes," mesenchymal stem cells of bone marrow origin that participate in wound repair (11, 12).

In early lesions of NSF, collagen bundles may be quite narrow, with abundant edema fluid and/or mucin separating them. Procollagen I positivity is already present, but noted inconspicuously in the perinuclear cytoplasm of the bland dermal fibrocytes. In more advanced disease, collagen bundles become thicker (still generally maintaining clefts of separation between their neighbors) and the cytoplasm of the fibrocytes becomes plump and intensely procollagen I positive (13). The dermis is always involved by the histopathological pattern noted above, while the epidermis is not typically affected by NSF, although some degree of basilar pigmentation and epidermal acanthosis may be noted in advanced disease (13). The subcutaneous septa are markedly widened. In these deeper NSF foci, the widened septa are collagenized in the same manner as described above (13).

Other occasional findings may be a combination of epithelioid CD68-positive histiocytes in the subcutaneous septa, multinucleated giant cells, osteoclast-like giant cells, foci of osteoid deposition, and/or calcified bone spicules (13). Increased numbers of factor XIIIa positive dendritic cells or a coexpression of factor XIIIa and CD68 in the same cell have been observed as well. Vascularity is not typically prominent, although some cases of NSF show evidence of angiogenesis. Microthrombi and vasculitis have never been observed (13). The fibrotic process may extend through the fascia and into the underlying skeletal muscle that can be swelling and hardened as well (13). Patients suspected of NSF should be fully assessed by an experienced dermatologist.

How to minimize the risk of NSF

Step 1: Identify patients at risk

The first step should be to identify patients at risk for NSF, that is, those patients that suffer from severe (stages 4 and 5) chronic kidney disease, that is, GFR below 30 mL/min/1.73 m^2, independently of their age, race or gender or acute kidney injury (14). The risk of NSF development in patients with GFR between 30 and 44 mL/min/1.73 m^2 (stage 3b) is much smaller, but the American College of Radiology Subcommittee on MR Safety recommends to manage this group of patients as those with stage 4 or 5 chronic kidney disease, since GFR determinations may fluctuate from one day to the next (14). Therefore, it is important to identify patients with GFR<45 mL/min/1.73 m^2.

The level of GFR should be estimated from prediction equations that take into account the serum creatinine concentration and some or all of the following variables: age, gender, race, and body size (14). Many experts (including the American College of Radiology Subcommittee on MR Safety) have recommended that an estimated GFR be obtained within six weeks of anticipated GBCA injection in patients who might have reduced renal function. It has been suggested that this would include any patient with a history of renal disease (including a solitary kidney, renal transplant, or renal neoplasm), anyone over the age of 60 years, and with a history of hypertension or diabetes mellitus (14).

The most widely used equations for adult patients are the Modification of Diet in Renal Disease (MDRD) study equation (15) and the Cockcroft-Gault formula (16). Even if both equations provide a marked improvement over serum creatinine alone (17), the MDRD Study equation may perform better than the Cockroft-Gault formula, but the data are very limited (18-20). Both prediction equations assume that the amount of creatinine produced by the patient is equal to the amount being removed by the kidneys. Therefore, both equations are not suitable if renal function is in an unstable condition—that is, in patients with acute renal failure or on dialysis. Results may also deviate from true values in patients with exceptional dietary intake (e.g., vegetarian diet, high protein diet, creatine supplements), extremes of body composition (e.g., very lean, obese, paraplegia), or severe liver disease. Among children, the Schwartz formula provides a clinically useful estimate of GFR (21).

Step 2: Assess risk-benefit of contrast-enhanced MRI in patients at risk

A patient at risk of NSF should receive a GBCA only when a risk–benefit assessment for that particular patient indicates that the benefit of doing so clearly outweighs the potential risk(s). The risk-benefit evaluation should be made by the radiologist in conjunction with the referring physician(s) and should be properly a prospectively documented. History of previous exposures to GBCAs or other factors that are thought to act as possible co-triggers of the disease, such as metabolic acidosis, vascular surgery, thrombotic events, etc. should be taken into account during the risk–benefit assessment of each individual patient.

Patients, or parents or guardians in case of minors, should be properly informed of the benefits, risks, and diagnostic alternatives, based on all the information available at that time, and provide their consent in writing.

Step 3: Perform any unenhanced MR sequence that may be helpful before injecting the contrast agent

In the United States, the Food and Drug Administration has requested the prescribing information of all GBCAs to be revised by adding a black boxed warning, according to which the use of GBCAs in risk patients should be avoided, unless the diagnostic information is essential and not available with non-contrast enhanced MRI. Therefore, the MR exam should be properly monitored. All unenhanced MR sequences that may be helpful to make a diagnosis should be performed, and the images evaluated by an experienced radiologist, in order to ensure that the administration of a GBCA is still deemed necessary.

Step 4: Do not expose at risk patients to high doses of GBCAs

If the use of a GBCA is still deemed necessary, use the lowest dose needed to reliably provide the diagnostic information being clinically sought. According to boxed warning required by the FDA, the recommended doses should never be exceeded and dosing should not be repeated.

Which agent should be used?

In the USA, as in Europe and Japan, some GBCAs (gadodiamide, Omniscan; gadopentetate dimeglumine, Magnevist; gadoversetamide, OptiMARK) are specifically contraindicated for use in patients at risk of NSF (22). The American College of Radiology recommends to never use these agents in patients with GFR <45 mL/min and in patients with known or suspected acute kidney injury, regardless of calculated GFR values (14). Features of acute kidney injury consist of rapid (over hours to days) and usually reversible decrease in kidney function, commonly in the setting of surgery, severe infection, injury, or drug-induced kidney toxicity (22).

The other approved agents (Ablavar, gadofosveset trisodium; Eovist, gadoxetate disodium; MultiHance, gadobenate dimeglumine; ProHance, gadoteridol) should be used in patients at risk of NSF only if the diagnostic information is essential and not available with non-contrast enhanced MRI or other imaging modalities.

What to do after the MRI exam?

The usefulness of hemodialysis in the prevention of NSF is unknown. However, to enhance and speed up the GBCA elimination, many experts recommend that consideration be given to the performance of several dialysis sessions following GBCA administration in patients with end-stage renal disease on chronic dialysis, with use of prolonged dialysis times and increased flow rates and volumes to assist in the process of GBCA clearance (14). Peritoneal dialysis provides much less potential NSF risk reduction compared to hemodialysis and should not be considered protective (14).

Patients at risk of NSF should be followed up at least for one year after a contrast-enhanced MR exam, to promptly identify any symptom or sign suggestive of NSF and confirm or rule out a diagnosis of NSF. Should a new diagnosis of NSF be made, it is recommended that all the regulatory authorities in the United States, Canada, Europe, Asia and other countries be properly notified.

Additional Information to Consider

A study conducted by Nandwana, et al. (23) was performed to determine the incidence of NSF in patients at high risk, that is, patients with end-stage renal disease (ESRD) who had received MultiHance as part of a pre-transplant recipient evaluation screening for abnormalities which could compromise renal transplant outcome. The study population included patients not undergoing dialysis as well as those undergoing hemodialysis or peritoneal dialysis. Enrollment included 401 patients of which 303 (75.5%) were currently undergoing dialysis. For the remaining 98 (24.4%) patients not undergoing dialysis, the mean eGFR was 17 mL/min/1.73 m^2. Patients underwent a combined MR imaging and MR angiography of the abdomen and pelvis. Following the institution's standard protocol, each patient received a total of 0.15 mmol/kg of MultiHance, a dose 50% higher than the approved dose of 0.10 mmol/kg. The mean volume administered during the index MR examination was 24 mL. A total of 66 patients underwent additional examinations with MultiHance. For this group the mean total cumulative dose of MultiHance was 47 mL. Each patient's electronic medical records including pathology, transplant notes, progress notes, consultation notes (with and without skin examinations) and additional patient communication were evaluated for NSF or NSF-like symptoms. The study found no case even suggestive of NSF after a mean follow up period of more than two years.

In another study, Shaffer, et al. (24), assessed renal safety of MRI with the administration of MultiHance in patients with decompensated cirrhosis awaiting liver transplantation. The study population included 352 patients of whom 70 (20%) had renal insufficiency defined as pre-dose serum creatinine values $\geq$ 1.5mg/dL, and 64 (18.2%) who had Chronic Kidney Disease defined as serum creatinine >1.5mg/dL for $\geq$ 3 months. For the entire population, the pre-dose serum creatinine values ranged from 0.360 to 4.860 mg/dL. Following the institution's protocol, patients received half the approved dose of MultiHance (0.05 mmol/kg) for their abdominal MRI examination. There were no incidences of NSF reported among these 352 cases over a follow up period of 25.8 months.

REFERENCES

1. Cowper SE, et al. Scleromyxoedema-like cutaneous disease in renal-dialysis patients. Lancet 2000;356:1000–1001.

2. Cowper SE, Boyer PJ. Nephrogenic systemic fibrosis: An update. Curr Rheumatol Rep 2006;8:151–157.

3. DeHoratius D, Cowper SE. Nephrogenic systemic fibrosis: An emerging threat among renal patients. Semin Dial 2006;19:191-194.

4. Introcaso CE, et al. Nephrogenic fibrosing dermopathy/nephrogenic systemic fibrosis: A case series of nine patients and review of the literature. Int J Dermatol 2007;6:447–452.

5. Mendoza FA, et al. Description of 12 cases of nephrogenic fibrosing dermopathy and review of the literature. Semin Arthritis Rheum 2006;35: 238-249.

6. Gibson SE, et al. Multiorgan involvement in nephrogenic fibrosing dermopathy; an autopsy case and review of the literature. Arch Path Lab Med 2006;130:209-212.

7. Keyrouz S, Rudnicki SA. Neuromuscular Involvement in nephrogenic systemic fibrosis. J Clin Neuromusc Dis 2007;9:297–302.

8. Ting WW, et al. Nephrogenic fibrosing dermopathy with systemic involvement. Arch Dermatol 2003;139:903–9.

9. Knopp EA, Cowper SE. Nephrogenic systemic fibrosis: Early recognition and treatment. Semin Dial 2008;21:123-8.

10. Cowper SE: Nephrogenic fibrosing dermopathy: The first 6 years. Curr Opin Rheumatol 2003;15:785–790.

11. Cowper SE, et al. Nephrogenic fibrosing dermopathy. Amer J Dermatopathol 2001;23:383–393.

12. Bucala R. Circulating fibrocytes: Cellular basis for NSF. J Am Coll Radiol 2008;5:36-39.

13. Cowper SE, et al., Clinical and histological findings in nephrogenic systemic fibrosis. Eur J Radiol 2008;66:191-9.

14. ACR Manual on Contrast Media - Version 7, 2010.

15. Levey AS, et al. A more accurate method to estimate glomerular filtration rate from serum creatinine: A new prediction equation. Modification of Diet in Renal Disease Study Group. Ann Intern Med 1999;130:461–470.

16. Cockcroft DW, Gault MH. Prediction of creatinine clearance from serum creatinine. Nephron 1976;16:31–41.

17. Levey AS, et al. National Kidney Foundation. National Kidney Foundation practice guidelines for chronic kidney disease: Evaluation, classification, and stratification. Ann Intern Med 2003;139:137–147. (Erratum in Ann Intern Med 2003; 139:605)

18. Stevens LA, et al. Impact of creatinine calibration on performance of GFR estimating equations in a pooled individual patient database. Am J Kidney Dis 2007;50:21–35.

19. Levey AS, et al. Chronic Kidney Disease Epidemiology Collaboration. Expressing the Modification of Diet in Renal Disease Study equation for estimating glomerular filtration rate with standardized serum creatinine values. Clin Chem 2007;53:766–772.

20. Levey AS, et al. Chronic Kidney Disease Epidemiology Collaboration. Using standardized serum creatinine values in the modification of diet in renal disease study equation for estimating glomerular filtration rate. Ann Intern Med 2006;145:247–254.

21. Schwartz GJ, et al. A simple estimate of glomerular filtration rate in children derived from body length and plasma creatinine. Pediatrics 1976;58:259–263.

22. http://www.fda.gov/Drugs/DrugSafety/ucm223966.htm

23. Nandwana SB, et al. Gadobenate dimeglumine administration and nephrogenic systemic fibrosis: Is there a real risk in patients with impaired renal function. Radiology 2015;15:741-747.

24. Shaffer KM, et al. The renal safety of intravenous gadolinium enhanced magnetic resonance imaging in patients awaiting liver transplantation. Liver Transplantation 2015;21:1340-6.

Pregnant Patients and MR Procedures

Magnetic resonance (MR) imaging has been used to evaluate obstetrical, placental, and fetal abnormalities in pregnant patients for more than 30 years. MR imaging is recognized as a beneficial diagnostic tool and is utilized to assess a wide range of diseases and conditions that affect the pregnant patient as well as the fetus.

Initially, there were substantial technical problems with the use of MR imaging primarily due to image degradation from fetal motion. However, several technological improvements, including the development of high-performance gradient systems and rapid pulse sequences, have provided major advances especially useful for imaging the pregnant patient and the fetus. Thus, MR imaging examinations for obstetrical and fetal applications may now be accomplished routinely in the clinical setting.

PREGNANCY AND MR SAFETY

The use of diagnostic imaging is often required in pregnant patients. Thus, it is not surprising that the question of whether or not a patient should undergo an MR examination during pregnancy will often arise. Safety issues include possible bioeffects of the static magnetic field of the MR system, risks associated with exposure to the gradient magnetic fields, the potential adverse effects of radiofrequency (RF) energy, and possible adverse effects related to the combination of these three electromagnetic fields.

MR environment-related risks are difficult to assess for pregnant patients due to the number of possible permutations of the various factors that are present in this setting (e.g., differences in field strengths, pulse sequences, exposure times, etc.). This becomes even more complicated since new hardware and software is developed for MR systems on an on-going basis.

There have been a number of laboratory and clinical investigations conducted to determine the effects of using MR imaging during pregnancy. Most of the laboratory studies showed no evidence of injury or harm to the fetus, while a few studies reported adverse outcomes for laboratory animals. However, whether or not these findings can be extrapolated to human subjects is debatable.

By comparison, there have been studies performed in pregnant human subjects exposed to MR imaging or the MR environment. Each investigation reported no adverse outcomes for the subjects. For example, Baker, et al. (1994) reported no demonstrable increase in disease, disability, or hearing loss in 20 children examined *in utero* using echo-planar MRI for suspected fetal compromise. Myers, et al. (1998) reported no significant reduction in fetal growth vs. matched controls in 74 volunteer subjects exposed *in utero* to echo-planar MRI performed at 0.5-Tesla. A survey of reproductive health among 280 pregnant MR healthcare professionals performed by Kanal, et al. (1993) showed no substantial increase in common adverse reproductive outcomes. Choi, et al. (2015) reported on a series of 15 patients exposed to MRI during the first trimester. Patients were prospectively followed up until the completion of their pregnancy during which there were no abnormalities attributed to MRI. Ray, et al. (2016) reported that exposure to MRI during the first trimester of pregnancy compared with nonexposure was not associated with increased risk of harm to the fetus or in early childhood. These studies provide evidence regarding the safety of MRI in first-trimester, pregnant women.

There has been on-going concern that acoustic noise associated with MRI may impact the fetus. Reeves, et al. (2010) conducted an investigation to establish whether fetal exposure to the operating noise of 1.5-T MR imaging causes cochlear injury and subsequent hearing loss in neonates. The findings in this study provided evidence that exposure of the fetus to 1.5-T MR imaging during the second and third trimesters is not associated with an increased risk of substantial neonatal hearing impairment. In another study, Strizek, et al. (2015) reported no adverse effects of exposure to 1.5-T MRI *in utero* on neonatal hearing function.

With regard to the publications to date, there are discrepancies with respect to the experimental findings of the effects of electromagnetic fields used for MR procedures and the pertinent safety aspects of pregnancy. These discrepancies may be explained by a variety of factors, including the differences in the scientific methodology used, the type of organism examined, and the variance in exposure duration, as well as the conditions of the exposure to the electromagnetic fields. Additional investigations are warranted before the risks associated with exposure to MR procedures can be absolutely known and properly characterized.

GUIDELINES FOR THE USE OF MR PROCEDURES IN PREGNANT PATIENTS

As stated in the Policies, Guidelines, and Recommendations for MR Imaging Safety and Patient Management issued by the Safety Committee of the Society for Magnetic Resonance Imaging in 1991, "MR imaging may be used in pregnant women if other nonionizing forms of diagnostic imaging are inadequate or if the examination provides important information that would otherwise require exposure to ionizing radiation (e.g., fluoroscopy, CT, etc.). Pregnant patients should be informed that, to date, there has been no indication that the use of clinical MR imaging during pregnancy has produced deleterious effects." This policy has been adopted by the American College of Radiology and is considered to be the "standard of care" with respect to the use of MR procedures in pregnant patients, regardless of the trimester. Importantly, this information applies to MR systems operating up to and including 3-Tesla.

Thus, MR procedures may be used in pregnant patients to address important clinical problems or to manage potential complications for the patient or fetus. The decision to utilize an MR procedure in a pregnant patient involves answering a series of important questions that will help to address risk versus benefit including, the following:

- Is sonography satisfactory for diagnosis?
- Is the MR procedure appropriate to address the clinical question?
- Is obstetrical intervention prior to the MR procedure a possibility? That is, is termination of pregnancy a consideration? Is early delivery a consideration?

With regard to the use of an MR procedure in a pregnant patient, this diagnostic technique should not be withheld for the following cases:

- Patients with active brain or spine signs and symptoms requiring imaging.
- Patients with cancer requiring diagnostic imaging.
- Patients with chest, abdomen, and pelvic signs and symptoms of active disease when sonography is non-diagnostic.
- Patients with cases of suspected fetal anomalies or complex fetal disorders.

REFERENCES

Abdelazim IA, et al. Complementary roles of prenatal sonography and magnetic resonance imaging in diagnosis of fetal renal anomalies. Aust N Z J Obstet Gynaecol 2010;50:237-41.

ACR–SPR Practice Parameter for the Safe and Optimal Performance of Fetal Magnetic Resonance Imaging (MRI) Res. 13 – 2010, Amended 2014. American College of Radiology (acr.org), Reston, VA.

Ain DL, et al. Cardiovascular imaging and diagnostic procedures in pregnancy. Cardiol Clin 2012;30:331-41.

Baker PN, et al, A three-year follow-up of children imaged in utero with echo-planar magnetic resonance. Am J Obstet Gynecol 1994;170:32-33.

Baron KT, et al. Comparing the diagnostic performance of MRI versus CT in the evaluation of acute nontraumatic abdominal pain during pregnancy. Emerg Radiol 2012;19:519-25.

Beddy P, et al. Magnetic resonance imaging for the evaluation of acute abdominal pain in pregnancy. Semin Ultrasound CT MR 2010;31:433-41.

Benson RC, Colletti PM, Platt LD, et al. MR imaging of fetal anomalies. Am J Roentgenol 1991;156:1205-1207.

Blondiaux E, Garel C. Fetal cerebral imaging - ultrasound vs. MRI: An update. Acta Radiol 2013;54:1046-54.

Bouyssi-Kobar M, et al. Fetal magnetic resonance imaging: Exposure times and functional outcomes at preschool age. Pediatr Radiol 2015;45:1823-30.

Brown CEL, Weinreb JC. Magnetic resonance imaging appearance of growth retardation in a twin pregnancy. Obstet Gynecol 1988;71:987.

Carnes KI, Magin RL. Effects of in utero exposure to 4.7 T MR imaging conditions on fetal growth and testicular development in the mouse. Magn Reson Imaging 1996;14:263.

Chen MM, et al. Guidelines for computed tomography and magnetic resonance imaging use during pregnancy and lactation. Obstet Gynecol 2008;112 (2 Pt 1):333-40.

Choi JS, et al. A case series of 15 women inadvertently exposed to magnetic resonance imaging in the first trimester of pregnancy. J Obstet Gynaecol 2015;35:871-2.

Ciet P, Litmanovich DE. MR safety issues particular to women. Magn Reson Imaging Clin N Am 2015;23:59-67.

Colletti PM. Computer-assisted imaging of the fetus with magnetic resonance imaging. Comput Med Imaging Graph 1996;20:491.

Colletti PM, Platt LD. When to use MRI in obstetrics. Diag Imaging 11, 84, 1989.

Colletti PM, Sylvestre PB. Magnetic resonance imaging in pregnancy. MRI Clin N Am 1994;2:291.

Derntl B, et al. Stress matters! Psychophysiological and emotional loadings of pregnant women undergoing fetal magnetic resonance imaging. BMC Pregnancy Childbirth 2015;15:25.

De Wilde JP, et al. A review of the current use of magnetic resonance imaging in pregnancy and safety implications for the fetus. Prog Biophys Mol Biol 2005;87:335-353.

Dinh DH, et al. The use of magnetic resonance imaging for the diagnosis of fetal intracranial anomalies. Child Nerv Syst 1990;6:212.

Dunn RS, Weiner SN. Antenatal diagnosis of sacrococcygeal teratoma facilitated by combined use of Doppler sonography and MR imaging. Am J Roentgenol 1991;156:1115.

Fitamorris-Glass R, Mattrey RF, Cantrell CJ. Magnetic resonance imaging as an adjunct to ultrasound in oligohydramnio. J Ultrasound Med 1989:8:159.

Fraser R. Magnetic resonance imaging of the fetus. Initial experience [letter]. Gynecol Obstet Invest 1990;29:255.

Garcia-Bournissen F, Shrim A, Koren G. Safety of gadolinium during pregnancy. Can Fam Physician 2006;52:309-10.

Gardens AS, et al. Fast-scan magnetic resonance imaging of fetal anomalies. Br J Obstet Gynecol 1991;98:1217-1222.

Habib VV, et al. Early indicators of cervical insufficiency assessed using magnetic resonance imaging of the cervix during pregnancy. J Matern Fetal Neonatal Med 2015;28;626-31.

Hand JW, et al. Prediction of specific absorption rate in mother and fetus associated with MRI examinations during pregnancy. Magn Reson Med 2006;55:883-893.

Hand JW, et al. Numerical study of RF exposure and the resulting temperature rise in the foetus during a magnetic resonance procedure. Phys Med Biol 2010;55:913-30.

Heinrichs WL, et al. Midgestational exposure of pregnant BALB/c mice to magnetic resonance imaging conditions. Magnetic Resonance Imaging 1988;6:305.

Hill MC, et al. Prenatal diagnosis of fetal anomalies using ultrasound and MRI. Radiol Clin North Am 1988;26:287-307.

Horvath L, Seeds JW. Temporary arrest of fetal movement with pancuronium bromide to enable antenatal magnetic resonance imaging of holosencephaly. Am J Roentgenol, 1989;6:418-420.

Huisman TA. Fetal magnetic resonance imaging. Semin Roentgenol 2008;43:314-36.

Jackson HA, Panigrahy A. Fetal magnetic resonance imaging: The basics. Pediatr Ann 2008;37:388-93.

Junkermann H. Indications and contraindications for contrast-enhanced MRI and CT during pregnancy. Radiologe 2007;47:774-7.

Expert Panel on MR Safety, Kanal E, Barkovich AJ, Bell C, et al. ACR guidance document on MR safe practices: 2013. J Magn Reson Imag 2013;37:501-30.

Kanal E, Gillen J, Evans J, Savitz D, Shellock FG. Survey of reproductive health among female MR workers. Radiology 1993;187:395-399.

Kanal E, Shellock FG, Sonnenblick D. MRI clinical site safety: Phase I results and preliminary data. Magn Reson Imaging 1988:7, Suppl 1:106.

Kay HH, Herfkens RJ, Kay BK. Effect of magnetic resonance imaging on Xenopus laevis embryogenesis. Magn Reson Imaging 1988;6:501-6.

Kikuchi S, et al. Temperature elevation in the fetus from electromagnetic exposure during magnetic resonance imaging. Phys Med Biol 2010;55:2411-26.

Krishnamurthy U, et al. MR imaging of the fetal brain at 1.5 T and 3.0 T field strengths: Comparing specific absorption rate (SAR) and image quality. J Perinat Med 2015;43:209-20.

Kok RD, et al. Absence of harmful effects of magnetic resonance exposure at 1.5 T in utero during the third trimester of pregnancy: A follow-up study. Magnetic Resonance Imaging 2004;22:851-4.

Krishnamurthy U, et al. MR imaging of the fetal brain at 1.5T and 3.0T field strengths: Comparing specific absorption rate (SAR) and image quality. J Perinat Med 2015;43:209-20.

Lee JW, et al. Genotoxic effects of 3 T magnetic resonance imaging in cultured human lymphocytes. Bioelectromagnetics 2011;32:535-42.

Leithner K, et al. Psychological reactions in women undergoing fetal magnetic resonance imaging. Obstet Gynecol 2008;111(2 Pt 1):396-402.

Lenke RR, et al. Use of pancuronium bromide to inhibit fetal movement during magnetic resonance imaging. J Reprod Med 34,315-317, 1989.

Levine D. Obstetric MRI. J Magn Reson Imag 2006;24:1-15.

Malko JA, et al. Search for influence of 1.5 T magnetic field on growth of yeast cells. Bioelectromagnetics 1987;15:495.

Manganaro L, et al. Magnetic resonance imaging of fetal heart: Anatomical and pathological findings. J Matern Fetal Neonatal Med 2014;27:1213-9.

Mansfield P, et al. Study of internal structure of the human fetus in utero at 0.5-T. Br J Radiol 1990;13:314-318.

Masselli G, et al. Acute abdominal and pelvic pain in pregnancy: MR imaging as a valuable adjunct to ultrasound? Abdom Imaging 2011;36:596-603.

McCarthy SM, et al. Uterine neoplasms: MR imaging. Radiology 1989:170:125.

McRobbie D, Foster MA. Pulsed magnetic field exposure during pregnancy and implications for NMR foetal imaging. A study with mice. Magn Reson Imaging 1985;3:231.

Myers C, et al. Failure to detect intrauterine growth restriction following in utero exposure to MRI. Br J Radiol 1998;71:549.

Murbach M, et al. Pregnant women models analyzed for RF exposure and temperature increase in 3T RF shimmed birdcages. Magn Reson Med 2017;77:2048-2056.

Murakami J, et al. Fetal developmet of mice following intrauterine exposure to a static magnetic field of 6.3-T. Magn Reson Imaging 1992;10:433.

Nara VR, et al. Effects of a 1.5T static magnetic field on spermatogenesis and embryogenesis in mice. Invest Radiology 1996;31:586.

Oto A. MR imaging evaluation of acute abdominal pain during pregnancy. Magnetic Resonance Imaging Clin N Am 2006;14:489-501.

Palacios-Jaraquemada JM, et al. MRI in the diagnosis and surgical management of abnormal placentation. Acta Obstet Gynecol Scand 2013;92:392-7.

Patenaude Y, et al. The use of magnetic resonance imaging in the obstetric patient. J Obstet Gynaecol Can 2014;36:349-55.

Ray JG, et al. Association between MRI exposure during pregnancy and fetal and childhood outcomes. JAMA. 2016;316:952-61.

Reeves MJ, et al. Neonatal cochlear function: Measurement after exposure to acoustic noise during in utero MR imaging. Radiology 2010;257:802-809.

Renfroe S, et al. Role of serial MRI assessment in the management of an abdominal pregnancy. BMJ Case Rep 2013;bcr2013200495.

Ruckhäberle E, et al. *In vivo* intrauterine sound pressure and temperature measurements during magnetic resonance imaging (1.5 T) in pregnant ewes. Fetal Diagn Ther 2008;24:203-10.

Semere LG, et al. Neuroimaging in pregnancy: A review of clinical indications and obstetric outcomes. J Matern Fetal Neonatal Med 2013;26:1371-9.

Shellock FG, Crues JV. MR procedures: Biologic effects, safety, and patient care. Radiology 2004;232:635-652.

Shellock FG, Kanal E. Policies, guidelines, and recommendations for MR imaging safety and patient management. J Magn Reson Imaging 1991;1:97.

Shellock FG, Kanal E. Chapter 4, Magnetic resonance procedures and pregnancy. In, Magnetic Resonance Bioeffects, Safety, and Patient Management. Second Edition, Lippincott-Ravin, Philadelphia, New York, 1996, pp. 49.

Smith FW, et al. Nuclear magnetic resonance imaging – a new look at the fetus. Br J Gynaecol 1985;92:1024-1033.

Smith FW, Sutherland HW. Magnetic resonance imaging: The use of the inversion recovery sequence to display fetal morphology. Br J Radiol 1988;61:338-341.

Sohlberg S, et al. Placental perfusion in normal pregnancy and early and late preeclampsia: A magnetic resonance imaging study. Placenta 2014;35:202-6.

Stark DD, et al. Pelvimetry by magnetic resonance imaging. Am J Roentgenol 1985;144:947-950.

Strizek B, et al. Safety of MR imaging at 1.5 T in fetuses: A retrospective case-control study of birth weights and the effects of acoustic noise. Radiology 2015;275:530-7.

Takahashi K, et al. Establishing measurements of subcutaneous and visceral fat area ratio in the early second trimester by magnetic resonance imaging in obese pregnant women. J Obstet Gynaecol Res 2014;40:1304-7.

Tesky GC, et al. Survivability and long-term stress reactivity levels following repeated exposure to nuclear magnetic resonance imaging procedures in rats. Physiol Chem Phys Med NMR 1987;19:43.

Tirada N, et al. Imaging pregnant and lactating patients. Radiographics 2015;35:1751-65.

Tocchio S, et al. MRI evaluation and safety in the developing brain. Semin Perinatol 2015;39:73-104.

Tyndall DA. MRI effects on the teratogenicity of x-irradiation in the C57BL/6J mouse. Magn Reson Imaging 1990;8:423.

Tyndall RJ, Sulik KK. Effects of magnetic resonance imaging on eye development in the C57BL/6J mouse. Teratology 1991;43:263

Tyndall DA. MRI effects on craniofacial size and crown-rump length in C57BL/6J mice in 1.5T fields. Oral Surg Oral Med Oral Pathol 1993;76: 65.

Yip YP, et al. Effects of MR exposure at 1.5 T on early embryonic development of the chick. J Magn Reson Imaging 1994;4:742.

Yip YP, et al. Effects of MR exposure on axonal outgrowth in the sympathetic nervous system of the chick. J Magn Reson Imaging 1995;4:457.

Yip YP, et al. Effects of MR exposure on cell proliferation and migration of chick motor neurons. J Magn Reson Imaging 1994;4:799.

Vadeyar SH, et al. Effect of fetal magnetic resonance imaging on fetal heart rate patterns. Am J Obstet Gynecol 2000;182:666.

Webb JA, et al. Members of Contrast Media Safety Committee of European Society of Urogenital Radiology (ESUR). The use of iodinated and gadolinium contrast media during pregnancy and lactation. Eur Radiol 2005;15:1234-40.

Weinreb JC, et al. Pelvic masses in pregnant patients, MR and US imaging. Radiology 1986;159:717.

Weinreb JC, et al. Magnetic resonance imaging in obstetric diagnosis. Radiology 1985;154:157-161.

Wenstrom KD, et al. Magnetic resonance imaging of fetuses with intracranial defects. Obstet Gynecol 1991;77:529-532.

Wieseler KM, et al. Imaging in pregnant patients: Examination appropriateness. Radiographics 2010;30:1215-29.

Wilcox A, et al. Incidence of early loss of pregnancy. New Engl J Med 1988;319:189-194.

Williamson RA, et al. Magnetic resonance imaging of anomalous fetuses. Obstet Gynecol 1989;73:952-956.

Zahedi Y, et al. Impact of repetitive exposure to strong static magnetic fields on pregnancy and embryonic development of mice. J Magn Reson Imag 2014;39:691-9.

Zaun G, et al. Repetitive exposure of mice to strong static magnetic fields in utero does not impair fertility in adulthood but may affect placental weight of offspring. J Magn Reson Imaging 2014;39:683-90.

Pregnant Technologists and Other Healthcare Workers in the MR Environment

Due to the concern with regard to pregnant technologists and other healthcare workers in the MR environment, a survey of reproductive health among female MR system operators was conducted by Kanal, et al. (1993). Questionnaires were sent to female MR technologists and nurses at the majority of the MRI facilities in the United States. The questionnaire addressed menstrual and reproductive experiences as well as work activities. This study attempted to account for known potential confounding variables (e.g., age, smoking, alcohol use, etc.) for this type of data.

Of the 1,915 completed questionnaires analyzed, there were 1,421 pregnancies: 280 occurred while working as an MR employee (technologist or nurse), 894 while employed at another job, 54 as a student, and 193 as a homemaker. Five categories were analyzed that included spontaneous abortion rate, pre-term delivery (less than 39 weeks), low birth weight (less than 5.5 pounds), infertility (taking more than eleven months to conceive), and gender of the offspring.

The data indicated that there were no statistically significant alterations in the five areas studied for MR healthcare professionals relative to the same group studied when they were employed elsewhere, prior to becoming MR healthcare employees. Additionally, adjustment for maternal age, smoking, and alcohol use failed to markedly change any of the associations. Menstrual regularity, menstrual cycle, and related topics were also examined in this study. These included inquiries regarding the number of days of menstrual bleeding, the heaviness of the bleeding, and the time between menstrual cycles.

Admittedly, this is a difficult area to objectively examine because it depends on both subjective memory and the memory of the respondent for a given topic. Subjective memory is often inadequate. Nevertheless, the data suggested that there were no clear correlations between MR workers and specific modifications of the menstrual cycle.

The findings from this extensive epidemiological investigation were reassuring insofar as that there did not appear to be deleterious effects from exposure to the static magnetic field of the MR system. Therefore, a policy is recommended that permits pregnant technologists and healthcare workers to perform MR procedures, as well as to enter the MR system room, and attend to the patient during pregnancy, regardless of the trimester. Importantly, technologists and healthcare workers should not remain within the MR system room or bore of the MR system during the actual operation of the scanner.

This particular recommendation is especially important for those healthcare professionals involved in patient management or interventional MR-guided examinations and procedures, since it may be necessary to be directly exposed to the MR system's electromagnetic fields at levels similar to those used for patients. These recommendations are not based on indications of adverse effects, but rather, from a conservative point of view because there is insufficient information pertaining to the bioeffects of the other electromagnetic fields used during MRI to permit unnecessary exposures.

REFERENCES

Evans JA, et al. Infertility and pregnancy outcome among magnetic resonance imaging workers. J Occu Med 1993;12:1191-1195.

International Commission on Non-Ionizing Radiation Protection (ICNIRP) statement, medical magnetic resonance procedures: Protection of patients. Health Physics 2004;87:197-216.

Kanal E, Gillen J, Evans J, Savitz D, Shellock FG. Survey of reproductive health among female MR workers. Radiology 1993;187:395-399.

Shellock FG. Magnetic Resonance Procedures: Health Effects and Safety. CRC Press, LLC, Boca Raton, FL, 2001.

Shellock FG, Kanal E. Policies, guidelines, and recommendations for MR imaging safety and patient management. J Magn Reson Imag 1991;1:97-101.

Prevention of Missile Effect Accidents

The "missile effect" refers to the capability of the fringe field of an MR system to attract a ferromagnetic object, drawing it rapidly into the scanner by considerable force. The missile effect can pose a significant risk to the patient inside the MR system and/or anyone in the path of the projectile. Furthermore, considerable damage to the MR system may result due to the impact of ferromagnetic objects. Therefore, a strict policy must be established by the MRI facility to detect metallic objects prior to allowing individuals or patients to enter the MR environment. In addition, to guard against accidents from projectiles, the immediate area around the MR system should be clearly demarcated, labeled with appropriate danger signs, and secured by trained staff aware of proper MR safety procedures.

For patients preparing to undergo MR examinations, all metallic or other potentially problematic personal belongings and devices (i.e. hearing aids, analog watches, beepers, cell phones, jewelry, etc.) must be removed as well as clothing items that have metallic fasteners or other metallic components (e.g., clothing with metallic threads). One of the most effective means of preventing a ferromagnetic object from a patient inadvertently becoming a missile and to ensure that no inappropriate objects enter the MR environment is to require the patient to wear a gown or scrubs without pockets for the MR examination.

Non-ambulatory patients must only be allowed to enter the area of the MR system using a nonferromagnetic wheelchair or nonferromagnetic gurney. Wheelchairs and gurneys should also be inspected for the presence of a ferromagnetic oxygen tank, IV pole, sand bag (which may have metal shot), or other similar problematic component or accessory before allowing the patient into the MR setting. Fortunately, there are many commercially-available, specially-designed devices that are appropriate for use to transport and support patients in the MR environment.

Any individual accompanying the patient must be required to remove all metallic objects or other problematic items before entering the MR area and should undergo a careful and thorough screening procedure. All hospital and outside personnel that may need to enter the MR environment periodically or in response to an emergency (e.g., custodial staff, maintenance workers, housekeeping staff, bioengineers, nurses, security officers, fire fighters, etc.) should also undergo MRI screening and be educated about the potential hazards associated with the MR system. These individuals should, likewise, be instructed to remove inappropriate objects before entering the MR environment.

Many serious incidents have occurred when individuals who were unaware of the potentially dangerous aspects of the MR system entered the MR environment with items such as steel oxygen tanks, wheel chairs, scissors, hand guns, monitors, and other similar objects.

In 2001, the first fatal accident occurred that illustrated the importance of careful attention to preventing ferromagnetic objects from entering the MR environment. In this widely publicized incident, a young patient suffered a blow to the head from a ferromagnetic oxygen tank that became a projectile in the presence of a 1.5-Tesla MR system.

While MR safety guidelines and procedures are well known, accidents related to the missile effect continue to occur. Guidelines for preventing these hazards are presented in **Table 1**.

Table 1. Guidelines for preventing hazards related to missile effects.*

1) Appoint an MRI safety officer or other appropriately trained person to be responsible for ensuring that proper procedures are in effect, enforced, and updated to ensure safety in the MR environment.

2) Establish and routinely review safety policies and procedures and assess the level of compliance by all staff members.

3) Provide all MR staff, along with other personnel who may need to enter the MR environment (e.g., transport personnel, security officers, housekeeping staff, maintenance workers, fire department personnel, etc.) with formal training on MR safety. This should be done especially for new employees and repeated on a regular basis (i.e. yearly).

4) Emphasize to all personnel that the MR system's powerful static magnetic field is always "on" and treat the MR environment, accordingly.

5) Don't allow equipment and devices containing ferromagnetic components into the MR environment, unless they have been tested and labeled "MR Safe" or "MR Conditional".

6) Adhere to the restrictions provided by suppliers regarding the use of MR Safe and/or MR Conditional equipment and devices in the MR environment.

7) Maintain a list of MR Safe and MR Conditional equipment, including restrictions for use. This list should be kept and updated in every MRI facility by the MR safety officer (refer to **www.MRIsafety.com** for comprehensive information).

8) Bring a non-ambulatory patient into the MR environment using a nonmagnetic wheelchair or gurney. Ensure that no oxygen tanks, IV poles, sandbags with metal shot, or other ferromagnetic objects are concealed under blankets or sheets or stowed away on the transport equipment.

9) Carefully screen all individuals and patients entering the MR environment to identify magnetic objects in their bodies (e.g., implants, bullets, shrapnel, etc.), on their bodies (e.g., hair pins, brassieres, buttons, zippers, jewelry, clothing with metallic threads), or attached to their bodies (e.g., body piercing jewelry, body modification implants, halo vests, cervical fixation devices, external fixation systems, prosthetic appliances). Ferromagnetic objects on or attached to the bodies of patients, family members, or staff members should be removed, if feasible, before the individuals enter the MR environment. Additional attention must also be given to items that are made from conducting metals, as these may pose hazards under certain conditions.

10) Have patients wear hospital gowns or scrubs without pockets and metallic fasteners for MR procedures. Clothing that contains metallic objects or threads that may pose a hazard in the MR environment.

11) Consider utilizing a ferromagnetic detection system as an important tool to help prevent projectile accidents.

[*Adapted and published permission from ECRI Institute Report, 2001 and Shellock FG, 2001. Reviewed and updated 2018.]

REFERENCES

Chaljub G, et al. Projectile cylinder accidents resulting from the presence of ferromagnetic nitrous oxide or oxygen tanks in the MR suite. Am J Roentgenol 2001;177:27-30.

Colletti PM. Size "H" oxygen cylinder: Accidental MR projectile at 1.5-Tesla. J Magn Reson Imag 2004;19:141-143.

ECRI Institute. Patient death illustrates the importance of adhering to safety precautions in magnetic resonance environments. ECRI Institute, Plymouth Meeting, PA, Aug. 6, 2001.

ECRI Institute. Best ferromagnetic detectors: Ratings for 7 products from Kopp Development, Mednovus, and Metrasens. Health Devices 2011;40:6-30

Expert Panel on MR Safety, Kanal E, Barkovich AJ, Bell C, et al. ACR guidance document on MR safe practices: 2013. J Magn Reson Imag 2013;37:501-30.

International Commission on Non-Ionizing Radiation Protection (ICNIRP) statement, medical magnetic resonance procedures: Protection of patients. Health Physics 2004;87:197-216.

Joint Commission on Accreditation of Healthcare Organizations, USA. Preventing accidents and injuries in the MRI suite. Sentinel Event Alert. 2008;Feb 14:1-3.

Lee CH, et al. Management of a sandbag accident in an MRI unit. Magn Reson Imaging 2015;33:1187-9.

Shellock FG, Crues JV, Editors. MRI Bioeffects, Safety, and Patient Management. Biomedical Research Publishing Group, Los Angeles, CA, 2014.

Tsai LL, et al. A practical guide to MR imaging safety: What radiologists need to know. Radiographics 2015;35:1722-37.

Weidman EK, et al. MRI safety: A report of current practice and advancements in patient preparation and screening. Clin Imaging 2015;39:935-7.

Signs to Help Control Access to the MR Environment

To guard against accidents and injuries to patients and other individuals as well as damage to magnetic resonance (MR) systems, the general and immediate areas associated with the scanner (also referred to as the MR environment) must have supervised and controlled access. Supervised and controlled access involves having MR safety-trained personnel present at all times during the operation of the facility to ensure that no unaccompanied or unauthorized individuals are allowed to enter the MR environment. MR safety-trained personnel must be responsible for performing comprehensive screening of patients and other individuals before allowing them to enter the MR system room. The area should be secured and/or controlled by appropriate means when MR safety-trained personnel are not present.

Importantly, it is necessary to educate and train individuals who need to enter the MR environment on a regular basis, those working on an intermittent basis, or responding to an emergency including custodial workers, transporters, security personnel, firefighters, nurses, anesthesiologists, and paramedics regarding the potential hazards related to the powerful magnetic field of the MR system. Unfortunately, even with proper MR safety procedures in place, many individuals and patients have inadvertently "wandered" unattended into the MR setting, and these situations have resulted in problematic or serious consequences.

As a means of helping to control access to the MR environment, the area must be clearly demarcated and labeled with prominently displayed signs to make individuals and patients aware of the risks associated with the MR system. Access to the MR environment must also be monitored and controlled on a continuous basis.

Signs with appropriate content and information were designed to promote a safe MR environment. According to the U.S. Food and Drug Administration document entitled, Guidance for the Submission Of Premarket Notifications for Magnetic Resonance Diagnostic Devices (issued November 14, 1998), Attachment B, states: "The controlled access area should be labeled "Danger - High Magnetic Field" at all entries." Also, this FDA document indicates, "Operators should be warned by appropriate signs about the presence of magnetic fields and their force and torque on magnetic materials, and that loose ferrous objects should be excluded."

"DANGER" Sign

In consideration of the above, the sign used for the MRI environment states: **DANGER**! Additionally, to inform everyone about the powerful static magnetic field associated with the MR system, especially individuals unacquainted with MR technology, the following information is prominently shown on this sign:

RESTRICTED ACCESS
STRONG MAGNETIC FIELD
THIS MAGNET IS ALWAYS ON!

With respect to the information for implants and devices, in addition to cardiac pacemakers, implantable cardioverter defibrillators (ICDs) are potentially hazardous for patients and individuals in the MR environment. Therefore, this information is included on the sign used for the MR environment. The peer-reviewed literature has reported that many types of metallic implants are acceptable for patients undergoing MR procedures, while others are not. Therefore, this information is clarified on the current sign, with individuals and patients informed to consult MRI professionals if there are questions regarding this matter, as follows:

"Persons with certain metallic, electronic, magnetic, or mechanically-activated implants, devices, or objects may not enter this area. Serious injury may result. <u>Do not enter</u> this area if you have any question regarding an implant, device, or object. Consult the MRI Technologist or Radiologist."

Finally, the sign also states:

"Objects made from ferrous materials must not be taken into this area. Serious injury or property damage may result. Electronic objects such as hearing aids, cell phones, and beepers may also be damaged."

Many individuals fail to realize that the MR system's static magnetic field is always on. In fact, investigations of accidents that involved relatively large ferromagnetic objects like oxygen cylinders, chairs, IV poles, and wheelchairs revealed that the offending personnel thought that the powerful magnetic field was activated *only* during the MR procedure. Therefore, a smaller sign or decal is particularly useful to emphasize the potentially hazardous nature of the MR environment, which states:

DANGER! THIS MAGNET IS ALWAYS ON!

Sign Placement. The strategic placement of signs in and around the MR environment is crucial to ensure that all individuals and patients see them before entering this area. In general, a sign should be placed on the door or entrance to MR system room and near or on the doorframe to be viewed by individuals and patients, especially if the door to the MR system room is open.

[*To obtain the afore-mentioned signs designed to help control access to the may be found at MRI Equip, www.mriequip.com and other distributors of MRI specialty products. In addition, signs for use in the MRI area may be downloaded for free from the website for the Institute of Physics and Engineering in Medicine, www.ipem.ac.uk]

REFERENCE

U. S. Department Of Health and Human Services, Center for Devices and Radiological Health Food and Drug Administration, the document entitled, Guidance for the, Submission Of Premarket Notifications for Magnetic Resonance Diagnostic Devices, Issued November 14, 1998.

Spatial Gradient Magnetic Field: How This Information is Applied to Labeling of Medical Implants and Devices*

[*Excerpted with permission from, Regarding the Value Reported for the Term "Spatial Gradient Magnetic Field" and How This Information Is Applied to Labeling of Medical Implants and Devices, Shellock FG, Kanal E, Gilk TB. Am J Roentgenol, 2011;196:142-145. To obtain the full-length article visit *www.IMRSER.org*.]

Differences in interpretations of testing and reporting criteria, methodologies, and perhaps even concerns about manufacturer legal liability have created a contemporary environment in which questions and confusion abound in the magnetic resonance imaging (MRI) industry. Of particular concern regarding the management of patients with implants and devices in the MRI environment is the disparities in the way that the spatial gradient magnetic field information is presented.

The intensity of the static magnetic field around an MR system varies with respect to the distance from the scanner. This so-called "fringe-field" of the MR system creates a "spatial gradient magnetic field". By definition, the spatial gradient magnetic field is a magnetic field that varies in intensity over distance. The spatial gradient magnetic field should not be confused with the time-varying, gradient magnetic fields produced by the gradient coils that are used during the imaging process for spatial encoding of the MRI signals.

The spatial gradient of the magnetic field produces an attractive displacement (or translational) force on ferromagnetic objects placed into the static magnetic field of the MR system (1-4). Importantly, the MRI-specific labeling that is used for medical implants and devices typically provides information for the "highest spatial gradient magnetic field" at which the medical device was tested and that is allowed for the object to be exposed to in order to ensure the safety of the patient relative to the device's translational attraction (1-6). The assessment of translational attraction (or displacement force) is just one aspect of implant testing that is performed when evaluating a medical device (1-5).

In most cases, the Food and Drug Administration (FDA) accepts the determination of translational attraction for a medical device that is conducted according to the procedure described by the American Society for Testing and Materials (ASTM) International Designation. F 2052, Standard test method for measurement of magnetically induced displacement force on passive implants in the magnetic resonance environment. Using this technique, a test apparatus with a protractor (also called the "fixture") is placed in an MR system with a horizontal magnetic field at the point of the highest "accessible" spatial gradient magnetic field (6). In general, the highest spatial gradient magnetic field used to assess translational attraction for a medical device is located off-axis, at a side-wall and near the opening of the bore of the scanner (1, 3). [Alternatively, the medical device is assessed for translational attraction at the point where the highest deflection angle occurs in association with the particular MR system used for the assessment.] The angular "deflection" of the device from the vertical is measured and the translational attraction is calculated (6).

Notably, the placement of the test fixture (apparatus with the protractor) in the MR system is at a position where it can be utilized properly (i.e. securely positioned) for the test procedure. This is almost always a worst-case position of greatest attractive force that the patient with the device will "pass through" when entering the bore of the MR system for an examination.

With regard to the translational attraction measurement for a medical device, if the deflection angle is less than 45-degrees, and the magnetic force is in the horizontal direction, the deflection force is less than the gravitational force associated with the device's weight and it is assumed that any risk imposed by the application of the magnetically-induced deflection force is no greater than any risk imposed by normal daily activity in the Earth's gravitational field (4, 6). However, even if a device exceeds 45-degrees of deflection, it may still be acceptable for a patient undergoing an MRI examination if sufficient counter-forces are present (e.g., from sutures, scarring, tissue in-growth, etc.) that prevent it from being moved or dislodged (3).

There is confusion about the term "spatial gradient magnetic field" (or "highest spatial gradient" or "magnetic spatial gradient") and how this parameter is reported for a given MR system relative to this term's use in the labeling of a medical device. [Note: The term "spatial gradient magnetic field" may also be misunderstood because some MRI professionals see the term "gradient" and presume that it refers to the "time-varying or gradient magnetic fields" (dB/dt) used for spatial location in association with MR imaging (2).] The term "spatial gradient magnetic field" refers to the rate at which the static magnetic field strength changes over space or distance per unit length. This parameter is indicated as dB/dx, using the units of Tesla/meter or gauss/centimeter.

According to test reports and resulting labeling for many implants tested at 3-Tesla, the highest "accessible" spatial gradient magnetic field of 720-gauss/cm was determined using highly involved methodology for the 3-Tesla MR system used for the measurements of translational attraction. (Researchers and MRI professionals, however, must typically rely on the magnitude and location of the spatial gradient magnetic field as it is provided by the MR system manufacturer.) To test the device, the apparatus with the protractor was placed at that position (720-gauss/cm) to measure the deflection angle. This information (i.e. the value for the highest spatial gradient magnetic field) is reported in the labeling for the device. Thus, the MRI-specific labeling would then state that the acceptable static magnetic field information for a given implant would be, as follows (2):

- 3-Tesla or less
- Highest spatial gradient magnetic field of 720-gauss/cm or less

To date, the Food and Drug Administration has approved MRI-specific labeling for more than three thousand medical devices according to the above-described process, especially with regard to how the displacement force is determined [i.e. by following the procedure described in the ASTM document (6)] and with respect to how the findings are presented in the labeling (i.e. reporting the value for the highest spatial gradient magnetic field that was used for the determination of the deflection angle for the medical device, which was based on where the apparatus with the protractor was positioned). Furthermore, the ASTM document that addresses the measurement of translational attraction for a medical device clearly states to report "10.1.7....the magnitude of the spatial gradient of the magnetic field, at the test location." That is why this particular spatial gradient magnetic field value has been used in the FDA-approved MRI labeling for thousands of medical devices. Of note is that the reported results describe the MR system variables under which the implant or device was tested and do not necessarily represent the safety threshold for translational forces.

Recently, MR system manufacturers have provided data to MRI professionals pertaining to the "spatial gradient magnetic field" values for a given scanner, including information for the highest spatial gradient magnetic field. Presumably, this was done in an effort to help address the case when a patient presents with a medical device that has labeling stating the "highest spatial gradient magnetic field" value permitted for that implant and that parameter is unknown for a specific MR system. The format, values, locations for measurement, and presentation of these reported MR system values have varied, and even conflicted between and within the MR system vendors that have provided these data.

Considerable confusion has inadvertently arisen as a result of these recently reported spatial gradient magnetic field values. The reason for this misunderstanding is simple: the location, and, therefore, the values, of the highest spatial gradient magnetic field measured and reported by the MR system manufacturers is not the same as that which is utilized for the location at which the implant/device displacement force testing was performed. To elaborate, the location of measurement of the highest spatial gradient magnetic field that is used when evaluating the displacement force for a medical implant or device (i.e. the place in the MR system where the apparatus with the protractor is positioned; which is generally off-axis, near the opening of the bore of the scanner) is not necessarily the same as the location where the MR system manufacturer measures the scanner's highest spatial gradient magnetic field.

The MR system manufacturer may have performed the measurement with the covers or shroud removed from the MR system, and/or without the patient table present. This permits access to stronger static magnetic fields and spatial gradient magnetic fields and, thus, can result in a greater measured value for the "highest spatial gradient magnetic field" as it is reported by the manufacturer. This region and, therefore, the measured value, however, is not one that can be reached by a patient with an implant and, thus, it does not represent a reasonable assessment of risk exposure for that situation.

We recognize that the values reported for the regions not normally accessible to patients may have significance or relevance for MR system manufacturers and their manufacturing and/or service employees. Nevertheless, from the point of view of clinical patient care, these "patient inaccessible regions" and the spatial gradient magnetic field values reported for them are of no particular benefit. Indeed, reporting these values seems to have resulted in confusion.

Furthermore, making decisions regarding the patients with implants or devices based on these higher spatial gradient magnetic field values measured in patient inaccessible regions might inadvertently lead to canceling requested and needed clinical MRI examinations for patients with devices tested and cleared to the patient accessible region's translational forces – but not to those higher values reported at patient inaccessible regions.

Clinical personnel responsible for assessing the labeling that states the "MR Conditional" aspects of an implant or device, rated as acceptable to a value of 720 gauss/cm, when their MR system by the specifications provided by the MR system manufacturer is identified as having a maximum value 200 gauss/cm higher (e.g., 900 gauss/cm), may refuse to scan the patient with the implant on that MR system which, ironically, is equivalent to the scanner used to demonstrate safety relative to translational attraction for the implant!

While the value for the highest spatial gradient magnetic field that the MR system manufacturer reports for a given scanner does not have direct relevance to a patient with a medical device, if the MR system manufacturer provides measurements that are obtained in radial increments from that position, these values may be useful for managing patients with medical implants and devices, if the position used to perform the deflection angle test on the device was known.

Because of the discrepancy between the MR system manufacturer's reported value for the highest spatial gradient magnetic field for a given scanner and the highest "accessible" spatial magnetic gradient value used for medical device testing that has led to confusion and frustration when MRI professionals must consider how to manage patients presented with MRI labeling information, we strongly recommend that standardization is necessary. Notably, it would be helpful and appropriate for all MR system manufacturers to report the greatest static magnetic field strength as well as the highest spatial gradient magnetic field values in regions that are readily accessible by patients and/or healthcare professionals working around an "intact" (i.e. with the covers or shroud not removed) MR system.

In order to accomplish such a task, the FDA needs to understand the nature of the present problems related to the MRI specific labeling for implants and devices, develop an appropriate strategy to address this matter, and implement a solution in a timely manner.

Clinical Implications. For today, a recognition that the spatial gradient magnetic field values provided by the MR system manufacturers may differ (i.e. typically the values are higher) from those at which the implant might have undergone testing for translational attraction is the first step towards understanding the important issues presented in this *Editorial Commentary*. Hopefully, this information will enable an appropriate determination of the risk-benefit for the management of patients with implants.

If the deflection angle information for the implant can be obtained from the device manufacturer, and the deflection angle value was somewhat trivial (e.g., 15-degrees or lower) for the specific MR system to be used for the examination, it would be reasonable to expect that a minor variation in the highest spatial gradient magnetic field value reported by the MR system manufacturer (i.e. compared to that reported in the labeling for the device) would not produce a clinically significant difference in the safety outcome. Of course, an entirely different conclusion might be reached if the translational attraction testing documented a significant deflection angle for the implant.

Conclusions. There are *two different positions* where the highest spatial gradient magnetic field may be measured and reported. One, the highest "patient accessible" spatial gradient magnetic field, which pertains to that used for the deflection angle test for a medical implant or device and through which a patient with an implant or device may pass. The other, the scanner's highest spatial gradient magnetic field, as reported in the specifications for the magnet of a given scanner, that reports the region of greatest dB/dx regardless of its accessibility to patients or healthcare providers. The values measured by the MR system manufacturers are inherently higher than those reported and used in the labeling of medical devices are of dubious clinical value, and should be replaced, or at the very least supplemented, with the greatest dB/dx values reachable or accessible by patients and healthcare professionals.

IMPORTANT NOTE: Recently, the Food and Drug Administration has approved MRI labeling pertaining to spatial gradient magnetic field values that have been calculated (or extrapolated) to higher values for implants and devices based on information for the measured deflection angles. There may or may not be an indication in the MRI labeling that the higher spatial gradient magnetic field value was calculated (or extrapolated) for a given implant or device.

REFERENCES

(1) American Society for Testing and Materials (ASTM) International Designation: F 2503. Standard Practice for Marking Medical Devices and Other Items for Safety in the Magnetic Resonance Environment. West Conshohocken, PA.

(2) Shellock FG, Woods TO, Crues JV. MRI labeling information for implants and devices: Explanation of terminology. Radiology 2009;253:26-30.

(3) Shellock FG. Reference Manual for Magnetic Resonance Safety Implants and Devices: 2014 Edition. Biomedical Research Publishing Group, Los Angeles, CA, 2014.

(4) Woods TO. Standards for medical devices in MRI: Present and future. J Magn Reson Imag 2007;26:1186-1189.

(5) www.MRIsafety.com

(6) American Society for Testing and Materials (ASTM) International Designation. F 2052. Standard test method for measurement of magnetically induced displacement force on passive implants in the magnetic resonance environment. West Conshohocken, PA.

Tattoos, Permanent Cosmetics, and Other Makeup

Traditional (i.e. decorative) and cosmetic tattoo procedures have been performed for thousands of years. Cosmetic tattoos or "permanent cosmetics" are used to reshape, recolor, recreate, or modify eye shadow, eyeliner, eyebrows, lips, beauty marks, and cheek blush. Additionally, permanent cosmetics are used aesthetically to enhance nipple-areola reconstruction procedures and for other applications.

Unfortunately, there is confusion regarding the overall safety aspects of permanent cosmetics. For example, based on a few reports of symptoms localized to the tattooed area during MR imaging, radiologists have refused to perform examinations on individuals with permanent cosmetics, particularly tattooed eyeliner. This undue and unwarranted concern for possible adverse events prevents patients with cosmetic tattoos access to an important diagnostic imaging technique.

While it is well-known that permanent cosmetics and decorative tattoos may cause artifacts and may be associated with relatively minor, short-term cutaneous reactions, the exact frequency and severity of soft tissue reactions or other problems related to MR imaging, while unknown, is considered to be quite low.

Tope and Shellock (2002) conducted a study to determine the frequency and severity of adverse events associated with MR imaging in a population of subjects with permanent cosmetics. A questionnaire was distributed to clients of cosmetic tattoo technicians. This survey asked subjects for demographic data, information about their tattoos, and for their experiences during MR imaging procedures. Results from 1,032 surveys were tabulated. One hundred thirty-five (13.1%) study subjects underwent MR imaging after having permanent cosmetics applied. Only two individuals (1.5%) experienced problems associated with MR imaging. One subject reported a sensation of "slight tingling" and the other reported a "burning" sensation. Both incidents were transient and did not prevent the MR procedures from being performed. Based on these findings and additional information in the peer-reviewed literature, it appears that MR imaging may be performed in patients with permanent cosmetics without serious soft tissue reactions or adverse events.

Therefore, the presence of permanent cosmetics should not prevent a patient from undergoing MR imaging.

Before undergoing an MR procedure, the patient should be asked if he or she has ever had a permanent coloring technique (i.e. tattooing) applied to the body. This includes cosmetic applications such as eyeliner, lip-liner, lip coloring, as well as decorative designs. This question is necessary because of the associated imaging artifacts and, more importantly, because a small number of patients (fewer than 10 documented cases) have experienced transient skin irritation, cutaneous swelling, or heating sensations at the site of the permanent colorings in association with MR procedures (review of Medical Device Reports, 1985 to 2012).

Interestingly, decorative tattoos tend to cause worse problems (including first- and second-degree burns) for patients undergoing MR imaging compared to those that have been reported for cosmetic tattoos. With regard to decorative tattoos, a letter to the editor described a second-degree burn that occurred on the skin of the deltoid from a decorative tattoo. The authors suggested that "the heating could have come either from oscillations of the gradients or, more likely from the RF-induced electrical currents". However, the exact mechanisms responsible for complications or adverse events in the various cases that have occurred related to decorative tattoos is unknown.

Additionally, Kreidstein, et al. (1997) reported that a patient experienced a sudden burning pain at the site of a decorative tattoo while undergoing MR imaging of the lumbar spine using a 1.5-Tesla MR system. Swelling and erythema was resolved within 12 hours, without evidence of permanent sequelae. The tattoo pigment used in this case was ferromagnetic, which possibly explained the symptoms experienced by the patient. Surprisingly, in order to permit the MRI examination, an excision of the tattooed skin was performed.

The authors of this report stated, "Theoretically, the application of a pressure dressing of the tattoo may prevent any tissue distortion due to ferromagnetic pull". (However, this relatively benign procedure was not attempted for this patient.) The authors also indicated that, "In some cases, removal of the tattoo may be the most practical means of allowing MRI".

Kanal and Shellock (1998) commented on this report in a letter to the editor, suggesting that the response to this situation was "rather aggressive". Clearly the trauma, expense, and morbidity associated with excision of a tattoo far exceed those that may be associated with ferromagnetic tattoo interactions. A firmly applied pressure bandage may be used if there is concern related to "movement" of the ferromagnetic particles in the tattoo pigment. Additionally, direct application of a cold compress to the site of a tattoo would likely mitigate any heating sensation that may occur in association with MR imaging.

Artifacts. Imaging artifacts associated with permanent cosmetics and certain types of eye makeup, hair products (e.g., hair loss concealers), and finger nail polishes have been reported. These artifacts are predominantly associated with the presence of pigments that use iron oxide or other type of metal and occur in the immediate area of the applied pigment or material. Therefore, tattoo-related and makeup-related MR imaging artifacts should not prevent a diagnostically adequate MR imaging procedure from being performed, especially because the careful selection of imaging parameters may minimize artifacts related to metallic materials. Of course, whenever possible, the hair product or other offending cosmetic should be thoroughly removed prior to the MRI examination if the area of interest is in or around where the metal-based pigment has been applied.

This is particularly important when a tattoo or metal-based cosmetic product is located in the imaging area interest. For example, Weiss, et al. (1989) reported that heavy metal particles used in the pigment base of mascara and eyeliner tattoos have a paramagnetic effect that causes alteration of the local magnetic field in adjacent tissues. Changes in the MR signal pattern may result in distortion of the globes. In some cases, the artifact and distortion may mimic actual ocular disease, such as a ciliary body melanoma or cyst.

GUIDELINES AND RECOMMENDATIONS

In consideration of the available literature and experience pertaining to MR procedures and patients with permanent cosmetics and tattoos, guidelines to manage these individuals include, the following:

1) The screening form used for patients should include a question to identify the presence of permanent cosmetics or decorative tattoos.
2) Before undergoing an MR procedure, the patient should be asked if he or she had a permanent coloring technique (i.e. tattooing) applied to any part of the body. This includes cosmetic applications such as eyeliner, lip-liner, lip coloring, as well as decorative designs.
3) The patient should be informed of the potential risks associated with the site of the tattoo.
4) The patient should be advised to immediately inform the MRI technologist regarding any unusual sensation felt at the site of the tattoo in association with the MR procedure.

5) The patient should be closely monitored using visual and auditory means throughout the operation of the MR system to ensure safety. In the event that the patient reports a problem, the MR examination must be stopped immediately and an investigation must be conducted to ensure patient safety.

6) As a precautionary measure, a cold compress (e.g., ice bag) may be applied to the tattoo site during the MR procedure.

In addition to the above, information and recommendations have been provided for patients by the United States Food and Drug Administration, Center for Food Safety and Applied Nutrition, Office of Cosmetics and Colors Fact Sheet, as follows: "… the risks of avoiding an MRI when your doctor has recommended one are likely to be much greater than the risks of complications from an interaction between the MRI and tattoo or permanent makeup. Instead of avoiding an MRI, individuals who have tattoos or permanent makeup should inform the radiologist or technician of this fact in order to take appropriate precautions, avoid complications, and assure the best results."

REFERENCES

Becker H. The use of intradermal tattoo to enhance the final result of nipple-areola reconstruction. Plast Reconstr Surg 1986;77:673.

Carr JJ. Danger in performing MR imaging on women who have tattooed eyeliner or similar types of permanent cosmetic injections. Am J Roentgenol 1995;165:1546-1547.

Chenji S, et al. Hair product artifact in magnetic resonance imaging. Magn Reson Imaging 2017;35:1-3.

DeBoer S, et al. Body piercing/tattooing and trauma diagnostic imaging: Medical myths vs realities. J Trauma Nurs 2007;14:35-8.

Escher KB, Shellock FG. Evaluation of MRI artifacts at 3-Tesla for 38 commonly used cosmetics. Magnetic Resonance Imaging 2013;31:778-782.

Gomey M. Tattoo pigments, patient clothing, and magnetic resonance imaging. Risk Management Bulletin #12748-8/95, The Doctors' Company, Napa, CA. August, 1995.

Halder RM, et al. Micropigmentation for the treatment of vitiligo. J Dermatol Surg Oncol 1989;15:1092-1098.

Jackson JG, Acker H. Permanent eyeliner and MR imaging. (letter) Am J Roentgenol 1987;149:1080.

Expert Panel on MR Safety, Kanal E, Barkovich AJ, Bell C, et al. ACR guidance document on MR safe practices: 2013. J Magn Reson Imag 2013;37:501-30.

Kanal E, Shellock FG. MRI interaction with tattoo pigments. (letter) Plast Reconstr Surg 1998;101:1150-1151.

Klitscher D, et al. MRT-induced burns in tattooed patients. Case report of a traumatic surgery patient. Unfallchirurg 2005;108:410-414.

Kreidstein ML, et al. MRI interaction with tattoo pigments: Case report, pathophysiology, and management. Plast Reconstr Surg 1997;99:1717-1720.

Laumann AE, Derick AJ. Tattoos and body piercings in the United States: A national data set. J Am Acad Dermatol 2006;55:413-21.

Lund A, et al. Tattooing of eyelids: Magnetic resonance imaging artifacts. Ophthalmic Surg 1986;17:550-553.

Morishita Y, et al. Influence of mechanical effect due to MRI-magnet on tattoo seal and eye makeup. Nippon Hoshasen Gijutsu Gakkai Zasshi 2008;64:587-90.

Noureddine Y, et al. Experience with magnetic resonance imaging of human subjects with passive implants and tattoos at 7T: A retrospective study. MAGMA 2015;28:577-90.

Offret H, et al. Permanent cosmetics and magnetic resonance imaging. J Fr Ophtalmol 2009;32:131.e1-3.

Ross JR, Matava MJ. Tattoo-induced skin "burn" during magnetic resonance imaging in a professional football player: A case report. Sports Health 2011;3:431-4.

Sacco D, et al. Artifacts caused by cosmetics in MR imaging of the head. Am J Roentgenol 1987;148:1001-1004.

Shellock FG, Crues JV, Editors. MRI Bioeffects, Safety, and Patient Management. Biomedical Research Publishing Group, Los Angeles, CA, 2014.

Tattoos. FDA Medical Bulletin 1994;24:8.

Tope WD, Shellock FG. Magnetic resonance imaging and permanent cosmetics (tattoos): Survey of complications and adverse events. J Magn Reson Imag 2002;15:180-184.

Vahlensieck M. Tattoo-related cutaneous inflammation (burn grade I) in a mid-field MR scanner. (letter) Eur Radiol 2000;10:97.

Wagle WA, Smith M. Tattoo-induced skin burn during MR imaging. (letter) Am J Roentgenol 2000;174:1795.

Weiss RA, et al. Mascara and eye-lining tattoos: MRI artifacts. Ann Ophthalmology 1989;21:129-131.

Terminology for Implants and Devices

MRI Labeling Information for Implants and Devices: Explanation of Terminology*

Summary Statement. This Editorial presents the recommendations from the Food and Drug Administration for MR safety terminology and labeling for medical devices and provides an explanation of how this information is applied.

The magnetic resonance (MR) environment may pose risks or problems to patients with certain implants and other medical devices primarily due to factors that include electromagnetic field interactions, MRI-related heating, and the creation of artifacts (1-5). In addition, for electrically-activated implants and other medical devices, there are concerns that the MR system may affect the operation of the medical device and/or to induce currents in the device (1-3, 5). With the growing use of MRI in the 1990s, the Food and Drug Administration (FDA) recognized the need for standardized tests to address MRI safety issues for implants and other medical devices (4, 6). Thus, over the years, test methods have been developed by various organizations including the American Society for Testing and Materials (ASTM) International (formerly the American Society for Testing and Materials), with an ongoing commitment to ensure patient safety in the MR environment (7-10).

The FDA is responsible for reviewing the MR terminology and labeling that manufacturers provide to their devices. The MR terminology, as it pertains to performing MR examinations in patients with implants and other medical devices, has continued to evolve to keep pace with advances in MRI technology (4, 6, 11). Unfortunately, members of the MRI community frequently do not always understand the terms that are used and are often confused by the conditions that are specified in "MR Conditional" labeling. This lack of understanding may result in patients with implants being exposed to potentially hazardous MRI conditions or in inappropriately preventing them from undergoing needed MRI examinations. Importantly, there is now new labeling terminology, which is associated with expanded labeling information. Therefore, the goal of this *Editorial* is to present background information about the terms used for MRI labeling of implants and other medical devices, to define the current terms, and to illustrate the use of the new labeling by providing a sample label with a detailed explanation of how the terminology is used.

Prior Terminology

In 1997, the FDA's Center for Devices and Radiological Health (CDRH) first proposed terms to be used to label MRI information for medical devices, which was presented in the draft document, "A Primer on Medical Device Interactions with Magnetic Resonance Imaging Systems" (6). These terms were defined, as follows (6):

MR Safe: This term indicates that the device, when used in the MR environment, has been demonstrated to present no additional risk to the patient, but may affect the quality of the diagnostic information.

MR Compatible: This term indicates that the device, when used in the MR environment, is MR Safe and has been demonstrated to neither significantly affect the quality of the diagnostic information nor have its operations affected by the MR device.

This document further stated that, "The use of the terms, "MR Compatible" and "MR Safe" without specification of the MR environment in which the device was tested should be avoided since interpretation of these claims may vary and are difficult to substantiate rigorously. Statements such as "intended for use in the MR environment" or similar claims along with appropriate qualifying information are preferred (i.e. test conditions should be specifically stated) (6)." Here, the term "MR environment" encompasses the static, gradient (time-varying), and RF electromagnetic fields that may impact an implant or device.

Using this terminology, MRI testing of an implant or device for "MR safety" involved *in vitro* assessments of static magnetic field interactions, MRI-related heating, and, in some cases, induced electrical currents (i.e. from gradient magnetic fields), while "MR compatibility" testing required all of these as well as characterization of artifacts. In addition, it may have been necessary to evaluate the effect of various MRI conditions on the functional or operational aspects of an implant or device (2, 3, 4, 6, 7-10).

Revised Terminology

In time, it became apparent that the terms, "MR Safe" and "MR Compatible" were confusing and often used interchangeably or incorrectly (2-4, 11, 12). In particular, the terms were sometimes used without including the list of conditions for which the device had been demonstrated to be safe, in some cases inappropriately giving the impression that the device is "safe" or "compatible" in all MR environments. Therefore, in an effort to develop more appropriate terminology and, more importantly, because the misuse of these terms could result in serious accidents for patients and others in the MR environment, the MR Task Group of ASTM International Committee F04 on Medical and Surgical Materials and Devices developed standard ASTM F2503 which includes a new set of MR labeling terms with associated icons (4). The new terms defined in ASTM F2503 (released in August 2005) and currently recognized by the FDA are (11, 13), as follows:

MR Safe - an item that poses no known hazards in all MRI environments. Using the terminology, "MR Safe" items are nonconducting, nonmetallic items such as a plastic Petri dish. An item may be determined to be MR Safe by providing a scientifically based rationale rather than test data.

MR Conditional - an item that has been demonstrated to pose no known hazards in a specified MR environment with specified conditions of use. "Field" conditions that define the MR environment include static magnetic field strength, spatial gradient, dB/dt (time rate of change of the magnetic field), radio frequency (RF) fields, and specific absorption rate (SAR). Additional conditions, including specific configurations of the item (e.g., the routing of leads used for a neurostimulation system), may be required.

For MR Conditional items, the item labeling includes results of testing sufficient to characterize the behavior of the item in the MR environment. In particular, testing for items that may be placed in the MR environment should address magnetically induced displacement force and torque, and RF heating. Other possible safety issues include but are not limited to, thermal injury, induced currents/voltages, electromagnetic compatibility, neurostimulation, acoustic noise, interaction among devices, and the safe functioning of the item and the safe operation of the MR system. Any parameter that affects the safety of the item should be listed and any condition that is known to produce an unsafe condition must be described.

MR Unsafe - an item that is known to pose hazards in all MRI environments. MR Unsafe items include magnetic items such as a pair of ferromagnetic scissors.

Associated Icons. In addition to the terms, MR Safe, MR Conditional, and MR Unsafe, the ASTM International MR marking standard introduced corresponding icons, consistent with international standards for colors and shapes of safety signs (13). These icons are intended for use on items that may be brought into or near the MR environment as well as in product labeling for implants and other medical devices. The icons may be reproduced in color or in black and white. However, the use of color is encouraged because of the added visibility (13).

The "MR Safe" icon consists of the letters 'MR' in green in a white square with a green border, or the letters 'MR' in white within a green square. The "MR Conditional" icon consists of the letters 'MR' in black inside a yellow triangle with a black border. The "MR Unsafe" icon consists of the letters 'MR' in black on a white field inside a red circle with a diagonal red band. Importantly, for "MR Conditional" items, the item's labeling must include the parameters and results used for testing that are sufficient to characterize the behavior of the item in the MRI environment (13).

Further details and a comprehensive discussion of the labeling applied to passive implants are presented in the recent FDA document, "Guidance for Industry and FDA Staff - Establishing Safety and Compatibility of Passive Implants in the Magnetic Resonance (MR) Environment" (11).

Use of Terminology: Reasons for Confusion

Because of the variety of MR systems and MR conditions in clinical use today (e.g., ranging from 0.2- to 9.4-Tesla), the current terminology is intended help elucidate labeling matters for medical devices and other items that may be used in the MR environment to ensure the safe use of MRI technology. However, it should be noted that this updated terminology has not been applied *retrospectively* to the many implants and devices that previously received FDA approved labeling using the terms "MR Safe" or "MR Compatible" (in general, this applies to those objects tested prior to the release of the ASTM International standard for labeling, around August 2005).

Therefore, this important point must be understood to avoid undue confusion regarding the matter of the labeling that has been applied to previously tested implants (i.e. labeled as "MR safe" or "MR Compatible") versus those that have recently undergone MRI testing (i.e. now labeled as "MR Conditional")(2, 3).

The labeling for medical devices that were **appropriately** labeled using the historical definitions for MR Safe or MR Compatible, **including the list of conditions** for which the device has been determined to be safe or compatible, is still accurate. Indeed, part of the confusion that exists on this matter is due to the coexistence of the newer terminology with the prior labeling terminology.

In order to eliminate this ongoing confusion, in 2005 FDA recognized the new set of terms in ASTM F2503 and asks manufacturers to use them for all new products. When manufacturers make a submission to FDA for an existing device, FDA requests the manufacturers of these previously approved devices update their labeling to use the new MR safety terminology. Labeling information for implants and other medical devices has been compiled and is available in published and on-line formats (2, 14). Specific testing and labeling for active implants (e.g., those involving electronics) is currently being developed by an ISO (International Standards Organization) – IEC (International Electrotechnical Commission) joint working group.

MR Conditional Labeling Information: Explanation of the Content

In addition to the frequent problems associated with understanding the MRI labeling, the actual content of the label is often misunderstood with respect to the conditions indicated for a given implant that is labeled "MR Conditional". Therefore, the following is an example of "MR Conditional" labeling for an implant, *Example Implant*, along with an explanation of the content, provided for each aspect of the label (1-4, 11, 13) (**Table 1**):

MRI Information

Non-clinical testing has demonstrated the Example Implant is MR Conditional. It can be scanned safely under the following conditions:

-Static magnetic field of 3-Tesla

This is the static magnetic field for which the implant gave acceptable test results, generally the largest static magnetic field used for testing the implant. In some cases the labeling will state, "Static magnetic field of 3-Tesla or less" or "Static magnetic field of 3-Tesla, *only*" or *"static magnetic field of 1.5-Tesla or 3-Tesla."* Therefore, carefully reading and implementing this portion of the labeling for the implant is advised in order to avoid possible injuries to patients.

-Spatial gradient magnetic field of 720-gauss/cm.

This is a frequently misinterpreted parameter because the MRI user sees the term "gradient field" and presumes that it refers to the time-varying or gradient fields used during MR imaging. However, the term, "**spatial** gradient magnetic field" for medical device labeling relates to the rate at which the static magnetic field strength changes over space per unit length (thus, indicated as dB/dx or, in this case, as 720-gauss/cm for this example). Notably, the point of the highest spatial magnetic gradient is the position where translational attraction (i.e. determined using the deflection angle method) is typically assessed for an implant or device, according to ASTM F2052. The MR system manufacturer is able to provide spatial gradient magnetic field information for a particular MR system or it may determined using a Gauss meter.

-Maximum MR system reported, whole body averaged specific absorption rate (SAR) of 2-W/kg for 15-minutes of scanning.

Confusion commonly exists with respect to this stated parameter insofar as the term "scanning" is presumed to apply to the entire MRI procedure when, in fact, it applies to only each particular pulse *sequence* (or "per pulse sequence") that is used and, of course, multiple sequences are utilized when performing the MRI examination. Therefore, to adequately safeguard the patient, the whole body averaged SAR for each scan sequence must be maintained at or below 2-W/kg for each scan sequence.

-In non-clinical testing, the Example Implant produced a temperature rise of less than 2.0°C at a maximum MR system reported, whole body averaged specific absorption rate (SAR) of 2- W/kg for 15 minutes of MR scanning in a (static magnetic field strength _____) (model _____) (MR system manufacturer _____) (software version _____) MR scanner.

The labeling for the implant has additional information with respect to the temperature rise that is associated with certain MRI parameters, that is based on the findings obtained in the MRI-related heating test. Therefore, as seen in this example, the expected "worst case" temperature rise is 2.0 degrees C or less during MRI performed at a whole body averaged SAR of 2-W/kg for 15-min., using a particular MR system type (i.e. with the make, model, and software of the scanner indicated). The MR system reported, whole body averaged SAR of 2-W/kg is the level specified in the ASTM F2182 and is the level commonly reported in device labeling, although higher or lower SAR levels may also be indicated. (It should be noted that, in this labeling section, certain labels for implants and other medical devices may state that this information applies to the use of a particular type of transmit RF coil that should be used, such as a transmit body or transmit head RF coil.)

Image Artifact

MR image quality may be compromised if the area of interest is in the same area or relatively close to the position of the device. Therefore, it may be necessary to optimize MR imaging parameters for the presence of this implant.

This is a common statement for many different implants and devices. Since the size of the artifact for an implant or device may impact the diagnostic use of MR imaging, information is typically provided in the label that characterizes the size and shape of the artifacts associated with certain pulse sequences (e.g., T1-weighted spin echo and gradient echo), according to ASTM F2119 or an equivalent method. For devices with a lumen (e.g., stent), the labeling may indicate whether the lumen is obscured by the size of the artifact.

The FDA also recommends that the patient register the conditions under which their MR Conditional implant can be scanned safely with the MedicAlert Foundation or other equivalent organization, so that the device labeling may include contact information for MedicAlert (11).

Table 1. Example of MRI labeling information for a medical implant or device.

MRI Information

Non-clinical testing has demonstrated the Example Implant is MR Conditional. It can be scanned safely under the following conditions:

- Static magnetic field of 3-Tesla.
- Spatial gradient magnetic field of 720-gauss/cm.
- Maximum MR system reported, whole body averaged specific absorption rate (SAR) of 2-W/kg for 15-minutes of scanning.
- In non-clinical testing, the Example Implant produced a temperature rise of less than 2.0°C at a maximum MR system reported, whole body averaged specific absorption rate (SAR) of 2- W/kg for 15 minutes of MR scanning in a (static magnetic field strength _____) (model _____) (MR system manufacturer _____) (software version _____) MR scanner.

Image Artifact

MR image quality may be compromised if the area of interest is in the same area or relatively close to the position of the device. Therefore, it may be necessary to optimize MR imaging parameters for the presence of this implant.

Summary and Conclusions

This Editorial presents current FDA recommendations for MR safety terminology and labeling for implants and other medical devices and provides an explanation of how this information may be applied. Notably, the specific content of the MR labeling may take other forms (especially for electrically active implants and devices) as the format continues to be refined by the FDA in an ongoing effort to properly communicate this information to ensure patient safety.

IMPORTANT NOTE: Recently, the Food and Drug Administration has approved MRI labeling pertaining to spatial gradient magnetic field values that have been calculated (or extrapolated) to higher values for implants and devices based on information for the measured deflection angles. There may or may not be an indication in the MRI labeling that the higher spatial gradient magnetic field value was calculated (or extrapolated) for a given implant or device.

REFERENCES

(1) Shellock FG, Crues JV. MR procedures: Biologic effects, safety, and patient care. Radiology 2004;232:635-652.

(2) Shellock FG. Reference Manual for Magnetic Resonance Safety Implants and Device: 2009 Edition. Biomedical Research Publishing Group, Los Angeles, CA, 2009.

(3) Shellock FG, Spinazzi A. MRI safety update: 2008, Part 2, Screening patients for MRI. Am J Roentgenol 2008;191:12-21.

(4) Woods TO. Standards for medical devices in MRI: Present and future. J Magn Reson Imag 2007;26:1186-9.

(5) Levine GN, Gomes AS, Arai AE, Bluemke DA, Flamm SD, Kanal E, Manning WJ, Martin ET, Smith JM, Wilke N, Shellock FG. Safety of magnetic resonance imaging in patients with cardiovascular devices: An American Heart Association Scientific Statement from the Committee on Diagnostic and Interventional Cardiac Catheterization. Circulation 2007; 116:2878-2891.

(6) United States Food and Drug Administration, Center for Devices and Radiological Health, A Primer on Medical Device Interactions with MRI Systems. http://www.fda.gov/cdrh/ode/primerf6.html 1997.

(7) American Society for Testing and Materials (ASTM) International, Designation: ASTM F2052 - 06e1, Standard Test Method for Measurement of Magnetically Induced Displacement Force on Medical Devices in the Magnetic Resonance Environment. ASTM International, West Conshohocken, PA.

(8) American Society for Testing and Materials (ASTM) International, Designation: ASTM F2213-06, Standard Test Method for Measurement of Magnetically Induced Torque on Medical Devices in the Magnetic Resonance Environment. ASTM International, West Conshohocken, PA.

(9) American Society for Testing and Materials (ASTM) International, Designation: ASTM F2119 – 07, Standard Test Method for Evaluation of MR Image Artifacts from Passive Implants. ASTM International, West Conshohocken, PA.

(10) American Society for Testing and Materials (ASTM) International, Designation: ASTM F2182 - 02a, Standard Test Method for Measurement of Radio Frequency Induced Heating Near Passive Implants During Magnetic Resonance Imaging. ASTM International, West Conshohocken, PA.

(11) Guidance for Industry and FDA Staff - Establishing Safety and Compatibility of Passive Implants in the Magnetic Resonance (MR) Environment. Document issued on: August 21, 2008; http://www.fda.gov/cdrh/osel/guidance/1685.html

(12) Shellock FG, Crues JV. Commentary: MR safety and the American College of Radiology White Paper. Am J Roentgenol 2002;178:1349-1352.

(13) American Society for Testing and Materials (ASTM) International, Designation: F2503-08, Standard Practice for Marking Medical Devices and Other Items for Safety in the Magnetic Resonance Environment. ASTM International, West Conshohocken, PA.

(14) http://www.mrisafety.com/ accessed June, 2009.

[*Portions of this content were excerpted with permission from Shellock FG, Woods TO, Crues JV. MRI Labeling Information for Implants and Devices: Explanation of Terminology. Radiology 2009;253:26-30. The full-length article may be downloaded at www.IMRSER.org]

The Joint Commission: Excerpts Pertaining to Requirements for MRI Safety*

[*Frank G. Shellock, Ph.D. - Member, The Joint Commission's Ionizing Radiation & Magnetic Resonance Imaging Expert Panel]

Standard EC.02.01.01
The organization manages safety and security risks.
Elements of Performance for EC.02.01.01

Applicable to Ambulatory Care Centers
A 14. The organization manages magnetic resonance imaging (MRI) safety risks associated with the following:
Or
Applicable to Hospitals and Critical Access Hospitals
A 14. The [critical access] hospital manages magnetic resonance imaging (MRI) safety risks associated with the following:

- Patients who may experience claustrophobia, anxiety, or emotional distress
- Patients who may require urgent or emergent medical care
- Patients with medical implants, devices, or imbedded metallic foreign objects (such as shrapnel)
- Ferromagnetic objects entering the MRI environment
- Acoustic noise

Applicable to Ambulatory Care Centers
A 16. The organization manages magnetic resonance imaging (MRI) safety risks by doing the following:
Or
Applicable to Hospitals and Critical Access Hospitals
A 16. The [critical access] hospital manages magnetic resonance imaging (MRI) safety risks by doing the following:

- Restricting access of everyone not trained in MRI safety or screened by staff trained in MRI safety from the scanner room and the area that immediately precedes the entrance to the MRI scanner room.
- Making sure that these restricted areas are controlled by and under the direct supervision of staff trained in MRI safety.
- Posting signage at the entrance to the MRI scanner room that conveys that potentially dangerous magnetic fields are present in the room. Signage should also indicate that the magnet is always on except in cases where the MRI system, by its design, can have its magnetic field routinely turned on and off by the operator.

Standard HR.01.05.03
Staff participate in ongoing education and training.
Elements of Performance for HR.01.05.03
Applicable to Ambulatory Care Centers
C 25. The organization verifies and documents that technologists who perform magnetic resonance imaging (MRI) examinations participate in ongoing education that includes annual training on safe MRI practices in the MRI environment, including the following:
Or
Applicable to Hospitals and Critical Access Hospitals
C 25. The [critical access] hospital verifies and documents that technologists who perform magnetic resonance imaging (MRI) examinations participate in ongoing education that includes annual training on safe MRI practices in the MRI environment, including the following:

- Patient screening criteria that address ferromagnetic items, electrically conductive items, medical implants and devices, and risk for Nephrogenic Systemic Fibrosis (NSF).
- Proper patient and equipment positioning activities to avoid thermal injuries.
- Equipment and supplies that have been determined to be acceptable for use in the MRI environment (MR Safe or MR Conditional).
- MRI safety response procedures for patients who require urgent or emergent medical care.
- MRI system emergency shutdown procedures, such as MRI system quench and cryogen safety procedures.
- Patient hearing protection.
- Management of patients with claustrophobia, anxiety, or emotional distress.

Using Ferromagnetic Detection Systems in the MRI Environment

A ferromagnetic detection system (FMDS) is available for use in the MRI environment. Various versions of the FMDS currently exist and include a portal system, pillar device, or a handheld version. These devices are specially designed to only detect ferromagnetic objects. Other materials, such as aluminum and copper are nonferromagnetic and, therefore, are not detected by an FMDS. For example, an FMDS will detect a steel gas cylinder and indicate a positive alarm but it will not detect or alarm on an aluminum one. Thus, the FMDS will only alarm on potentially dangerous objects relative to issues related to magnetic field interactions. Utilizing an FMDS in the MRI environment is recommended by several influential organizations concerned with MRI safety, including the American College of Radiology (ACR) and the Joint Commission.

As the name suggests, ferromagnetic detection systems selectively detect ferromagnetic objects, ignoring nonferromagnetic items. Because only ferromagnetic objects pose a missile-related hazard, an FMDS detects threats and works by monitoring the ambient magnetic field using magnetic sensors. The ambient field is a combination of the fringe field of the magnet and the Earth's magnetic field plus the contribution from architectural steel and any other stationary steel objects in the vicinity. A ferromagnetic object distorts the ambient field in its vicinity. If it is brought close to an FMDS, the distortion is detected as a changing magnetic field and an alert is triggered.

Importantly, an FMDS ignores static magnetic fields (i.e. magnetic fields that do not change with time). In practice, this means that the FMDS is only sensitive to changing magnetic fields, or moving ferromagnetic objects. The FMDS is insensitive to a stationary ferromagnetic object, so if an object is placed near to the FMDS it will be detected as it is put in place but thereafter ignored, until it is moved again. The reason for this is that the ambient magnetic fields are very large compared with the magnetic perturbations caused by ferromagnetic objects, and it is difficult to measure tiny changes on a large background field. The large static background is therefore removed by the FMDS by filtering it out, irrespective of whichever components make up that static magnetic field including the magnet of the MR system, the Earth's magnetic field, or a metal cabinet next to the FMDS.

For a handheld FMDS, the object may be stationary but the FMDS is moved, so it is the relative motion that is important when using this type of device. A stationary FMDS detects moving ferromagnetic objects only.

Overall, the use of a stationary FMDS significantly enhances the safety level of MRI facilities, although non-ideal aspects of the current systems can impact the day-to-day activity of the MRI staff members, especially the MRI technologists. The individuals who are believed to cause most missile-related accidents are non-MRI workers who enter the MR system room. While MRI technologists may not be able to constantly supervise and control access to the MR system room, an FMDS can accomplish this and, thus, provides a warning to a person entering when the door is unsupervised. If non-technologists cause "alarms", they should be trained to seek the advice of an MRI technologist before entering the MR system room.

When an FMDS alarms, its purpose is to prompt the MRI technologist to investigate. As an example, an MRI technologist pushes an MR Conditional gurney into the room and the alarm sounds, as always, because the gurney has ferromagnetic components. The correct response of the MRI technologist is to stop and to perform a final check of the gurney. Is the gurney acceptable to use with this particular MR system? Is there an oxygen cylinder or IV pole present that is MR Unsafe? Is there a ferromagnetic object under the sheets? The incorrect response is to ignore the alarm because an MR Conditional gurney will always trigger an alarm. Many accidents have occurred because of ferromagnetic items being placed on top of gurneys or underneath sheets. In this case, the alarm from the FMDS acts as a reminder to do a final check.

The Patient Screening Process Using an FMDS. Screening the patient using an FMDS is an additional step in the screening process and is the last step before the MRI examination. It is important to note that it is not a replacement for any aspect of the screening procedure but rather it is an addendum that adds a final objective check prior to performing MRI. This type of screening normally takes less than one minute to complete provided that there is no positive alarm. It takes somewhat longer to use a handheld FMDS because it has to be manually scanned over the entire area of the patient's body. Ideally, there will be a line at the bottom of the screening questionnaire that records the result of FMDS screening and any observations or actions as a result.

If a patient passes the FMDS screening without a detection occurring (i.e. no positive alarm), this should be documented on the screening form and the patient may then proceed with the MRI examination. If an alarm occurs, then the patient must be investigated for the presence of a ferromagnetic object and it should be removed (if possible). Once this has been done, the patient should be re-screened using the FMDS. If a ferrous object cannot be found, the FMDS screening should be repeated in case the original result was a false alarm. For genuine alarms that cannot be resolved, the MRI technologist must then suspect the possibility that the ferromagnetic object is internal, being either an implant or a foreign body. The patient's history should then be thoroughly checked before proceeding to MRI.

Using a Wall-Mounted or Piller FMDS Versus a Handheld FMDS. The use of a wall-mounted FMDS provides head-to-toe, whole-body screening that is easy to accomplish and fast to perform for cooperative ambulatory patients. For non-ambulatory patients the only means of screening with a wall-mounted FMDS is to use a ferrous-free gurney or wheelchair and perform a "drive-by" in two directions parallel to the FMDS, pushed by a ferrous-free MRI technologist. However, this process will not provide the close range required to detect the smallest objects, but is nonetheless useful for the detection of larger personal items.

The use of a handheld FMDS is somewhat similar to using a standard handheld metal detector (e.g., the type used at airports), insofar as it must be swept or scanned over the surface of the body at close range, usually within 5-cm of the surface. The sensing area is quite small (approximately 5-cm x 9-cm) so care must be taken to ensure that screening occurs with no gaps while maintaining a relatively short, stand-off distance. Due to this being a manual process, the quality and reliability of the screening depends on the person performing the scan using the handheld FMDS.

Staff members may be reluctant to screen an intimate patient area, such as the groin. Notably, the only available handheld FMDS at this time has a strong permanent magnet within it to boost the magnetization of ferrous objects. Because of this, this type of handheld FMDS should not be used close the eyes or near cardiac pacemakers or other similar implanted devices in case the magnetic field poses possible problems. A handheld FMDS can be used for a non-ambulatory patient on an MR Conditional gurney or wheelchair, as opposed to ferrous-free ones. With a gurney, the patient needs to turn over from one side to the other to get full coverage. With a wheelchair, it is more difficult to get full coverage unless the patient can stand for a short while.

Using an FMDS to Screen for Metallic Implants, Devices, and Foreign Bodies. The question surrounding the detection of ferromagnetic implants, devices, and foreign bodies is a topic with growing international interest, as reported by Shellock and Karacozoff (2013). Currently, the use of a patient screening FMDS is not approved by a governmental entity or organization and, thus, it is not intended to be used for the specific purpose of detecting implanted objects. However, because human flesh is effectively transparent to ferromagnetic detection, the distinction between *ex vivo* and *in vivo* ferromagnetic objects is merely one of range. To date, studies on implant detection have been conducted as well as on foreign bodies. The results indicate that patient screening using an FMDS is capable of detecting many *in vivo* ferromagnetic objects, which has important implications for patient safety in the MRI environment.

[Excerpted from *Using Ferromagnetic Detection Systems in the MRI Environment* by Mark N. Keene, Ph.D., in MRI Bioeffects, Safety, and Patient Management, F.G. Shellock and J.V. Crues, Editors. Biomedical Research Publishing Group, Los Angeles, CA, 2014. Reviewed and updated 2018.]

REFERENCES

ECRI Institute, Health Devices. 2010 Top 10 Technology Hazards; November 2009;38:No.11:1-10.

Gianesin B, et al. Characterization of ferromagnetic or conductive properties of metallic foreign objects embedded within the human body with magnetic iron detector (MID): Screening patients for MRI. Magn Reson Med 2015;73:2030-7.

Guttler FV, et al. Whole-body ferromagnetic detector systems in clinical MRI. Radiologe 2015;55:649-53.

Joint Commission. Preventing accidents and injuries in the MRI suite. Sentinel Event Alert, Issue 38, February 14, 2008.

Kanal E, Barkovich AJ, Bell C, et al. ACR guidance document on MR safe practices: 2013. J Magn Reson Imag 2013;37:501-530.

James CA, Karacozoff AM, Shellock FG. Undisclosed and undetected foreign bodies during MRI screening resulting in a potentially serious outcome. Magnetic Resonance Imaging 2013;31:630-633.

Karacozoff AM, Shellock FG. Armor-piercing bullet: 3-Tesla MRI findings and identification by a ferromagnetic detection system. Military Medicine 2013;178:e380- e385.

Kopp Development, Inc., www.koppdevelopment.com

Metrasens Ltd., www.metrasens.com

Mednovus Inc., www.mednovus.com

Shellock FG, Karacozoff AM. Detection of implants and other objects using a ferromagnetic detection system: Implications for patient screening prior to MRI. Am J Roentgenol 2013;201:720-725.

SECTION II

MR Procedures and Implants, Devices, and Materials

General Information

Magnetic resonance (MR) procedures may be contraindicated for patients primarily because of risks associated with movement or dislodgment of a ferromagnetic biomedical implant or device. There are other possible hazards and problems related to the presence of a metallic object that include excessive heating, the induction of currents (e.g., in materials that are conductors), changes in the operational aspects of the device, and the difficulty in interpretation of the MR images or the misinterpretation of an imaging artifact as an abnormality.

Magnetic Field Interactions. Numerous studies have assessed magnetic field interactions for implants and other items by measuring translational attraction, torque or other interactions associated with the static magnetic fields of MR systems. These investigations demonstrated that, for certain implants, MR procedures may be performed safely in patients with metallic objects that are nonferromagnetic or "weakly" ferromagnetic (i.e. only minimally attracted by the magnetic field in relation to its *in vivo* application), such that the associated magnetic field interactions are insufficient to move or dislodge them, *in situ*. Furthermore, the "intended *in vivo* use" of the implant or device must be taken into consideration, because this can impact whether or not a given object is safe for a patient undergoing an MR procedure. Notably, sufficient counter-forces may exist to retain even a ferromagnetic implant, *in situ*.

In general, each implant or other item (particularly those made from unknown materials) should be evaluated using *ex vivo* techniques before allowing an individual or patient with the object to enter the MR environment and/or before performing the MR procedure. By following this guideline, the magnetic qualities of an object may be determined so that a competent decision can be made concerning possible risks associated with exposure to the MR system. Because movement or dislodgment of an implanted metallic object in a patient undergoing an MR procedure is the primary mechanism responsible for an injury, this aspect of testing is considered to be of utmost importance and should involve the use of an MR system operating at an appropriate static magnetic field strength. It is also be necessary to assess MRI-related heating for the implant or device.

Various factors influence the risk of performing an MR procedure in a patient with a metallic object including the strength of the static magnetic field, the magnetic susceptibility of the object, the mass of the object, the geometry of the object, the location and orientation of the object *in situ*, the presence of retentive mechanisms (i.e. fibrotic tissue, sutures, etc.) and the length of time the object has been implanted. These factors should be carefully considered before subjecting a patient or individual with a ferromagnetic object to an MR procedure or allowing entrance to the MR environment. This is particularly important if the object is located in a potentially dangerous area of the body such as a vital neural, vascular, of soft tissue structure where movement or dislodgment could injure the patient.

Furthermore, in certain cases, there is a possibility of changing the operational or functional aspects of the implant or device as a result of exposure to the electromagnetic fields of the MR system. Therefore, this important aspect must be evaluated using comprehensive testing techniques to verify that specific MR conditions will not impact the operation of the device.

Patients with certain implants or devices that have relatively strong ferromagnetic qualities may be safely scanned using MR procedures because the objects are held in place by sufficient retentive forces that prevent them from being moved or dislodged with reference to the "intended *in vivo* use" of an implant or device. For example, there is an interference screw (i.e. the Perfix Interference Screw) used for reconstruction of the anterior cruciate ligament that is highly ferromagnetic. However, once this implant is screwed into the patient's bone, this prevents it from being moved, even if the patient is exposed to a 1.5-Tesla MR system. Other implants that exhibit substantial ferromagnetic qualities may likewise be safe for patients undergoing MR procedures under highly specific conditions as a result of the presence of counter-forces that prevent movement of these objects.

MR systems with very low (0.2-Tesla or less) or very high (9.4-Tesla) static magnetic fields are currently used for clinical and research applications. Considering that most metallic objects evaluated for magnetic field interactions were assessed at 1.5-Tesla, an appropriate variance or modification of the information provided regarding the safety of performing an MR procedure in a patient with a metallic object may exist when an MR system with a lower or higher static magnetic field strength is used. That is, it may be acceptable to adjust safety recommendations depending on the static magnetic field strength and other aspects of a given MR system. Obviously, performing an MR procedure using a 0.2-Tesla MR system has different risk implications for a patient with a ferromagnetic object compared with using a 9.4-Tesla MR system.

Lenz Effect. In 1835, Heinrich Lenz stated the law that an electric current induced by a changing magnetic field will flow such that it will create its own magnetic field that opposes the magnetic field that created it. These opposing fields, which occupy the same space at the same time, result in a pair of forces. The more current that is generated, the greater the force that opposes it. The so-called "Lenz Effect" occurs with electrically conductive materials (i.e. not just ferromagnetic materials) that develop eddy currents in the presence of high-field-strength static magnetic fields, such as those associated with MR systems.

Forces described by the Lenz Effect may restrict movement for metallic objects (e.g., for an aluminum oxygen tank) or compromise the function of certain implants in the MRI setting, such as those with moving metallic parts. This may be a concern for prosthetic heart valves that have leaflets or discs, especially if the implant is used for mitral valve replacement, where the range of pressures that are present are relatively low (higher pressures are more likely to overcome any significant Lenz Effect).

Condon and Hadley (2000) first reported the theoretical possibility of electromagnetic interaction with heart valve prostheses that contain metallic disks or leaflets. In theory, "resistive pressure" may develop with the potential to inhibit both the opening and closing aspects of a mechanical heart valve prosthesis that has leaflets or disks.

Edwards, et al. (2015) conducted an *in vitro* study of the occurrence of Lenz-related forces on various heart valve prostheses at 1.5-Tesla and assessed the risk of the impedance of valve function. The findings provided evidence of the Lenz Effect on certain cardiac valve prostheses exposed to the static magnetic field, which resulted in functional valve impedance and a potentially increased risk of valve regurgitation. While further evaluation of this phenomenon may be warranted, to date, the Lenz Effect has not been observed in association with clinical MR examinations nor has it posed additional risks for patients with certain heart valve prostheses (i.e. those with metallic leaflets or disks) undergoing MRI.

Heating. Temperature increases produced in association with MR procedures have been studied using *ex vivo* techniques to evaluate various metallic implants, devices, and objects with a variety of sizes, shapes, and material compositions. In general, reports have indicated that only minor temperature changes occur in association with MR procedures involving relatively small metallic objects that are "passive" implants (i.e. those that are not electronically-activated), including implants such as aneurysm clips, hemostatic clips, prosthetic heart valves, vascular access ports, and similar devices. Therefore, heat generated during an MR procedure involving a patient with a "small" metallic passive implant does not appear to be a substantial hazard. In fact, to date, there has been no report of a patient being seriously injured as a result of excessive heat that developed in a relatively small passive metallic implant or device during an MR procedure.

MRI-related heating is potentially problematic for implants and devices that have an elongated shape or those that form a conducting loop of a certain diameter. For example, substantial heating can occur under some MR conditions for objects that form resonant conducting loops or for elongated implants (e.g., leads, wires, etc.) that form resonant antennae.

Induced Electrical Currents. The potential for MR procedures to injure patients by inducing electrical currents in conductive materials or devices such as gating leads, indwelling catheters with metallic components (e.g., thermodilution catheters, intracranial pressure monitoring catheters, etc.), guidewires, cardiac pacemaker leads, neurostimulation system leads, disconnected or broken surface coils, external fixation devices, cervical fixation devices, cochlear implants, infusion pumps, or improperly used physiologic monitors has been previously reported. Recommendations have been presented to protect patients from injuries related to induced currents that may develop during MR procedures.

Artifacts. The type and extent of artifacts caused by the presence of metallic implants, materials, and devices have been described and tend to be easily recognized on MR images. Artifacts and image distortion associated with metallic objects are predominantly caused by a disruption of the local magnetic field that perturbs the relationship between position and frequency. Additionally, artifacts associated with metallic objects may be caused by gradient switching due to the generation of eddy currents.

The relative amount of artifact seen on an MR image is dependent on the magnetic susceptibility, quantity, shape, orientation, and position of the object in the body as well as the technique used for imaging (i.e. the specific pulse sequence parameters) and the image processing method. An artifact caused by the presence of a metallic object in a patient during MR imaging is seen typically as a signal void or loss and may include a local or regional distortion of the image. In some cases, there may be areas of high signal intensity seen along the edge of a signal void or when there is an abrupt change in the shape of the object (e.g., the tip of a biopsy needle).

Information Pertaining to Implants, Materials, Devices and Objects. The information contained in this textbook is a compilation of the current data available relative to the assessment of magnetic field interactions, MRI-related heating, and other tests conducted on implants and devices and is based on published reports in the peer-reviewed literature as well as other sources. This compilation also includes unpublished data acquired from *ex vivo* testing performed on implants and devices using standardized or well-accepted techniques. Furthermore, MRI-related information obtained from manufacturers (e.g., the *Product Insert* or *Instructions for Use, IFU*, information) is provided for various implants and devices.

Although every attempt was made to provide comprehensive and accurate information, there are many other implants, devices, and objects that remain to be evaluated with regard to the MR environment. In addition, new or updated information may exist for a given implant, especially those that are electronically-activated (i.e. active devices), since the procedures used to assess these devices continue to evolve. Therefore, to ensure the safety of an individual or patient in the MR environment or undergoing an MR procedure, MR healthcare professionals should follow the guideline whereby MR examinations should only be performed in a patient with a metallic object that has been previously tested and demonstrated to be safe or otherwise acceptable. A similar guideline should be followed with regard to whether or not to allow an individual with an implant or device to enter the MR environment. Finally, for electronically-activated implants, the most current safety guidelines must be obtained and followed. Therefore, the MR healthcare professional is advised to confirm the latest MRI labeling information with the respective manufacturer prior to performing an MRI examination on the patient.

Terminology Applied to Implants and Devices

To ensure proper understanding of the terminology applied to implants and devices, please review section, **Terminology for Implants and Devices.**

REFERENCES

American Society for Testing and Materials (ASTM) International, Designation: F2503. Standard Practice for Marking Medical Devices and Other Items for Safety in the Magnetic Resonance Environment. ASTM International, West Conshohocken, PA.

American Society for Testing and Materials (ASTM) International, Designation: F 2052. Standard test method for measurement of magnetically induced displacement force on passive implants in the magnetic resonance environment. ASTM International, West Conshohocken, PA.

Arena L, Morehouse HT, Safir J. MR imaging artifacts that simulate disease: How to recognize and eliminate them. Radiographics 1995;15:1373-1394.

Calcagnini G, et al. *In vitro* investigation of pacemaker lead heating induced by magnetic resonance imaging: Role of implant geometry. J Magn Reson Imag 2008;28:879-86.

Condon B, Hadley DM. Potential MR hazard to patients with metallic heart valves: The Lenz effect. J Magn Reson Imag 2000;12:171-176.

Davis PL, et al. Potential hazards in NMR imaging: Heating effects of changing magnetic fields and RF fields on small metallic implants. Am J Roentgenol 1981;137:857-860.

Dempsey MF, Condon B, Hadley DM. Investigation of the factors responsible for burns during MRI. J Magn Reson Imag 2001;13:627-631.

Diaz F, Tweardy L, Shellock FG. Cervical fixation devices: MRI issues at 3-Tesla. Spine 2010;35:411-5.

Dietrich O, et al. Artifacts in 3-T MRI: Physical background and reduction strategies. Eur J Radiol 2008;65:29-35.

Edwards MB, et al. In vitro assessment of the Lenz effect on heart valve prostheses at 1.5 T. J Magn Reson Imaging 2015;41:74-82.

Feng DX, et al. Evaluation of 39 medical implants at 7.0 T. Br J Radiol, 2015;88(1056):20150633.

Graf H, Steidle G, et al. Metal artifacts caused by gradient switching. Magnetic Resonance in Medicine 2005;54;231-234.

Golestanirad L, et al. Comprehensive analysis of Lenz effect on the artificial heart valves during magnetic resonance imaging. Progress In Electromagnetics Research 2012;128:1-17.

Hargreaves BA, et al. Metal-induced artifacts in MRI. Am J Roentgenol 2011;197:547-55.

Expert Panel on MR Safety, Kanal E, Barkovich AJ, Bell C, et al. ACR guidance document on MR safe practices: 2013. J Magn Reson Imag 2013;37:501-30.

Koch KM, et al. Magnetic resonance imaging near metal implants. J Magn Reson Imag 2010;32:773-87.

Levine GN, et al. Safety of magnetic resonance imaging in patients with cardiovascular devices: An American Heart Association scientific statement from the Committee on Diagnostic and Interventional Cardiac Catheterization. Circulation 2007;116:2878-2891.

Masaki F, et al. Iatrogenic second-degree burn caused by a catheter encased tubular braid of stainless steel during MRI. Burns 2007;33:1077-9.

Muranaka H, et al. Evaluation of RF heating due to various implants during MR procedure. Magn Reson Med Sci 2011;10:11-9.

Nordbeck P, et al. Spatial distribution of RF-induced E-fields and implant heating in MRI. Magn Reson Med 2008;60:312-9.

Nordbeck P, et al. Measuring RF-induced currents inside implants: Impact of device configuration on MRI safety of cardiac pacemaker leads. Magn Reson Med 2009;61:570-8.

Nordbeck P, et al. Impact of imaging landmark on the risk of MRI-related heating near implanted medical devices like cardiac pacemaker leads. Magn Reson Med 2011;65:44-50.

Nyenhuis JA, et al. Heating near implanted medical devices by the MRI RF-magnetic field. IEEE Trans Magn 1999;35:4133-4135.

Nyenhuis JA, Park SM, Kamondetdacha R, Amjad A, Shellock FG, Rezai A. MRI and implanted medical devices: Basic interactions with an emphasis on heating. IEEE Transactions on Device and Materials Reliability 2005;5:467-478.

Pietryga JA, et al. Invisible metallic microfiber in clothing presents unrecognized MRI risks for cutaneous burns. Am J Neuroradiol 2013;34:E47-50.

Rezai AR, Baker K, Tkach J, Phillips M, Hrdlicka G, Sharan A, Nyenhuis J, Ruggieri P, Henderson J, Shellock FG. Is magnetic resonance imaging safe for patients with neurostimulation systems used for deep brain stimulation (DBS)? Neurosurgery 2005;57:1056-1062.

Roguin A, et al. Magnetic resonance imaging in individuals with cardiovascular implantable electronic devices. Europace 2008;10:336-46.

Schenck JF. Chapter 1, Health Effects and Safety of Static Magnetic Fields. In: Magnetic Resonance Procedures: Health Effects and Safety. CRC Press, LLC, Boca Raton, FL, 2001; pp. 1-31.

Shellock FG, Crues JV, Editors. MRI Bioeffects, Safety, and Patient Management. Biomedical Research Publishing Group, Los Angeles, CA, 2014.

Shellock FG. Guest Editorial. Comments on MRI heating tests of critical implants. J Magn Reson Imag 2007;26:1182-1185.

Shellock FG. Excessive temperature increases in pacemaker leads at 3-T MR imaging with a transmit-received head coil. Radiology 2009;251:948-949.

Shellock FG. Biomedical implants and devices: Assessment of magnetic field interactions with a 3.0-Tesla MR system. J Magn Reson Imag 2002;16:721-732.

Shellock FG. MR safety update 2002: Implants and devices. J Magn Reson Imag 2002;16:485-496.

Shellock FG, Crues JV. High-field strength MR imaging and metallic biomedical implants: An *ex vivo* evaluation of deflection forces. Am J Roentgenol 1988;151:389-392.

Shellock FG, Crues JV. MR procedures: Biologic effects, safety, and patient care. Radiology 2004;232:635-652.

Shellock FG, Kanal E, Gilk T. Regarding the value reported for the term "spatial gradient magnetic field" and how this information is applied to labeling of medical implants and devices. Am J Roentgenol 2011;196:142-145.

Shellock FG, et al. MRI and orthopedic implants used for anterior cruciate ligament reconstruction: Assessment of ferromagnetism and artifacts. J Magn Reson Imag 1992;2:225-228.

Shellock FG, Spinazzi A. MRI Safety Update: 2008, Part 2, Screening patients for MRI. Am J Roentgenol 2008;191:12-21.

Shellock FG, et al. Aneurysm clips: Evaluation of magnetic field interactions and translational attraction using "long-bore" and "short-bore" 3.0-Tesla MR systems. Am J Neuroradiology 2003;24:463-471.

Shellock FG, et al. Cardiac pacemakers, ICDs, and loop recorder: Evaluation of translational attraction using conventional ("long-bore") and "short-bore" 1.5- and 3.0-Tesla MR systems. Journal of Cardiovascular Magnetic Resonance 2003;5:387-397.

Shellock FG, Woods TO, Crues JV. MRI labeling information for implants and devices: Explanation of terminology. Radiology 2009;253:26-30.

Smith CD, et al. Chapter 16. Health effects of induced electrical currents: Implications for implants. In: Magnetic resonance: Health Effects and Safety, FG Shellock, Editor, CRC Press, Boca Raton, FL, 2001; pp. 393-413.

Stradiotti P, et al. Metal-related artifacts in instrumented spine. Techniques for reducing artifacts in CT and MRI: State of the art. Eur Spine J 2009;18 Suppl 1:102-8.

Woods TO. Guidance for Industry and FDA Staff - Establishing Safety and Compatibility of Passive Implants in the Magnetic Resonance (MR) Environment, 2008.

Woods TO. Standards for medical devices in MRI: Present and future. J Magn Reson Imag 2007;26:1186-9.

Yang CW, et al. Magnetic resonance imaging of artificial lumbar disks: Safety and metal artifacts. Chin Med J (Engl) 2009;20;122:911-6.

Zanchi MG, et al. An optically coupled system for quantitative monitoring of MRI-induced RF currents into long conductors. IEEE Trans Med Imag 2010;29:169-78.

3-Tesla MR Safety Information for Implants and Devices

Because previous investigations performed to evaluate MR safety issues for implants and devices used mostly scanners with static magnetic fields of 1.5-Tesla or less, it is crucial to perform *ex vivo* testing at 3-Tesla to determine possible risks for these objects with respect to magnetic field interactions and heating. Importantly, a metallic object that displayed "weakly" ferromagnetic qualities at 1.5-Tesla may exhibit substantial magnetic field interactions at 3-Tesla or higher.

Furthermore, for elongated devices or those that form a loop of a certain diameter, the effects of MRI-related heating may be substantially different at 3-Tesla/128-MHz versus, for example, 1.5-Tesla/64-MHz. Evidence from an *ex vivo* study conducted by Shellock, et al. (2005) reported that significantly *less* MRI-related heating occurred at 3-Tesla/128-MHz (MR system reported, whole body averaged SAR, 3-W/kg) versus 1.5-Tesla/64-MHz (MR system reported, whole body averaged SAR, 1.4-W/kg) for a pacemaker lead not connected to a pulse generator (same lead length, positioning in the phantom, etc.). This phenomenon, whereby less heating was observed at 3-Tesla/128-MHz versus 1.5-Tesla/64-MHz, has also been observed for external fixation devices, Foley catheters with temperature sensors, neurostimulation systems, relatively long peripheral vascular stents, and other objects (Unpublished Observations, F.G. Shellock, 2011). Therefore, it is crucial to conduct *ex vivo* testing to assess magnetic field interactions as well as MRI-related heating to identify potentially hazardous implants prior to subjecting patients to an MR examination at 3-Tesla.

Magnetic Field Interactions at 3-Tesla. From a magnetic field interaction consideration, translational attraction and/or torque may cause movement or dislodgment of a ferromagnetic implant resulting in an uncomfortable sensation or injury. Translational attraction is dependent on the strength of the static magnetic field, the spatial gradient magnetic field, the mass of the object, the shape of the object, and its magnetic susceptibility. The effects of translational attraction on external and implanted ferromagnetic objects are predominantly responsible for serious hazards in the immediate area of the MR system. That is, as one moves closer to the MR system or is moved into the scanner for an examination. An evaluation of torque is also important for a metallic object, especially if it has an elongated configuration. Qualitative and quantitative techniques have been used to determine magnetic field-related torque for implants and devices at 3-Tesla.

From a practical consideration, in addition to the findings for translational attraction and torque, the "intended *in vivo* use" of the implant or device must be considered as well as mechanisms that may provide retention of the object *in situ* (e.g., implants or devices held in place by sutures, granulation or ingrowth of tissue, fixation devices, or by other means) with regard to potential risks for the metallic object (for further information on this topic, please refer to the section, **General Information**).

Long-Bore vs. Short-Bore 3-Tesla MR Systems. Different magnet designs exist for commercially available 3-Tesla MR systems, including configurations that are older "long-bore" scanners and "short-bore" systems. Because of physical differences in the position and magnitude of the highest spatial gradient magnetic fields for different magnets, measurements of deflection angles for implants using long-bore vs. short-bore MR systems can produce substantially different results for deflection angle measurements (i.e. translational attraction), as reported by Shellock, et al. Studies conducted using 3-Tesla MR systems indicated that, in general, there were significantly ($p<0.01$) higher deflection angles measured for implants using short-bore vs. the long-bore MR systems. The differences in deflection angle measurements for the metallic objects were related to differences in the highest spatial gradient magnetic fields for short-bore versus long-bore scanners.

The safety implications are primarily for magnetic field-related translational attraction with respect to short-bore versus long-bore 3-Tesla MR systems. For example, the deflection angle measured for an implant on a short-bore can be substantially higher (and, thus, potentially unsafe from a magnetic field interaction consideration) compared to the deflection angle measured on a long-bore MR system. Therefore, safety information for measurements of magnetic field interactions for metallic objects must be considered with regard to the specific type of MR system used for the evaluation or, more accurately, with respect to the level of the highest spatial gradient magnetic field that was used for the test.

Lenz Effect. In 1835, Heinrich Lenz stated the law that an electric current induced by a changing magnetic field will flow such that it will create its own magnetic field that opposes the magnetic field that created it. These opposing fields, which occupy the same space at the same time, result in a pair of forces. The more current that is generated, the greater the force that opposes it. The so-called "Lenz Effect" occurs with electrically-conductive materials (i.e. not just ferromagnetic materials) that develop magnetic field eddy currents in the presence of high-field-strength static magnetic fields, such as those associated with MR systems.

Forces described by the Lenz Effect may restrict movement for metallic objects (e.g., for an aluminum oxygen tank) or compromise the function of certain implants in the MRI setting, such as those with moving metallic parts. This may be a concern for prosthetic heart valves that have leaflets or discs, especially if the implant is used for mitral valve replacement, where the range of pressures that are present are relatively low (higher pressures are more likely to overcome any significant Lenz Effect). Importantly, the Lenz Effect is proportional to the strength of the static magnetic field.

Condon and Hadley (2000) first reported the theoretical possibility of electromagnetic interaction with heart valve prostheses that contain metallic disks or leaflets. In theory, "resistive pressure" may develop with the potential to inhibit both the opening and closing aspects of a mechanical heart valve prosthesis that has leaflets or disks.

Edwards, et al. (2015) conducted an *in vitro* study of the occurrence of Lenz-related forces on various heart valve prostheses at 1.5-Tesla and assessed the risk of the impedance of valve function. The findings provided evidence of the Lenz Effect on certain cardiac valve prostheses exposed to the static magnetic field, which resulted in functional valve impedance and a potentially increased risk of valve regurgitation. While further evaluation of this phenomenon may be warranted, to date, the Lenz Effect has not been observed in association with clinical MR examinations with respect of causing harm nor has it posed additional risks for patients with certain heart valve prostheses (i.e. those with metallic leaflets or disks) undergoing MRI.

Heating of Implants and Devices at 3-Tesla/128-MHz. *Ex vivo* testing has been used to evaluate MRI-related heating for various metallic implants, materials, devices, and objects of a variety of sizes, shapes, and metallic compositions. In general, reports have indicated that only minor temperature changes occur in association with MR procedures involving metallic objects that are relatively small passive implants (e.g., those that are not electronically-activated). Therefore, heat generated during an MR procedure performed at 3-Tesla/128-MHz on a patient with a relatively small, passive metallic implant does not appear to be a substantial hazard.

However, because excessive heating and burns have occurred in implants and devices that have elongated configurations or that form conducting loops of certain diameter, patients with these objects should not undergo MR procedures at 3-Tesla until *ex vivo* heating assessments are performed to determine the relative risks. *Ex vivo* investigations have demonstrated that excessive heating may occur for some implants related to MRI performed at 3-Tesla/128-MHz under certain operating conditions.

REFERENCES

American Society for Testing and Materials (ASTM) International Designation: F 2052. Standard test method for measurement of magnetically induced displacement force on passive implants in the magnetic resonance environment. West Conshohocken, PA.

Bottomley PA, Kumar A, et al. Designing passive MRI-safe implantable conducting leads with electrodes. Med Phys 2010;37:3828-43.

Condon B, Hadley DM. Potential MR hazard to patients with metallic heart valves: The Lenz effect. J Magn Reson Imag 2000;12:171-176.

Dempsey MF, Condon B, Hadley DM. Investigation of the factors responsible for burns during MRI. J Magn Reson Imag 2001;13:627-631.

Diaz F, Tweardy L, Shellock FG. Cervical fixation devices: MRI issues at 3-Tesla. Spine 2010;35:411-5.

Edwards MB, et al. Mechanical testing of human cardiac tissue: Some implications for MRI safety. J Cardiovasc Magn Resonance 2005;7:835-840.

Edwards MB, et al. In vitro assessment of the lenz effect on heart valve prostheses at 1.5 T. J Magn Reson Imaging 2015;41:74-82.

Gimbel JR. Magnetic resonance imaging of implantable cardiac rhythm devices at 3-Tesla. Pacing Clin Electrophysiol 2008;31:795-801.

Golestanirad L, et al. Comprehensive analysis of Lenz effect on the artificial heart valves during magnetic resonance imaging. Progress In Electromagnetics Research 2012;128:1-17.

Hennemeyer CT, et al. *In vitro* evaluation of platinum Guglielmi detachable coils at 3-T with a porcine model: Safety issues and artifacts. Radiology 2001;219:732-737.

Kakizawa Y, et al. Cerebral aneurysm clips in the 3-Tesla magnetic field. Laboratory investigation. J Neurosurg 2010;113:859-69.

Martin AD, et al. Safety evaluation of titanium middle ear prostheses at 3-Tesla. Otolaryngol Head Neck Surg 2005;132:537-42.

Nyehnuis JA, et al. Heating near implanted medical devices by the MRI RF-magnetic field. IEEE Trans Magn 1999;35:4133-4135.

Schenck JF. Chapter 1, Health Effects and Safety of Static Magnetic Fields. In: Magnetic Resonance Procedures: Health Effects and Safety. CRC Press, LLC, Boca Raton, FL, 2001; pp. 1-31.

Shellock FG. Biomedical implants and devices: Assessment of magnetic field interactions with a 3.0-Tesla MR system. J Magn Reson Imag 2002;16:721-732.

Shellock FG. Begnaud J, Inman DM. VNS Therapy System: *In vitro* evaluation of MRI-related heating and function at 1.5- and 3-Tesla. Neuromodulation 2006;9:204-213.

Shellock FG. Forder J. Drug eluting coronary stent: *In vitro* evaluation of magnetic resonance safety at 3-Tesla. Journal of Cardiovascular Magnetic Resonance 2005;7:415-419.

Shellock FG, Woods TO, Crues JV. MRI labeling information for implants and devices: Explanation of terminology. Radiology 2009;253:26-30.

Shellock FG, Kanal E, Gilk T. Regarding the value reported for the term "spatial gradient magnetic field" and how this information is applied to labeling of medical implants and devices. Am J Roentgenol 2011;196:142-145.

Shellock FG, Gounis M, Wakhloo A. Detachable coil for cerebral aneurysms: *In vitro* evaluation of magnet field interactions, heating, and artifacts at 3-Tesla. American Journal of Neuroradiology 2005;26:363-366.

Shellock FG, et al. Cardiac pacemakers, ICDs, and loop recorder: Evaluation of translational attraction using conventional ("long-bore") and "short-bore" 1.5- and 3.0-Tesla MR systems. Journal of Cardiovascular Magnetic Resonance 2003;5:387-397.

Shellock FG, et al. Aneurysm clips: Evaluation of magnetic field interactions and translational attraction using "long-bore" and "short-bore" 3.0-Tesla MR systems. American Journal of Neuroradiology 2003;24:463-471.

Shellock FG, Valencerina S. Septal repair implants: Evaluation of MRI safety at 3-Tesla. Magnetic Resonance Imaging 2005;23:1021-1025.

Shellock FG, Valencerina S, Fischer L. MRI-related heating of pacemaker at 1.5- and 3-Tesla: Evaluation with and without pulse generator attached to leads. Circulation 2005;112;Supplement II:561.

Shellock FG. Valencerina S. *In vitro* evaluation of MR imaging issues at 3-T for aneurysm clips made from MP35N: Findings and information applied to 155 additional aneurysm clips. Am J Neuroradiol 2010;31:615-619

Smith CD, et al. Interactions of MRI magnetic fields with elongated medical implants. J Appl Physics 2000;87:6188-6190.

Sommer T, et al. High field MR imaging: Magnetic field interactions of aneurysm clips, coronary artery stents and iliac artery stents with a 3.0 Tesla MR system. Rofo 2004;176:731-8.

Woods TO. Standards for medical devices in MRI: Present and future. J Magn Reson Imag 2007;26:1186-9.

Woods TO. Guidance for Industry and FDA Staff - Establishing Safety and Compatibility of Passive Implants in the Magnetic Resonance (MR) Environment. Document issued on: August 21, 2008.

ActiFlo Indwelling Bowel Catheter System

The ActiFlo Indwelling Bowel Catheter System (also known as the Zassi Bowel Management System, Hollister, Libertyville, IL) is intended for diversion of fecal matter to minimize external contact with the patient's skin, to facilitate the collection of fecal matter for patients requiring stool management, to provide access for colonic irrigation and to administer enema or medications. This system consists the catheter, the collection bag, and the irrigation bag. The ActiFlo Indwelling Bowel Catheter System allows stool to drain directly from the rectum into a closed or drainable collection bag.

MRI Information

The ActiFlo Indwelling Bowel Catheter System was determined to be MR Conditional:

Non-clinical testing demonstrated that this product is MR Conditional according to the following conditions:

- Static magnetic field of 3-Tesla or less
- Highest spatial gradient magnetic field of 720-gauss/cm

Important note: A metallic spring used for this device is located outside of the patient's body during the intended *in vivo* use of this product. Therefore, the only possible MRI-related issue pertains to magnetic field interactions. Heating and artifacts are of no concern. Therefore, the assessment of magnetic field interactions for this product specifically involved evaluations of translational attraction and torque in relation to exposure to a 3-Tesla MR system, *only.*

REFERENCE

www.hollister.co.za/us/

ActiPatch

ActiPatch (BioElectronics, Frederick, MD) is a medical, drug-free device that delivers pulsed electromagnetic frequency therapies to accelerate healing of soft tissue injuries. The ActiPatch has an embedded battery-operated microchip that delivers continuous pulsed therapy to reduce pain and swelling.

MRI and the ActiPatch

The ActiPatch must be removed prior to performing an MRI procedure to prevent possible damage to this device and the potential risk of excessive heating.

REFERENCE

www.bielcorp.com

Alsius Intravascular Temperature Management

Alsius Corporation (a Zoll Corporation, Chelmsford, MA) products are designed for placement in the central venous system. Via a proprietary, "closed loop" internal cooling circuit, the catheter cools or warms the patient's blood as it circulates past the catheter. The catheters (Cool Line, Icy, and Fortius) are attached to the CoolGard 3000 Thermal Regulation System. This is an electronic cooling system that regulates the cooling performance of the catheter via remote sensing of the patient's temperature. Alsius catheters are also designed to facilitate critical care management with features similar to those found in conventional central venous catheters.

CoolGard 3000. All Alsius heat exchange catheters connect to the CoolGard 3000 Thermal Regulation System, which achieves and maintains a target temperature input by the user. It remotely senses changes in patient core temperature and automatically adjusts the temperature of the circulating saline within the catheter (0 to 42 degrees C), providing consistent maintenance of temperature.

Cool Line Catheter. The Cool Line Catheter is inserted into the subclavian or jugular vein and resides in the superior vena cava. The Cool Line Catheter combines temperature control and central venous catheter capabilities.

Icy Catheter. The Icy catheter is inserted into the femoral vein and resides in the inferior vena cava.

Fortius Catheter. The Fortius catheter is inserted percutaneously into the femoral vein residing in the inferior vena cava, just below the heart. The Fortius catheter provides maximum heat exchange power with minimum time to target temperature.

MRI Information

The following models of Alsius Heat Exchange catheters have been determined to be MR Safe:

1) Cool Line
2) Icy
3) Fortius

Magnetic resonance imaging (MRI) procedures must be performed according to the following guidelines:

Through non-clinical testing, these catheters were shown to be MR Safe* at a field strength of 1.5 Tesla or less and a maximum whole body averaged specific absorption rate (SAR) of 2.0 W/kg for 20 minutes of MRI. MRI at 1.5-Tesla (highest spatial gradient magnetic field, 2.4 Tesla/meter) or less may be performed immediately following the insertion of the one of these catheters.

MR image quality may be compromised if the area of interest is in the exact same area or relatively close to the position of these catheters. Therefore, it may be necessary to optimize the MRI parameters for the presence of these metallic devices.

IMPORTANT NOTE: The Alsius CoolGard 3000 system is not MRI Safe nor Compatible nor intended for use in an MRI environment. The Catheter should be disconnected from the System prior to moving the patient to the MRI facility.

[*Note the use of the term "MR Safe". These products underwent testing and labeling prior to the implementation of the current terminology. For further explanation, please refer to section: **Terminology for Implants and Devices.**]

REFERENCES

www.alsius.com
www.zoll.com

Ambulatory Infusion Systems

Ambulatory Infusion Systems (Smiths Medical) are designed to help healthcare providers administer medications accurately, monitor patient's response to therapy, stimulate early clinical assessment and facilitate patient recovery. These devices include, the following:

CADD – 1 Ambulatory Infusion Pump

CADD – Legacy 1 Ambulatory Infusion Pump

CADD – Legacy Ambulatory Infusion Pump

CADD – Legacy PCA Ambulatory Infusion Pump

CADD – Legacy PLUS Ambulatory Infusion Pump

CADD – Micro Ambulatory Infusion Pump

CADD – MS 3 Ambulatory Infusion Pump

CADD – PCA Ambulatory Infusion Pump

CADD – PLUS Ambulatory Infusion Pump

CADD – Prizm PCS Ambulatory Infusion Pump

CADD – Prizm PCS II Ambulatory Infusion Pump

CADD – Prizm VIP Ambulatory Infusion Pump

CADD – Solis Ambulatory Infusion Pump

CADD – TPN Ambulatory Infusion Pump

MRI Information
Regarding the pump used for each device, the Operator's Manual states: "Magnetic fields produced by magnetic resonance imaging (MRI) equipment may adversely affect the operation of the pump. Remove the pump from the patient during MRI procedures and keep it at a safe distance from magnetic energy."

REFERENCE

www.smiths-medical.com

Aneurysm Clips

The surgical management of intracranial aneurysms and arteriovenous malformations (AVMs) by the application of aneurysm clips is a well-established procedure. The presence of an aneurysm clip in a patient referred for an MR procedure represents a situation that requires the utmost consideration because of the associated risks.

Certain types of intracranial aneurysm clips (e.g., those made from martensitic stainless steels such as 17-7PH or 405 stainless steel) are a contraindication to the use of MR procedures because excessive, magnetically induced forces can displace these implants and cause serious injury or death. By comparison, aneurysm clips classified as "nonferromagnetic" or "weakly ferromagnetic" (e.g., those made from Phynox, Elgiloy, austentitic stainless steels, titanium alloy, or commercially pure titanium) are acceptable for patients undergoing MR examinations.

[For the sake of discussion, the term "weakly magnetic" refers to metal that may demonstrate some extremely low ferromagnetic qualities using highly sensitive measurements techniques (e.g., vibrating sample magnetometer, superconducting quantum interference device or SQUID magnetometer, etc.) and, thus, may not be technically referred to as being "nonmagnetic." All metals possess some degree of magnetism, such that no metal is entirely nonmagnetic.]

MR procedures have been used to evaluate patients with certain types of aneurysm clips. Becker, et al. (1988), using MR systems that ranged from 0.35 to 0.6-Tesla, studied three patients with nonferromagnetic aneurysm clips (one patient, Yasargil, 316 LVM stainless steel; two patients, Vari-Angle McFadden, MP35N; 316 LVM) and one patient with a ferromagnetic aneurysm clip (Heifetz aneurysm clip) without incident. Dujovny, et al. (1985) similarly reported no adverse effects in patients with nonferromagnetic aneurysm clips that underwent procedures using 1.5-Tesla MR systems.

Pride, et al. (2000) performed a study in patients with nonferromagnetic aneurysm clips that underwent MR imaging. There were no adverse outcomes for the patients, confirming that MR procedures can be performed safely in patients with nonferromagnetic clips. Brothers, et al. (1990) also demonstrated that MR imaging at 1.5-Tesla can be performed safely in patients with nonmagnetic aneurysm clips. This report was particularly important because, according to Brothers, et al. (1990), MR imaging was found to be better than CT in the postoperative assessment of aneurysm patients, especially with regard to showing small zones of ischemia.

To date, only one ferromagnetic aneurysm clip-related fatality has been reported in the peer-reviewed literature. According to this report, the patient became symptomatic at a distance of approximately 1.2-meters from the bore of the MR system, suggesting that translational attraction of the aneurysm clip was likely responsible for dislodgment of this implant.

This incident was the result of erroneous information pertaining to the type of aneurysm clip that was present in the patient. That is, the clip was thought to be a nonmagnetic Yasargil aneurysm clip (Aesculap Inc., Central Valley, PA) and turned out to be a magnetic Vari-Angle clip (Codman & Shurtleff, Randolf, MA).

There has never been a report of an injury to a patient or individual in the MR environment related to the presence of an aneurysm clip made from a nonmagnetic or "weakly" magnetic material. In fact, there have been cases in which patients with ferromagnetic aneurysm clips (based on the extent of the artifact seen during MR imaging or other information) have undergone MR procedures without sustaining injuries (Personal communications, D. Kroker, 1995; E. Kanal, 1996; A. Osborne, 2002).

In these cases, the aneurysm clips were exposed to magnetic-induced translational attraction and torque associated with MR systems operating at 1.5-Tesla or less. Although these cases do not prove safety, they do demonstrate the difficulty of predicting the outcome for patients with ferromagnetic aneurysm clips that undergo MR procedures. Variables to consider include the size, shape (especially the length of the blade), mass, and material of the aneurysm clip.

There is controversy regarding the amount of ferromagnetism that needs to be present in an aneurysm clip to constitute a hazard for a patient in the MR environment. Consequently, this issue has not only created problems for MR healthcare professionals but for manufacturers of aneurysm clips, as well.

For example, MR healthcare professionals performing tests on aneurysm clips similar to the method described in the report by Kanal, et al. (1996) identified the presence of magnetic field interactions and returned several clips made from Phynox to the manufacturer (Personal Communication, Aesculap, Inc., South San Francisco, CA, 1997). However, the testing method used by Kanal, et al. (1996) was admittedly crude and developed to primarily obtain rapid, qualitative screening data for large numbers of aneurysm clips to determine if quantitative assessments were necessary. Importantly, the testing technique used by Kanal, et al. (1996) may be problematic and yield spurious results, especially if the aneurysm clip has a shape or configuration that is somewhat "unstable" (Unpublished Observations, F.G. Shellock, 1997). For example, aneurysm clips with blades that are bayonet, curved, or angled shapes are less stable on a piece of plate glass (i.e. using the testing method described by Kanal, et al.) when placed in certain orientations compared with aneurysm clips with straight blades.

A variety of more appropriate testing techniques have been developed and utilized over the years to evaluate the relative amount of ferromagnetism present for implants and devices prior to allowing patients with these objects to enter the MR environment. In 2002, the American Society for Testing and Materials (ASTM) provided recommendations for testing passive implants that involves the use of the deflection angle test, originally described by New, et al., to assess translational attraction. Additionally, the U.S. Food and Drug Administration recommends that an evaluation of torque should be performed on aneurysm clips. Thus, procedures such as the deflection angle test and some form of evaluation of torque (qualitative or quantitative) are the most appropriate means of determining which specific aneurysm clip may present a hazard to a patient or individual in the MR environment.

Aneurysm Clips and MRI Procedures: Guidelines. The following guidelines are recommended with regard to performing an MR procedure in a patient or before allowing an individual with an aneurysm clip into the MR environment:

1) Specific information (i.e. manufacturer, type or model, material, lot and serial numbers) about the aneurysm clip must be known, especially with respect to the material used to make the aneurysm clip, so that only patients or individuals with nonferromagnetic or weakly ferromagnetic clips are allowed into the MR environment. The manufacturer provides this information in the labeling of the aneurysm clip. The implanting surgeon is responsible for properly recording and communicating this information in the patient's or individual's records.

2) An aneurysm clip that is in its original package and made from Phynox, Elgiloy, MP35N, titanium alloy, commercially pure titanium or other material known to be nonferromagnetic or weakly ferromagnetic does not need to be evaluated for ferromagnetism.

Aneurysm clips made from nonferrromagnetic or "weakly" ferromagnetic materials in original packages do not require testing of ferromagnetism because the manufacturers ensure the pertinent MR safety or conditional aspects of these clips and, therefore, are responsible for the accuracy of the labeling.

3) If the aneurysm clip is not in its original package and/or properly labeled, it should undergo testing for magnetic field interactions following appropriate testing procedures to determine if it is safe.

4) The radiologist and implanting surgeon are responsible for evaluating the information pertaining to the aneurysm clip, verifying its accuracy, obtaining written documentation, and deciding to perform the MR procedure after considering the risk vs. benefit aspects for a given patient.

5) Consideration must be give to the static magnetic field strength that is to be used for the MRI procedure and the strength of the static magnetic field used to test magnetic field interactions for the aneurysm clip in question.

MRI at 3-Tesla and Aneurysm Clips. Many aneurysm clips have been tested for magnetic field interactions in association with 3-Tesla MR systems (refer to **The List** for information for aneurysm clips tested at 3-Tesla). Findings for these specific implants indicated that they either exhibited no magnetic field interactions or relatively minor or "weak" magnetic field interactions. Accordingly, these particular aneurysm clips are considered acceptable for patients undergoing MR procedures using MR systems operating at 3-Tesla or less.

Yasargil Aneurysm Clips (Information dated 11/11/09 - Aesculap Inc., Center Valley, PA)

Aesculap currently markets two lines of YASARGIL aneurysm clips, one from a cobalt-chrome alloy ("Phynox") and one from a titanium alloy. Phynox clips have been available since 1983 and have catalog numbers that begin with "FE". Titanium clips have been available since 1997 and have catalog numbers that begin with "FT". All "FE" and "FT" model YASARGIL aneurysm clips are non-ferromagnetic and may be safely exposed to MRI. Both implant materials have been tested and proven MR Safe as per ASTM-2052-02 up to 3.0 Tesla*.

Prior to 1985, Aesculap distributed various models of aneurysm clips manufactured from stainless steel. These aneurysm clips were identified with the letters "FD" and have not been proven safe under exposure to MRI. For this reason, **Aesculap does not recommend the use of MRI**

on a patient implanted with a YASARGIL aneurysm clip identified with the letters "FD".

For additional information, please refer to the following three scientific publications:

1)   Dujovny, M., et. al. (1985). *Aneurysm clip motion during magnetic resonance imaging: In vivo experimental study with metallurgical factor analysis, Journal of Neurosurgery 17(4), 543-548.*

2)   *Shellock, F.G, Kanal, E. (1998). Aneurysm clips: Evaluation of MR imaging artifacts at 1.5. Radiology, 209(2), 563-566.*

3)   Romner, B., et. al. (1989). *Magnetic resonance imaging and aneurysm clips, Journal of Neurosurgery, 70(3), 426-431.*

*These Aesculap devices were cleared by FDA as "MR Safe" per ASTM 2052-02. Due to a change in definition within this standard (F 2503 2005-08), these devices are now termed as "MR Conditional" by ASTM. The FDA has not mandated a revision to our labeling because the device material and performance have not changed.

Aneurysm Clips, Codman & Shurtleff, Inc., a Johnson & Johnson Company

Three different MP35N aneurysm clips (Codman Slim-Line Aneurysm Clip, Straight, Blade length 25-mm; Codman Slim-Line Aneurysm Clip Graft, 5-mm Diameter x 5-mm width; Codman Slim-Line Aneurysm Clip, Reinforcing 30-degree angle, 6-mm x 18-mm; Codman & Shurtleff, Inc., a Johnson & Johnson Company) underwent MRI testing that represented the largest mass for 155 additional clips made from MP35N. The clips were evaluated at 3-Tesla for magnetic field interactions, heating, and artifacts. Each aneurysm clip showed relatively minor magnetic field interactions that will not cause movement *in situ*. Heating was not excessive (highest temperature change, < 1.8°C). Artifacts may create issues if the area of interest is in the same area or close to the aneurysm clip. The results of this investigation demonstrated that it would be acceptable (i.e. "MR Conditional" using current terminology) for patients with these aneurysm clips to undergo MRI at 3-Tesla or less. Notably, in consideration of the sizes of the clips that underwent testing, these findings pertain to 155 additional aneurysm clips made from the same material including, the following:

Codman Slim-Line Aneurysm Clip
Codman AVM Micro Clip
Codman Slim-Line Aneurysm Clip Graft
Codman Slim-Line Mini Aneurysm Clip
Codman Slim-Line Temporary Vessel Aneurysm Clip

The following information is the MRI labeling for these aneurysm clips approved by the Food and Drug Administration:

Magnetic Resonance Imaging Information

Non-clinical testing of representative configurations of **Codman Slim-Line Aneurysm, Mini, Micro and Graft Clips** (Codman Slim-Line Clips) up to 25-mm in blade length has demonstrated that they are **MR Conditional.** A patient with one such clip up to 25-mm in blade length (i.e. Codman Slim-Line Aneurysm, Mini, Micro and Graft Clips (Codman Slim-Line Clips) can be scanned safely, immediately after placement under the following conditions.

3.0 Tesla Systems:

- Static magnetic field of 3.0 Tesla.
- Spatial gradient magnetic field of 720 gauss/cm or less.
- Maximum MR system reported, whole-body-averaged specific absorption rate (SAR) of 3.0 W/kg for 15 minutes of scanning (i.e. per pulse sequence).

MRI Related Heating

MRI related heating was assessed for the representative configurations of the Codman clips (up to 25-mm in blade length) following guidelines provided in ASTM F2182. A maximum temperature change equal to or less than 1.8°C was observed during testing (parameters listed below).

Parameters:

- Maximum MR system-reported, whole-body-averaged SAR of 3.0 W/kg (associated calorimetry measured whole body averaged value of 2.8 W/kg).
- 15-minute duration MR scanning (i.e. per pulse sequence).
- 3 Tesla MR System (EXCITE MR Scanner, Software G3 .0-052B, General Electric Healthcare, Milwaukee, WI) using a transmit/receive RF body coil.

Artifact Information

Artifacts were assessed for representative clip configurations using T1-weighted spin echo (T1-SE) and gradient echo (GRE) pulse sequences following methods similar to the guidelines provided in ASTM F2119-07. The 25-mm blade-length aneurysm clip imaged using a GRE pulse sequence produced an artifact that extended approximately 5-cm from the clip in the parallel (long-axis) imaging plane. The void size corresponding to this artifact was approximately 1251-mm^2. MR image quality may be compromised if the area of interest is in the exact location or within a few centimeters of the Codman Slim-Line Clip. In general, the GRE pulse sequence produced larger artifacts than the T1-SE sequence for each clip. However, MRI artifacts can be minimized by careful selection of pulse sequence parameters.

MRI at 8.0-Tesla and Aneurysm Clips. *Ex vivo* testing has been conducted to identify potentially hazardous implants and devices using an 8-Tesla MR system. The first investigation of this type was conducted by Kangarlu and Shellock.

Twenty-six different aneurysm clips were tested for magnetic field interactions using previously-described techniques. These implants were specifically selected for this investigation because they represent various types of clips used for temporary or permanent treatment of aneurysms or arteriovenous malformations. Additionally, these aneurysm clips were reported to be safe for patients undergoing MR procedures using MR systems with static magnetic field strengths of 1.5-Tesla or less.

According to the results, six aneurysm clips (i.e. type, model, blade length) made from stainless steel alloy (Perneczky) and Phynox (Yasargil, Models FE 748 and FE 750) displayed deflection angles above 45 degrees (i.e. referring to the guideline stated by the American Society for Testing and Materials, ASTM) and relatively high qualitative torque values. These findings indicated that these specific aneurysm clips may be unsafe for individuals or patients in an 8.0-Tesla or higher MR environment.

Aneurysm clips made from commercially pure titanium (Spetzler), Elgiloy (Sugita), titanium alloy (Yasargil, Model FE 750T), and MP35N (Sundt) displayed deflection angles less than 45 degrees (i.e. referring to the ASTM guideline) and qualitative torque values that were relatively minor. Accordingly, these aneurysm clips are considered to be acceptable for patients or individuals exposed to an 8.0-Tesla MR system.

As previously indicated, at 1.5-Tesla, aneurysm clips that are considered to be acceptable for patients or others in the MR environment include those made from commercially pure titanium, titanium alloy, Elgiloy, Phynox, and austentic stainless steel. By comparison, findings from the 8.0-Tesla study indicated that deflection angles for the aneurysm clips made from commercially pure titanium and titanium alloy ranged from 5 to 6 degrees, suggesting that these aneurysm clips would be safe for patients or individuals in the 8.0-Tesla MR environment. However, deflection angles for aneurysm clips made from Elgiloy ranged from 36 to 42 degrees, such that further consideration must be given to the specific type of Elgiloy clip that is present. For example, an Elgiloy clip that has a greater mass (e.g., due to a longer blade length) than those tested in this study may exceed a deflection angle of 45 degrees (i.e. referring to the ASTM guideline of 45 degrees or less being acceptable for translational attraction) in association with an 8.0-Tesla MR system.

Depending on the actual dimensions and mass, an aneurysm clip made from Elgiloy may or may not be acceptable for a patient or individual in the 8.0-Tesla MR environment. Notably, the results of this investigation are specific to the types of intracranial aneurysm clips that underwent testing (i.e. with regard model, shape, size, blade length, material, etc.) as well as the spatial gradient magnetic field associated with the 8.0-Tesla MR system.

Effects of Long-Term and Multiple Exposures to the MR System. MR testing procedures used for aneurysm clips, if performed routinely prior to implantation, would result in the reintroduction of aneurysm clips into strong magnetic fields several times prior to use in the patient. Furthermore, there are patients with implanted aneurysm clips previously designated as "MR Safe" or "MR Conditional" that have undergone repeated exposures to strong magnetic fields during follow-up MR examinations.

A concern has emerged that a potential alteration in the magnetic properties of pre- or post-implanted aneurysm clips may occur due to long-term or multiple exposures to strong magnetic fields. Long-term or multiple exposures to strong magnetic fields (such as those associated with MR imaging systems) have been suggested to grossly "magnetize" aneurysm clips, even if they are made from nonferromagnetic or weakly ferromagnetic materials. This theoretical problem could present a substantial hazard to an individual in the MR environment. Therefore, an *in vitro* investigation was conducted by Kanal and Shellock to study intracranial aneurysm clips prior to and following long-term and multiple exposures to 1.5-Tesla MR systems. This was done to quantify possible alterations in the magnetic properties of these aneurysm clips.

Aneurysm clips made from Elgiloy, Phynox, titanium alloy, commercially pure titanium, and austenitic stainless steel were tested in association with long-term and multiple exposures to 1.5-Tesla MR systems. The findings indicated a lack of response to the magnetic field exposure conditions that were used. Accordingly, long-term or multiple exposures to 1.5-Tesla MR systems should not result in significant changes in their magnetic properties.

Artifacts Associated with Aneurysm Clips. An additional problem related to aneurysm clips is that artifacts produced by these metallic implants may substantially detract from the diagnostic aspects of MR procedures. MR imaging, MR angiography, and functional MRI are frequently used to evaluate the brain or cerebral vasculature of patients with aneurysm clips. For example, to reduce morbidity and mortality after subarachnoid hemorrhage, it is imperative to assess the results of the surgical treatment of cerebral aneurysms.

The extent of the artifact produced by an aneurysm clip will have a direct effect on the diagnostic aspects of the MR procedure. Therefore, an investigation was conducted to characterize artifacts associated with aneurysm clips made from nonferromagnetic or weakly ferromagnetic materials. Five different aneurysm clips made from five different materials were evaluated in this investigation, as follows:

1) Yasargil, Phynox (Aesculap, Inc., Central Valley, PA),
2) Yasargil, titanium alloy (Aesculap, Inc., Central Valley, PA),
3) Sugita, Elgiloy (Mizuho American, Inc., Beverly, MA),
4) Spetzler Titanium Aneurysm Clip, commercially pure titanium (Elekta Instruments, Inc., Atlanta, GA), and
5) Perneczky, cobalt alloy (Zepplin Chirurgishe Instrumente, Pullach, Germany).

These aneurysm clips were selected for testing because they are made from nonferromagnetic or weakly ferromagnetic materials. These aneurysm clips were previously reported to be acceptable for patients in the 1.5-Tesla MR environment and, as such, are often found in patients referred for MR procedures.

Artifact testing revealed that the size of the signal voids were directly related to the type of material (i.e. the magnetic susceptibility) used to make the particular clip. Arranged in decreasing order of artifact size, the materials responsible for the artifacts associated with the aneurysm clips were, as follows: Elgiloy (Sugita), cobalt alloy (Perneczky), Phynox (Yasargil), titanium alloy (Yasargil), and commercially pure titanium (Spetzler). These results have implications when one considers the various critical factors that are responsible for the decision to use a particular type of aneurysm clip (e.g., size, shape, closing force, biocompatibility, corrosion resistance, material-related effects on diagnostic imaging examinations, etc.).

An aneurysm clip that causes a relatively large artifact is less desirable because it can impact the diagnostic capabilities of the MR procedure if the area of interest is in the immediate location of where the aneurysm clip was implanted. Fortunately, aneurysm clips exist that are made from materials (i.e. commercially pure titanium and titanium alloy) that created minimal artifacts.

Burtscher, et al. (1998) conducted additional artifact research with the intent of determining the extent to which titanium aneurysm clips could improve the quality of MR imaging compared to stainless steel aneurysm clips and to assess whether the artifacts could be reduced by controlling MR imaging parameters. The results indicated that the use of titanium aneurysm clips reduced MR artifacts by approximately 60% compared to stainless steel aneurysm clips. MR imaging artifacts were further reduced by using spin echo pulse sequences with high bandwidths or, if necessary, gradient echo pulse sequences with a low echo times (TE).

REFERENCES

American Society for Testing and Materials (ASTM) Designation: F 2052. Standard test method for measurement of magnetically induced displacement force on passive implants in the magnetic resonance environment. ASTM, West Conshohocken, PA.

Becker RL, Norfray JF, Teitelbaum GP, et al. MR imaging in patients with intracranial aneurysm clips. Am J Roentgenol 1988;9:885-889.

Brothers MF, et al. MR imaging after surgery for vertebrobasilar aneurysm. Am J Neuroradiol 1990;11:149-161.

Brown MA, Carden JA, Coleman RE, et al. Magnetic field effects on surgical ligation clips. Magnetic Resonance Imaging 1987;5:443-453.

Burtscher IM, et al. Aneurysm clip MR artifacts. Titanium versus stainless steel and influence of imaging parameters. Acta Radiology 1998;39:70-76.

Dujovny M, et al. Aneurysm clip motion during magnetic resonance imaging: In vivo experimental study with metallurgical factor analysis. Neurosurgery 1985;17:543-548.

FDA stresses the need for caution during MR scanning of patients with aneurysm clips. In: Medical Devices Bulletin, Center for Devices and Radiological Health. March, 1993;11:1-2.

Johnson GC. Need for caution during MR imaging of patients with aneurysm clips [Letter]. Radiology 1993;188:287.

Kakizawa Y, et al. Cerebral aneurysm clips in the 3-tesla magnetic field. Laboratory investigation. J Neurosurg 2010;113:859-69.

Expert Panel on MR Safety, Kanal E, Barkovich AJ, Bell C, et al. ACR guidance document on MR safe practices: 2013. J Magn Reson Imag 2013;37:501-30.

Kanal E, Shellock FG. MR imaging of patients with intracranial aneurysm clips. Radiology 1993;187:612-614.

Kanal E, Shellock FG. Aneurysm clips: Effects of long-term and multiple exposures to a 1.5-Tesla MR system. Radiology 1999;210:563-565.

Kanal E, Shellock FG, Lewin JS. Aneurysm clip testing for ferromagnetic properties: Clip variability issues. Radiology 1996;200:576-578.

Kangarlu A, Shellock FG. Aneurysm clips: Evaluation of magnetic field interactions with an 8.0-T MR system. J Magn Reson Imag 2000;12:107-111.

Khursheed F, et al. Artifact quantification and tractography from 3T MRI after placement of aneurysm clips in subarachnoid hemorrhage patients. BMC Med Imaging 2011;11:19.

Klucznik RP, et al. Placement of a ferromagnetic intracerebral aneurysm clip in a magnetic field with a fatal outcome. Radiology 1993;187:855-856.

Lauer UA, et al. Radio frequency versus susceptibility effects of small conductive implants-a systematic MRI study on aneurysm clips at 1.5 and 3 T. Magnetic Resonance Imaging 2005;23:563-9.

McFadden JT. Magnetic resonance imaging and aneurysm clips. J Neurosurg 2012;117:1-11.

New PFJ, et al. Potential hazards and artifacts of ferromagnetic and nonferromagnetic surgical and dental materials and devices in nuclear magnetic resonance imaging. Radiology 1983;147:139-148.

Olsrud J, et al. Magnetic resonance imaging artifacts caused by aneurysm clips and shunt valves: Dependence on field strength (1.5 and 3 T) and imaging parameters. J Magn Reson Imag 2005;22:433-7.

Pride GL, et al. Safety of MR scanning in patients with nonferromagnetic aneurysm clips. J Magn Reson Imag 2000;12:198-200.

Shellock FG, Crues JV, Editors. MRI Bioeffects, Safety, and Patient Management. Biomedical Research Publishing Group, Los Angeles, CA, 2014.

Shellock FG. Biomedical implants and devices: Assessment of magnetic field interactions with a 3.0-Tesla MR system. J Magn Reson Imag 2002;16:721-732.

Shellock FG, et al. Aneurysm clips: Evaluation of magnetic field interactions and translational attraction using "long-bore" and "short-bore" 3.0-Tesla MR systems. American Journal of Neuroradiology 2003;24:463-471.

Shellock FG, Crues JV. High-field strength MR imaging and metallic biomedical implants: An *ex vivo* evaluation of deflection forces. Am J Roentgenol 1988;151:389-392.

Shellock FG, Crues JV. Aneurysm clips: Assessment of magnetic field interaction associated with a 0.2-T extremity MR system. Radiology 1998;208:407-409.

Shellock FG, Kanal E. Aneurysm clips: Evaluation of MR imaging artifacts at 1.5-Tesla. Radiology 1998;209:563-566.

Shellock FG, Kanal E. Yasargil aneurysm clips: Evaluation of interactions with a 1.5-Tesla MR system. Radiology 1998;207:587-591.

Shellock FG, Shellock VJ. MR-compatibility evaluation of the Spetzler titanium aneurysm clip. Radiology 1998;206:838-841.

Shellock FG. Valencerina S. *In vitro* evaluation of MR imaging issues at 3-T for aneurysm clips made from MP35N: Findings and information applied to 155 additional aneurysm clips. Am J Neuroradiol 2010;31:615-619.

Argus II Retinal Prosthesis System

The MRI labeling for the Argus II Retinal Prosthesis System (Second Sight Medical Products, Inc., www.2-sight.com) is, as follows:

WARNINGS

The Argus II Implant has been classified as an MR Conditional device. Individuals with an Argus II Implant may undergo a magnetic resonance imaging (MRI) procedure ONLY if it is performed using a 1.5 or 3.0 Tesla MRI System and ONLY following the MRI Instructions provided later in this insert. Individuals with an Argus II Implant should not enter a room housing an MRI System that has a rating other than 1.5 or 3.0 Tesla, even if the Argus II System is not being used. The external equipment (i.e. the VPU and glasses) should remain outside the MR system room, as severe harm to people in the MR system room could occur. If any pain is experienced during the MRI procedure the patient should be instructed to notify the technician immediately.

Information about Specific Procedures

Magnetic Resonance Imaging (MRI) – Refer to the Warnings section above and the MRI Information section below for more information about MRI.

MRI INFORMATION

The Argus II Implant is MR Conditional according to the terminology specified in the American Society for Testing and Materials (ASTM) International, Designation: F2503, Standard Practice for Marking Medical Devices and Other Items for Safety in the Magnetic Resonance Environment. Non-clinical testing demonstrated that the Argus II Implant meets the MR Conditional classification.

WARNING
Do NOT take the Argus II VPU or glasses into the MR system room. The VPU and glasses are MR Unsafe. The VPU and glasses were not tested in the MRI environment and are not permitted to be worn by the patient in the MR system room. Severe harm to the patient and/or damage to the external equipment may occur.

An individual with an Argus II Implant may safely undergo an MRI procedure under the conditions specified below:

- Static magnetic field of 1.5-Tesla or 3-Tesla
- Maximum spatial gradient magnetic field of 720-gauss/cm
- Maximum MR system reported, whole body averaged specific absorption rate (SAR) of 2-W/kg for 15 minutes of scanning (i.e. per pulse sequence)
- Normal Operating Mode of operation for the MR system

MRI-Related Heating, 1.5-Tesla

In non-clinical testing, the Argus II Implant produced the following temperature rise during MRI performed for 15-min of scanning (i.e. per pulse sequence) in the 1.5-Tesla (1.5-Tesla/64-MHz, Symphony, Siemens Medical Solutions, Erlangen, Germany) MR system: Highest temperature change was +0.6°C.

Therefore, the MRI-related heating for the Argus II Implant at 1.5-Tesla using a transmit/receive RF body coil at an MR system reported whole body averaged SAR of 3.5-W/kg indicated that the greatest amount of heating that occurred in association with these specific conditions was equal to or less than +0.6°C.

MRI-Related Heating, 3-Tesla

In non-clinical testing, the Argus II Implant produced the following temperature rise during MRI performed for 15-min of scanning (i.e. per pulse sequence) in a 3-Tesla (3-Tesla/128-MHz, Excite, HDx, Software 14X.M5, General Electric Healthcare, Milwaukee, WI) MR system: Highest temperature change was +2.1°C.

Therefore, the MRI-related heating for the Argus II Implant at 3-Tesla using a transmit/receive RF body coil at an MR system reported whole body averaged SAR of 2.9-W/kg indicated that the greatest amount of heating that occurred in association with these specific conditions was equal to or less than +2.1°C.

Artifact Information

MR image quality may be compromised if the area of interest is in the exact same area or relatively close to the position of the Argus II Implant. Therefore, optimization of MR imaging parameters to compensate for the presence of the implant may be necessary.

During the MRI Procedure

The MRI technologist should tell the patient to notify the MRI system operator if pain or unusual sensation occurs during the MRI examination. If the patient experiences any pain or unusual sensation, the MRI procedure should be stopped immediately and the source of the problem should be investigated.

Device Functionality

In non-clinical MRI tests, the Argus II implant was exposed to eight different pulse sequences using 1.5-T/64MHz (Symphony, Siemens Medical Solution, Erlangen, Germany) and 3.0-T/128MHz (Excite, HDx, Software 14X.M5, General Electric Healthcare, Milwaukee, WI) MR systems. The results indicated that exposing the Argus II implant to these MRI conditions did not damage or alter the function of the device nor did it have adverse effects on the device's functionality. However, it is strongly recommended that the Argus II Implant be tested by a qualified clinician or Second Sight personnel as soon as possible following an MRI procedure to confirm that it is still functioning properly.

Additional MRI labeling information exists. Contact Second Sight Medical Products, Inc., www.2-sight.com for more information.

[MR healthcare professionals are advised to contact the respective manufacturer in order to obtain the latest safety information to ensure patient safety relative to the use of an MR procedure.]

REFERENCES

Castaldi E, et al. Visual BOLD response in late blind subjects with Argus II Retinal Prosthesis. PLoS Biol 2016;14:e1002569.

Second Sight Medical Products, Inc., www.2-sight.com

Weiland JD, Faraji B, Greenberg RJ, Humayun MS, Shellock FG. Assessment of MRI issues for the Argus II retinal prosthesis. Magnetic Resonance Imaging 2012;30:382-389.

Baha, Bone Conduction Implant

The Baha, Bone Conduction Implant is MR Conditional. Comprehensive labeling information must be reviewed to ensure patient safety.

Carefully review the latest MRI labeling conditions and guidelines at: www.cochlear.com.

Note to MR Healthcare Professionals: Different MRI guidelines exist for different countries. Therefore, use the appropriate information for your country.

[MR healthcare professionals are advised to contact the respective manufacturer in order to obtain the latest safety information to ensure patient safety relative to the use of an MR procedure.]

REFERENCE

www.cochlear.com

Biopsy Needles, Markers, and Devices

Magnetic resonance (MR) imaging may be used to guide tissue biopsy and apply markers. These specialized procedures require tools that are acceptable for use with MR systems. Many commercially available biopsy needles, markers, and devices (e.g., guidewires, stylets, marking wires, marking clips, biopsy guns, etc.) have undergone MRI evaluations with respect to safety issues and artifacts. The results indicated that many of the commercially available tools are not useful for MR-guided biopsy procedures due to the presence of excessive ferromagnetism and the associated artifacts that may limit or obscure the area of interest. Fortunately, several needles, markers, and devices have been developed using materials with low magnetic susceptibility specifically for utilization in MR-guided procedures.

Although most of the biopsy guns tested for magnetic field interactions and artifacts were found to be ferromagnetic, since these are not used in the immediate area of the target tissue, artifacts associated with these devices are unlikely to affect the resulting images during MR-guided biopsy procedures. Nevertheless, the presence of ferromagnetism may preclude the optimal use of most various guns or similar devices in the MR environment, especially at 3-Tesla. Currently, there are several commercially available biopsy devices, including vacuum-assisted systems, that have been developed specifically for use in MR-guided procedures.

REFERENCES

Causer PA, Piron CA, Jong RA, et al. MR imaging-guided breast localization system with medial or lateral access. Radiology 2006;240:369-79.

Chen X, et al. MRI-guided breast biopsy: Clinical experience with 14-gauge stainless steel core biopsy needle. Am J Roentgenol 2004;182:1075-80.

Daniel BL, et al. An MRI-compatible semiautomated vacuum-assisted breast biopsy system: Initial feasibility study. J Magn Reson Imag 2005;21:637-44.

Hall WA, Galicich W, Bergman T, Truwit CL. 3-Tesla intraoperative MR imaging for neurosurgery. J Neurooncol 2006;77:297-303.

Karacozoff AM, Shellock FG. Fiducial marker for lung lesion: *In vitro* assessment of MRI issues at 3-Tesla. Am J Roentgenol 2013;200:1234-7.

Kerimaa P, et al. MRI-guided biopsy and fine needle aspiration biopsy (FNAB) in the diagnosis of musculoskeletal lesions. Eur J Radiol 2013;82:2328-33.

Lehman CD, et al. MR imaging-guided breast biopsy using a coaxial technique with a 14-gauge stainless steel core biopsy needle and a titanium sheath. Am J Roentgenol 2003;181:183-5.

Lewin JS, et al. Needle localization in MR-guided biopsy and aspiration: Effect of field strength, sequence design, and magnetic field orientation. Am J Roentgenol 1996;166:1337-1341.

Lufkin R, Layfield L. Coaxial needle system of MR- and CT-guided aspiration cytology. J Computer Assist Tomogr 1989;13:1105-1107.

Lufkin R, Teresi L, Hanafee W. New needle for MR-guided aspiration cytology of the head and neck. Am J Roentgenol 1987;149:380-382.

Moscatel M, Shellock FG, Morisoli S. Biopsy needles and devices: Assessment of ferromagnetism and artifacts during exposure to a 1.5-Tesla MR system. J Magn Reson Imag 1995;5:369-372.

Shellock FG, Cronenweth C. Assessment of MRI issues at 3-Tesla for a new metallic tissue marker. International Journal of Breast Cancer 2015;823759.

Shellock FG, Crues JV, Editors. MRI Bioeffects, Safety, and Patient Management. Biomedical Research Publishing Group, Los Angeles, CA, 2014.

Shellock FG, Kanal E. Magnetic Resonance: Bioeffects, Safety, and Patient Management. Second Edition, Lippincott-Raven Press, New York, 1996.

Shellock FG, Shellock VJ. Additional information pertaining to the MR-compatibility of biopsy needles and devices. J Magn Reson Imag 1996;6:411.

Shellock FG, Shellock VJ. Metallic marking clips used after stereotactic breast biopsy: *Ex vivo* testing of ferromagnetism, heating, and artifacts associated with MRI. Am J Roentgenol 1999;172:1417-1419.

Thomas C, et al. Carbon fibre and nitinol needles for MRI-guided interventions: First *in vitro* and *in vivo* application. Eur J Radiol 2011;79:353- 358.

Veltman J, et al. Magnetic resonance-guided biopsies and localizations of the breast: Initial experiences using an open breast coil and compatible intervention device. Invest Radiol 2005;40:379-84.

Zangos S, et al. MR-compatible assistance system for punction in a high-field system: Device and feasibility of transgluteal biopsies of the prostate gland. Eur Radiol 2007;17:1118-24.

Bone Fusion Stimulator/Spinal Fusion Stimulator

The implantable bone fusion or spinal fusion stimulator is designed for use as an adjunct therapy to a spinal fusion procedure.

The SpF-XL IIb and SpF PLUS-Mini Implantable Spinal Fusion Stimulators (EBI, LLC and Biomet, Inc.) are MR Conditional at 1.5-Tesla/64-MHz. Comprehensive labeling information must be reviewed to ensure patient safety.

Carefully review the latest MRI labeling conditions and guidelines at: www.biomet.com.

[MR healthcare professionals are advised to contact the respective manufacturer in order to obtain the latest safety information to ensure patient safety relative to the use of an MR procedure.]

REFERENCES

Chou C-K, McDougall JA, Chan KW. RF heating of implanted spinal fusion stimulator during magnetic resonance imaging. IEEE Trans Biomed Engineering 1997;44:357-373.

Shellock FG, Crues JV, Editors. MRI Bioeffects, Safety, and Patient Management. Biomedical Research Publishing Group, Los Angeles, CA, 2014.

Shellock FG, Hatfield M, Simon BJ, Block S, Wamboldt J, Starewicz PM, Punchard WFB. Implantable spinal fusion stimulator: Assessment of MRI safety. J Magn Reson Imag 2000;12:214-223.

www.biomet.com

Bravo pH Monitoring System

Indications for Use. The Bravo pH Monitoring System with Accessories (Medtronic, Inc. and Given Imaging) is intended for measurement of gastroesophageal pH and monitoring gastric reflux. The pH probe (capsule) can be delivered and placed endoscopically or with standard manometric procedures. The pH Software Analysis Program is intended to record, store, view and analyze gastroesophageal pH data.

Warnings and Precautions. Potential complications associated with gastrointestinal endoscopy include but are not limited to: perforation, hemorrhage, aspiration, fever, infection, hypertension, respiratory arrest, cardiac arrhythmia or arrest. Potential complications associated with nasal intubation include but are not limited to: sore throat, trauma to nasopharynx or bloody nose. Complications associated with the Bravo System include premature detachment of the capsule, failure of the capsule to slough off in a timely period, or discomfort associated with the capsule requiring endoscopic removal.

The Bravo pH Capsule with Delivery System is a single use, disposable device. Reuse or any other misuse of a Bravo pH Capsule with Delivery System will result in an increased potential for damage to the device and ancillary equipment.

Prior to use, all equipment for the procedure should be examined carefully to verify proper function.

MRI Information
Patients are restricted from undergoing an MRI study within 30 days of the Bravo procedure.

[MR healthcare professionals are advised to contact the respective manufacturer in order to obtain the latest safety information to ensure patient safety relative to the use of an MR procedure.]

REFERENCES

www.givenimaging.com
www.medtronic.com

Breast Tissue Expanders and Implants

Adjustable breast tissue expanders and mammary implants are utilized for breast reconstruction following mastectomy, for the correction of breast and chest-wall deformities and underdevelopment, for tissue defect procedures, and for cosmetic augmentation. These devices are typically equipped with either an integral injection site or a remote injection dome that is utilized to accept a needle for placement of saline for expansion of the prosthesis intra-operatively and/or postoperatively.

There are many different types of breast tissue expanders. For example, the Becker and the Siltex prostheses provide a choice of a standard injection dome or a micro-injection dome. The Radovan expander is indicated for temporary implantation only. The injection port for this device contains 316L stainless steel to guard against piercing the injection port by the needle used to fill the implant. In this case, 316L stainless steel does not pose a serious hazard for a patient undergoing MRI.

Notably, there are various breast tissue expanders that have *magnetic* ports to allow for a more accurate detection of the injection site. These devices are substantially attracted to the static magnetic fields of MR systems and, therefore, may be uncomfortable, injurious, or contraindicated for patients undergoing MR procedures. One such device is the Contour Profile Tissue Expander (Mentor, Santa Barbara, CA), which contains a magnetic injection dome and is considered to be unsafe (i.e. MR Unsafe) for an MR examination.

Breast tissue expanders with magnetic ports produce relatively large artifacts on MR images and, therefore, assessment of the breast using MRI is problematic. Various manufacturers make these particular implants.

Importantly, there may be a situation during which a patient is referred for MR imaging for the determination of breast cancer or a breast implant rupture, such that the presence of the metallic artifact could obscure the precise location of the abnormality. In view of this possibility, it is recommended that a patient with a breast tissue expander that has a metallic component be identified prior to MRI so that the radiologist is aware of the potential problems related to the generation of artifacts as well as a possible injury

McGhan Medical Breast Tissue Expanders and MRI Issues. McGhan Medical Breast Tissue Expanders are intended for temporary subcutaneous implantation to develop surgical flaps and additional tissue coverage (Product Information documents, McGhan Medical/INAMED Aesthetics; Allergan, Inc.). These breast tissue expanders are constructed from silicone elastomer and consist of an expansion envelope with a textured surface, and a MAGNA-SITE integrated injection site. The expanders are available in a wide range of styles and sizes to meet diverse surgical needs. Specific styles include: Style 133 FV with MAGNA-SITE injection site, Style 133 LV with MAGNA-SITE injection site, Style 133 MV with MAGNA-SITE injection site, and Style 133 V with MAGNA-SITE injection site.

The MAGNA-SITE injection site and MAGNA-FINDER external locating device contain rare-earth, permanent magnets for an accurate injection system. When the MAGNA-FINDER is passed over the surface of the tissue being expanded, its rare-earth, permanent magnet indicates the location of the MAGNA-SITE injection site.

The Product Information documents for these breast tissue expanders states: "DO NOT use MAGNA-SITE expanders in patients who already have implanted devices that would be affected by a magnetic field (e.g., pacemakers, drug infusion devices, artificial sensing devices). DO NOT perform diagnostic testing with Magnetic Resonance Imaging (MRI) in patients with MAGNA-SITE expanders in place."

Furthermore, in the Warnings section of the Product Information document, the following is indicated: "Diagnostic testing with Magnetic Resonance Imaging (MRI) is contraindicated in patients with MAGNA-SITE expanders in place. The MRI equipment could cause movement of the MAGNA-SITE breast tissue expander, and result in not only patient discomfort, but also expander displacement, requiring revision surgery. In addition, the MAGNA-SITE magnet could interfere with MRI detection capabilities."

Therefore, MR procedures are deemed unsafe for patients with these specific breast tissue expanders.

Zegzula and Lee (2001) presented a case of bilateral tissue expander infusion port dislodgment associated with an MRI examination. The report involved a 56-year-old woman that underwent bilateral mastectomy and immediate reconstruction with McGhan BIOSPAN tissue expanders. As noted, these implants contain the "MAGNA-SITE" components. Several weeks postoperatively the patient underwent MR imaging of her spine. Subsequently, the infusion ports could not be located with the finder magnet (used to re-fill the tissue expander). A chest radiograph was obtained that demonstrated bilateral dislodgment of the infusion ports. Surgical removal and replacement of the tissue expanders were required. This incident emphasizes that all patients undergoing tissue expansion with implants that contain magnetic ports should be thoroughly warned about the potential hazards of MRI and managed appropriately.

In another incident involving a tissue expander, Duffy and May (1995) reported a case of a woman who developed a burning sensation at the site of the tissue expander during an MR procedure. The sensation resolved rapidly once the scan was discontinued. The implications of the symptoms in this case are unclear.

By comparison, a study conducted by Thimmappa, et al. (2016) indicated that it is possible to safely perform MRI exams safely at 1.5-Tesla in patients with certain breast tissue expanders by following special precautions. Nevertheless, a patient with a tissue expander that requires an MR procedure should be alerted to the possibility of localized symptoms in the region of the implant during scanning as well as other possible problems related to exposure to the powerful static magnetic field of the MR system.

Breast Tissue Expander with Remote Port. A recent investigation performed by Linnemeyer H, et al. (2014) evaluated MRI issues (i.e. magnetic field interactions, heating, and artifacts) at 3-Tesla for a breast tissue expander with a remote port. The breast tissue expander, Integra Breast Tissue Expander, (Model 3612-06 with Standard Remote Port, PMT Corporation, Chanhassen, MN) underwent evaluations for magnetic field interactions (translational attraction and torque), MRI-related heating, and artifacts using standardized techniques. The findings indicated that a patient with this breast tissue expander with a remote port may safely undergo MRI at 3-Tesla or less under the conditions used for this investigation.

Importantly, the findings reported by Linnemeyer H, et al. (2014) are highly specific to the particular tissue expander with remote port that underwent testing and the MR conditions that were used for the evaluation. Other similar products exist from various manufacturers but it is unknown how these devices respond relative to the use of MRI.

REFERENCES

Duffy FJ Jr, May JW Jr. Tissue expanders and magnetic resonance imaging: The "hot" breast implant. Ann Plast Surg 1995;5:647-9.

Fagan LL, Shellock FG, Brenner RJ, Rothman B. *Ex vivo* evaluation of ferromagnetism, heating, and artifacts of breast tissue expanders exposed to a 1.5-T MR system. J Magn Reson Imag 1995;5:614-616.

Liang MD, Narayanan K, Kanal E. Magnetic ports in tissue expanders: A caution for MRI. Magnetic Resonance Imaging 1989;7:541-542.

Linnemeyer H, Shellock FG, Ahn CY. *In vitro* assessment of MRI issues at 3-Tesla for a breast tissue expander with a remote port. Magn Reson Imaging 2014;32:297-302.

Nava MB, et al. Effects of the magnetic resonance field on breast tissue expanders. Aesthetic Plast Surg 2012;36:901-7.

Product Information, Style 133 Family of Breast Tissue Expanders with Magna-Site Injection Sites, McGhan Medical/INAMED Aesthetics, Santa Barbara, CA.

Product Information, Directions for Use, Style 133V Series Tissue Expander Matrix, With Magna-Site Injection Sites, Allergan, Inc.

Thimmappa ND, Shellock FG, Giangarra C, Ahan CY, Prince MR, Levine JL. Breast tissue expanders with magnetic ports: *In vitro* testing and clinical experience at 1.5-Tesla Proceedings of the International Society for Magnetic Resonance in Medicine 2013;21:3456.

Thimmappa ND, et al. Breast tissue expanders with magnetic ports: Clinical experience at 1.5 T. Plastic and Reconstructive Surgery 2016:1171-78.

Zegzula HD, Lee WP. Infusion port dislodgment of bilateral breast tissue expanders after MRI. Ann Plast Surg 2001;46:46-8.

Cardiac Pacemakers and Implantable Cardioverter Defibrillators

Cardiac pacemakers and implantable cardioverter defibrillators (ICDs) are crucial implanted devices for patients with heart conditions and serve to maintain quality of life and substantially reduce morbidity. Expanded indications for cardiac pacemakers and ICDs (e.g., heart failure, obstructive sleep apnea, and other conditions) emphasize that an increasing number of patients will be treated with these devices. Currently, these cardiovascular implants are considered a relative contraindication for patients referred for MR procedures. Additionally, individuals with cardiac pacemakers and ICDs should be prevented from entering the MR environment because of potential risks unless, of course, the cardiac device is MR Conditional.

Conventional cardiac pacemakers and ICDs have been suggested to present potential problems to patients undergoing MR procedures from various mechanisms, including:

1) Movement and/or vibration of the pulse generator or lead(s)
2) Temporary or permanent modification of the function (i.e. damage) of the device
3) Inappropriate sensing, triggering, or activation of the device
4) Excessive heating of the leads
5) Induced currents in the leads
6) Electromagnetic interference

The effects of the MR environment and MR procedures on the functional and operational aspects of cardiac pacemakers and ICDs vary, depending on several factors including the type of device, how the device is programmed, the static magnetic field strength of the MR system, and the imaging conditions used for the procedure (i.e. the anatomic region imaged relative to the transmit RF coil, type of transmit RF coil used, the pulse sequence, amount of radiofrequency energy used, etc.). Notably, much of the data concerning the deleterious effects of MRI on cardiac pacemakers involved the use of older versions (i.e. pre-1996) of these devices.

Many compelling reports have been published concerning "modern-day" pacemakers (i.e. devices with decreased ferromagnetic components and more sophisticated circuitry) that indicate that certain patients may undergo MR examinations without harmful effects by following specific guidelines to minimize or prevent risks. Thus, there is evidence that it may be possible to perform MR procedures safely in patients with cardiovascular devices under highly controlled conditions (see below). Alternatively, as previously mentioned, MR Conditional cardiac pacing systems now exist that were specifically-designed to provide a high margin of safety for patients referred for MR procedures. Some of these cardiac devices are approved for both 1.5-Tesla and 3-Tesla scanners.

Implantable cardioverter defibrillators (ICDs) are medical devices designed to automatically detect and treat episodes of ventricular fibrillation, ventricular tachycardias, bradycardia, and other conditions. When a problem is identified, the device can deliver defibrillation, cardioversion, antitachycardia pacing, bradycardia pacing, or other therapy.

In general, exposure to an MR system or to an MR procedure has similar effects on an ICD as those previously described for a cardiac pacemaker. However, there are several unique aspects of ICDs that impact the possible safe performance of MR procedures in patients with these devices. Therefore, patients and individuals with these cardiac devices are generally not allowed to enter the MR environment. In addition, since ICDs have electrodes placed in the myocardium, patients are typically not permitted to undergo MR examinations because of the inherent risks related to the presence of these conductive materials.

Similar to cardiac pacemakers, it is anticipated that, in lieu of developing a truly acceptable ICD for the MR environment, safety criteria may be determined for "modern-day" ICDs that entail using specialized programming, monitoring procedures, and MR conditions to allow patients to undergo MR examinations safely. Several studies have described patients with ICDs examined by MR imaging without serious problems with the caveat that ICDs, in fact, tend to be more problematic than pacemakers relative to the use of MR examinations. Notably, potential problems remain even for "modern" cardiac pacemakers and ICDs as indicated by reports by Gimbel (2009) and Mollerus, et al. (2009), such that extreme caution must be exercised when scanning patients with these devices. Alternatively, as previously mentioned, MR Conditional ICDs now exist that were specifically-designed for patients referred for MR procedures, including those that are approved for use with 1.5-Tesla and 3-Tesla MR systems.

Evidence for Performing MR Procedures Safely in Nonpacemaker Dependent Patients

Harmful effects related to performing MRI procedures in patients with cardiac pacemakers have been documented. In virtually every case involving a fatality, the patient apparently entered the MR environment without the staff knowing a conventional cardiac pacemaker was present. Importantly, these deaths were poorly characterized, no electrocardiographic findings were available for review, it was unknown whether these patients were pacemaker dependent, and the actual causes or mechanisms of death were not confirmed or otherwise verified. By comparison, no irreversible harm has been reported when patients with cardiac pacemakers were carefully monitored during MR procedures and/or the devices underwent programming prior to the scans.

Regardless of the known hazards of subjecting a patient with a cardiac pacemaker to the MR environment, numerous patients (3,000+, Unpublished observations, various investigators) have now undergone MR imaging during purposeful, monitored procedures performed for necessary diagnostic examinations. These patients were safely and successfully imaged using MR systems operating at static magnetic fields ranging from 0.2- to 3-Tesla without serious adverse events.

In consideration of the above, there is evidence from *in vitro*, laboratory, and clinical studies that strict restrictions prohibiting MR procedures in patients with "modern" cardiac pacemakers and ICDs should be reconsidered. Similar to performing MR procedures in patients with other "active" devices (e.g., bone fusion stimulators, cochlear implants, neurostimulation systems, programmable injusion pumps, etc.), scanning patients with cardiac pacemakers and ICDs involves following highly specific procedures to ensure patient safety.

Interestingly, a study by Gimbel (2008) reported scanning patients with cardiac pacemakers at 3-Tesla with no restrictions placed on pacemaker dependency, region scanned, device type, or manufacturer. This limited experience suggested that patients may undergo carefully tailored 3-Tesla MRI examinations when pre-MRI programming of the device occurs in conjunction with extensive monitoring, supervision, and follow-up.

Guidelines for Performing MRI in Nonpacemaker Dependent Patients

Guidelines have been presented by Martin, et al. (2004), Roquin, et al. (2004), Loewy, et al. (2004), the American College of Radiology (2007) and the American College of Cardiology/American Heart Association (2007) and others with regard to performing MR procedures in nonpacemaker dependent patients. These guidelines include, the following:

- Establish a risk-benefit ratio for the patient
- Obtain written and verbal informed consent
- Pretest pacemaker functions using appropriate equipment outside of the MR environment
- A cardiologist/electrophysiologist should decide whether it is necessary to program the pacemaker prior to the MR examination
- A cardiologist/electrophysiologist with Advanced Cardiac Life Support (ACLS) training must be in attendance for the entire MRI examination
- The patient should be monitored continuously during the MR procedure using proper procedures and technology (e.g., blood pressure, pulse rate, oxygen saturation, and ECG)
- Appropriate personnel, a crash cart, and a defibrillator must be available throughout the procedure to address an adverse event
- Maintain visual and voice contact throughout the procedure with the patient
- Instruct the patient to alert the MR system operator of any unusual sensations or problems so that, if necessary, the MR system operator can immediately terminate the procedure
- After the MRI examination, a cardiologist/electrophysiologist should interrogate the pacemaker to confirm that the function is consistent with the pre-MR procedure state

Magnetic Field Interactions at 1.5- and 3-Tesla for Cardiac Pacemakers and ICDs

As previously discussed, one important safety aspect of the MR environment on cardiac pacemakers and ICDs is related to magnetic field interactions. Component parts of pacemakers and ICDs, such as batteries, reed-switches, or transformer core materials may contain ferromagnetic materials. Therefore, substantial magnetic field interactions may exist, causing these implants to move or be uncomfortable for patients or individuals. Therefore, as an important part of evaluating pacemakers and ICDs, tests for magnetic field interactions have been conducted using MR systems operating at static magnetic field strengths ranging from 0.2-Tesla (i.e. the dedicated-extremity MR system) to 3-Tesla.

Luechinger, et al. (2001) investigated magnetic field interactions for thirty-one cardiac pacemakers and thirteen ICDs in association with exposure to a 1.5-Tesla MR system (Gyroscan ACS NT, Philips Medical

Systems, Best, The Netherlands). The investigators reported that "newer" cardiac pacemakers had relatively low magnetic force values compared to older devices. With regard to ICDs, with the exception of one newer model (GEM II, 7273 ICD, Medtronic, Inc.), all ICDs showed relatively high magnetic field interactions. Luechinger, et al. concluded that modern-day pacemakers present no safety risk with respect to magnetic field interactions at 1.5-Tesla, while ICDs could pose problems due to strong magnet-related mechanical forces.

The use of 3-Tesla MR systems for brain, musculoskeletal, body, cardiovascular, and other applications has become routine in many clinical settings. Because previous investigations performed to determine MR safety for pacemakers and ICDs used MR systems with static magnetic fields of 1.5-Tesla or less, it is crucial to perform *ex vivo* testing at 3-Tesla to characterize magnetic field-related safety for these implants, with full appreciation that additional safety issues exist for these devices, as described-above.

A critical aspect of determining magnetic field interactions for metallic implants involves the measurement of translational attraction. Translational attraction is assessed for metallic implants using the standardized deflection angle test recommended by the American Society for Testing and Materials (ASTM) International. According to ASTM International guidelines, the deflection angle for an implant or device is generally measured at the point of the "highest spatial gradient" for the specific MR system used for testing. Notably, the deflection angle test is commonly performed as an integral part of safety testing for metallic implants and devices.

Various types of magnets exist for commercially available 1.5- and 3-Tesla MR systems, including magnet configurations that are used for conventional "long-bore" scanners and newer "short-bore" systems. Because of physical differences in the position and magnitude of the highest spatial gradient for different magnets, measurements of deflection angles for implants using long-bore vs. short-bore MR systems can produce substantially different results for magnetic field-related translational attraction, as reported by Shellock, et al. (2003).

The implications are primarily for magnetic field-related translational attraction with regard to long-bore vs. short-bore 3-Tesla MR systems (with short-bore scanners producing greater translational attraction for a given implant). Therefore, a study was conducted on fourteen different cardiac pacemakers and four ICDs to evaluate translational attraction for these devices in association with long-bore and short-bore 1.5- and 3-

Tesla MR systems. Deflection angles were measured based on guidelines from the ASTM International.

In general, deflection angles for the cardiovascular implants that underwent evaluation were significantly ($p<0.01$) higher on 1.5- and 3-Tesla short-bore scanners compared to long-bore MR systems. For the 1.5-Tesla MR systems, three cardiac pacemakers (Cosmos, Model 283-01 Pacemaker, Intermedics, Inc., Freeport, TX; Nova Model 281-01 Pacemaker, Intermedics, Inc., Freeport, TX; Res-Q ACE, Model 101-01 Pacemaker; Intermedics, Inc., Freeport, TX) exhibited deflection angles greater than 45 degrees (i.e. exceeding the recommended ASTM International criteria) on both long-bore and short-bore 1.5-Tesla MR systems. The findings indicated that these devices are potentially problematic for patients from a magnetic field interaction consideration.

With regard to the 3-Tesla MR systems, seven implants exhibited deflection angles greater than 45 degrees on the long-bore 3-Tesla scanner, while 13 exhibited deflection angles greater than 45 degrees on the short-bore 3-T MR system (refer to **The List** for information on the cardiac pacemakers and ICDs that underwent testing). Importantly, the findings for magnetic field-related translational attraction were substantially different comparing the long-bore (i.e. lower values) and short-bore (i.e. higher values) MR systems.

As stated, other factors exist that may impact MRI issues for these conventional cardiac pacemakers and ICDs. Therefore, regardless of the fact that magnetic field interactions may not present a risk for some of the cardiovascular devices that have been tested, the other potentially hazardous mechanisms must also be considered carefully for these devices.

MR Conditional Cardiac Devices

As a result of considerable design changes, many MR Conditional cardiac pacing systems and implantable cardioverter defibrillators (ICDs, as well as cardiac monitors, are available for patients referred for MR examinations including those manufacturered by Abbott/St.Jude Medical, Biotronic, Boston Scientific, Medtronic, Inc., and Sorin/LivaNova. For additional information pertaining to these MR Conditional cardiac devices, please refer to the pertinent sections in this textbook and visit the websites of the aforementioned manufacturers. For those interested in the latest comprehensive information on this important topic, please refer to the recent publication, "2017 HRS expert consensus statement on magnetic resonance imaging and radiation exposure in patients with cardiovascular implantable electronic devices" (Indik JH, et al. 2017).

Important Note to MR Healthcare Professionals: Different MRI guidelines may exist for different countries. Therefore, use the appropriate information for your country.

[MR healthcare professionals are advised to contact the respective manufacturer in order to obtain the latest safety information to ensure patient safety relative to the use of an MR procedure.]

REFERENCES

Acha MR, et al. Increased perforation risk with an MRI-conditional pacing lead: A single-center study. Pacing Clin Electrophysiol 2015;38:334-42.

Achenbach S, et al. Effects of magnetic resonance imaging on cardiac pacemakers and electrodes. Am Heart J 1997;134:467-473.

Ahmed FZ, et al. Not all pacemakers are created equal: MRI conditional pacemaker and lead technology. J Cardiovasc Electrophysiol 2013;24:1059-65.

Ainslie M, et al. Cardiac MRI of patients with implanted electrical cardiac devices. Heart 2014;100:363-9.

Alagona P, et al. Nuclear magnetic resonance imaging in a patient with a DDD pacemaker. Pacing Clin Electrophysiol 1989;12:619 (letter).

Al-Wakeel N, et al. Cardiac MRI in patients with complex CHD following primary or secondary implantation of MRI-conditional pacemaker system. Cardiol Young 2016;26:306-14.

American Society for Testing and Materials (ASTM) Designation: F2052. Standard test method for measurement of magnetically induced displacement force on passive implants in the magnetic resonance environment. West Conshohocken, PA.

Anfinsen OG, et al. Implantable cardioverter defibrillator dysfunction during and after magnetic resonance imaging. Pacing Clin Electrophysiol 2002;25:1400-1402.

Awad K, et al. Clinical safety of the Iforia ICD System in patients subjected to thoracic spine and cardiac 1.5T MRI scanning conditions. Heart Rhythm 2015;12:2155-61.

Baikoussis NG, et al. Safety of magnetic resonance imaging in patients with implanted cardiac prostheses and metallic cardiovascular electronic devices. Ann Thorac Surg 2011;91:2006-11.

Bailey SM, et al. Magnetic resonance imaging (MRI) of the brain in pacemaker dependent patients. Pacing and Clinical Electrophysiology 2005;2:S128.

Bailey WM, et al. Clinical safety of the ProMRI pacemaker system in patients subjected to thoracic spine and cardiac 1.5-T magnetic resonance imaging scanning conditions. Heart Rhythm 2016;13(2):464-71.

Barbier T, et al. An RF-induced voltage sensor for investigating pacemaker safety in MRI. MAGMA 2014;27:539-49.

Baser K, et al. High ventricular lead impedance of a DDD pacemaker after cranial magnetic resonance imaging. Pacing Clin Electrophysiol 2012;35:e251-3.

Bertelsen L, et al. Safety of magnetic resonance scanning without monitoring of patients with pacemakers. Europace 2017;19:818-823.

Bhachu DS, Kanal E. Implantable pulse generators (pacemakers) and electrodes: Safety in the magnetic resonance imaging scanner environment. J Magn Reson Imag 2000;12:201-204.

Bhandiwad AR, et al. Cardiovascular magnetic resonance with an MR compatible pacemaker. J Cardiovasc Magn Reson 2013;15:18.

Boilson BA, et al. Safety of magnetic resonance imaging in patients with permanent pacemakers: A collaborative clinical approach. J Interv Card Electrophysiol 2012;33:59-67

Bonnet CA, Elson JJ, Fogoros RN. Accidental deactivation of the automatic implantable cardioverter defibrillator. Am Heart J 1990;3:696-697.

Bovenschulte H, et al. MRI in patients with pacemakers: Overview and procedural management. Dtsch Arztebl Int 2012;109:270-5.

Buendía F, et al. Nuclear magnetic resonance imaging in patients with cardiac pacing devices. Rev Esp Cardiol 2010;63:735-9.

Buendía F, et al. Cardiac magnetic resonance imaging at 1.5 T in patients with cardiac rhythm devices. Europace 2011;13:533-8.

Burke PT, et al. A protocol for patients with cardiovascular implantable devices undergoing magnetic resonance imaging (MRI): Should defibrillation threshold testing be performed post-(MRI). J Interv Card Electrophysiol 2010;28:59-66.

Cadieu R, et al. Central nervous system MRI and cardiac implantable electronic devices. J Neuroradiol 2017;44:1-9.

Calcagnini G, et al. *In vitro* investigation of pacemaker lead heating induced by magnetic resonance imaging: Role of implant geometry. J Magn Reson Imag 2008;28:879-86.

Chow GV, et al. MRI for patients with cardiac implantable electrical devices. Cardiol Clin 2014;32:299-304.

Cohen JD, et al. Determining the risks of magnetic resonance imaging at 1.5 Tesla for patients with pacemakers and implantable cardioverter defibrillators. Am J Cardiol 2012;110:1631-6.

Colletti PM, Shinbane JS, Shellock FG. "MR-conditional" pacemakers: The radiologist's role in multidisciplinary management. Am J Roentgenol 2011;197:W457-9.

Corzani A, et al. Clinical management of electromagnetic interferences in patients with pacemakers and implantable cardioverter-defibrillators: Review of the literature and focus on magnetic resonance conditional devices. J Cardiovasc Med 2015;16:704-13.

Dandamudi S, et al. The safety of cardiac and thoracic magnetic resonance imaging in patients with cardiac implantable electronic devices. Acad Radiol 2016;23:1498-1505.

Del Ojo JL, et al. Is magnetic resonance imaging safe in cardiac pacemaker recipients? Pacing Clin Electrophysiol 2005;28:274-8.

Duru F, et al. Pacing in magnetic resonance imaging environment: Clinical and technical considerations on compatibility. Eur Heart J 2001;22:113-124.

Duru F, Luechinger R, Candinas R. MR imaging in patients with cardiac pacemakers. Radiology 2001;219:856-858.

Erlebacher JA, Cahill PT, Pannizzo F, Knowles RJR. Effect of magnetic resonance imaging on DDD pacemakers. Am J Cardio 1986;57:437-440.

Expert Panel on MR Safety, Kanal E, Barkovich AJ, Bell C, et al. ACR guidance document on MR safe practices: 2013. J Magn Reson Imag 2013;37:501-30.

Fanourgiakis J, Kanoupakis E. Cardiac rhythm management devices in a magnetic resonance environment. Expert Rev Med Devices 2014;11:199-203.

Faris OP, Shein M. Food and Drug Administration perspective: Magnetic resonance imaging of pacemaker and implantable cardioverter-defibrillator patients. Circulation 2006;114:1232-1233.

Ferreira AM, et al. MRI-conditional pacemakers: Current perspectives. Med Devices 2014;7:115-124.

Fetter J, et al. The effects of nuclear magnetic resonance imagers on external and implantable pulse generators. Pacing Clin Electrophysiol 1984;7:720-727.

Fiek M, et al. Complete loss of ICD programmability after magnetic resonance imaging. Pacing Clin Electrophysiol 2004;27:1002-4.

Forleo GB, et al. Clinical and electrical performance of currently available MRI-safe pacing systems. Do all devices perform in the same way? Int J Cardiol 2013;167:2340-1.

Fontaine JM, et al. Rapid ventricular pacing in a pacemaker patient undergoing magnetic resonance imaging. Pacing Clin Electrophysiol 1998;21:1336-1339.

Forleo GB, et al. Safety and efficacy of a new magnetic resonance imaging-compatible pacing system: Early results of a prospective comparison with conventional dual-chamber implant outcomes. Heart Rhythm 2010;7:750-4

Friedman HL, et al. Magnetic resonance imaging in patients with recently implanted pacemakers. Pacing Clin Electrophysiol 2013;36:1090-5.

Garcia-Bolao I, et al. Magnetic resonance imaging in a patient with a dual chamber pacemaker. Acta Cardiol 1998;53:33-35.

Gimbel JR. Unexpected asystole during 3T magnetic resonance imaging of a pacemaker dependent patient with a 'modern' pacemaker. Europace 2009;11:1241-2.

Gimbel JR. Unexpected pacing inhibition upon exposure to the 3T static magnetic field prior to imaging acquisition: What is the mechanism? Heart Rhythm 2011;8:944-5.

Gimbel JR. Letter to the Editor. Pacing Clin Electrophysiol 2003;26:1.

Gimbel JR. Magnetic resonance imaging of implantable cardiac rhythm devices at 3-Tesla. Pacing Clin Electrophysiol 2008;31:795-801.

Gimbel JR. The safety of MRI scanning of pacemakers and ICDs: What are the critical elements of safe scanning? Ask me again at 10,000. Europace 2010;12:915-7.

Gimbel JR, et al. Safe performance of magnetic resonance imaging on five patients with permanent cardiac pacemakers. Pacing Clin Electrophysiol 1996;19:913-919.

Gimbel JR, et al. Outcome of magnetic resonance imaging (MRI) in selected patients with implantable cardioverter defibrillators (ICDs). Pacing Clin Electrophysiol 2005;28:270-3.

Gimbel JR, et al. Randomized trial of pacemaker and lead system for safe scanning at 1.5 Tesla. Heart Rhythm 2013;10:685-91.

Gimbel JR, et al. MRI conditional devices, safety, and access; Choose wisely and when you come to the fork in the road, take it. Pacing Clin Electrophysiol 2015;38:1373-6.

Gold MR, et al. Preclinical evaluation of implantable cardioverter-defibrillator developed for magnetic resonance imaging use. Heart Rhythm 2015;12:631-8.

Gold MR, et al. Full-body MRI in patients with an implantable cardioverter-defibrillator: Primary results of a randomized study. J Am Coll Cardiol 2015;65:2581-8.

Goldsher D, et al. Magnetic resonance imaging for patients with permanent pacemakers: Initial clinical experience. Isr Med Assoc J 2006;8:91-94.

Goldsher D, et al. Successful cervical MR scan in a patient several hours after pacemaker implantation. Pacing Clin Electrophysiol 2009;32:1355-6.

Halshtok O, et al. Pacemakers and magnetic resonance imaging: No longer an absolute contraindication when scanned correctly. Isr Med Assoc J. 2010;12:391-5.

Harden SP. MRI conditional pacemakers: The start of a new era. Br J Radiol 2011;84:773-4.

Hawryluk L, et al. The use of 1.5 T magnetic resonance imaging for therapeutic decisions in patients with cardiac implantable electronic devices and significant neurological, neurosurgical and neuro-oncology diagnostic indications. Neurol Neurochir Pol 2015;49:16-23.

Hayes DL, et al. Effect of 1.5 Tesla nuclear magnetic resonance imaging scanner on implanted permanent pacemakers. J Am Coll Cardiol 1987;10:782-786.

Heatlie G, Pennell DJ. Cardiovascular MR at 0.5-T in five patients with permanent pacemakers. J Cardiovasc Magn Reson 2007;9:15-9.

Higgins JV, et al. Safety and outcomes of magnetic resonance imaging in patients with abandoned pacemaker and defibrillator leads. Pacing Clin Electrophysiol 2014;37:1284-90.

Holmes DJ, et al. The effects of magnetic resonance imaging on implantable pulse generators. Pacing Clin Electrophysiol 1986;9:360-370.

Horwood L, et al. Magnetic resonance imaging in patients with cardiac implanted electronic devices: Focus on contraindications to magnetic resonance imaging protocols. Europace 2017;19:812-817.

Inbar S, et al. Case report: Nuclear magnetic resonance imaging in a patient with a pacemaker. Am J Med Sci 1993;3:174-175.

Indik JH, et al. 2017 HRS expert consensus statement on magnetic resonance imaging and radiation exposure in patients with cardiovascular implantable electronic devices. Heart Rhythm 2017;14:e97-e153.

Irnich W, et al. Do we need pacemakers resistant to magnetic resonance imaging? Europace 2005;7:353-65.

International Commission on Non-Ionizing Radiation Protection (ICNIRP) statement, medical magnetic resonance procedures: Protection of patients. Health Physics 2004;87:197-216.

Ipek EG, Nazarian S. Safety of implanted cardiac devices in an MRI environment. Curr Cardiol Rep 2015;17:605.

Ishibashi K, et al. Clinical utility of a magnetic resonance-conditional pacemaker in a patient with cardiac sarcoidosis. Intern Med 2013;52:1341-5.

Jung W, et al. Safe magnetic resonance image scanning of the pacemaker patient: Current technologies and future directions. Europace 2012;14:631-7.

Jung W, et al. MRI and implantable cardiac electronic devices. Curr Opin Cardiol 2015;30:65-73.

Junttila MJ, et al. Safety of serial MRI in patients with implantable cardioverter defibrillators. Heart. 2011;97:1852-6.

Kaasalainen T, et al. MRI with cardiac pacing devices - safety in clinical practice. Eur J Radiol 2014;83:1387-95.

Kaasalainen T, et al. Cardiac MRI in patients with cardiac pacemakers: Practical methods for reducing susceptibility artifacts and optimizing image quality. Acta Radiol 2016;57:178-87.

Kanal E, Barkovich AJ, et al. ACR guidance document for safe MR practices: 2007. Am J Roentgenol 2007;188:1447-1474.

Khan JN, et al. MRI-safe pacemakers and reduction of cardiac MRI artefacts with right-sided implantation. Eur Heart J Cardiovasc Imaging 2013;14:830.

Klein-Wiele O, et al. Feasibility and safety of adenosine cardiovascular magnetic resonance in patients with MR conditional pacemaker systems at 1.5 Tesla. J Cardiovasc Magn Reson 2015;17:112.

Korutz AW, et al. Pacemakers in MRI for the neuroradiologist. AJNR Am J Neuroradiol 2017 (In press).

Kypta A, et al. Clinical safety of an MRI conditional implantable cardioverter defibrillator system: A prospective monocenter ICD-magnetic resonance imaging feasibility study (MIMI). J Magn Reson Imaging 2016;43:574-84.

Langman DA, Finn JP, Ennis D. Abandoned pacemaker leads are a potential risk for patients undergoing MRI. Pacing Clin Electrophysiol 2011;34:1051-3.

Langman DA, et al. Pacemaker lead tip heating in abandoned and pacemaker-attached leads at 1.5 Tesla MRI. J Magn Reson Imag 2011;33:426-31.

Langman DA, et al. The dependence of radiofrequency induced pacemaker lead tip heating on the electrical conductivity of the medium at the lead tip. Magn Reson Med 2012;68:606-13.

Lauck G, et al. Effects of nuclear magnetic resonance imaging on cardiac pacemakers. Pacing Clin Electrophysiol 1995;18:1549-55.

Levine PA. Industry Viewpoint: St. Jude Medical: Pacemakers, ICDs and MRI. Pacing and Clinical Electrophysiology 2005;28:266.

Levine GN, Gomes AS, Arai AE, Bluemke DA, Flamm SD, Kanal E, Manning WJ, Martin ET, Smith JM, Wilke N, Shellock FG. Safety of magnetic resonance imaging in patients with cardiovascular devices: An American Heart Association scientific statement from the Committee on Diagnostic and Interventional Cardiac Catheterization. Circulation 2007;116:2878-2891.

Lobodzinski SS. Recent innovations in the development of magnetic resonance imaging conditional pacemakers and implantable cardioverter-defibrillators. Cardiol J 2012;19:98-104.

Loewy J, Loewy A, Kendall EJ. Reconsideration of pacemakers and MR imaging. Radiographics 2004;24:1257-1268.

Lowe MD, et al. Safe use of MRI in people with cardiac implantable electronic devices. Heart 2015;101:1950-3.

Luechinger RC. Safety Aspects of Cardiac Pacemakers in Magnetic Resonance Imaging. Swiss Institute of Technology, Zurich, Dissertation, 2002.

Luechinger RC, et al. Pacemaker reed-switch behavior in 0.5, 1.5, and 3.0 Tesla magnetic resonance units: Are reed switches always closed in strong magnetic fields? Pacing Clin Electrophysiol 2002;25:1419-1423.

Luechinger RC, et al. Force and torque effects of a 1.5 Tesla MRI scanner on cardiac pacemakers and ICDs. Pacing Clin Electrophysiol 2001;24:199-205.

Luechinger RC, et al. *In vivo* heating of pacemaker leads during magnetic resonance imaging. Eur Heart J 2005;26:376-83.

Lowe MD, et al. Safe use of MRI in people with cardiac implantable electronic devices. Heart 2015;101:1950-3.

Macfie CC, et al. Planned magnetic resonance imaging for a patient with a permanent pacemaker *in situ* with suspected spontaneous intracranial hypotension. Br J Anaesth 2013;111:1033-4.

Maglia G, et al. Assessing access to MRI of patients with magnetic resonance-conditional pacemaker and implantable cardioverter defibrillator systems: The Really ProMRI study design. J Cardiovasc Med 2015;16:715-20.

Martin TE, Coman JA, Shellock FG, Pulling C, Fair R, Jenkins K. Magnetic resonance imaging and cardiac pacemaker safety at 1.5-Tesla. Journal of the American College of Cardiology 2004;43:1315-1324.

Mason S, et al. Real world MRI experience with non-conditional and conditional cardiac rhythm devices after MagnaSafe. J Cardiovasc Electrophysiol 2017 (In press).

Mattei E, et al. Role of the lead structure in MRI-induced heating: *In vitro* measurements on 30 commercial pacemaker/defibrillator leads. Magn Reson Med 2012;67:925-35.

Mattei E, et al. Impact of capped and uncapped abandoned leads on the heating of an MR conditional pacemaker implant. Magn Reson Med 2015;73:390-400.

Mattei E, et al. Wrong detection of ventricular fibrillation in an implantable cardioverter defibrillator caused by the movement near the MRI scanner bore. Conf Proc IEEE Eng Med Biol Soc 2015;2015:7200-3.

Medtronic, Inc., www.medtronic.com/mri

Miller JD, et al. Implantable electronic cardiac devices and compatibility with magnetic resonance imaging. Journal of the American College of Cardiology 2016:1590–8.

Mollerus M, et al. Ectopy in patients with permanent pacemakers and implantable cardioverter-defibrillators undergoing an MRI scan. Pacing Clin Electrophysiol 2009;32:772-8.

Mollerus M, et al. Magnetic resonance imaging of pacemakers and implantable cardioverter-defibrillators without specific absorption rate restrictions. Europace 2010;12:947-51.

Moss AJ, Kutyifa V. Safe MRI in patients with an upgraded (conditional) implantable cardioverter-defibrillator: The beneficial tip of a troublesome iceberg. J Am Coll Cardiol 2015;65:2589-90.

Muehling OM, et al. Immediate and 12 months follow up of function and lead integrity after cranial MRI in 356 patients with conventional cardiac pacemakers. J Cardiovasc Magn Reson 2014;16:39.

Naehle CP, et al. Evaluation of cumulative effects of MR imaging on pacemaker systems at 1.5 Tesla. Pacing Clin Electrophysiol 2009;32:1526-35.

Naehle CP, et al. Safety of brain 3-T MR imaging with transmit-receive head coil in patients with cardiac pacemakers: Pilot prospective study with 51 examinations. Radiology 2008;249:991-1001.

Naehle CP, et al. Magnetic resonance imaging at 1.5-T in patients with implantable cardioverter-defibrillators. J Am Coll Cardiol 2009;54:549-55.

Naehle CP, et al. Safety, feasibility, and diagnostic value of cardiac magnetic resonance imaging in patients with cardiac pacemakers and implantable cardioverters/defibrillators at 1.5 T. Am Heart J 2011;161:1096-105.

Nakai T, et al. MRI mode programming for safe magnetic resonance imaging in patients with a magnetic resonance conditional cardiac device. Int Heart J 2016;57:173-6.

Nazarian S, Halperin HR. How to perform magnetic resonance imaging on patients with implantable cardiac arrhythmia devices. Heart Rhythm 2009;6:138-43.

Nazarian S, et al. Clinical utility and safety of a protocol for noncardiac and cardiac magnetic resonance imaging of patients with permanent pacemakers and implantable-cardioverter defibrillators at 1.5 Tesla. Circulation 2006;114:1277-1284.

Nazarian S, et al. A prospective evaluation of a protocol for magnetic resonance imaging of patients with implanted cardiac devices. Ann Intern Med 2011;155:415-424.

Nazarian S, et al. Utilization and likelihood of radiologic diagnostic imaging in patients with implantable cardiac defibrillators. J Magn Reson Imaging 2016;43:115-27.

Nordbeck P, et al. Measuring RF-induced currents inside implants: Impact of device configuration on MRI safety of cardiac pacemaker leads. Magn Reson Med 2009;61:570-8.

Nordbeck P, et al. Impact of imaging landmark on the risk of MRI-related heating near implanted medical devices like cardiac pacemaker leads. Magn Reson Med 2011;65:44-50.

Nordbeck P, et al. Reducing RF-related heating of cardiac pacemaker leads in MRI: Implementation and experimental verification of practical design changes. Magn Reson Med 2012;68:1963-72.

Nordbeck P, et al. Magnetic resonance imaging safety in pacemaker and implantable cardioverter defibrillator patients: How far have we come? Eur Heart J 2015;36:1505-11.

Nordbeck P, et al. Magnetic resonance imaging safety in pacemaker and implantable cardioverter defibrillator patients: how far have we come? Eur Heart J 2015;36:1505-11.

Ono M, et al. Feasibility, safety, and potential demand of emergent brain magnetic resonance imaging of patients with cardiac implantable electronic devices. J Arrhythm 2017;33:455-458.

Pavlicek W, Geisinger M, et al. The effects of nuclear magnetic resonance on patients with cardiac pacemakers. Radiology 1983;147:149-153.

Pfeil A, et al. Compatibility of temporary pacemaker myocardial pacing leads with magnetic resonance imaging: An *ex vivo* tissue study. Int J Cardiovasc Imaging 2012;28:317-326.

Pulver AF, et al. Safety and imaging quality of MRI in pediatric and adult congenital heart disease patients with pacemakers. Pacing Clin Electrophysiol 2009;32:450-6.

Quarta G, et al. Cardiovascular magnetic resonance in cardiac sarcoidosis with MR conditional pacemaker *in situ*. J Cardiovasc Magn Reson 2011;13:26.

Raj V, et al. MRI and cardiac pacing devices - beware the rules are changing. Br J Radiol 2011;84:857-9.

Roguin A, et al. Magnetic resonance imaging in individuals with cardiovascular implantable electronic devices. Europace 2008;10:336-46.

Roguin A, et al. Cardiac magnetic resonance imaging in a patient with implantable cardioverter-defibrillator. Pacing Clin Electrophysiol 2005;28:336-8.

Roguin A, et al. Modern pacemaker and implantable cardioverter-defibrillator systems can be MRI-safe. Circulation 2004;110:475-482.

Russo RJ. Determining the risks of clinically indicated nonthoracic magnetic resonance imaging at 1.5 T for patients with pacemakers and implantable cardioverter-defibrillators: rationale and design of the MagnaSafe Registry. Am Heart J 2013;165:266-72.

Russo RJ, et al. Assessing the risks associated with MRI in patients with a pacemaker or defibrillator. N Engl J Med 2017;376:755-764.

Sabzevari K, et al. Provision of magnetic resonance imaging for patients with 'MR-conditional' cardiac implantable electronic devices: An unmet clinical need. Europace 2017;19:425-431.

Santini L, et al. Evaluating MRI-compatible pacemakers: Patient data now paves the way to widespread clinical application? Pacing Clin Electrophysiol 2013;36:270-8.

Sasaki T, et al. Quantitative assessment of artifacts on cardiac magnetic resonance imaging of patients with pacemakers and implantable cardioverter defibrillators. Circ Cardiovasc Imaging 2011;4:662-70.

Savouré A, et al. The Kora Pacemaker is safe and effective for magnetic resonance Imaging. Clin Med Insights Cardiol 2015;9:85-90.

Schmiedel A, et al. Magnetic resonance imaging of the brain in patients with cardiac pacemakers. *In-vitro-* and *in-vivo*-evaluation at 1.5 Tesla. Rofo 2005;177:731-44.

Shellock FG. Guest Editorial. Comments on MRI heating tests of critical implants. J Magn Reson Imag 2007;26:1182-1185.

Shellock FG. Excessive temperature increases in pacemaker leads at 3-T MR imaging with a transmit-received head coil. Radiology 2009;251:948-949.

Shellock FG. Cardiac pacemakers: Growing evidence for MRI safety. Signals, No. 48, Issue 1, pp. 14-15, 2004.

Shellock FG, Crues JV. MR procedures: Biologic effects, safety, and patient care. Radiology 2004;232:635-652.

Shellock FG, Fieno DS, et al. Cardiac pacemaker: *In vitro* assessment of MR safety at 1.5-Tesla. American Heart Journal 2006;151:436-443.

Shellock FG, Fischer L, Fieno DS. Cardiac pacemakers and implantable cardioverter defibrillators: *In vitro* evaluation of MRI safety at 1.5-Tesla. Journal of Cardiovascular Magnetic Resonance 2007;9:21-31.

Shellock FG, et al. Cardiac pacemakers and implantable cardiac defibrillators are unaffected by operation of an extremity MR system. Am J Roentgenol 1999;72:165-170.

Shellock FG, Tkach JA, Ruggieri PM, Masaryk TJ. Cardiac pacemakers, ICDs, and loop recorder: Evaluation of translational attraction using conventional ("long-bore") and "short-bore" 1.5- and 3.0-Tesla MR systems. Journal of Cardiovascular Magnetic Resonance 2003;5:387-397.

Shellock FG, Valencerina S, Fischer L. MRI-related heating of pacemaker at 1.5- and 3-Tesla: Evaluation with and without pulse generator attached to leads. Circulation 112;Supplement II:561, 2005.

Shenthar J, et al. MRI scanning in patients with new and existing CapSureFix Novus 5076 pacemaker leads: Randomized trial results. Heart Rhythm 2015;12:759-65.

Shinbane J, Colletti P, Shellock FG. MR in patients with pacemakers and ICDs: Defining the issues. Journal of Cardiovascular Magnetic Resonance 2007;9:5-13.

Shinbane J, Colletti P, Shellock FG. MR imaging in patients with pacemakers and other devices: Engineering the future. Journal of the American College of Cardiology Imaging 2012;5:332-3.

Shinbane J, Colletti P, Shellock FG. Magnetic resonance imaging in patients with cardiac pacemakers: Era of "MR conditional" designs. Journal of Cardiovascular Magnetic Resonance 2011;197:W457-9.

Soejima K, et al. Safety evaluation of a leadless transcatheter pacemaker for magnetic resonance imaging use. Heart Rhythm 2016;13:2056-63.

Sommer T, Vahlhaus C, et al. MR imaging and cardiac pacemakers: *In vitro* evaluation and *in vivo* studies in 51 patients at 0.5 T. Radiology 2000;215:869-879.

Sommer T, et al. Strategy for safe performance of extrathoracic magnetic resonance imaging at 1.5 Tesla in the presence of cardiac pacemakers in non-pacemaker-dependent patients: A prospective study with 115 examinations. Circulation 2006;114:1285-92.

Sommer T, et al. German Roentgen Society Statement on MR Imaging of Patients with Cardiac Pacemakers. Rofo 2015;187:777-787.

Strach K, et al. Low-field magnetic resonance imaging: Increased safety for pacemaker patients? Europace 2010;12:952-60.

Sutton R, Kanal E, Wilkoff BL, et al. Safety of magnetic resonance imaging of patients with a new Medtronic EnRhythm MRI SureScan pacing system: Clinical study design. Trials 2008;9:68.

Tandri H, et al. Determinants of gradient field-induced current in a pacemaker lead system in a magnetic resonance imaging environment. Heart Rhythm 2008;5:462-8.

Ubee SS, et al. Implications of pacemakers and implantable cardioverter defibrillators in urological practice. J Urol 2011;186:1198-205.

Vahlhaus C, et al. interference with cardiac pacemakers by magnetic resonance imaging: Are there irreversible changes at 0.5 Tesla? Pacing Clin Electrophysiol 2001;24(Pt. I):489-95.

van der Graaf AW, et al. MRI and cardiac implantable electronic devices: Current status and required safety conditions. Neth Heart J 2014;22:269-76.

Verma A, et al. Canadian Heart Rhythm Society and Canadian Association of Radiologists consensus statement on magnetic resonance imaging with cardiac implantable electronic devices. Can J Cardiol 2014;30:1131-41.

Weishaupt D, et al. Pacemakers and magnetic resonance imaging: Current status and survey in Switzerland. Swiss Med Wkly 2011;141:w13147.

Wilkoff BL, et al. Magnetic resonance imaging in patients with a pacemaker system designed for the magnetic resonance environment. Heart Rhythm 2011;8:65-73.

Wilkoff BL, et al. EnRhythm MRI SureScan Pacing System Study Investigators. Magnetic resonance imaging in patients with a pacemaker system designed for the magnetic resonance environment. Heart Rhythm 2011;8:65-73.

Wilkoff BL, et al. Safe MRI scanning of patients with cardiac rhythm devices: A role for computer modeling. Heart Rhythm 2013;10:1815-21.

Wollmann C, et al. Safe performance of magnetic resonance imaging on a patient with an ICD. Pacing Clin Electrophysiol 2005;28:339-42.

Wollmann CG, et al. Clinical routine implantation of a dual chamber pacemaker system designed for safe use with MRI: A single center, retrospective study on lead performance of Medtronic lead 5086MRI in comparison to Medtronic leads 4592-53 and 4092-58. Herzschrittmacherther Elektrophysiol 2011;22:233-6, 239-42.

Wollmann CG, et al. Monocenter feasibility study of the MRI compatibility of the Evia pacemaker in combination with Safio S pacemaker lead. J Cardiovasc Magn Reson 2012;14:67.

Wollman CG, et al. Safe performance of magnetic resonance of the heart in patients with magnetic resonance conditional pacemaker systems: the safety issue of the ESTIMATE study. J Cardiovasc Magn Reson 2014;16:30.

Zikria JF, et al. MRI of patients with cardiac pacemakers: A review of the medical literature. Am J Roentgenol 2011;196:390-401.

Zimmermann BH, Faul DD. Artifacts and hazards in NMR imaging due to metal implants and cardiac pacemakers. Diagn Imaging Clin Med 1984;53:53-56.

Cardiac Pacemakers, Implantable Cardioverter Defibrillators, and Other Cardiac Devices: MR Conditional Versions – Abbott/St. Jude Medical

Abbott/St. Jude Medical has a variety of MR Conditional cardiac pacemakers, implantable cardioverter defibrillators (ICDs) and other cardiac devices. For a full listing of MR Conditional cardiac devices, visit www.sjm.com.

Important Note to MR Healthcare Professionals: Different MRI guidelines may exist for different countries. Therefore, use the appropriate information for your country.

[MR healthcare professionals are advised to contact the respective manufacturer in order to obtain the latest safety information to ensure patient safety relative to the use of an MR procedure.]

REFERENCE

St. Jude Medical, www.sjm.com

Cardiac Pacemakers, Implantable Cardioverter Defibrillators, and Other Cardiac Devices: MR Conditional Versions – Biotronik

Biotronik has a variety of MR Conditional versions of cardiac pacemakers, implantable cardioverter defibrillators (ICDs) and other cardiac devices. For a full listing of MR Conditional cardiac devices, visit www.biotronik.com.

Important Note to MR Healthcare Professionals: Different MRI guidelines may exist for different countries. Therefore, use the appropriate information for your country.

[MR healthcare professionals are advised to contact the respective manufacturer in order to obtain the latest safety information to ensure patient safety relative to the use of an MR procedure.]

REFERENCE

Biotronik, www.biotronik.com

Cardiac Pacemakers, Implantable Cardioverter Defibrillators, and Other Cardiac Devices: MR Conditional Versions – Boston Scientific

Boston Scientific has a variety of MR Conditional versions of cardiac pacemakers, implantable cardioverter defibrillators (ICDs) and other cardiac devices. For a full listing of MR Conditional cardiac devices visit www.bostonscientific.

Important Note to MR Healthcare Professionals: Different MRI guidelines may exist for different countries. Therefore, use the appropriate information for your country.

[MR healthcare professionals are advised to contact the respective manufacturer in order to obtain the latest safety information to ensure patient safety relative to the use of an MR procedure.]

REFERENCES

Boston Scienfitic, www.bostonscientific.com
Boston Scientific, www.bostonscientific.com/imageready

Cardiac Pacemakers, Implantable Cardioverter Defibrillators, and Other Cardiac Devices: MR Conditional Versions – Medtronic, Inc.

Medtronic, Inc. has a variety of MR Conditional versions of cardiac pacemakers, implantable cardioverter defibrillators (ICDs) and other cardiac devices. For a full listing of MR Conditional devices, visit www.medtronic/mri.

Important Note to MR Healthcare Professionals: Different MRI guidelines may exist for different countries. Therefore, use the appropriate information for your country.

[MR healthcare professionals are advised to contact the respective manufacturer in order to obtain the latest safety information to ensure patient safety relative to the use of an MR procedure.]

REFERENCE

Medtronic, Inc., www.medtronic/mri

Cardiac Pacemakers, Implantable Cardioverter Defibrillators, and Other Cardiac Devices: MR Conditional Versions – Sorin/LivaNova

Sorin/LivaNova has a variety of MR Conditional versions of cardiac pacemakers, implantable cardioverter defibrillators (ICDs) and other cardiac devices. For a full listing of MR Conditional devices, visit www.livanova.sorin.com.

Important Note to MR Healthcare Professionals: Different MRI guidelines may exist for different countries. Therefore, use the appropriate information for your country.

[MR healthcare professionals are advised to contact the respective manufacturer in order to obtain the latest safety information to ensure patient safety relative to the use of an MR procedure.]

REFERENCE

Sorin, www.livanova.sorin.com

Cardiovascular Catheters and Accessories

Cardiovascular catheters and accessories are indicated for use in the assessment and management of critically-ill or high-risk patients including those with acute heart failure, cardiogenic shock, severe hypovolemia, complex circulatory abnormalities, acute respiratory distress syndrome, pulmonary hypertension, certain types of arrhythmias and other serious conditions. In these cases, cardiovascular catheters are used to measure intravascular pressures, intracardiac pressures, cardiac output, and oxyhemoglobin saturation. Secondary indications include venous blood sampling and therapeutic infusion of solutions or medications. In addition, some cardiovascular catheters are designed for temporary cardiac pacing and intra-atrial or intraventricular electrocardiographic monitoring.

Because patients with cardiovascular catheters and associated accessories may require evaluation using MR procedures or these devices may be considered for use during MR-guided or interventional procedures, it is imperative that a thorough *ex vivo* assessment of MRI issues be conducted to ascertain the potential risks. For example, MR imaging, angiography, and spectroscopy procedures may play an important role in the diagnostic evaluation of the seriously ill patients. Furthermore, the performance of certain MR-guided procedures may require the utilization of cardiovascular catheters and accessories to monitor patients during biopsies, interventions, or treatments.

There is one report of a cardiovascular catheter, the Swan-Ganz Triple Lumen Thermodilution Catheter, that "melted" in a patient undergoing MR imaging. It was postulated that the high-frequency electromagnetic fields induced heating of either the wires within the thermodilution catheter or the radiopaque material used in the construction of the catheter. Thus, there are realistic concerns pertaining to the use of similar catheter devices in patients undergoing MR examinations. This incident suggests that patients with this catheter or a similar device that has conductive wires or other component parts, could be potentially injured during an MR examination.

Excessive heating of implants or devices made from conductive materials has been reported to be a hazard for patients who undergo MR procedures. This is particularly a problem for a device that is a certain length or in the form of a loop or coil of a certain diameter because current can be induced during MR imaging, resulting in a serious injury.

A case report by Masaki, et al. (2007) described an iatrogenic second-degree burn caused by a catheter (percutaneous transluminal coronary angioplasty or PTCA) encased by tubular, braided stainless steel. The presence of this PTCA catheter caused a superficial burn of the abdomen during an MRI procedure performed at 1.5-Tesla and further illustrates the potential risks associated with cardiovascular catheters that are made from conducting, metallic materials.

Because of possible deleterious and unpredictable effects, patients referred for MR procedures with cardiovascular catheters and accessories that have internally or externally-positioned conductive wires or similar components should not undergo MR procedures without a thorough assessment of risk versus benefit because of the possible associated risks, unless findings from MR imaging tests demonstrate otherwise. Further support of this recommendation is based on the fact that inappropriate use of monitoring devices during MR procedures is often the cause of patient injuries. For example, burns have resulted in association with the use MR examinations and certain devices that utilize conductive wires.

[MR healthcare professionals are advised to contact the respective manufacturer in order to obtain the latest safety information to ensure patient safety relative to the use of an MR procedure.]

REFERENCES

Dempsey MF, Condon B, Hadley DM. Investigation of the factors responsible for burns during MRI. J Magn Reson Imag 2001;13:627-631.

ECRI Institute, Health devices alert. A new MRI complication? May 27, 1988.

Elbes D, et al. Magnetic resonance imaging-compatible circular mapping catheter: An in vivo feasibility and safety study. Europace 2017;19:458-464.

Masaki F, Shuhei Y, Riko K, Yohjiro M. Iatrogenic second-degree burn caused by a catheter encased tubular braid of stainless steel during MRI. Burns 2007;33:1077-9.

Owens S, et al. Evaluation of epidural and peripheral nerve catheter heating. Reg Anesth Pain Med 2014;39:534-9.

Ratnayaka K, et al. Real-time MRI-guided right heart catheterization in adults using passive catheters. Eur Heart J 2013;34:380-9.

Shellock FG, Crues JV, Editors. MRI Bioeffects, Safety, and Patient Management. Biomedical Research Publishing Group, Los Angeles, CA, 2014.

Shellock FG, Kanal E. Magnetic Resonance: Bioeffects, Safety, and Patient Management. Second Edition, Lippincott-Raven Press, New York, 1996.

Shellock FG, Shellock VJ. Cardiovascular catheters and accessories: *Ex vivo* testing of ferromagnetism, heating, and artifacts associated with MRI. J Magn Reson Imag 1998;8:1338-1342.

Shellock FG, Valencerina S, Fischer L. MRI-related heating of pacemaker at 1.5- and 3-Tesla: Evaluation with and without pulse generator attached to leads. Circulation 2005;112;Supplement II:561.

Carotid Artery Vascular Clamps

A carotid artery vascular clamp is a medical device that is surgically placed around the carotid artery and used to temporarily block blood flow through the carotid artery in order to treat a cerebral aneurysm. To date, each carotid artery vascular clamp tested in association with a 1.5-Tesla MR system displayed positive magnetic field interactions. However, only the Poppen-Blaylock carotid artery vascular clamp is considered contraindicated for patients undergoing MR procedures due to the existence of substantial ferromagnetism. The other carotid artery clamps were considered safe for patients exposed to MR systems operating at 1.5-Tesla or less because they were deemed "weakly" ferromagnetic. With the exception of the Poppen-Blaylock clamp, patients with the other carotid artery vascular clamps that have been evaluated for magnetic field interactions have been imaged by MR systems with static magnetic fields up to 1.5-Tesla without experiencing discomfort or neurological sequelae.

REFERENCES

Shellock FG, Crues JV, Editors. MRI Bioeffects, Safety, and Patient Management. Biomedical Research Publishing Group, Los Angeles, CA, 2014.

Shellock FG, Kanal E. Magnetic Resonance: Bioeffects, Safety, and Patient Management. Second Edition, Lippincott-Raven Press, New York, 1996.

Teitelbaum GP, Lin MCW, Watanabe AT, et al. Ferromagnetism and MR imaging: Safety of carotid vascular clamps. Am J Neuroradiol 1990;11:267-272.

Celsius Control System or Temperature Modulation Therapy

The **Celsius Control System** (or **Temperature Modulation Therapy**, Zoll) provides physicians with state-of-the-art, endovascular technology that can safely and rapidly lower the patient's body temperature, precisely maintain a chosen target temperature, and rewarm the patient to normothermic levels.

Medical research suggests there are a number of potential clinical applications for the Celsius Control System such as inducing mild hypothermia in surgery, stroke, and heart attack or for temperature control in surgical and critical care procedures.

The Celsius Control System consists of an endovascular catheter, console and proprietary disposables. The distal portion of the catheter incorporates a flexible Temperature Control Element (TCE) that is cooled or warmed with saline solution circulated in a closed-loop manner from the console. When placed in the inferior vena cava, the TCE exchanges thermal energy directly with the blood, resulting in cooling or warming of the downstream organs and body. The Celsius Control System does not infuse fluid into the patient, nor is blood circulated outside of the body.

Celsius Control System
The Celsius Control System consists of a disposable endovascular heat transfer catheter, administration cassette, and a console. The distal portion of the catheter (10.7 Fr. and 14 Fr.) has a flexible, metallic temperature control element (TCE) that is cooled or warmed by sterile saline circulated within it from the Celsius Control Console. The administration cassette connects the catheter to the console, maintaining the sterility of the saline conduit. The TCE does not expand inside the body so the outer diameter of the TCE will remain consistent throughout the entire cooling/warming procedure unlike balloon based cooling systems which expand to outer diameters of 24 Fr.-47 Fr. during use.

Accutrol Catheter
The Accutrol Catheter contains an integrated temperature sensor, which can accurately determine the patient's core body temperature within

0.1°C of pulmonary artery temperature. The proprietary, novel Accutrol software control algorithm provides automated body temperature control. The Accutrol system eliminates the need to place bladder or rectal probes, which can be slow to react to actual decreases in core body temperature, may be uncomfortable to the patient, and time-consuming to place. The Accutrol catheter is beneficial in the critical care environment where gradual rewarming may be warranted.

Standard Catheter
The Standard catheter incorporates the same design features as the Accutrol catheter including performance attributes. However, an external core temperature feedback probe is required for operation.

MAGNETIC RESONANCE IMAGING (MRI)

The Celsius Control Catheter is "MR Conditional" according to the American Society for Testing and Materials (ASTM) International, Designation: F2503. Standard Practice for Marking Medical Devices and Other Items for Safety in the Magnetic Resonance Environment. The Celsius Control Catheter demonstrates no known hazards when a "head-only" MRI procedure is performed according to the conditions stated in this labeling.

It is important to read and understand this document in its entirety before conducting a head-only MRI (magnetic resonance imaging) procedure on a patient with an indwelling Celsius Control Catheter. Failure to strictly adhere to these guidelines may result in serious injury to the patient. This information applies to the following INNERCOOL Therapies products:

Catalog No.
11-10-65-1 Celsius Control Standard Catheter 10.7 Fr.
11-14-65-1 Celsius Control Standard Catheter 14 Fr.
11-10-65-2 Celsius Control Accutrol Catheter 10.7 Fr.
11-14-65-2 Celsius Control Accutrol Catheter 14 Fr.

Warnings
-Disconnect Celsius Control Catheter from the Celsius Control Console completely prior to entering the MRI environment. Failure to do so may result in serious injury to the patient. It is not possible to continue therapy with the system during an MRI procedure.

-This labeling information applies to "head-only" MRI procedures conducted using a 1.5-Tesla transmit/receive RF head coil or a transmit RF body/receive-only head coil, *ONLY*.

MRI examinations of other parts of the body are strictly prohibited with the Celsius Control Catheter *in situ.*

-Testing has not been performed using other MR systems operating at other static magnetic field strengths (i.e. 1.5-Tesla, *only*) and, therefore, other scanners should not be used to perform an MRI examination on a patient who has an indwelling Celsius Control Catheter.

-The Celsius Control Catheter must be properly positioned per the directions for use with the catheter introduced through the femoral vein of either the left or right groin of the patient and advanced into the IVC such that the catheter is parallel to the bore of the MR system. Do not perform the MRI examination with the Celsius Control Catheter placed in any other configuration. Failure to follow this guideline may result in serious injury to the patient.

-Using the transmit/receive RF head coil, do not exceed an MR system reported, whole body averaged specific absorption rate (SAR) greater than 0.4-W/Kg.

-Using the transmit RF body coil/receive-only head coil, do not exceed an MR system reported, whole body averaged SAR of greater than 3.5-W/Kg.

Overview
The Celsius Control Catheter has undergone extensive *in vitro* testing to demonstrate that, by following specific guidelines, it is safe to perform a head-only MRI procedure on a patient with this device in a 1.5-Tesla MR system, ONLY. Variability among MR systems, differences in how scanners estimate or calculate specific absorption rates (SAR) cannot be simulated comprehensively using *in vitro* techniques. This document outlines recommended guidelines and specific conditions under which the Celsius Control Catheter has been shown to pose minimal risk to a patient undergoing a head only MRI procedure. Deviation from these guidelines may increase the potential for serious harm to the patient. MRI conditions utilizing MR systems with higher or lower static magnetic fields have not been assessed for the Celsius Control Catheter and, as such, must be avoided to ensure patient safety. The user of this information assumes full responsibility for the consequences of conducting a MRI examination on a patient with an indwelling Celsius Control Catheter.

Magnetic Field Interactions
Translation Attraction and Torque. Magnetic materials contained within an implanted or indwelling device may experience translational or rotational forces when brought into the static magnetic field of a MRI system. The Celsius Control Catheter contains relatively minor magnetic

materials. *In vitro* testing demonstrated that the Celsius Control Catheter is not substantially affected by translational attraction and torque related to exposure to a 1.5-Tesla MR system.

MRI-Related Heating
Under certain conditions, RF fields generated by MRI can induce substantial currents in metallic components contained within medical device products. This may rapidly produce significant heating of a device. Failure to follow the recommendations contained in this communication may result in the generation of thermal lesions and serious patient harm. *In vitro* testing demonstrated that the Celsius Control Catheter is not substantially affected by the RF fields related to exposure to a 1.5-Tesla MR system under the conditions used for testing.

MRI Artifacts
The presence of the Celsius Control Catheter will cause moderate artifacts on the MR image depending on the pulse sequence parameters used for MRI. However, the artifacts are confined to the position of the Celsius Control Catheter and, as such, will not affect the diagnostic use of MR imaging for head only MRI examinations.

Procedure
In addition to standard safety procedures for MRI, the following precautions must be followed specific to the Celsius Control Catheter:

1) Inform the patient of the potential risks of undergoing a MRI procedure with the Celsius Control Catheter.
2) Disconnect all cables and patient monitoring devices attached to the Celsius Control Catheter prior to transporting the patient into the MRI environment.
3) The MRI procedure must be performed using a 1.5-Tesla MR system, *only*.
4) MRI examinations must be performed to image the *head only.* Use only the following types of radio frequency (RF) coils for the MRI procedure:
   a) Transmit/receive RF head coil
   b) Transmit body RF coil/receive-only head coil.
5) Using the transmit/receive RF head coil, do not exceed an MR system reported SAR of 0.4-W/kg. Using the transmit RF body coil/receive-only RF head coil, do not exceed an MR system reported SAR of 3.5-W/kg.
6) It is important to place the Celsius Control Catheter in a specific geometry to minimize the potential for excessive heating during the MRI procedure. The Celsius Control Catheter must be properly positioned as per the directions for use with the catheter introduced

through the femoral vein of either the left or right groin of the patient and advanced into the IVC such that the catheter is parallel to the bore of the MR system (but not touching the bore of the MR system). Do not perform the MRI examination with the Celsius Control Catheter placed in any other configuration. Failure to follow this guideline may result in serious injury to the patient.

7) Ensure that the proper patient weight is used for the SAR calculations. Verify that the MRI system has appropriately calculated and updated the SAR value after all parameter changes have been made.

8) A knowledgeable MRI expert (e.g., MRI physicist, MRI-trained radiologist, etc.) must verify that all set-up steps and settings have been properly implemented and checked prior to performing the head only MRI procedure.

9) Verify that all proposed MRI examination parameters and conditions for the Celsius Control Catheter comply with the instructions described herein. If they do not comply, do not perform the head only MRI procedure.

10) Provide the patient with a means by which he/she can alert the MR system operator during the MRI procedure if any discomfort or unusual sensations should occur.

11) Monitor the patient continuously during the head only MRI examination and be prepared respond or to terminate the MRI procedure immediately in the event of a complaint.

12) Determine if the patient has any other implants or conditions that would prohibit or contraindicate a head only MRI examination. Do not conduct a head only MRI examination if any conditions or implanted devices that would prohibit or contraindicate a MRI are present.

[MR healthcare professionals are advised to contact the manufacturer to ensure that the latest safety information is obtained and carefully followed in order to ensure patient safety relative to the use of an MR procedure.]

REFERENCE

www.zoll.com

Cerebrospinal Fluid (CSF) Shunt Valves and Accessories

Hydrocephalus is the accumulation of cerebrospinal fluid in the brain resulting from increased production, or more commonly, pathway obstruction or decreased absorption of fluid. Cerebrospinal fluid (CSF) shunts have been used for decades for the treatment of hydrocephalus. A CSF shunt involves establishing an accessory pathway for the movement of CSF to bypass an obstruction of the natural pathways.

The shunt is positioned to enable the CSF to be drained from the cerebral ventricles or sub-arachnoid spaces into another absorption site (e.g., the right atrium of the heart or the peritoneal cavity) through a system of small catheters. A regulatory device, such as a valve, may be inserted into the pathway of the catheters. In general, the valve keeps the CSF flowing away from the brain and moderates the pressure or flow rate. Some valves are fixed pressure valves (i.e. monopressure valves) and others have adjustable or programmable settings. The drainage system using catheters and valves enables the excess CSF within the brain to be evacuated and, thereby, the pressure within the cranium to be reduced.

There are many different types of CSF shunt valves and associated accessories used for treatment of hydrocephalus. For shunt valves that utilize magnetic components, highly specific safety guidelines must be followed in order to perform MRI procedures safely in patients with these devices. Findings from a study conducted by Mirzayan, et al. (2012) at 7-Tesla indicated that a certain programmable CSF shunt valve may be compromised by exposure to this very high-field-strength MR system.

The following content provides information for several different CSF shunt valve products. Information for many other types of shunt valves may be found by visiting www.MRIsafety.com and referring to **The List.**

CODMAN CERTAS Programmable Valve, CSF Shunt Valve Description. CODMAN CERTAS Programmable Valve, CSF Shunt Valve (Codman, a Johnson & Johnson Company) is a programmable CSF shunt valve.

Warnings

- The use of Magnetic Resonance (MR) systems operating at 3-Tesla or less will not damage the valve mechanism and testing shows that the valve is resistant to unintended changes in the setting. However, it is recommended that the clinician confirm the valve setting after a magnetic resonance imaging (MRI) procedure.

- The valve setting is adjusted with the application and manipulation of strong magnets. A change to the valve setting is unlikely to occur under normal circumstances. However, magnetic fields should not be placed in close proximity to the valve due to the possibility of an unintentional setting change.

- Read the *MRI Information* before performing an MRI procedure on a patient implanted with the valve.

Magnetic Resonance Imaging (MRI) Information

The CODMAN CERTAS Therapy Management System (TMS) is considered "MR Unsafe" in accordance with the American Society for Testing and Materials (ASTM) Standard F2503-05. Do not use the TMS in the MR suite. The CODMAN CERTAS Programmable Valve contains small metallic parts that are insulated and isolated from patient tissue by nonmetallic, nonconducting materials. There is no metal in contact with the patient. Non-clinical testing has demonstrated that the CODMAN CERTAS Programmable Valve is considered "MR Conditional" in accordance with ASTM F2503 and it can be scanned safely under the following conditions and specific guidelines at any time after implantation:

Conditions

- Static magnetic field of 3-Tesla or less.
- Highest spatial gradient magnetic field of 720-gauss/cm or less.
- The MR system can be operated in either of the following modes:

- **Normal Operating Mode** (i.e. mode of operation of the MR EQUIPMENT in which none of the outputs has a value that might cause physiological stress to PATIENTS) only with a maximum whole-body averaged specific absorption rate of 2.0-W/kg.

- **First Level Controlled Operating Mode** (i.e. mode of operation of the MR EQUIPMENT in which one or more outputs reach a value that might cause physiological stress to PATIENTS that needs to be controlled by MEDICAL SUPERVISION) with a whole-body-averaged specific absorption rate of 4.0 W/kg.

Specific Guidelines. It is recommended that the valve setting be verified after the MRI procedure (see *Post Implantation Adjustment Procedure* Steps 1 through 3 in the ***Instructions for Use***).

MRI TESTING INFORMATION

Static Magnetic Field. Translational attraction and torque associated with a 3 Tesla or lower field strength MR system are at levels that are less than those related to gravity and will not pose an additional hazard or risk to the patient in an MRI environment at 3 Tesla or less.

MRI-Related Heating. In non-clinical testing, the valve produced a temperature rise of 1.8 degrees C at a maximum MR system reported whole-body-averaged specific absorption rate (SAR) of 3.0 W/kg as assessed by calorimetry for 15 minutes of MR scanning (per pulse sequence) in a 3 T EXCITE MR Scanner, HDx, Software 14X.M5, General Electric Healthcare, Milwaukee, WI, USA.

MRI Artifacts. Artifacts were assessed using T1-weighted spin echo (SE) and gradient echo (GRE) pulse sequences. The details of these pulse sequences and the corresponding artifact sizes are listed in Table 2 (please refer to ***Instructions for Use***). MR image quality might be compromised if the area of interest is in the exact location or relatively close to the location of the CODMAN CERTAS Programmable Valve. However, MRI artifacts can be minimized by careful selection of pulse sequence parameters. **Note:** The maximum artifact size, as seen on the gradient echo pulse sequence, extends approximately 15-mm relative to the size and shape of the valve.

Codman Hakim Precision Valve, CSF Shunt Valve

Description. The CODMAN HAKIM Precision Fixed Pressure Valve (CSF shunt valve, Codman, a Johnson & Johnson Company) offers five distinct and narrow bandwidths to assure the correct pressure setting for each individual case. It also uses the proven ball and cone technology to insure that each pressure range is correct within a +/-10mm H2O variance. The CODMAN HAKIM Precision Fixed Pressure Valve is available in eight basic configurations, and each of these configurations can be purchased with a unitized distal catheter or as a valve only.

The Codman Hakim Precision CSF Shunt Valve (CSF shunt valve, Codman, a Johnson & Johnson Company) is "MR Conditional" according to ASTM F2503. The valve demonstrates no known hazards when an MRI is performed under the following conditions:

- MRI can be performed at any time after implantation
- Use an MR system with a static magnetic field of 3-T or less

- Use an MR System with a spatial gradient of 720 gauss/cm or less
- Limit the exposure to RF energy to a whole-body-averaged specific absorption rate (SAR) of 3 W/kg for 15 minutes (per pulse sequence)

MR image quality may be compromised if the area of interest is relatively close to the device. Distortion may be seen at the boundaries of the artifact. Therefore, optimization of the MR imaging parameters may be necessary.

CODMAN HAKIM Programmable Valves

Description. The CODMAN HAKIM Programmable Valve (CSF shunt valve, Codman, a Johnson & Johnson Company) includes a valve mechanism that incorporates a flat 316L stainless steel spring in which the calibration is accomplished by a combination between a pillar and a micro-adjustable telescoping fulcrum. The valve chassis is made of titanium. The ball and cone are manufactured from synthetic ruby. Intraventricular pressure is maintained at a constant level by the ball and cone valve seat design.

The pressure setting of the spring in the inlet valve unit is noninvasively adjusted by the use of an external programmer, which activates the stepper motor within the valve housing. The programmer transmits a codified magnetic signal to the motor allowing eighteen pressure settings, ranging from 30 mm to 200 mm H_2O (294 to 1960 Pa) in 10 mm (98 Pa) increments. These are operating pressures of the valve unit and have been determined with a flow rate of 15 to 25 ml H_2O per hour.

The valve is classified by its working pressure with a specified flow rate and not by the opening and closing pressures. The pressure that a valve sustains with a given flow is the parameter that reflects the working pressure of the valve once it is implanted. Before shipment, each valve is calibrated with special equipment: Duplication of these test procedures cannot be accomplished in the operating room.

Indications. The CODMAN HAKIM Programmable Valves are implantable devices that provide constant intraventricular pressure and drainage of CSF for the management of hydrocephalus.

Programmable Valve Configurations

- In-line with SIPHONGUARD Device
- In-line
- Right Angle with SIPHONGUARD Device

- Right Angle
- Cylindrical with Prechamber
- Cylindrical
- Micro with RICKHAM Reservoir
- Micro

CODMAN HAKIM In-line and Right Angle Valves include a programmable valve with a low profile and flat bottom, and an in-line or right angle integral reservoir with or without SIPHONGUARD.

CODMAN HAKIM Cylindrical Valves include a programmable valve, a pumping chamber, and an outlet valve available with or without a prechamber.

CODMAN HAKIM Micro Valves include a programmable valve with or without an integral RICKHAM reservoir.

WARNINGS. Subjecting the valve to strong magnetic fields may change the setting of the valve.

- The use of Magnetic Resonance (MR) systems up to 3-Tesla will not damage the valve mechanism, but may change the setting of the valve. Confirm the valve setting after an MRI procedure.
- Common magnets greater than 80 gauss, such as household magnets, loudspeaker magnets, and language lab headphone magnets may affect the valve setting when placed close to the valve.
- Magnetic fields generated from microwaves, high-tension wires, electric motors, transformers, etc., do not affect the valve setting.

Read the *MRI Information* before performing an MRI procedure on a patient implanted with the programmable valve.

MRI Information

The CODMAN HAKIM Programmable Valve (CSF shunt valve, Codman, a Johnson & Johnson Company) is "MR Conditional" according to ASTM F 2503. The valve demonstrates no known hazards when an MRI is performed under the following conditions:

- MRI can be performed at any time after implantation
- Use an MR system with a static magnetic field of 3 T or less
- Use an MR System with a spatial gradient of 720 gauss/cm or less
- Limit the exposure to RF energy to a whole-body-averaged specific absorption rate (SAR) of 3 W/kg for 15 minutes

- Verify the valve setting after the MRI procedure (see *Programming the Valve*)

In non-clinical testing, the valve produced a temperature rise of 0.4-degrees C at a maximum whole-body-averaged specific absorption rate (SAR) of 3-W/kg for 15 minutes of MR scanning in a 3-T Excite General Electric MR scanner.

MR image quality may be compromised if the area of interest is relatively close to the device. Distortion may be seen at the boundaries of the artifact. Therefore, optimization of the MR imaging parameters may be necessary.

The following table provides a comparison between the signal void and imaging pulse sequence at 3-Tesla:

Signal Void	Pulse Sequence	Imaging Plane
1,590-mm^2	T1-weighted, spin echo	Parallel
1,022-mm^2	T1-weighted, spin echo	Perpendicular
2,439-mm^2	Gradient echo	Parallel
2,404-mm^2	Gradient echo	Perpendicular

Delta Shunt Assembly

The Delta Shunt Assembly (Medtronic Neurosurgery, www.medtronic.com) combines the Delta valve with an integral, open-end, radiopaque peritoneal catheter. All Delta shunt assemblies incorporate the same product features as the Delta valves. These include injectable reservoir domes, occluders for selective flushing, and a completely nonmetallic design. The valves are fabricated of dissimilar materials - polypropylene and silicone elastomer - reducing the chance of valve sticking and deformation. The normally closed Delta chamber mechanism minimizes over-drainage by utilizing the principles of hydrodynamic leverage. Because of the nonmetallic design, the Delta shunt is safe for patients undergoing MRI procedures.

proGAV Programmable Valve

The programmable valve, proGAV (Aesculap, Inc. and B. Braun), has magnetic components used for the programming mechanism. This device underwent evaluation relative to the use of a 3-Tesla MR system (i.e. tested for magnetic field interactions, heating, artifacts, and functional alterations). In consideration of the results of these tests, in order to take proper precautions to ensure patient safety, the following guidelines are recommended for scanning a patient with this device:

1) A patient with the programmable valve, proGAV, may undergo MRI at 3-T or less immediately after implantation.
2) Prior to MRI, the programmable valve setting should be determined by appropriate personnel using proper equipment.
3) The exposure to RF energy should be limited to a whole body averaged SAR of 2.1-W/kg for 15-min. (i.e. per pulse sequence).
4) After MRI, the proGAV programmable valve setting should be determined and re-set, as needed.

Pulsar Valve

The Pulsar Valve (Sophysa, Inc.) for CSF drainage is a monopressure valve. Its principal is based on the play of a silicone membrane, calibrated in low, medium, or high pressure, ensuring a proximal regulation of CSF flow through the shunt system. The Pulsar Valve is safe for patients undergoing MRI procedures.

Sophy Mini Monopressure Valve

The Sophy Mini Monopressure Valve (Sophysa, Inc.) for CSF drainage has a ball-in-cone mechanism. This device is safe for patients undergoing MRI procedures.

Strata, Strata II, and Strata NSC Programmable CSF Shunt Valves

MRI Information

The Strata, Strata NSC, and Strata II Programmable CSF shunt valves (Medtronic Neurosurgery, www.medtronic.com) are Magnetic Resonance Conditional (MR Conditional) in accordance with ASTM F2503. MRI systems of up to 3.0-Tesla may be used any time after implantation and will not damage the Strata, Strata NSC, or Strata II valve mechanisms, but can change the performance level setting. The performance level setting should always be checked before and after MRI exposure. The results of the tests performed to assess magnetic field interactions, artifacts, and heating, indicated the presence of the valves evaluated should present no substantial risk to a patient undergoing an MRI procedure using the following conditions:

- Static magnetic field of 3.0 Tesla or less
- Spatial gradient magnetic field of 720 gauss/cm or less
- Radio Frequency (RF) Fields with an average Specific Absorption Rate (SAR) of 3 W/kg for 15 minutes. Using the GE 3T Excite HD MRI System, the valve experienced a maximum temperature change of 0.4°C over a 15 minute exposure period. The table below provides maximum signal voids (artifact sizes)

for standard imaging pulse sequences at 3 Tesla per ASTM F2119.

Signal Void	Pulse Sequence	Imaging Plane
35.16-cm^2	T1-weighted, spin echo	Parallel
33.03-cm^2	T1-weighted, spin echo	Perpendicular
75.91-cm^2	Gradient echo	Parallel
66.55-cm^2	Gradient echo	Perpendicular

Adjustment Kits

Do **NOT** take the Adjustment Tool into an MRI facility as these magnets could potentially be a safety hazard to the patient and/or user. Proximity to MRI suite may impede the mechanism in the Indicator Tool due to the field strength of an MRI magnet. Move out of the vicinity prior to attempting to verify a valve setting.

SOPHY Adjustable Pressure Valve

The principle of the SOPHY Adjustable Pressure Valve (Sophysa, Inc.) resides in the variation in pressure exerted on a ball by a semi-circular spring at various points along its circumference. The spring is attached to a magnetic rotor whose position can be noninvasively altered using an adjustment magnet. A series of indentations allows a variety of positions to be selected, each position representing a different pressure setting. The valve's ball-in-cone mechanism maintains the selected pressure constant without significant drift.

Because a magnetic component is associated with this device, special MR safety precautions exist for scanning patients with the SOPHY Adjustable Pressure Valve, as follows:

- The pressure settings should always be checked in case of shock on the implantation site.
- Changing pressure settings must only be performed by a neurosurgeon.
- The patient must be advised that carrying his Patient Identification Card is important and necessary for the follow-up of the clinical conditions.
- Patients undergoing MRI exposure should be advised that they might feel a small yet harmless effect due to MRI.
- The pressure settings should always be checked before and after MRI exposure, or after strong magnetic field exposure.

- The patient must be advised that in the case of implantation on the skull vibrations due to CSF flow may be perceived.
- Patients with implanted valve systems must be kept under close observation for symptoms of shunt failure.

[MR healthcare professionals are advised to contact the respective manufacturer in order to obtain the latest safety information to ensure patient safety relative to the use of an MR procedure.]

REFERENCES

Akbar M, et al. Adjustable cerebrospinal fluid shunt valves in 3.0-Tesla MRI: A phantom study using explanted devices. Rofo. 2010;182:594-602.

Anderson RCE, et al. Adjustment and malfunction of a programmable valve after exposure to toy magnets. J Neurosurg (Pediatrics) 2004;101:222-225.

Capitanio JF, et al. Prosepective study to evaluate rate and frequency of perturbations of implanted programmable Hakim Codman Valve after 1.5-Tesla magnetic resonance imaging. World Neurosurg 2016;88:297-9.

Codman, a Johnson and Johnson Company, www.depuysynthes.com

Fransen P. Transcutaneous pressure-adjustable valves and magnetic resonance imaging: An *ex vivo* examination of the Codman-Medos programmable valve and the Sophy adjustable pressure valve. Neurosurgery 1998;42:430.

Fransen P, Dooms G, Thauvoy C. Safety of the adjustable pressure ventricular valve in magnetic resonance imaging: Problems and solutions. Neuroradiology 1992;34:508-509.

Inoue T, et al. Effect of 3-Tesla magnetic resonance imaging on various pressure programmable shunt valves. J Neurosurg 2005;103(2 Suppl):163-5.

Krishnamurthy S, et al. Radiation risk due to shunted hydrocephalus and the role of MR imaging-safe programmable valves. AJNR 2013;34:695-7. Lindner D, et al. Effect of 3-T MRI on the function of shunt valves--evaluation of Paedi GAV, Dual Switch and proGAV. Eur J Radiol 2005;56:56-9.

Lollis SS, et al. Programmable CSF shunt valves: radiographic identification and interpretation. Am J Neuroradiol 2010;31:1343-6.

Ludemann W, et al. Reliability of a new adjustable shunt device without the need for readjustment following 3-Tesla MRI. Childs Nerv Syst 2005;21:227-229.

Medtronic, Inc. www.medtronic.com ,

Mirzayan MJ, et al. MRI safety of a programmable shunt assistant at 3 and 7 Tesla. Br J Neurosurg 2012;26:397-400.

Miwa K, Kondo H, Sakai N. Pressure changes observed in Codman-Medos programmable valves following magnetic exposure and filliping. Childs Nerv Syst 2001;17:150-153.

Moghtader D, et al. Assessment of MRI issues for a new cerebral spinal fluid shunt, gravitational valve (GV). Magnetic Resonance Imaging 44;2017:8-14.

Ortler M, et al. Transcutaneous pressure-adjustable valves and magnetic resonance imaging: An *ex vivo* examination of the Codman-Medos programmable valve and the Sophy adjustable pressure valve. Neurosurgery 1997;40:1050-1057.

Schneider T, et al. Electromagnetic field hazards involving adjustable shunt valves in hydrocephalus. J Neurosurg 2002;96:331-334.

Shellock FG. MR safety and Cerebral Spinal Fluid Shunt (CSF) Valves. Signals, No. 51, Issue 4, pp. 10, 2004.

Shellock FG, Bedwinek A, Oliver-Allen M, Wilson SF. Assessment of MRI issues for a 3-T "immune" programmable CSF shunt valve. Am J Roentgenol 2011;197:202-7.

Shellock FG, et al. Programmable CSF shunt valve: *In vitro* assessment of MRI safety at 3-Tesla. American Journal of Neuroradiology 2006;27:661-665.

Shellock FG, Wilson SF, Mauge CP. Magnetically-programmable shunt valve: MRI at 3-Tesla. Magnetic Resonance Imaging 2007;25:1116-21.

Sophysa, Cerebral Spinal Fluid Shunt Valves and Accessories, www.sophysa.com

Toma AK, et al. Adjustable shunt valve-induced magnetic resonance imaging artifact: A comparative study. J Neurosurg 2010;113:74-8.

Watanabe A, et al. Overdrainage of cerebrospinal fluid caused by detachment of the pressure control cam in a programmable valve after 3-Tesla magnetic resonance imaging. J Neurosurg 2010;112:425-7.

Zabramski JM, et al. 3T magnetic resonance imaging testing of externally programmable shunt valves. Surg Neurol Int 2012;3:81.

Zemack G, Romner B. Seven years of clinical experience with the programmable Codman Hakim valve: A retrospective study of 583 patients. J Neurosurg 2000;92:941-8.

Cochlear Implants

Cochlear implants are electronically-activated or "active" devices. Consequently, an MR procedure may be contraindicated for a patient with this type of implant because of the possibility of injuring the patient and/or altering or damaging the function of the device. In general, patients and other individuals with cochlear implants should be prevented from entering the MR environment unless specific guidelines exist to ensure safety for these devices.

Investigations have been conducted to determine if there are situations and specific conditions for a patient with a cochlear implant to safely undergo an MR procedure. These studies have resulted in highly specific guidelines that must be followed in order to safely perform MR examinations in patients with certain cochlear implants. Notably, some cochlear implants require the use of a 0.2-Tesla or 0.3-Tesla MR system, *only,* as part of the guidelines. In other cases, the magnet associated with the cochlear implant may require removal prior to the MRI examination and the replacement following the scan.

Recently, cochlear implants have received approval of MR Conditional labeling at 1.5- and 3-Tesla, some of which do not require the removal of the implanted magnets prior to MRI procedures but do require the use of specialized compression bandages. In certain cases where the magnet remains in place, patients have experienced uncomfortable sensations in association with MRI which have prevented the completion of the exams. Notably, when the magnet of the cochlear implant remains in place, the image quality will be compromised due to the presence of substantial signal loss related to the presence of the magnet.

Additional MRI concerns include possible demagnetization of the internal magnet associated with the cochlear implant by exposure to the powerful static magnetic field of the MR system, as well as the substantial artifacts that exist if the internal magnet remains in place during an MRI examination.

The content below presents information for certain cochlear implants. Additional information may be obtained from the respective company website.

HiRes 90K Cochlear Implant, HiRes 90K ADVANTAGE Cochlear Implant, Advanced Bionics Corporation

The HiRes 90K Cochlear Implant, HiRes 90K ADVANTAGE Cochlear Implant (Advanced Bionics) are MR Conditional. Comprehensive labeling information must be reviewed to ensure patient safety.

Carefully review the latest MRI labeling conditions and guidelines at: www.advancedbionics.com

[MR healthcare professionals are advised to contact the manufacturer to ensure that the latest safety information is obtained and carefully followed in order to ensure patient safety relative to the use of an MR procedure.]

Cochlear Implants, MED-EL Corporation

The following cochlear implants from MED-EL Coporation are MR Conditional:

MED-EL COMBI 40+ Cochlear implant

MED-EL CONCERT Cochlear Implant

MED-EL CONCERT PIN Cochlear Implant

MED-EL PULSAR Cochlear Implant

MED-EL SONATA Cochlear Implant

MED-EL SYNCHRONY Cochlear Implant

MED-EL SYNCHRONY PIN Cochlear Implant

Comprehensive labeling information must be reviewed to ensure patient safety.

Carefully review the latest MRI labeling conditions and guidelines at: www.medel.com

Note to MR Healthcare Professionals: Different MRI guidelines exist for different countries. Therefore, use the appropriate information for your country.

[MR healthcare professionals are advised to contact the manufacturer to ensure that the latest safety information is obtained and carefully followed in order to ensure patient safety relative to the use of an MR procedure.]

Cochlear Nucleus Implants, Cochlear Corporation

Certain Cochlear Nucleus Implants are MR Conditional. Comprehensive labeling information must be reviewed to ensure patient safety.

Carefully review the latest MRI labeling conditions and guidelines at: www.cochlear.com

Note to MR Healthcare Professionals: Different MRI guidelines exist for different countries. Therefore, use the appropriate information for your country.

[MR healthcare professionals are advised to contact the manufacturer to ensure that the latest safety information is obtained and carefully followed in order to ensure patient safety relative to the use of an MR procedure.]

REFERENCES

Bao G, et al. Cochlear implant patients underwent successful MRI examination after local bandaging: A case report. Lin Chung Er Bi Yan Hou Tou Jing Wai Ke Za Zhi 2012;26:759.

Broomfield SJ, et al. Cochlear implants and magnetic resonance scans: A case report and review. Cochlear Implants Int 2013;14:51-5.

Carlson ML, et al. Magnetic resonance imaging with cochlear implant magnet in place: Safety and imaging quality. Otol Neurotol 2015;36:965-71.

Chou H-K, et al. Absence of radiofrequency heating from auditory implants during magnetic resonance imaging. Bioelectromagnetics 1995;16:307-316.

Cuda D, et al. Focused tight dressing does not prevent cochlear implant magnet migration under 1.5 Tesla MRI. Acta Otorhinolaryngol Ital 2013;33:133-6.

Deneuve S, et al. Cochlear implant magnet displacement during magnetic resonance imaging. Otol Neurotol 2008;29:789-190.

Doshi J, et al. Magnetic resonance imaging and bone anchored hearing implants: Pediatric considerations. Int J Pediatr Otorhinolaryngol 2014;78:277-9.

Dubrulle F, et al. Cochlear implant with a non-removable magnet: Preliminary research at 3-T MRI. Eur Radiol 2013;23:1510-8.

Freden Jansson KJ, et al. MRI induced torque and demagnetization in retention magnets for a bone conduction implant. IEEE Trans Biomed Eng 2014;61:1887-93.

Gubbels SP, McMenomey SO. Safety study of the Cochlear Nucleus 24 device with internal magnet in the 1.5 Tesla magnetic resonance imaging scanner. Laryngoscope 2006;116:865-71.

Hassepass F, et al. Magnet dislocation: An increasing serious complication following MRI in patients with cochlear implants. Rofo 2014;186:680-5.

Hassepass F, et al. Revision surgery due to magnet dislocation in cochlear implant patients: An emerging complication. Otol Neurotol 2014;35:29-34.

Heller JW, et al. Evaluation of MRI compatibility of the modified nucleus multi-channel auditory brainstem and cochlear implants. Am J Otol 1996;17:724-729.

Jansson KJ, et al. MRI induced torque and demagnetization in retention magnets for a bone conduction implant. IEEE Trans Biomed Eng 2014;61:1887-93.

Jeon JH, et al. Reversing the polarity of a cochlear implant magnet after magnetic resonance imaging. Auris Nasus Larynx 2012;39:415-7.

Kanal E. Magnetic resonance imaging in cochlear implant recipients: Pros and cons. JAMA Otolaryngol Head Neck Surg 2015;141:52-3.

Kim JH, et al. Magnetic resonance imaging compatibility of the polymer-based cochlear implant. Clin Exp Otorhinolaryngol 2012;5:S19-23.

Kim BG, et al. Adverse events and discomfort during magnetic resonance imaging in cochlear implant recipients. JAMA Otolaryngol Head Neck Surg 2015;141:45-52.

Kong Sk, et al. The reversed internal magnet of cochlear implant after magnetic resonance imaging. Am J Otolaryngol 2014;35:239-41.

Majdani O, et al. Artifacts caused by cochlear implants with non-removable magnets in 3T MRI: Phantom and cadaveric studies. Eur Arch Otorhinolaryngol 2009;266:1885-90.

Majdani O, et al. Demagnetization of cochlear implants and temperature changes in 3.0T MRI environment. Otolaryngol Head Neck Surg 2008;139:833-9.

Migirov L, et al. Magnet removal and reinsertion in a cochlear implant recipient undergoing brain MRI. J Otorhinolaryngol Relat Spec 2013;75:1-5.

Nospes S, et al. Magnetic resonance imaging in patients with magnetic hearing implants: Overview and procedural management. Radiologe 2013;53:1026-32.

Ouayoun M, et al. Nuclear magnetic resonance and cochlear implant. Ann Otolaryngol Chir Cervicofac 1997;114:65-70.

Ozturk E, et al. A rare complication of cochlear implantation after magnetic resonance imaging: Reversion of the magnet. J Craniofac Surg 2017 (In press).

Sharon JD, et al. Magnetic resonance imaging at 1.5 Tesla with a cochlear implant magnet in place: Image quality and usability. Otol Neurotol 2016;37:1284-90.

Teissl C, et al. Cochlear implants: *In vitro* investigation of electromagnetic interference at MR imaging-compatibility and safety aspects. Radiology 1998;208:700-708.

Teissl C, et al. Magnetic resonance imaging and cochlear implants: Compatibility and safety aspects. J Magn Reson Imag 1999;9:26-38.

Todt I, et al. MRI artifacts and cochlear implant positioning at 3 T in vivo. Otol Neurotol 2015;36:972-6.

Todt I, et al. Pain free 3 T MRI scans in cochlear implantees. Otol Neurotol 2017 (In press).

Wagner F, et al. Significant artifact reduction at 1.5 T and 3 T MRI by the use of a cochlear implant with removable magnet: An experimental human cadaver study. PLoS One 2015;10:e0132483.

Walton J, et al. MRI without magnet removal in neurofibromatosis type 2 patients with cochlear and auditory brainstem implants. Otol Neurotol 2014;35:821-5.

Young NM, et al. Magnetic resonance imaging of cochlear implant recipients. Otol Neurotol 2016;37:665-71.

Codman Microsensor ICP (Intracranial Pressure) Monitor Transducer

The Codman Microsensor Intracranial Pressure (ICP) Monitor Transducer and associated system components (Codman) monitors intracranial pressure directly at the source: subdural, parenchymal or intraventricular. The Codman Microsensor Intracranial Pressure (ICP) Monitor Transducer is MR Conditional. Comprehensive labeling information must be reviewed to ensure patient safety.

Carefully review the latest MRI labeling conditions and guidelines to ensure patient safety.

Important Note to MR Healthcare Professionals: Different MRI guidelines may exist for different countries. Therefore, use the appropriate information for your country.

[MR healthcare professionals are advised to contact the respective manufacturer in order to obtain the latest safety information to ensure patient safety relative to the use of an MR procedure.]

REFERENCE

Depuy Synthes, www.depuysynthes.com

Coils, Stents, Filters, and Grafts

Coils, stents, filters and vascular grafts have been evaluated relative to the use of MR systems. Several of these demonstrated magnetic field interactions. Fortunately, the devices that exhibited positive magnetic field interactions typically become incorporated securely in tissue within six weeks after implantation due to ingrowth and other mechanisms. Therefore, for most coils, filters, stents and grafts that have been tested, it is unlikely that these implants would become moved or dislodged as a result of exposure to MR systems operating at 1.5-Tesla or less. Additionally, many of these items have been evaluated at 3-Tesla (see below). MRI-related heating may also be of concern for certain configurations or shapes for coils, stents, filters, and vascular grafts. To date, there has been no reported case of excessive heating in association with MRI and these types of implants.

Many coils, filters, stents and grafts are made from nonferromagnetic materials, such as the LGM IVC filter (Vena Tech) used for caval interruption and the Wallstent biliary endoprosthesis (Schneider, Inc.) used for treatment of biliary obstruction. As such, these implants are acceptable for patients undergoing MR procedures relative to the use of the particular field strength utilized in the *ex vivo* testing (for specific information, see **The List**). Notably, it is unnecessary to wait after surgery to perform an MR procedure in a patient with a "passive" metallic implant that is made from a nonmagnetic material (see **Guidelines for the Management of the Post-Operative Patient Referred for a Magnetic Resonance Procedure**). In fact, there are reports in the peer-reviewed literature that describe placement of vascular stents or other similar devices using MR-guidance at 1.5-Tesla and 3-Tesla. Interestingly, some of these vascular implants (e.g., vascular stent grafts and stainless steel embolization coils) display high magnetic field interactions in association with 1.5- and 3-Tesla MR systems, yet have MR Conditional labeling approved by the Food and Drug Administration.

Patients with the specific coils, stents, filters and vascular grafts indicated in **The List** have had procedures using MR systems operating at static magnetic field strengths of 3-Tesla or less without reported injuries or other problems.

A study by Taal, et al. (1997) supports the fact that not all stents are safe for patients undergoing MR procedures. This investigation was performed to evaluate potential problems for four different types of stents: the Ultraflex (titanium alloy), the covered Wallstent (Nitinol), the Gianturco stent (Cook), and the modified Gianturco stent (Song) - the last two are made from stainless steel. Taal, et al. reported "an appreciable attraction force and torque" found for both types of Gianturco stents. Taal, et al. stated, "the Gianturco (Cook) stent pulled toward the head with a force of 7 g…however, it is uncertain whether this is a potential risk for dislodgment." In consideration of these results, the investigators advised, "…specific information on the type of stent is necessary before a magnetic resonance imaging examination is planned."

MRI at 3-Tesla and Coils, Stents, Filters and Vascular Grafts. Different coils, stents, filters and vascular grafts have been evaluated at 3-Tesla. Of these implants, two displayed magnetic field interactions that exceeded the American Society for Testing and Materials (ASTM) International guideline for safety (i.e. the deflection angles were greater than 45 degrees). However, similar to other comparable implants, tissue ingrowth and other mechanims are sufficient to prevent them from posing a substantial risk to a patient or individual in the 3-Tesla MR environment. Please refer to **The List** for specific information related to coils, stents, filters and vascular grafts.

Imporant Note: For additional information, please refer the section: **Guidelines for the Management of Patients with Coronary Artery Stents Referred for MRI Procedures**.

REFERENCES

Ahmed S, Shellock FG. Magnetic resonance imaging safety: Implications for cardiovascular patients. Journal of Cardiovascular Magnetic Resonance 2001;3:171-181.

Audet-Griffin A, Pakbaz S, Shellock FG. Evaluation of MRI issues for a new, liquid embolic device. J Neurointervent Surg 2014;6:624-629.

Bueker A, et al. Real-time MR fluoroscopy for MR-guided iliac artery stent placement. J Magn Reson Imag 2000;12:616-622.

Cook Medical, www.cookmedical.com

Girard MJ, et al. Wallstent metallic biliary endoprosthesis: MR imaging characteristics. Radiology 1992;184:874-876.

Green SR, Gianchandani YB. Wireless magnetoelastic monitoring of biliary stents. Journal of Microelectromechanical Systems 2009;18:64-78.

Hennemeyer CT, et al. *In vitro* evaluation of platinum Guglielmi detachable coils at 3-T with a porcine model: Safety issues and artifacts. Radiology 2001;219:732-737.

Hiramoto JS, et al. Long-term outcome and reintervention after endovascular abdominal aortic aneurysm repair using the Zenith stent graft. J Vasc Surg 2007;45:461-452.

Hiramoto JS, et al. The effect of magnetic resonance imaging on stainless-steel Z-stent-based abdominal aortic prosthesis. J Vasc Surg 2007;45:472-474.

Hug J, et al. Coronary arterial stents: Safety and artifacts during MR imaging. Radiology 2000;216:781-787.

Karacozoff AM, Shellock FG, Wakhloo AK. A next-generation, flow-diverting implant used to treat brain aneurysms: *In vitro* evaluation of magnetic field interactions, heating and artifacts at 3-T. Magnetic Resonance Imaging 2013;31:145-9.

Kaya MG, et al. Long-term clinical effects of magnetic resonance imaging in patients with coronary artery stent implantation. Coron Artery Dis 2009; 20:138-42.

Kiproff PM, et al. Magnetic resonance characteristics of the LGM vena cava filter: Technical note. Cardiovasc Intervent Radiol 1991;14:254-255.

Leibman CE, et al. MR imaging of inferior vena caval filter: Safety and artifacts. Am J Roentgenol 1988;150:1174-1176.

Manke C, et al. MR imaging-guided stent placement in iliac arterial stenoses: A feasibility study. Radiology 2001;219:527-534.

Marshall MW, et al. Ferromagnetism and magnetic resonance artifacts of platinum embolization microcoils. Cardiovasc Intervent Radiol 1991;14:163-166.

Nehra A, et al. MR safety and imaging of Neuroform Stents at 3-T. Am J Neuroradiol 2004;25:1476-1478.

Patel M, et al. Acute myocardial infarction: Safety of cardiac MR imaging after percutaneous revascularization with stents. Radiology 2006;240:674-680.

Porto I, et al. Safety of magnetic resonance imaging one to three days after bare metal and drug-eluting stent implantation. Am J Cardiol 2005;96:366-8.

Rutledge JM, et al. Safety of magnetic resonance immediately following Palmaz stent implant: A report of three cases. Catheter Cardiovasc Interv 2001;53:519-523.

Shellock FG. MR Safety at 3-Tesla: Bare Metal and Drug Eluting Coronary Artery Stents. Signals No. 53, Issue 2, pp. 26-27, 2005.

Shellock FG. Biomedical implants and devices: Assessment of magnetic field interactions with a 3.0-Tesla MR system. J Magn Reson Imag 2002;16:721-732.

Shellock FG, Detrick MS, Brant-Zawadski M. MR-compatibility of the Guglielmi detachable coils. Radiology 1997;203:568-570.

Shellock FG. Forder J. Drug eluting coronary stent: *In vitro* evaluation of magnetic resonance safety at 3-Tesla. Journal of Cardiovascular Magnetic Resonance 2005;7:415-419.

Shellock FG, Giangarra CJ. Assessment of 3-Tesla MRI issues for a bioabsorbable, coronary artery scaffold with metallic markers. Magnetic Resonance Imaging 2014;32:163-167.

Shellock FG, Gounis M, Wakhloo A. Detachable coil for cerebral aneurysms: *In vitro* evaluation of magnet field interactions, heating, and artifacts at 3-Tesla. Am J Neuroradiol 2005;26:363-366.

Shellock FG, Shellock VJ. Stents: Evaluation of MRI safety. Am J Roentgenol 1999;173:543-546.

Slesnick TC, et al. Safety of magnetic resonance imaging after implantation of stainless steel embolization coils. Pediatr Cardiol 2016;37:62-7.

Sommer T, et al. High field MR imaging: Magnetic field interactions of aneurysm clips, coronary artery stents and iliac artery stents with a 3.0 Tesla MR system. Rofo 2004;176:731-8.

Spuentrup E, et al. Magnetic resonance-guided coronary artery stent placement in a swine model. Circulation 2002;105:874-879.

Taal BG, et al. Potential risks and artifacts of magnetic resonance imaging of self-expandable esophageal stents. Gastrointestinal Endoscopy 1997;46;424-429.

Teitelbaum GP, et al. MR imaging artifacts, ferromagnetism, and magnetic torque of intravascular filters, stents, and coils. Radiology 1988;166:657-664.

Teitelbaum GP, et al. Ferromagnetism and MR imaging: Safety of cartoid vascular clamps. Am J Neuroradiol 1990;11:267-272.

Teitelbaum GP, Ortega HV, Vinitski S, et al. Low artifact intravascular devices: MR imaging evaluation. Radiology 1988;168:713-719.

Teitelbaum GP, et al. Evaluation of ferromagnetism and magnetic resonance imaging artifacts of the Strecker tantalum vascular stent. Cardiovasc Intervent Radiol 1989;12:125-127.

Titterington B, Shellock FG. A new vascular coupling device: Assessment of MRI issues at 3-Tesla. Magn Reson Imaging 2014;32:585-9.

Watanabe AT, Teitelbaum GP, Gomes AS, et al. MR imaging of the bird's nest filter. Radiology 1990;177:578-579.

Winter L, et al. On the RF heating of coronary stents at 7.0 Tesla MRI. Magn Reson Med 2015;74.

Dental Implants, Devices, and Materials

Many of the dental implants, devices, materials, and objects evaluated for ferromagnetic qualities exhibited measurable deflection forces (e.g., brace bands, brace wires, etc.) but only the ones with magnetically-activated components appear to present potential problems for patients during MR procedures (also, see **Magnetically-Activated Implants and Devices**). The issues that exist for magnetically-activated dental implants include possible demagnetization of the magnetic components and the substantial artifacts that the magnetic parts produce on MR imaging.

In general, most dental implants, devices, and materials made from ferromagnetic materials (with the exception of dental implants that incorporate magnetically-activated components) tend to be held in place with sufficient counter-forces to prevent them from causing problems related to movement or dislodgment in association with MR systems operating 3-Tesla or less. In addition, for the dental devices that have undergone evaluation, MRI-related heating does not appear to pose problems.

Wezel, et al. (2014) conducted an investigation to determine MRI issues for common dental retainer wires at 7-Tesla in terms of potential RF heating and magnetic susceptibility effects (i.e. artifacts). Electromagnetic simulations and experimental results were compared for dental retainer wires placed in tissue-mimicking phantoms. Simulations were then performed for a human model with dental wire in place. Additionally, image quality was evaluated for different scanning protocols and wires. The findings indicated that the simulations and experimental data in phantoms agreed well, with the length of the wire correlating to maximum heating in phantoms being approximately 47-mm. Even in that case, no substantial heating occurred when scanning within the specific absorption rate (SAR) guidelines for the head at 7-Tesla. Artifacts from the most ferromagnetic dental wire were not significant for any brain region. Wezel, et al. (2014) concluded that dental retainer wires appeared to be acceptable for patients undergoing MRI at 7-Tesla. Notably, these findings are specific to the wire types, configurations, and the particular MRI conditions that were used in this study.

REFERENCES

Ayyildiz S, et al. Radiofrequency heating and magnetic field interactions of fixed partial dentures during 3-Tesla magnetic resonance imaging. Oral Surg Oral Med Oral Pathol Oral Radiol 2013;116:640-7.

Blankenstein FH, et al. Signal loss in magnetic resonance imaging caused by intraoral anchored dental magnetic materials. Rofo 2006;178:787-93.

Duttenhoefer F, et al. Magnetic resonance imaging in zirconia-based dental implantology. Clin Oral Implants Res 2015;26:1195-202.

Gegauff A, et al. A potential MRI hazard: Forces on dental magnet keepers. J Oral Rehabil 1990;17:403-410.

Gorgulu S, et al. Effect of orthodontic brackets and different wires on radiofrequency heating and magnetic field interactions during 3-T MRI. Dentomaxillofac Radiol 2014;43:20130356.

Hasegawa M, et al. Radiofrequency heating of metallic dental devices during 3.0 T MRI. Dentomaxillofac Radiol 2013;42:20120234.

Hasegawa M, et al. 3-T MRI safety assessments of magnetic dental attachments and castable magnetic alloys. Dentomaxillofac Radiol 2015;44:20150011.

Hubalkova H, et al. Dental alloys and magnetic resonance imaging. Int Dent J 2006;56:135-41.

Ideta T, et al. Investigation of radio frequency heating of dental implants made of titanium in 1.5 Tesla and 3.0 Tesla magnetic resonance procedure: Measurement of the temperature by using tissue-equivalent phantom. Nihon Hoshasen Gijutsu Gakkai Zasshi 2013;69:521-8.

Klinke T, et al. Artifacts in magnetic resonance imaging and computed tomography caused by dental materials. PLoS One 2012;7:e31766.

Korn P, et al. MRI and dental implantology: Two which do not exclude each other. Biomaterials 2015;53:634-45.

Lissac MI, Metrop D, Brugigrad, et al. Dental materials and magnetic resonance imaging. Invest Radiol 1991;26:40-45.

Miyata K, et al. Radiofrequency heating and magnetically induced displacement of dental magnetic attachments during 3.0 T MRI. Dentomaxillofac Radiol 2012;41:668-74.

New PFJ, et al. Potential hazards and artifacts of ferromagnetic and nonferromagnetic surgical and dental materials and devices in nuclear magnetic resonance imaging. Radiology 1983;147:139-148.

Omatsu M, et al. Magnetic displacement force and torque on dental keepers in the static magnetic field of an MR scanner. J Magn Reson Imaging 2014;40:1481-6.

Oriso K, et al. Impact of the static and radiofrequency magnetic fields produced by a 7T MR imager on metallic dental materials. Magn Reson Med Sci 2015 2016;15:26-33.

Seong-Cheol P, et al. Magnetic resonance imaging distortion and targeting errors from strong rare earth metal magnetic dental implant requiring revision. Turk Neurosurg 2016 (In press).

Shellock FG. *Ex vivo* assessment of deflection forces and artifacts associated with high-field strength MRI of "mini-magnet" dental prostheses. Magnetic Resonance Imaging 1989;7 (Suppl 1):38.

Shellock FG, Crues JV, Editors. MRI Bioeffects, Safety, and Patient Management. Biomedical Research Publishing Group, Los Angeles, CA, 2014.

Shellock FG, Crues JV. High-field strength MR imaging and metallic biomedical implants: An *ex vivo* evaluation of deflection forces. Am J Roentgenol 1988;151:389-392.

Tymofiyeva O, et al. Influence of dental materials on dental MRI. Dentomaxillofac Radiol 2013;42:2012.

Wezel J, et al. Assessing the MR compatibility of dental retainer wires at 7 Tesla. Magn Reson Med 2014;72:1191-8.

Zho SY, et al. Artifact reduction from metallic dental materials in T1-weighted spin-echo imaging at 3.0 tesla. J Magn Reson Imaging 2013;37:471-8.

Diaphragms

A contraceptive diaphragm may have a metallic ring that maintains it in position during use. Thus, certain contraceptive diaphragms with metallic components may display positive magnetic field interactions in association with exposure to MR systems. Furthermore, because of the metallic parts associated with these devices, substantial artifacts may be found. MR examinations have been performed in patients with contraceptive diaphragm without complaints or adverse sensations related to movement or displacement. Furthermore, there is no danger of heating a contraceptive diaphragm during an MR procedure under conditions currently recommended by the United States Food and Drug Administration. Therefore, the presence of a contraceptive diaphragm is not a contraindication for a patient undergoing an MR examination using an MR system operating at 3-Tesla or less. Regardless of the afore-mentioned information, it is advisable to remove a contraceptive diaphragm prior to an MRI examination in order to avoid issues if the imaging area of interest is where the device is located.

REFERENCES

Shellock FG. Magnetic Resonance Procedures: Health Effects and Safety. CRC Press, LLC, Boca Raton, FL, 2001.

Shellock FG, Crues JV, Editors. MRI Bioeffects, Safety, and Patient Management. Biomedical Research Publishing Group, Los Angeles, CA, 2014.

Shellock FG, Kanal E. Magnetic Resonance: Bioeffects, Safety, and Patient Management. Second Edition, Lippincott-Raven Press, New York, 1996.

Dressings Containing Silver and MRI Procedures

Clarification: Antimicrobial Dressings Containing Silver Aren't Necessarily Hazardous during MR Scans*

[*ECRI Institute. Antimicrobial dressings containing silver may cause pain and burns during MR scans [Hazard Report and clarification]. Health Devices 2007 Jul;36:232-3 and 2008 Feb; 37:60-2. Copyright 2007, 2008 ECRI Institute. Content reprinted with permission.]

In our July 2007 issue, we published a Hazard Report titled "Antimicrobial Dressings Containing Silver May Cause Pain and Burns During MR Scans" in which we reported on a patient who suffered pain during a magnetic resonance (MR) scan. The patient was wearing dressings containing silver, which acts as an antimicrobial agent. We discussed the possibility that the silver in the dressings might have been heated by the radio-frequency (RF) energy that is present during any MR scan.

Our report on this incident has given some readers the impression that patients wearing dressings containing silver should never undergo MR scans. That is not the case. We are publishing this update to further explain the issue and clarify our recommendations. In particular, we want to make the following points clear:

First, the fact that a patient is wearing silver-containing dressings should not keep the patient from having an MR examination.

Second, the reason that some silver-containing dressings are contraindicated by the dressing manufacturer for use during MR scans is because they could produce artifacts and distortions in the MR image, not because of any risk they might pose to the patient (although such risk cannot be conclusively ruled out).

Third, the exact cause of the patient's pain in the reported incident was never determined; the silver-containing dressings are only one of the possible causes.

DISCUSSION

Our position on silver-containing dressings in MR scans. We believe that the presence of antimicrobial dressings containing silver should not disqualify a patient from undergoing an MR scan. We do advise, whenever feasible, that such dressings be removed before a scan and that the wound be washed with water to remove as many traces of silver as possible. The reason for doing so is to minimize any detrimental effects the silver might have on the quality of the image. If it isn't feasible to remove the dressings, we believe the scan should still be carried out.

However, clinicians should be aware that there may be a risk, albeit remote, that the silver in the dressing— some of which will have been absorbed into the wound and its exudate—could become heated by the RF energy present during the scan (see Possible Causes of Pain, below). As in any MR procedure, the patient should be monitored closely, and any report of unusual pain or heating should be promptly addressed, as described in our Recommendations.

Note that the dressings are only likely to be a concern if the dressed area will be included in the scanned area. If, for example, a head scan is being performed and there are silver-containing dressings on the patient's foot, there is probably no reason the dressings need to be disturbed.

Possible causes of pain.

In the reported incident, the patient was an amputee whose stump was being scanned. The stump had been covered with silver-containing dressings. During the MR acquisition, the patient experienced significant pain, and the scan was aborted.

A week later, the study was continued, after the dressing had been removed and the wound lightly washed with water at the advice of the dressing manufacturer. However, the patient still experienced significant pain, and the reporting hospital noted that the amputation stump retained a silvery sheen despite the washing. It was suspected that the MR energy had interacted with the silver. But no further testing was undertaken to verify that suspicion.

Silver is not ferromagnetic, so the patient's pain could not have been caused by any magnetic effects of the MR field on the silver. As discussed above, though, MR scans create RF energy, which can induce electrical currents within electrical conductors. These currents can cause heating and lead to patient burns. This has been previously reported by Wagle and Smith (2000) and Franiel, et al. (2006). However, empirical testing with implants and devices shows that excessive heating only occurs for those that have an elongated shape forming a closed loop of a certain diameter (Dempsey and Condon, 2001). In the case that we reported, it is conceivable that the silver formed a large conducting loop around the wound; but the large amount of silver that would be needed makes this unlikely. Also, although the patient felt a burning sensation, there were no visible signs of a burn. So the evidence is far from conclusive.

RECOMMENDATIONS

Until further empirical testing is done to establish the required conditions, if any, necessary to produce a heating effect, the following revised recommendations should be followed:

1) Alert MR healthcare workers that some silver-containing antimicrobial dressings are contraindicated for MR exams in order to avoid artifacts. Therefore, if contraindicated dressings are close to the region being scanned or within the transmit RF coil, they should be removed if possible. However, a patient wearing such a dressing should not be prevented from having an MR procedure.

2) In some cases, it may be possible to reapply the same dressing to the patient after the scan. Whether this can be done depends in part on the amount of exudates on the dressing. The decision to reapply a dressing must be made by qualified staff.

3) As with any MR procedure, the patient should be carefully monitored and instructed to immediately report any unusual pain or heating. All such cases should be investigated immediately. If it is not possible to determine the cause of the pain and alleviate the problem (e.g., by applying a cold compress), then the procedure should be abandoned.

4) Report any similar occurrences of patient pain or burns to the dressing manufacturer and to ECRI Institute. Full details of the procedure should be recorded, including the field strength, coil used, and scan parameters.

REFERENCES

Dempsey MF, Condon B. Thermal injuries associated with MRI. Clin Radiol 2001 Jun;56:457-65.

Franiel T, Schmidt S, Klingebiel R. First-degree burns on MRI due to nonferrous tattoos. Am J Roentgenol 2006;187(5):W556.

Tope WD, Shellock FG. Magnetic resonance imaging and permanent cosmetics (tattoos): Survey of complications and adverse events. J Magn Reson Imag 2002;15:180-4.

Wagle WA, Smith M. Tattoo-induced skin burn during MR imaging. Am J Roentgenol 2000;174:1795.

Wagner M, Lanfermann H, Zanella F. MR-induced burn-reaction in a female patient with "permanent make-up" Rofo 2006;178:728-30.

Yuh WT, Fisher DJ, Shields RK, Ehrhardt JC, Shellock FG. Phantom limb pain induced in amputee by strong magnetic fields. J Magn Reson Imag 1992;2:221-3.

Dressings Containing Silver and MRI Procedures: Aquacel AG

Aquacel Ag (ConvaTec, Skillman, New Jersey) is a dressing that contains ionic silver, which combines the antibacterial action of silver with a barrier dressing that utilizes Hydrofiber technology (E.R. Squibb & Sons, LLC, New Brunswick, NJ) to absorb large amounts of wound exudate without requiring frequent dressing changes.

Nyenhuis and Duan (2009) evaluated MRI issues for this dressing at 1.5- and 3-Tesla. Based on the findings, the Aquacel Ag wound dressing impregnated with ionic silver was reported to be "MR Safe" (i.e. an item that poses no known hazards in all MRI environments), particularly since it exhibited electric properties similar to human tissues. Therefore, an Aquacel Ag dressing may be left in place in a patient undergoing an MRI procedure.

REFERENCES

Nyenhuis J, Duan L. An evaluation of MRI safety and compatibility of a silver-impregnated antimicrobial wound dressing. J Am Coll Radiol 2009;6:500-5.

Shellock FG, Woods TO, Crues JV. MRI labeling information for implants and devices: Explanation of terminology. Radiology 2009;253:26-30.

Dressings Containing Silver and MRI Procedures: Mepilex Ag and Mepilex Border AG

Two different antimicrobial, silver-containing wound dressings Mepilex Ag and Mepilex Border AG (Molnlycke Health Care AB, Goteborg, Sweden) have undergone MRI testing at 3-Tesla that included evaluations of magnetic field interactions, heating, and artifacts. Additionally, conductivity (i.e. electrical resistance) measurements were performed on these dressings. There were no magnetic field interactions displayed by these dressings. In each case, MRI-related heating effects were at the same levels as the background temperature rises. The dressings did not create noticeable artifacts on the MR images. With regard to the conductivity assessments, the average resistance values were within acceptable limits.

Thus, the results demonstrated that these specific silver-containing wound dressings will not pose hazards or risks to patients and, therefore, are considered "MR Safe" according to the current labeling terminology used for medical products. Importantly, each dressing may be left in place when a patient undergoes an MRI examination.

REFERENCES

Escher KB, Shellock FG. Assessment of MRI issues at 3-Tesla for antimicrobial, silver-containing wound dressings. Ostomy Wound Management 2012;58:22-7.

Shellock FG, Woods TO, Crues JV. MRI labeling information for implants and devices: Explanation of terminology. Radiology 2009;253:26-30.

ECG (EKG) Electrodes

To ensure patient safety and proper recording of the electrocardiogram during an MRI procedure, it is advisable to only use electrocardiograph (ECG or EKG) electrodes tested specifically with regard to the factors that impact MRI safety issues and are recommended by the monitor's manufacturer. Tests should include an evaluation of magnetic field interactions, MRI-related heating, and characterization of artifacts.

Various ECG electrodes have been specially developed for use during MRI examinations to protect the patient from potentially hazardous conditions and to minimize MRI-related artifacts. **The List** provides a compilation of ECG electrodes that have been evaluated for MRI issues using MR systems operating with static magnetic fields of 1.5-Tesla and 3-Tesla. Importantly, these electrodes should be used according to the guidelines provided by the manufacturers of the ECG monitoring devices.

IMPORTANT NOTE: To ensure patient safety and proper recording of the electrocardiogram during an MRI procedure, it is important to use only electrocardiograph (EKG/ECG) electrodes tested specifically with regard to the MRI environment and recommended by the manufacturer for use with the respective the MR Conditional monitoring equipment.

ECG electrodes should only be used according to the specific guidelines provided by the manufacturers of the MR Conditional, monitoring systems.

To prevent injuries (e.g., burn), for a patient undergoing an MRI procedure, ECG electrodes must be removed if they are not connected to acceptable MR Conditional monitoring equipment.

REFERENCES

Shellock FG. MRI and ECG electrodes. Signals, No. 29, Issue 1, pp. 10-14, 1999.

Shellock FG. Magnetic Resonance Procedures: Health Effects and Safety. CRC Press, LLC, Boca Raton, FL, 2001.

Shellock FG, Crues JV, Editors. MRI Bioeffects, Safety, and Patient Management. Biomedical Research Publishing Group, Los Angeles, CA, 2014.

EmpowerMR Contrast Injection System

The **EmpowerMR Contrast Injection System** is uniquely designed for seamless integration within the magnetic resonance imaging (MRI) setting. This device has the following features:

- Virtually eliminates RF transients in the scanner room
- MR Conditional up to 7-Tesla
- The compact, rotating head adapts to workflow and the environment

The EmpowerMR Injector Head, which is MR Conditional, can be positioned on either the right or left side of the MR scanner, on either side of the patient gantry. The controls on the Injector Head should be outward facing to the clinician to ensure that the patient can be observed concurrently with the injector controls.

There is no minimum distance requirement within these locations to the exterior of the MR scanner, within these prescribed locations for static magnetic field strengths up to 7-Tesla.

Two system configurations are possible. The only difference between the two system configurations is the location of the Hydraulic Controller. In one configuration, the Hydraulic Controller is located in the Equipment Room and in the other it is located in the Control Room.

The Equipment Room is the preferred location due to the noise of the Hydraulic Controller. As a general rule, the Hydraulic Controller must be located beyond the ten gauss level.

REFERENCE

www.bracco.com

Epidural Pump, ambIT Infusion Pumps

The ambIT Infusion Pumps (Summit Medical Products) are used to infuse medication and/or fluids into patients primarily for pain management. Routes of delivery are generally intravenous, epidural and/or regional.

MRI Information
Warnings

Safety hazards such as under infusion may be associated with external radio frequency interference (RFI) or electromagnetic radiation. Typical equipment which may generate such radiation include X-ray machines, MRI equipment, and any other non-shielded electrical equipment.

REFERENCE

www.ambitpump.com

Essure Device

The Essure Device (Conceptus Incorported and Bayer) is a metallic implant developed for permanent female contraception. The presence of this implant is intended to alter the function and architecture of the fallopian tube, resulting in permanent contraception. The Essure Device is composed of 316L stainless steel, platinum, iridium, nickel-titanium alloy, silver solder, and polyethylene terephthalate (PET) fibers.

The MRI assessment of this device involved testing for magnetic field interactions (1.5-Tesla), heating, induced electrical currents, and artifacts using previously described techniques. There were no magnetic field interactions, the highest temperature changes were $\leq +0.6$ degrees C, and the induced electrical currents were minimal. Furthermore, artifacts should not create a substantial problem for diagnostic MR imaging unless the area of interest is in the exact same position as where this implant is located. Thus, the findings indicated that it is acceptable for a patient with the Essure Device to undergo an MR procedure at 1.5-Tesla or less.

MRI at 3-Tesla and the Essure Device. The Essure Device has been evaluated (i.e. tested for magnetic field interactions and MRI-related heating) at 3-Tesla and found to be acceptable for patients undergoing MR procedures at this static magnetic field strength.

REFERENCES

Essure, www.essure.com

Shellock FG. Biomedical implants and devices: Assessment of magnetic field interactions with a 3.0-Tesla MR system. J Magn Reson Imag 2002;16:721-732.

Shellock FG. New metallic implant used for permanent female contraception: Evaluation of MR safety. Am J Roentgenol 2002;178:1513-1516.

External Fixation Devices

Most orthopedic implants and materials do not pose substantial problems for patients undergoing MR procedures. However, because of the length of the implant and/or the formation of a conductive loop, MR examinations may be hazardous for certain orthopedic implants, including external fixation devices or systems.

External fixation systems comprise specially designed frames, clamps, rods, rod-to-rod couplings, pins, posts, fasteners, wire fixations, fixation bolts, washers, nuts, hinges, sockets, connecting bars, screws and other components used in orthopedic and reconstructive surgery. Indications for external fixation systems are varied and include the following treatment applications:

- Open or closed fractures fixation;
- Correction of pseudoarthroses of long bones (both congenital and acquired);
- Limb lengthening by metaphyseal or epiphyseal distraction;
- Correction of bony or soft tissue defects; and
- Correction of bony or soft tissue deformities.

The assessment of MRI issues for external fixation systems is especially challenging because of the myriad of possible components (many of which are made from conductive materials) and configurations used for these devices. The primary concern is MRI-related heating which is dependent on the particular aspects (e.g., the lengths of the component parts) of the external fixation system. Importantly, the MRI conditions (e.g., strength of the static magnetic field, frequency of the RF field, type of RF transmit coil, pulse sequence, body part imaged, position of the fixation device relative to the transmit RF coil, etc.) directly impact the safety aspects of scanning patients with external fixation systems.

For example, Luechinger, et al. (2007) used MRI to study "large orthopedic external fixation clamps and related components". Forces induced by a 3-Tesla MR scanner were compiled for newly designed nonmagnetic clamps and older clamps that contained ferromagnetic components. Heating trials were performed in 1.5- and 3-Tesla MR systems for two assembled external fixation frames. Forces acting on the newly designed clamps were more than a factor of two lower as the gravitational force on the devices whereas, magnetic forces on the older devices showed over 10 times the force induced by earth's acceleration of gravity. No torque effects could be found for the newly designed clamps.

Furthermore, the investigators recorded temperatures at the tips of Schanz screws in the 1.5-Tesla MR system and reported a rise of 0.7 degrees C for a pelvic frame and of 2.1 degrees C for a diamond knee bridge frame when normalized to a specific absorption rate (SAR) of 2-W/kg. The normalized temperature increases at 3-Tesla MR system were 0.9 degrees C for the pelvic frame and 1.1 degrees C for the knee bridge frame. Large external fixation frames assembled with the newly designed clamps (390 Series Clamps), carbon fiber reinforced rods, and implant quality 316L stainless steel Schanz screws met acceptable safety guidelines when tested at 3-Tesla. Notably, this information pertains to the specific configuration of the fixation devices that underwent testing relative to the MRI conditions that were used.

To ensure patient safety, guidelines for external fixation devices must be applied on a case-by-case and configuration-by-configuration basis. Therefore, MR healthcare professionals are referred to product labeling approved by the U.S. Food and Drug Administration or other notified body for a given external fixation system. Importantly, this information may only apply to a particular configuration for the external fixation device.

There are several external fixation systems with MR Conditional labeling that are acceptable for scanning patients as long as the frame is not in the bore of the MR system (i.e. located within the transmit RF body coil). For example, the Large External Fixator (Depuy Synthes, www.depuysynthes.com) has the following MR Conditional labeling:

Large External Fixator (external fixation system) devices used in a typical construct include clamps, rods and various attachments. A patient with a Synthes Large External Fixator frame may be scanned safely after placement of the frame under the following conditions:

- Static magnetic field of 1.5 Tesla or 3.0 Tesla when the fixator frame is positioned outside the MRI Bore at Normal Operator or in First Level Control Mode
- Highest spatial gradient magnetic field of 720 Gauss/cm or less
- Maximum MR system reported whole body averaged specific absorption rate (SAR) of 2 W/kg for the Normal Operating Mode and 4 W/kg for the First Level Controlled Mode for 15 minutes of scanning

- Use only whole body RF transmit coil, no other transmit coils are allowed, local receive only coils are allowed
- Specialty coils, such as knee or head coils, should not be used as they have not been evaluated for RF heating and may result in higher localized heating
- Do not place any radio frequency (RF) transmit coils over the Large External Fixator frame

Note: In nonclinical testing, the Large External Fixator frame was tested in several different configurations. This testing was conducted with the construct position 7 cm from within the outside edge of the MRI bore. The results showed a maximum observed heating for a pelvic frame of less than 1°C for 1.5 T and 3.0 T with a machine reported whole body averaged SAR of 2 W/kg.

Importantly, certain external fixation systems are labeled, MR Unsafe, such as the Hybrid Ring Fixator, External Fixation Recon System: The "Hybrid Ring Fixator" is MR Unsafe. Do not use this device in any MR environment. This device is known to pose hazards in all MR environments.

MRI Simulations and External Fixation Systems. Because external fixation systems have a variety of sizes, shapes, and component parts it is particularly challenging to assess MRI-related heating for these devices. An efficient means of addressing this issue is to conduct MRI simulations to predict the worst-case of MRI-induced heating for a particular external fixation system type under 1.5-T/64-MHz and 3-T/128-MHz conditions and then to apply the experimental test to validate the numerical results for worst-case heating by conducting MRI-related heating assessments, as described by Liu, et al. (2013).

Vibration Associated With MR Procedures. Graf, et al. (2006) reported that considerable torque may act on relatively large metallic implants due to eddy-current induction in associated with MR imaging. Larger implants (such as fixation devices) made from conducting materials are especially affected. Gradient switching was shown to produce fast alternating torque. Significant vibrations at off-center positions of the metal parts may explain why some patients with metallic implants may report feeling sensations of "heating" during MR examinations.

[MR healthcare professionals are advised to contact the respective manufacturer in order to obtain the latest safety information to ensure patient safety relative to the use of an MR procedure.]

REFERENCES

Depuy Synthes, www.depuysynthes.com

Elsissy P, et al. MRI evaluation of the knee with non-ferromagnetic external fixators: Cadaveric knee model. Eur J Orthop Surg Traumatol 2015;25:933.

Graf H, Lauer UA, Schick F. Eddy-current induction in extended metallic parts as a source of considerable torsional moment. J Magn Reson Imag 2006;23:585-590.

Hayden BL, et al. MRI of trauma patients treated with contemporary external fixation devices: A multi-center case series. J Orthop Trauma 2017 (In press).

Liu Y, et al. Numerical investigations of MRI RF field induced heating for external fixation devices. Biomed Eng Online 2013;12:12.

Liu Y, et al. Effect of insulating layer material on RF-induced heating for external fixation system in 1.5T MRI system. Electromagn Biol Med 2014;33:223-7.

Liu Y, Chen J, Shellock FG, Kainz W. Computational and experimental studies of an orthopedic implant: MRI-related heating at 1.5-Tesla/64-MHz and 3-Tesla/128-MHz. J Magn Reson Imaging 2013;37:491-497.

Luechinger R, Boesiger P, Disegi JA. Safety evaluation of large external fixation clamps and frames in a magnetic resonance environment. J Biomed Mater Res B Appl Biomater 2007;82:17-22.

Shellock FG. External Fixation Devices and MRI Safety. Signals, No. 56, Issue 1, pp. 15, 2006.

Foley Catheters With and Without Temperature Sensors

Foley catheters utilized to drain the bladder typically have no or few metallic components. Accordingly, these devices tend to be acceptable for patients undergoing MR procedures. However, certain Foley catheters have sensors to measure the temperature of the urine in the bladder, which is an appropriate means of determining "deep" body or core temperature. This type of Foley catheter usually has a thermistor or thermocouple located on or near the tip of the device and a wire that runs the length of the catheter to a connector that plugs into a temperature monitor. Sometimes an additional external cable is also used, which may or may not be removable. To date, a Foley catheter with a temperature sensor should never be connected to an external cable and/or the temperature monitor because this equipment has not been shown to be safe for patients undergoing MR examinations.

Several Foley catheters with temperature sensors have been evaluated for MRI issues by determining magnetic field interactions, heating, and artifacts. In general, the findings indicated that it would be acceptable to perform MR procedures in patients with certain Foley catheters with temperature sensors as long as specific recommendations and conditions are followed.

Similar to other devices with conductive components, the position of the wire and/or cable associated with the Foley catheter with a temperature sensor has an important effect on the amount of heating that develops during an MR procedure. Therefore, to prevent excessive heating associated with an MR examination, a Foley catheter with a temperature sensor must be positioned in a straight configuration (without a loop) down the center of the MR system and away from transmit RF coil or inside of the bore of the scanner. The metal connector, cable, or wire, must not touch the patient. Typical recommendations for the specific Foley catheters with temperature sensors that have undergone MRI testing include, the following:

1) If the Foley catheter with a temperature sensor has a removable connector cable or extension, it should be disconnected prior to the MR procedure.

2)   Remove all electrically conductive material from the bore of the MR system that is not required for the procedure (i.e. unused surface coils, cables, etc.).

3)   Keep electrically conductive material that must remain in the bore of the MR system from directly contacting the patient by placing insulation or space between the conductive material and the patient.

4)   Position the Foley catheter with a temperature sensor in a straight configuration down the center of the MR system table to prevent cross points, coils, and loops.

5)   Ensure that the connector, cable, or wire *does not touch the patient*.

6)   MR imaging should be performed using MR systems shown to be acceptable and safe for patients (e.g., operating at a specific static magnetic field and frequency, 1.5-Tesla/64-MHz, or other tested field strength/frequency level) and all pertinent safety guidelines must be followed.

7)   Follow the **Instructions for Use** for a given Foley catheter with a temperature sensor with regard to the MR system reported, whole body averaged specific absorption rate (SAR).

8)   Monitor the patient continuously using a verbal means (e.g., intercom).

9)   If the patient reports any unusual sensation, discontinue the MR procedure immediately.

Specific labeling instructions for a given Foley catheter with temperature sensor must be carefully followed. Importantly, not all Foley catheters with temperature sensors are acceptable for patients undergoing MR procedures.

An example of specific instructions for a Foley catheter with temperature sensor that has MRI labeling approved by the Food and Drug Administration is, as follows:

Foley Catheter with Temperature Sensor, Bardex Latex-Free Temperature-Sensing 400-Series Foley Catheter (C. R. Bard, Inc., www.bardmedical.com)

MRI Safety Instructions

Warning: This product should never be connected to the temperature monitor or connected to a cable during an MRI procedure. Failure to follow this guideline may result in serious injury to the patient. Refer to *Instructions for Use.* It is important to closely follow these specific conditions that have been determined to permit the examination to be conducted safely. Any deviation may result in a serious injury to the patient.

Non-clinical testing demonstrated that these Foley catheters with temperature sensors are MR Conditional. A patient with one of these devices can be scanned safely, immediately after placement under the following conditions:

- Static magnetic field of 1.5-Tesla or 3-Tesla with regard to magnetic field interactions.
- Spatial gradient magnetic field of 720-gauss/cm or less with regard to magnetic field interactions.
- Maximum MR system reported, whole-body-averaged specific absorption rate (SAR) of 3.5-W/kg at 1.5-Tesla or 3-W/kg at 3-Tesla for 15 minutes of scanning (i.e. per pulse sequence).

Importantly, the MRI procedure should be performed using an MR system operating at a static magnetic field strength of 1.5-Tesla or 3-Tesla, ONLY. The safe use of an MR system operating at lower or higher static magnetic field strength for a patient with a Foley catheter with temperature sensor has not been determined.

Special Instructions: The position of the wire of the Foley Catheter with Temperature Sensor has an important effect on the amount of heating that may develop during an MRI procedure. Accordingly, the Foley catheter with temperature sensor must be positioned in a straight configuration down the center of the patient table (i.e. down the center of the MR system without any loop) to prevent possible excessive heating associated with an MRI procedure.

Additional safety instructions include the following:

1) The Foley catheter with temperature sensor should not be connected to the temperature monitoring equipment during the MRI procedure.

2) If the Foley catheter with temperature sensor has a removable catheter connector cable, it should be disconnected prior to the MRI procedure.

3) Remove all electrically conductive material from the bore of the MR system that is not required for the procedure (i.e. unused surface coils, cables, etc.).

4) Keep electrically conductive material that must remain in the bore of the MR system from directly contacting the patient by placing thermal and/or electrical insulation (including air) between the conductive material and the patient.

5)   Position the Foley catheter with a temperature sensor in a straight configuration down the center of the patient table to prevent cross points and conductive coils or loops.

6)   The wire and connector of the Foley catheter with temperature sensor should not be in contact with the patient during the MRI procedure. Position the device, accordingly.

7)   MR imaging should be performed using an MR system with static magnetic strength of 1.5-Tesla or 3-Tesla, ONLY.

8)   At 1.5-Tesla, the MR system reported whole body averaged SAR should not exceed 3.5-W/kg for 15-min. of scanning (i.e. per pulse sequence).

9)   At 3-Tesla, the MR system reported whole body averaged SAR should not exceed 3-W/kg for 15-min of scanning (i.e. per pulse sequence).

In addition to the above, the **Guidelines to Prevent Excessive Heating and Burns Associated with Magnetic Resonance Procedures** should be considered and implemented.

[MR healthcare professionals are advised to contact the respective manufacturer in order to obtain the latest safety information to ensure patient safety relative to the use of an MR procedure.]

REFERENCES

Bard Medical, www.bardmedical.com

Dempsey MF, Condon B, Hadley DM. Investigation of the factors responsible for burns during MRI. J Magn Reson Imag 2001;13:627-631.

Shellock FG. Magnetic Resonance Procedures: Health Effects and Safety. CRC Press, LLC, Boca Raton, FL, 2001.

Shellock FG, Kanal E. Magnetic Resonance: Bioeffects, Safety, and Patient Management. Second Edition, Lippincott-Raven Press, New York, 1996.

Glaucoma Drainage Implants (Shunt Tubes)

A glaucoma drainage implant or device, also known as a shunt tube, is implanted to maintain an artificial drainage pathway to control intraocular pressure for patients with glaucoma. Intraocular pressure is lowered when aqueous humor flows from inside the eye through the tube into the space between the plate that rests on the scleral surface and surrounding fibrous capsule. The implantation of a glaucoma drainage device is used to treat glaucoma that is refractory to medical and standard surgical therapy. These are usually cases where standard drainage procedures have been unsuccessful or have a poor prognosis including failed trabeculectomy, juvenile glaucoma, neovascular glaucoma and glaucoma secondary to uveitis, traumatic glaucoma, cataract with glaucoma and high risk cases of primary glaucoma.

Importantly, for certain glaucoma drainage implants, radiographic findings may suggest the diagnosis of an orbital foreign body if the ophthalmic history is unknown, as reported by Ceballos and Parrish (2002). In this case report, a patient was denied an MRI examination for fear of dislodging an apparent "metallic foreign body." In fact, the patient had a Baerveldt glaucoma drainage implant that was mistakenly identified as an orbital metallic object based on its radiographic characteristics (i.e. due to the presence of barium-impregnated silicone).

At least one glaucoma drainage implant, the Ex-PRESS miniature glaucoma shunt (Optonol Ltd., Neve Ilan, Israel) is made from 316L stainless steel which, according to De Feo, et al. (2009), may affect MRI examinations of the optic nerve. Geffen, et al. (2010) reported that the Ex-PRESS glaucoma shunt is acceptable for patients undergoing MRI at 3-Tesla or less.

Many other glaucoma drainage implants are made from nonmetallic materials and are safe for patients undergoing MRI procedures. Commonly used devices that do not contain metal include, the following:

- Baerveldt glaucoma drainage implant (Pharmacia Co., Kalamazoo, MI)

- Krupin-Denver eye valve to disc implant (E. Benson Hood Laboratories, Pembroke, MA)
- Ahmed glaucoma valve (New World Medical, Rancho Cucamonga, CA)
- Molteno drainage device (Molteno Ophthalmic Ltd., Dunedin, New Zealand)
- Joseph valve (Valve Implants Limited, Hertford, England)

REFERENCES

Allemann R, et al. Ultra high-field magnetic resonance imaging of a glaucoma microstent. Curr Eye Res 2011;36:719-26.

Ceballos EM, Parrish RK. Plain film imaging of Baerveldt glaucoma drainage implants. American Journal of Neuroradiology 2002;23;935-937.

Dahan E, Carmichael TR. Implantation of a miniature glaucoma device under a scleral flap. J Glaucoma 2005;14:98-102.

De Feo F, et al. Magnetic resonance imaging in patients implanted with Ex-PRESS stainless steel glaucoma drainage microdevice. Am J Ophthalmol. 2009;147:907-11.

Geffen N, et al. Is the Ex-PRESS Glaucoma Shunt ,magnetic resonance imaging safe? J Glaucoma. 2010;19:116-118.

Hong CH, et al. Glaucoma drainage devices: A systematic literature review and current controversies. Surv Ophthalmol 2005;50:48-60.

Jeon TY, et al. MR imaging features of giant reservoir formation in the orbit: An unusual complication of Ahmed glaucoma valve implantation. Am J Neuroradiol 2007;28:1565-1566.

Mabray MC, et al. Ex-PRESS glaucoma filter: An MRI compatible metallic orbital foreign body imaged at 1.5 and 3T. Clin Radiol 2015;70:e28-34.

Seibold LK, et al. MRI of the Ex-PRESS stainless steel glaucoma drainage device. Br J Ophthalmol 2011;95:251-254.

Sidoti PA, Baerveldt G. Glaucoma drainage implants. Curr Opin Ophthalmol 1994;5:85-98.

Traverso CE, et al. Long term effect on IOP of a stainless steel glaucoma drainage implant (Ex-PRESS) in combined surgery with phacoemulsification. British Journal of Ophthalmology 2005;89:425-429.

Guidewires

Advances in interventional MR procedures have resulted in the need for guidewires that are acceptable for endovascular therapy, drainage procedures, and other similar applications. Conventional guidewires are made from stainless steel or Nitinol, materials known to be conductive. Accordingly, radiofrequency fields used for MR procedures may induce substantial currents in guidewires, leading to excessive temperature increases and potential injuries.

Liu, et al. (2000) studied the theoretical and experimental aspects of the RF heating resonance phenomenon of an endovascular guidewire. A Nitinol-based guidewire (Terumo, Tokyo, Japan) was inserted into a vessel phantom and imaged using 1.5-T and 0.2-T MR systems with continuous temperature monitoring at the guidewire tip. The guidewire was deployed in the phantom in a "straight" manner. Heating effects due to different experimental conditions were examined. A model was developed for the resonant current and the associated electric field produced by the guidewire acting as an antenna. Temperature increases of up to 17 degrees C were measured while imaging the guidewire at an off-center position in the 1.5-Tesla MR system. Power absorption produced by the resonating wire decreased as the repetition time was increased. No temperature rise was measured during MRI performed using the 0.2-Tesla MR system. Thus, considering the potential utility of low-field, open MR systems for MR-guided endovascular interventions, it is important to be aware of the safety of such applications for metallic guidewires and the potential hazards associated with using a guidewire with MR systems operating at higher static magnetic field strengths, including 3-Tesla.

An investigation conducted by Konings, et al. (2000) examined the radiofrequency (RF) heating of an endovascular guidewire frequently used in interventional MR procedures. A Terumo guidewire was partly immersed in an oblong saline bath to simulate an endovascular intervention. The temperature rise of the guidewire tip during MR imaging was measured using a Luxtron fluoroptic thermometry system. Starting from a baseline level of 26 degrees C, the tip of the guidewire reached temperatures up to 74 degrees C after 30 seconds of scanning using a 1.5-Tesla MR system. Touching the guidewire produced a skin burn.

The excessive heating of a linear conductor, like the guidewire that underwent evaluation, was explained by the resonating RF waves. According to Konings, et al. (2000), the capricious dependencies of this resonance phenomenon have potentially severe consequences for safety guidelines of interventional MR procedures involving guidewires.

Advances in guidewire designs reported by Kocaturk, et al. (2009) and Kramer, et al. (2009) have yielded guidewires that appear to be more acceptable for interventional MRI procedures with respect to both safety and visualization aspects.

REFERENCES

Buecker A. Safety of MRI-guided vascular interventions. Minim Invasive Ther Allied Technol 2006;15:65-70.

Etezadi-Amoli M, et al. Controlling radiofrequency-induced currents in guidewires using parallel transmit. Magn Reson Med 2015;74:1790-802.

Johnston T, et al. Intraoperative MRI: Safety. Neurosurg Clin N Am 2009;20:147-53.

Kocaturk O, et al. Whole shaft visibility and mechanical performance for active MR catheters using copper-nitinol braided polymer tubes. J Cardiovasc Magn Reson 2009;11:29.

Konings MK, Bartels LW, Smits HJ, Bakker CJ. Heating around intravascular guidewires by resonating RF waves. J Magn Reson Imag 2000;12:79-85.

Kramer NA, et al. Preclinical evaluation of a novel fiber compound MR guidewire *in vivo*. Invest Radiol 2009;44:390-7.

Liu CY, et al. Safety of MRI guided endovascular guidewire applications. Magn Reson Imaging 2000;12:75-8.

Schleicher KE, et al. Radial MRI with variable echo times: Reducing the orientation dependency of susceptibility artifacts of an MR-safe guidewire. MAGMA 2017 (In press).

Sonmez M, et al. MRI active guidewire with an embedded temperature probe and providing a distinct tip signal to enhance clinical safety. J Cardiovasc Magn Reson 2012;14:38.

van den Bosch MR, et al. New method to monitor RF safety in MRI-guided interventions based on RF induced image artefacts. Med Phys 2010;37:814-21.

Wolska-Krawczyk M, et al. Heating and safety of a new MR-compatible guidewire prototype versus a standard nitinol guidewire. Radiol Phys Technol 2014;7:95-101.

Halo Vests and Cervical Fixation Devices

Halo vests and cervical fixation devices are typically constructed from a combination of metallic components and other materials. Although some commercially available halo vests and cervical fixation devices are composed entirely of nonferromagnetic metals, there may be hazards due to excessive MRI-related heating that can be generated because of the conductive nature of the metallic parts. Additionally, there is a potential for the patient's tissue to be involved in part of a current loop, such that excessive heating and burns may occur. The currents generated within a "ring" or conductive loop is of additional concern because eddy current induction can cause image degradation. Adjusting the phase encoding direction of the pulse sequence so that it is parallel to the axis of the halo ring may reduce artifacts associated with eddy currents.

Serious injuries have occurred in patients with halo vests and cervical fixation devices that have undergone MR procedures. For example, Kim, et al. (2003) described a case of a patient that underwent MRI at 1.5-Tesla wearing a titanium-based halo vest system (the name, model and manufacturer of this device were not provided). After the MR procedure, substantial burns were evident on the scalp of the right two posterior skull pins. According to the report, "the stoic patient had clearly perceived significant burning pain during MR imaging, but did not notify the technicians."

Fortunately, several halo vests and cervical fixation devices have been specially designed to be acceptable for patients undergoing MR procedures at 1.5-Tesla and 3-Tesla (see **The List**).

Vibration Effects. A study was conducted to evaluate the possible heating of halo vests and cervical fixation devices during MR imaging performed at 1.5-Tesla MR system using a variety of pulse sequences. The data indicated that no substantial heating was detected for the specific devices tested. Of interest is that there appeared to be subtle, rapid motions of the halo ring associated with a magnetization transfer contrast (MTC) pulse sequence, as shown by recordings obtained using a motion sensitive, laser-Doppler flow monitor.

Apparently, the imaging parameters used for the MTC pulse sequence and other MR imaging techniques can produce sufficient vibration of the "halo" ring to create the sensation of heating. Accordingly, patients may interpret rapid movements or vibrations as a "heating" sensation. This is likely to occur when the vibration frequency is at a level that stimulates nerve receptors located in the subcutaneous region, which detect sensations of pain and temperature changes.

The aforementioned is a hypothesis based on the available experimental data and requires further investigation to substantiate this theory. However, additional support for this premise is provided in a report by Hartwell and Shellock (1997). In this case, a halo ring and vest (removed from a patient who complained of severe "burning" in a front skull pin during MR imaging) was evaluated for heating and other potential problems associated with MR imaging. This work was performed in conjunction with the neurosurgeon who applied the device to the patient. The halo ring and vest were connected similar to the manner used on the patient. A fluid-filled Plexiglas phantom was placed within the vest. The device was then placed in a 1.5-Tesla MR system and imaging was performed using the same parameters that were associated with the "burning" sensation experienced by the patient. The neurosurgeon remained inside of the MR system to visually observe the cervical fixation device and to maintain physical contact (i.e. touching the skull pins and other components of the cervical fixation device) during the MR procedure.

No perceivable temperature change was noted for the metallic components during MR imaging. However, the components (e.g., halo ring, vertical supports, vest bolts, etc.) vibrated substantially during MR imaging. Furthermore, when the skull pins were held firmly during the scan, there was a "drilling" sensation, which could be interpreted as a "burning" effect. Nevertheless, the skull pins remained cool to the touch throughout the MR procedure. Recent work conducted at 3-Tesla likewise supports the fact that substantial vibration can occur in cervical fixation devices (Unpublished observations, F.G. Shellock, 2009).

Graf, et al. (2006) reported that torque acting on relatively large metallic implants due to eddy-current induction in associated with MR imaging can be considerable. Larger implants (such as fixation devices) made from well-conducting materials are especially affected. Gradient switching was shown to produce fast alternating torque. Significant vibrations at off-center positions of the metal parts may explain why some patients with metallic implants sometimes report feeling heating sensations during MR examinations.

In consideration of the above, it is inadvisable to permit patients with certain cervical fixation devices to undergo MR procedures using an MTC pulse sequence or other similar pulse sequences until this problem can be further characterized to avoid unwanted patient responses, regardless of the lack of safety concern related to excessive heating. Importantly, the Instructions for Use (IFU) information provided by halo vest and cervical fixation device manufacturers should be carefully followed.

MRI at 3-Tesla and Cervical Fixation Devices. To date, several cervical fixation devices have undergone MRI testing at 3-Tesla. MRI information for these devices are, as follows:

'LiL Angel Pediatric Halo System with Jerome Halo Vest and Resolve Glass-composite Halo Ring and Resolve Ceramic-tipped Skull Pins

'LiL Angel Pediatric Halo System with Resolve Halo Vest and Resolve Glass-composite Halo Ring and Resolve Ceramic-tipped Skull Pins

Resolve Halo System with Jerome Halo Vest and Resolve Glass-composite Halo Ring and Resolve Ceramic-tipped Skull Pins

Resolve Halo System with Resolve Halo Vest and Resolve Glass-composite Halo Ring and Resolve Ceramic-tipped Skull Pins (Each product above is from OSSUR Reykjavik, Iceland and OSSUR AMERICAS, Aliso Viejo, CA)

Non-clinical testing has demonstrated that each product indicated above used as a cervical fixation or cervical traction device or system is *MR Conditional*. A patient with this system may undergo MRI safely under the following conditions:

- Static magnetic field of 3-Tesla or less
- Maximum spatial gradient magnetic field of 720 gauss/cm or less
- Maximum MR system reported, specific absorption rate (SAR) of 3.0 W/kg for 15 minutes of scanning (i.e. per pulse sequence)

In non-clinical testing, this system produced maximum temperature changes of 0.6 degrees C or less at a maximum MR system reported, specific absorption rate (SAR) of 3.0 W/kg for 15 minutes of MRI using a 3-Tesla MR system (Excite, Software G3.0-052B, General Electric Healthcare, Milwaukee, WI). MR image quality may be compromised if the area of interest is in the exact same area or relatively close to the position of the Skull Pins. Therefore, it may be necessary to optimize MR imaging parameters for the presence of these metallic objects.

Important Note: All of the materials used for the above products included metals with very low magnetic susceptibility (e.g., commercially pure titanium, titanium alloy, aluminum, etc.) or are nonmetallic and nonconductors. Accordingly, little or no substantial magnetic field interactions are present for these products in association with a 3-Tesla MR system.

PMT Halo System with Carbon Graphite Open Back Ring and Titanium Skull Pin (PMT Corporation, Chanhassen, MN)

Non-clinical testing has demonstrated that the PMT Halo System with Carbon Graphite Open Back Ring and Titanium Skull Pins used as a cervical fixation or cervical traction device or system is *MR Conditional*. A patient with this system may undergo MRI safely under the following conditions:

- Static magnetic field of 3-Tesla and 1.5-Tesla, only
- Maximum spatial gradient magnetic field of 720 gauss/cm or less
- Maximum MR system reported, specific absorption rate (SAR) of 3.0 W/kg for 15 minutes of scanning (i.e. per pulse sequence)

In non-clinical testing, this system produced maximum temperature changes of 0.5 degrees C or less at a maximum MR system reported, specific absorption rate (SAR) of 3.0 W/kg for 15 minutes of MRI using a 3-Tesla MR system (Excite, Software G3.0-052B, General Electric Healthcare, Milwaukee, WI). MR image quality may be compromised if the area of interest is in the exact same area or relatively close to the position of the Titanium Skull Pins. Therefore, it may be necessary to optimize MR imaging parameters for the presence of these metallic objects.

Important Note: All of the materials used for the above products included metals with very low magnetic susceptibility (e.g., commercially pure titanium, titanium alloy, aluminum, etc.) or are nonmetallic and nonconductors. Accordingly, little or no substantial magnetic field interactions are present for these products in association with the 3-Tesla MR system.

Bremer Halo Crown System with Bremer Air Flo Vest and Titanium Skull Pins (DePuy Spine Inc.)

Non-clinical testing has demonstrated that the Bremer Halo Crown System with Bremer Air Flo Vest and Titanium Skull Pins used as a cervical fixation or cervical traction device or system is *MR Conditional*. A patient with this system may undergo MRI safely under the following conditions:

- Static magnetic field of 3-Tesla or less
- Maximum spatial gradient magnetic field of 720 gauss/cm or less
- Maximum MR system reported, specific absorption rate (SAR) of 3.0 W/kg for 15 minutes of scanning (i.e. per pulse sequence)

In non-clinical testing, this system produced maximum temperature changes of 0.6 degrees C or less at a maximum MR system reported, specific absorption rate (SAR) of 3.0 W/kg for 15 minutes of MRI using a 3-Tesla MR system (Excite, Software G3.0-052B, General Electric Healthcare, Milwaukee, WI). MR image quality may be compromised if the area of interest is in the exact same area or relatively close to the position of the Titanium Skull Pins. Therefore, it may be necessary to optimize MR imaging parameters for the presence of these metallic objects.

Important Note: All of the materials used for the above products included metals with very low magnetic susceptibility (e.g., commercially pure titanium, titanium alloy, aluminum, etc.) or are nonmetallic and nonconductors. Accordingly, little or no substantial magnetic field interactions are present for these products in association with the 3-Tesla MR system.

Bremer 3D Halo Crown System with Bremer Air Flo Vest and Titanium Skull Pins (DePuy Spine Inc.)

Non-clinical testing has demonstrated that the Bremer 3D Halo Crown System with Bremer Air Flo Vest and Titanium Skull Pins used as a cervical fixation or cervical traction device or system is *MR Conditional*. A patient with this system may undergo MRI safely under the following conditions:

- Static magnetic field of 3-Tesla or less
- Maximum spatial gradient magnetic field of 720 gauss/cm or less
- Maximum MR system reported, specific absorption rate (SAR) of 3.0 W/kg for 15 minutes of scanning (i.e. per pulse sequence)

In non-clinical testing, this system produced maximum temperature changes of 0.6 degrees C or less at a maximum MR system reported, specific absorption rate (SAR) of 3.0 W/kg for 15 minutes of MRI using a 3-Tesla MR system (Excite, General Electric). MR image quality may be compromised if the area of interest is in the exact same area or relatively close to the position of the Titanium Skull Pins. Therefore, it may be necessary to optimize MR imaging parameters for the presence of these metallic objects.

Important Note: All of the materials used for the above products included metals with very low magnetic susceptibility (e.g., commercially pure titanium, titanium alloy, aluminum, etc.) or are nonmetallic and nonconductors. Accordingly, little or no substantial magnetic field interactions are present for these products in association with the 3-Tesla MR system.

[MR healthcare professionals are advised to contact the respective manufacturer in order to obtain the latest safety information to ensure patient safety relative to the use of an MR procedure.]

REFERENCES

Ballock RT, et al. The quality of magnetic resonance imaging, as affected by the composition of the halo orthosis. J Bone Joint Surg 1989;71-A:431-434.

Clayman DA, et al. Compatibility of cervical spine braces with MR imaging. A study of nine nonferrous devices. Am J Neuroradiol 1990;11:385-390.

Diaz F, Tweardy L, Shellock FG. Cervical fixation devices: MRI issues at 3-Tesla. Spine 2010;35:411-5.

Graf H, et al. Eddy-current induction in extended metallic parts as a source of considerable torsional moment. J Magn Reson Imag 2006;23:585-590.

Hartwell CG, Shellock FG. MRI of cervical fixation devices: Sensation of heating caused by vibration of metallic components. J Magn Reson Imag 1997;7:771.

Hua J, Fox RA. Magnetic resonance imaging of patients wearing a surgical traction halo. J Magn Reson Imag 1996;1:264-267.

Kim LJ, et al. Scalp burns from halo pins following magnetic resonance imaging. Case Report. Journal of Neurosurgery 2003;99:186.

Malko JA, Hoffman JC, Jarrett PJ. Eddy-current-induced artifacts caused by an "MR-compatible" halo device. Radiology 1989;173:563-564.

Shellock FG. MR imaging and cervical fixation devices: Assessment of ferromagnetism, heating, and artifacts. Magnetic Resonance Imaging 1996;14:1093-1098.

Shellock FG, Slimp G. Halo vest for cervical spine fixation during MR imaging. Am J Roentgenol 1990;154:631-632.

Hearing Aids and Other Hearing Systems

External hearing aids are included in the category of electronically-activated devices that may be found in patients referred for MR procedures. Exposure to the magnetic fields used for MR examinations can damage these devices. Therefore, a patient or other individual with an external hearing aid must not enter the MR system room. Fortunately, most external hearing aids can be readily identified and removed from the patient or individual to prevent damage associated with the MRI environment.

Other hearing devices may have external components as well as pieces that are surgically implanted. Hearing devices with external and internal components may be especially problematic for patients and individuals in relative to the use of MR procedures. Accordingly, patients and individuals with these particular hearing devices may not be allowed into the MR environment because of the risk of damage to the components. The manufacturers of these devices should be contacted for current MRI labeling information.

For information on other hearing systems, please refer to other sections, including: **Baha, Bone Conduction Implant**; **Cochlear Implants**, **Sophono Alpha Magnetic Implant;** and **InSound XT Series** and **Lyric Hearing Device**.

[MR healthcare professionals are advised to contact the respective manufacturer in order to obtain the latest safety information to ensure patient safety relative to the use of an MR procedure.]

REFERENCES

Azadarmaki R, et al. MRI information for commonly used otologic implants: review and update. Otolaryngol Head Neck Surg 2014;150:512-9.

Shellock FG. Magnetic Resonance Procedures: Health Effects and Safety. CRC Press, LLC, Boca Raton, FL, 2001.

Heart Valve Prostheses and Annuloplasty Rings

Many heart valve prostheses and annuloplasty rings have been evaluated for MR issues, especially with regard to the presence of magnetic field interactions associated with exposure to MR systems operating at field strengths of as high as 4.7-Tesla. Of these, the majority displayed measurable yet relatively minor magnetic field interactions. That is, because the attractive forces exerted on the heart valve prostheses and annuloplasty rings were minimal compared to the force exerted by the beating heart (i.e. approximately 7.2-N), to date, an MR procedure is not considered to be hazardous for a patient that has any heart valve prosthesis or annuloplasty ring tested relative to the field strength of the magnet (i.e. MR system) used for the evaluation. Importantly, this recommendation includes the Starr-Edwards Model Pre-6000 heart valve prosthesis previously suggested to be a potential risk for a patient undergoing an MR examination.

With respect to the clinical use of MR procedures, there has been no report of a patient incident or injury related to the presence of a heart valve prosthesis or annuloplasty ring. However, it should be noted that not all heart valve prostheses have been evaluated and at least one prototype (to date, not commercially available) exists that has magnetic components.

Heart Valve Prostheses and the Lenz Effect. Condon and Hadley (2000) reported the theoretical possibility of a previously unconsidered electromagnetic interaction with prosthetic heart valves that contain metallic disks or leaflets. Basically, any metal (i.e. not just ferromagnetic material) moving through a magnetic field will develop another magnetic field that opposes the primary magnetic field. This phenomenon is referred to as the "Lenz Effect". In theory, "resistive pressure" may develop in heart valve prostheses that have metallic disks or leaflets (note, at the present time, mostly tissue valves are used instead of those with metallic leaflets) with the potential to inhibit both the opening and closing aspects of the valve. The Lenz Effect is proportional to the strength of the static magnetic field. Accordingly, it has been suggested that there may be problems for patients with heart valves that have metallic discs or leaflets in association with MRI procedures, especially those performed at very high static magnetic fields.

Edwards, et al. (2015) conducted an *in vitro* study of the occurrence of Lenz-related forces on various heart valve prostheses at 1.5-Tesla and assessed the risk of the impedance of valve function. The findings provided evidence of the Lenz Effect on certain cardiac valve prostheses exposed to the static magnetic field, which resulted in functional valve impedance and a potentially increased risk of valve regurgitation. While further evaluation of this phenomenon may be warranted, to date, the Lenz Effect has not been observed in association with clinical MR examinations nor has it posed additional risks for patients with certain heart valve prostheses (i.e. those with metallic leaflets or disks) undergoing MRI.

Important Note: For additional information, refer to section: **Guidelines for the Management of Patients with Heart Valve Prostheses and Annuloplasty Rings Referred for MRI Procedures.**

REFERENCES

Ahmed S, Shellock FG. Magnetic resonance imaging safety: Implications for cardiovascular patients. Journal of Cardiovascular Magnetic Resonance 2001;3:171-181.

Condon B, Hadley DM. Potential MR hazard to patients with metallic heart valves: The Lenz effect. J Magn Reson Imag 2000;12:171-176.

Edwards MB, Taylor KM, Shellock FG. Prosthetic heart valves: Evaluation of magnetic field interactions, heating, and artifacts at 1.5-Tesla. J Magn Reson Imag 2000;12:363-369.

Edwards MB, et al. Mechanical testing of human cardiac tissue: Some implications for MRI safety. J Cardiovasc Magn Reson 2005;7:835-840.

Edwards MB, et al. In vitro assessment of the lenz effect on heart valve prostheses at 1.5 T. J Magn Reson Imaging 2015;41:74-82.

Frank H, Buxbaum P, Huber L, et al. *In vitro* behavior of mechanical heart valves in 1.5-T superconducting magnet. Eur J Radiol 1992;2:555-558.

Golestanirad L, et al. Comprehensive analysis of Lenz Effect on the artificial heart valves during magnetic resonance imaging. Progress In Electromagnetics Research 2012;128:1-17.

Hassler M, et al. Effects of magnetic fields used in MRI on 15 prosthetic heart valves. J Radiol 1986;67:661-666.

Levine GN, et al. Safety of magnetic resonance imaging in patients with cardiovascular devices: An American Heart Association scientific statement from the Committee on Diagnostic and Interventional Cardiac Catheterization. Circulation 2007;116:2878-2891.

Myers PO, et al. .Safety of magnetic resonance imaging in cardiac surgery patients: Annuloplasty rings, septal occluders, and transcatheter valves. Ann Thorac Surg 2012;93:1019.

Pruefer D, et al. *In vitro* investigation of prosthetic heart valves in magnetic resonance imaging: Evaluation of potential hazards. J Heart Valve Disease 2001;10:410-414.

Randall PA, et al. Magnetic resonance imaging of prosthetic cardiac valves *in vitro* and *in vivo*. Am J Cardiol 1988;62:973-976.

Saeedi M, Thomas A, Shellock FG. Evaluation of MRI issues at 3-Tesla for a transcatheter aortic valve replacement (TAVR) bioprosthesis. Magnetic Resonance Imaging 2015;33:497-501.

Shellock FG. Biomedical implants and devices: Assessment of magnetic field interactions with a 3.0-Tesla MR system. J Magn Reson Imag 2002;16:721-732.

Shellock FG. Prosthetic heart valves and annuloplasty rings: Assessment of magnetic field interactions, heating, and artifacts at 1.5-Tesla. Journal of Cardiovascular Magnetic Resonance 2001;3:159-169.

Shellock FG, Morisoli SM. *Ex vivo* evaluation of ferromagnetism, heating, and artifacts for heart valve prostheses exposed to a 1.5-Tesla MR system. J Magn Reson Imag 1994;4:756-758.

Shellock FG, Shellock VJ. MRI Safety of cardiovascular implants: Evaluation of ferromagnetism, heating, and artifacts. Radiology 2000;214:P19H.

Soulen RL. Magnetic resonance imaging of prosthetic heart valves [Letter]. Radiology 1986;158:279.

Soulen RL, Budinger TF, Higgins CB. Magnetic resonance imaging of prosthetic heart valves. Radiology 1985;154:705-707.

Hemostatic Clips, Other Clips, Fasteners, and Staples

Various hemostatic vascular clips, other types of clips, fasteners, and staples evaluated for magnetic field interactions were not attracted by static magnetic fields of MR systems operating at 3-Tesla or less. These implants were made from nonferromagnetic materials such as tantalum, commercially pure titanium, and nonferromagnetic forms of stainless steel. Additionally, some forms of ligating, hemostatic, or other types of clips are made from biodegradable materials. Therefore, patients that have the implants made from nonmagnetic or "weakly" magnetic materials listed in **The List** are not at risk for injury during MR procedures. Importantly, for the devices that have been tested to date, there has been no report of an injury to a patient in association with a hemostatic vascular clip, other type of clip, fastener, or staple associated with the MR environment. Patients with nonferromagnetic versions of these implants may undergo MR procedures immediately after they are placed.

Vascular grafts frequently have clips or fasteners applied that may present problems for MR imaging because of the associated artifacts. Weishaupt, et al. (2000) evaluated the artifact size on three-dimensional MR angiograms as well as the MR issues for 18 different commercially available hemostatic and ligating clips. All of the clips were acceptable or safe at 1.5-Tesla insofar as there was no substantial magnetic field interactions or heating measured for these implants.

Specific MRI-related labeling statements for certain hemostatic clips that require further attention during the pre-MRI screening procedure are, as follows:

Long Clip, HX-600-090L. The Long Clip HX-600-090L (Olympus Medical Systems Corporation) is indicated for placement within the gastrointestinal tract for the purpose of endoscopic marking, hemostasis, or closure of GI tract luminal perforations within 20-mm as a supplementary method. Currently, the Long Clip HX-600-090L is labeled, as follows: "Do not perform MRI procedures on patients who have clips placed within their gastrointestinal tracts. This could be harmful to the patient."

Additional information: Olympus endoscopic clips have been shown to remain in the patient an average of 9.4 days, but retention is based on a variety of factors and may result in a longer retention period. Prior to MRI, the physician should confirm there are no residual clips in the GI tract. The following techniques may be used for confirmation:

1) View the lesion under radiologic imaging. Olympus clip fixing devices are radiopaque. By using X-ray, the physician can determine if any residual clips are in the gastrointestinal tract. If no clips are evident under radiologic imaging, MRI may be accomplished.

2) Endoscopically examine the lesion. If no clips remain at the lesion, MRI may be accomplished.

QuickClip2, HX-201LR-135 & HX-201UR-135. The QuickClip2, HX-201LR-135 & HX-201UR-135 (Olympus Medical Systems Corporation) are indicated for placement within the gastrointestinal tract for the purpose of endoscopic marking, hemostasis, or closure of GI tract luminal perforations within 20-mm as a supplementary method. Currently, the QuickClip2 (HX-201LR-135 & HX-201UR-135) is labeled, as follows: "Do not perform MRI procedures on patients who have clips placed within their gastrointestinal tracts. This could be harmful to the patient."

Additional information: Olympus endoscopic clips have been shown to remain in the patient an average of 9.4 days, but retention is based on a variety of factors and may result in a longer retention period. Prior to MRI, the physician should confirm there are no residual clips in the GI tract. The following techniques may be used for confirmation:

1) View the lesion under radiologic imaging. Olympus clip fixing devices are radiopaque. By using X-ray, the physician can determine if any residual clips are in the gastrointestinal tract. If no clips are evident under radiologic imaging, MRI may be accomplished.

2) Endoscopically examine the lesion. If no clips remain at the lesion, MRI may be accomplished.

QuickClip2 Long, HX-201LR-135L & HX-201UR-135L. The QuickClip2 Long, HX-201LR-135L & HX-201UR-135L (Olympus Medical Systems Corporation) are indicated for placement within the gastrointestinal tract for the purpose of endoscopic marking, hemostasis, or closure of GI tract luminal perforations within 20-mm as a supplementary method. The QuickClip2 Long (HX-201LR-135L & HX-201UR-135L) is labeled, as follows: "Do not perform MRI procedures on patients who have clips placed within their gastrointestinal tracts. This could be harmful to the patient."

Additional information: Olympus endoscopic clips have been shown to remain in the patient an average of 9.4 days, but retention is based on a variety of factors and may result in a longer retention period. Prior to MRI, the physician should confirm there are no residual clips in the GI tract. The following techniques may be used for confirmation:

1) View the lesion under radiologic imaging. Olympus clip fixing devices are radiopaque. By using X-ray, the physician can determine if any residual clips are in the gastrointestinal tract. If no clips are evident under radiologic imaging, MRI may be accomplished.

2) Endoscopically examine the lesion. If no clips remain at the lesion, MRI may be accomplished.

TriClip Endoscopic Clipping Device. An investigation by Gill, et al. (2009) involving excised tissue exposed to a 1.5-Tesla MR system, reported that the TriClip (TriClip Endoscopic Clipping Device, Wilson-Cook Medical Inc., Winston-Salem, NC) demonstrated "detachment from gastric tissue". Therefore, the TriClip should be considered *"unsafe"* for MRI.

MRI at 3-Tesla and Hemostatic Clips, Other Clips, Fasteners, and Staples. At 3-Tesla, a variety of hemostatic clips, other clips, fasteners, and staples have been evaluated for MRI issues including magnetic field interactions and MRI-related heating. In general, these devices do not present an additional risk to patients undergoing MR procedures. For example, Gill and Shellock (2012) tested metallic skin closure staples and vessel ligation clips at 3-Tesla to characterize MRI issues in order to ensure patient safety. Clips were selected for testing that represented the largest metallic sizes made from materials with the highest magnetic susceptibilities among 61 other similar implants. Each surgical implant showed only minor magnetic field interactions and heating was not substantial. The results demonstrated that it would be acceptable for patients with these particular metallic surgical implants to undergo MRI at 3-Tesla or less. Because of the materials and dimensions of the skin closure staples and vessel ligation clips that underwent testing, the findings pertained to 61 additional similar implants. Refer to **The List** for specific information for other hemostatic clips, other clips, fasteners, and staples.

REFERENCES

Brown MA, et al. Magnetic field effects on surgical ligation clips. Magnetic Resonance Imaging 1987;5:443-453.

Barrafato D, Henkelman RM. Magnetic resonance imaging and surgical clips. Can J Surg 1984;27:509-512.

De Silva S, et al. Magnetic resonance imaging safety of surgical clips and staples. Anaesthesia 2015;70:1463.

Gill A, Shellock FG. Assessment of MRI issues at 3-Tesla for metallic surgical implants: Findings applied to 61 additional skin closure staples and vessel ligation clips. J Cardiovasc Magn Reson. 2012;14:3-7.

Gill KR, Pooley RA, Wallace MB. Magnetic resonance imaging compatibility of endoclips. Gastrointest Endosc 2009;70:532-6.

Mavrogenis G, et al. Hemostatic clips and magnetic resonance imaging. Are there any compatibility issues? Endoscopy 2013;45:933.

Raju GS. Endoclips for GI endoscopy. Gastrointestinal Endoscopy 2004;59:267-279.

Shellock FG. Hemostatic Clips and MRI Procedures: Some Safe...Some May Not Be. Signals No. 66, pp. 20-21, 2008.

Shellock FG, Crues JV, Editors. MRI Bioeffects, Safety, and Patient Management. Biomedical Research Publishing Group, Los Angeles, CA, 2014.

Shellock FG. MR imaging of metallic implants and materials: A compilation of the literature. Am J Roentgenol 1988;151:811-814.

Shellock FG. Biomedical implants and devices: Assessment of magnetic field interactions with a 3.0-Tesla MR system. J Magn Reson Imag 2002;16:721-732.

Shellock FG, Crues JV. High-field strength MR imaging and metallic biomedical implants: An *ex vivo* evaluation of deflection forces. Am J Roentgenol 1988;151:389-392.

Shellock FG, Morisoli S, Kanal E. MR procedures and biomedical implants, materials, and devices: 1993 update. Radiology 1993;189:587-599.

Shellock FG, Swengros-Curtis J. MR imaging and biomedical implants, materials, and devices: An updated review. Radiology 1991;180:541-550.

Weishaupt D, et al. Ligating clips for three-dimensional MR angiography at 1.5-T: *In vitro* evaluation. Radiology 2000;214:902-9.

InSound XT Series and Lyric Hearing Device

MRI Information
For the **InSound XT Series** and the **Lyric Hearing Device** (InSound Medical, Newark, CA), each hearing system must be removed prior to an MRI procedure. Furthermore, these devices are not allowed in the MR system room. Each device may be self-removed by the patient if an MRI examination is required.

[MR healthcare professionals are advised to contact the manufacturer to ensure that the latest safety information is obtained and carefully followed in order to ensure patient safety relative to the use of an MR procedure.]

REFERENCE

Senova, www.sonova.com

Insulin Pumps

An insulin pump allows the replacement of slow-acting insulin for basal needs with a continuous infusion of rapid-acting insulin. By using an insulin pump, the patient can typically match the dosage of insulin to lifestyle and activities, rather than adjusting those to the body's response to insulin injections. The advantages of using an insulin pump include the fact that it replaces the need for periodic injections by delivering rapid-acting insulin continuously throughout the day via a catheter, which greatly simplifies the management of diabetes.

There are two basic types of insulin pumps: one is used as an external device and the other is implanted. Both types currently pose hazards to patients referred to MRI procedures. For an external insulin pump, in general, the device typically needs to be removed and kept out of the MRI environment to ensure that there is no adverse impact on the functionality of the external pump. The information below provides examples of MRI information for several, commonly used insulin pumps. Note that many other external and implantable insulin pumps also exist.

Insulin Pumps, Animas Corporation

This MRI information pertains to the following insulin pumps from the Animas Corporation:

- Animas 2020 Insulin Pump
- IR Animas 1200
- IR 1000 Insulin Pump
- IR 1100 Insulin Pump
- IR 1200 Insulin Pump
- OneTouch Ping Insulin Pump

Each insulin pump indicated above should not be exposed to very strong electromagnetic fields, such as MRIs, RF welders, or magnets used to pick up automobiles. Very strong magnetic fields, such as that associated with MRI, can "magnetize" the portion of the insulin pump's motor that regulates insulin delivery and, thus, damage the device.

For the patient: If you plan to undergo an MRI, remove the insulin pump beforehand and keep it outside of the MR system room during the procedure.

If the pump is accidentally allowed into the MR system room, disconnect the pump immediately and contact Animas Pump Support for important instructions.

Precautions: If you are going to have diagnostic or surgical procedures that expose you to X-ray, CT scan, MRI or any other type of radiation therapy, you may need to remove your insulin pump (and meter-remote), and place them outside of the treatment area. For specific procedure information please refer to the instructions for use that accompanied your insulin pump. Consult your healthcare professional for direction in maintaining your blood glucose levels during these type of procedures.

For the Healthcare Professional: Do not bring the insulin pump into the MR system at any time. If the pump is accidentally allowed into the MR system room, disconnect the pump immediately and contact Animas Pump Support for important instructions.

Cozmo Pump, Infusion Pump, Smiths Medical

According to the User Manual for the Cozmo Pump which is a device used to administer insulin, the following is stated regarding MRI:

Caution: Avoid strong electromagnetic fields, like those present with Magnetic Resonance Imaging (MRI) and direct X-ray, as they can affect how the pump works. If you cannot avoid them, you must take the pump off.

Medtronic MiniMed 2007 Implantable Insulin Pump System, Medtronic, Inc.

The Medtronic 2007 Implantable Insulin Pump System may offer treatment advantages for diabetes patients who have difficulty maintaining consistent glycemic control. Patients that have not responded well to intensive insulin therapy, including multiple daily insulin injections or continuous subcutaneous insulin infusion using an external pump, may be primary candidates for the Medtronic MiniMed 2007 System. The Medtronic MiniMed 2007 System delivers insulin into the peritoneal cavity in short, frequent bursts or "pulses", similar to how pancreatic beta cells secrete insulin.

The Medtronic MiniMed 2007 Implantable Insulin Pump is designed to withstand common electrostatic and electromagnetic interference but must be removed prior to undergoing an MR procedure. Any magnetic field exceeding 600 gauss will interfere with the proper functioning of the pump for as long as the pump remains in that field. Fields much higher than that, such as those emitted by an MR system, may cause irreparable damage to the pump.

By comparison, infusion sets (MMT-11X, MMT-31X, MMT-32X, MMT-37X, MMT-39X) used with this device contain no metallic components and are safe to be used and can remain attached to the patient during an MR procedure. The only exceptions would be Polyfin infusion sets. Polyfin infusion sets (MMT-106 AND MMT-107, MMT-16X, MMT-30X, MMT-36X) have a surgical steel needle that remains in the subcutaneous tissue. These infusion sets should be removed prior to any MR procedure.

MiniMed Paradigm REAL-Time Insulin Pump and Continuous Glucose Monitoring System (Models 522, 722 and Revel Insulin Pumps), Medtronic, Inc.

MRI Information for Patients and Magnetic Fields

Do **not** use pump cases that have a magnetic clasp.

Do **not** expose your insulin pump to MRI equipment or other devices that generate very strong magnetic fields.

The magnetic fields in the immediate vicinity of these devices can damage the part of the pump's motor that regulates insulin delivery, possibly resulting in over-delivery and severe hypoglycemia.

Your pump must be removed and kept outside the room during magnetic resonance imaging (MRI) procedures.

If your pump is inadvertently exposed to a strong magnetic field, discontinue use and contact your local help line or representative for further assistance.

The insulin pump, transmitter, and sensor must be removed prior to entering the MRI environment.

MiniMed 530G System, Medtronic, Inc.

The MiniMed 530G system is intended for continuous delivery of basal insulin (at user selectable rates) and administration of insulin boluses (in user selectable amounts) for the management of diabetes mellitus in persons, sixteen years of age and older, requiring insulin as well as for the continuous monitoring and trending of glucose levels in the fluid under the skin. The MiniMed 530G system can be programmed to automatically suspend delivery of insulin for up to two hours when the sensor glucose value falls below a predefined threshold value.

MRI Information for the Patient

Exposure to magnetic fields and radiation. If you are going to have an X-ray, MRI, diathermy treatment, CT scan, or other type of exposure to radiation, take off your pump, sensor, transmitter, meter and remote control before entering a room containing any of these equipment. The magnetic fields and radiation in the immediate vicinity of these devices can make them nonfunctional or damage the part of the pump that regulates insulin delivery, possibly resulting in over delivery and severe hypoglycemia. If your pump is inadvertently exposed to a magnetic field, discontinue use and contact our 24 Hour HelpLine for further assistance.

DANA Diabecare IIS Insulin Pump and DANA Diabecare Insulin Infusion Pump (SOOIL Development Co., Ltd.)

The pump must not be used in the presence of intense electromagnetic fields, such as those generated by certain electrically powered medical devices. The pump should be removed prior to the user having a CT Scan, MRI or X-ray.

t:slim Insulin Pump, Tandem Diabetes Care, Inc.
MRI Information for the Patient: Radiology and Medical Procedures

If you are going to have an X-ray, computerized tomography (CAT) scan, magnetic resonance imaging (MRI), or other exposure to radiation, take off your t:slim Insulin Pump and remove it from the procedure room. If you have questions, contact Tandem Diabetes Care Customer Technical Support at 1-877-801-6901.

ACCU-CHEK Insulin Pump, All Models, Roche Diagnostics
MRI Information for the Patient: Do not use your pump around electromagnetic fields such as radar or antenna installations, high-voltage sources, X-Ray sources, MRI, CAT scan, and all other sources of electrical current as they may cause your pump not to work. Insulin delivery may stop and an error E7: ELECTRONIC ERROR may occur. Always stop and remove your pump before you enter these areas.

OmniPod Insulin Management System, Insulin Pump, Insulet Corporation

Controlling device must be removed before entering the MR system room.

[MRI healthcare professionals are advised to contact the respective manufacturer in order to obtain the latest safety information to ensure patient safety relative to the use of an MR procedure.]

REFERENCES

www.accu-chek.com
www.animascorp.com
www.medtronicdiabetes.com
www.myomnipod.com
www.smiths-medical.com
www.sooilusa.com
www.tandemdiabetes.com

Intrauterine Contraceptive Devices and Other Devices

Intrauterine contraceptive devices (IUD) may be made from nonmetallic materials (e.g., plastic) or a combination of nonmetallic and metallic materials. Copper is typically the metal used in an IUD, however, stainless steel or other metals may also be utilized. The "Copper T" and "Copper 7" both have a fine copper coil wound around a portion of the IUD. Testing conducted to determine MRI issues for the copper IUDs indicated that these objects are safe for patients in the MR environment using MR systems operating at 1.5-Tesla or less. This includes the Multiload Cu375, the Nova T (containing copper and silver), and the Gyne T IUDs. An artifact may be seen for the metallic component of the IUD, however, the extent of this artifact is relatively small because of the low magnetic susceptibility of copper.

Zieman and Kanal (2007) reported 3-Tesla MRI *in vitro* test results for the Copper T 380A IUD. No significant deflection, torque, heating or artifact was found. Thus, this IUD is acceptable for patients undergoing MRI at 3-Tesla or less.

Importantly, stainless steel IUDs exist and, to date, these devices have not undergone testing to determine if they are acceptable for patients in association with MR procedures.

The Mirena intrauterine system (IUS) is a hormone-releasing device that contains levonorgestrel to prevent pregnancy. This T-shaped device is made entirely from nonmetallic materials that include polyethylene, barium sulfate (i.e. which makes it radiopaque), and silicone. Therefore, the Mirena is safe for patients undergoing MR procedures using MR systems operating at all static magnetic field strengths.

The Implanon implant (Etonogestrel) is a single-rod, nonmetallic, subdermal device that offers women up to three years of contraceptive protection. This implant is acceptable for patients undergoing MR procedures at all static magnetic field strengths (i.e. it is MR Safe).

REFERENCES

Berger-Kulemann V, et al. Magnetic field interactions of copper-containing intrauterine devices in 3.0-Tesla magnetic resonance imaging: In vivo study. Korean J Radiol 2013;14:416-22.

Ciet P, Litmanovich DE. MR safety issues particular to women. Magn Reson Imaging Clin N Am 2015;23:59-67.

Correia L, et al. Magnetic resonance imaging and gynecological devices. Contraception 2012;85:538-43.

Hess T, Stepanow B, Knopp MV. Safety of intrauterine contraceptive devices during MR imaging. Eur Radiol 1996;6:66-68.

Implanon, www.implanon.com

Kido A, et al. Intrauterine devices and uterine peristalsis: Evaluation with MRI. Magnetic Resonance Imaging 2008;26:54-8.

Mark AS, Hricak H. Intrauterine contraceptive devices: MR imaging. Radiology 1987;162:311-314.

Mirena, www.mirena-us.com

Shellock FG. Magnetic Resonance Procedures: Health Effects and Safety. CRC Press, LLC, Boca Raton, FL, 2001.

Westerway SC, Picker R, Christie J. Implanon implant detection with ultrasound and magnetic resonance imaging. Aust NZ Obstet Gynaecol 2003;43:346-350.

Zhuang LQ, Yang BY. Comparison of clinical effects of stainless steel IUDs with and without copper. Shengzhi Yu Biun 1984;4:48-50.

Zieman M, Kanal E. Copper T 380A IUD and magnetic resonance imaging. Contraception 2007;75:93-5.

IsoMed Implantable Constant-Flow Infusion Pump

IsoMed: All models beginning with 8472
Medtronic, Inc.

The IsoMed Implantable Constant-Flow Infusion Pump (Medtronic, Inc.) is MR Conditional.

Comprehensive labeling information must be reviewed to ensure patient safety. Carefully review the latest MRI labeling conditions and guidelines at: www.medtronic.com/mri

Note: For a full listing of MR Conditional devices, visit www.medtronic.com/mri

Important Note to MR Healthcare Professionals: Different MRI guidelines may exist for different countries. Therefore, use the appropriate information for your country.

[MR healthcare professionals are advised to contact the respective manufacturer in order to obtain the latest safety information to ensure patient safety relative to the use of an MR procedure.]

REFERENCES

Medtronic, Inc., www.medtronic.com
Medtronic, Inc., www.medtronic.com/mri

MAGEC System
Nuvasive, Inc.

The MAGEC System (magnetically-controlled distraction rods) (Nuvasive, Inc.) offers a unique treatment for early onset scoliosis (EOS) by providing a noninvasive solution to manage growth and progression of spinal deformity in growing children. The system consists of an adjustable growing rod and an External Remote Controller (ERC) that features innovative magnetic technology allowing for noninvasive control of the implanted device. Other distraction-based treatments for EOS require on-going distraction surgeries throughout treatment. After an initial procedure to implant the MAGEC Rod, the device can be distracted or retracted during routine outpatient visits. The MAGEC System is designed to reduce the impact of EOS on the lives of patients and families by eliminating planned distraction surgeries and the risks associated with them while providing optimal clinical outcomes.

MRI Safety Information

Non-clinical testing demonstrated that the MAGEC System is MR Conditional. The following conditions must be followed:

A patient with this device can be scanned in an MR system meeting the following conditions:

- Static magnetic field of 1.5 Tesla (1.5 T)
- Maximum spatial field gradient of 3000 gauss/cm (30 T/m)
- Maximum MR system reported, whole body averaged specific absorption rate (SAR) of 0.5 W/kg at 1.5 T

Under the scan conditions defined above, the MAGEC system is expected to produce a maximum temperature rise of no greater than 3.7° C after 15 minutes of continuous scanning.

Caution: The RF heating behavior does not scale with static field strength. Devices that do not exhibit detectable heating at one field strength may exhibit high values of localized heating at another field strength.

- The patient should not be permitted to roll on the table, as this motion may cause unintended lengthening/shortening of the implant.
- The External Remote Controller, Manual Distractor, and Wand Magnet Locator are MR Unsafe. Do not bring them into the MRI scan room.
- In non-clinical testing, the image artifact caused by the MAGEC system extends beyond the imaging field of view when imaged with a gradient-echo pulse sequence in a 1.5 T MRI system. However, imaging in locations approximately 20 cm away from the actuator of the MAGEC System may produce images in which anatomical features may be discerned.

REFERENCE

Nuvasive, Inc., www.nuvasive.com

Magnetically-Activated Implants and Devices

Various types of implants incorporate magnets for a variety of reasons. For example, the magnet may be used to retain the implant in place (e.g., certain prosthetic devices), to guide a ferromagnetic object into a specific position, to permit the functional aspects of the implant, to change the operation of the implant (e.g., adjustable shunt valves), or to program the device (e.g., certain cardiac devices). Because there is a high likelihood of perturbing the function, demagnetizing, or displacing these implants, MR procedures typically should not be performed in patients with these implants or devices. However, in some cases, patients with magnetically-activated implants and devices may undergo MR procedures as long as certain precautions are followed. For example, see section entitled **Cerebrospinal Fluid (CSF) Shunt Valves and Accessories** and **MAGEC System.**

Implants and devices that use magnets (e.g., certain types of dental implants, magnetic sphincters, magnetic stoma plugs, magnetic ocular implants, otologic implants, and other similar devices) may be damaged by exposure to MR systems which, in turn, may necessitate surgery to replace or reposition them. For example, Schneider, et al. (1995) reported that an MR examination is capable of demagnetizing the permanent magnet associated with an otologic implant (i.e. the Audiant magnet). Obviously, this has important implications for patients undergoing MR procedures. Notably, cochlear implants often incorporate a magnetic component which may pose problems for the patient referred for an MRI examination. Please see the section entitled, **Cochlear Implants**.

Whenever possible, and if this can be done without risk to the patient, a magnetically-activated implant or device (e.g., an externally applied prosthesis or magnetic stoma plug) should be removed prior to the MR procedure. This may permit the examination to be performed safely. Knowledge of the specific aspects of the magnetically-activated implant or device is essential to recognize potential problems and to guarantee that an MR examination may be performed without risk.

Extrusion of an eye socket magnetic implant in a patient imaged with a 0.5-Tesla MR system has been described by Yuh, et al. (1991). This type of magnetic prosthesis was used in the patient after enucleation. For this prosthesis, a removable eye prosthesis adheres with a magnet of opposite polarity to a permanent implant sutured to the rectus muscles and conjunctiva by magnetic attraction through the conjunctiva. This "magnetic linkage" is intended to permit the eye prosthesis to move in a coordinated fashion with that of eye movement. In the reported incident, the static magnetic field of the MR system produced sufficient attraction of the ferromagnetic portion of the prosthesis to cause serious injury to the patient.

Certain dental prosthetic appliances utilize magnetic forces to retain the implant in place. The magnet may be contained within the prosthesis and attached to a ferromagnetic post implanted in the mandible or the magnetic component may be the implanted component. Therefore, whether or not an MR procedure may be performed without problems depends on the configuration of the magnetically-active dental implant and other factors.

REFERENCES

Blankenstein FH, et al. Signal loss in magnetic resonance imaging caused by intraoral anchored dental magnetic materials. Rofo 2006;178:787-93.

Cuda D, et al. Focused tight dressing does not prevent cochlear implant magnet migration under 1.5 Tesla MRI. Acta Otorhinolaryngol Ital 2013;33:133-6.

Gaston A, et al. External magnetic guidance of endovascular catheters with a superconducting magnet: Preliminary trials. J Neuroradiol 1988;15:137-147.

Hassepass F, et al. Magnet dislocation: An increasing serious complication following MRI in patients with cochlear implants. Rofo 2014;40:1481-6.

Hassepass F, et al. Revision surgery due to magnet dislocation in cochlear implant patients: An emerging complication. Otol Neurotol 2014;35:29-34.

Jansson KJ, et al. MRI induced torque and demagnetization in retention magnets for a bone conduction implant. IEEE Trans Biomed Eng 2014;61:1887-93.

Jeon JH, et al. Reversing the polarity of a cochlear implant magnet after magnetic resonance imaging. Auris Nasus Larynx 2012;39:415-7.

Kim BG, et al. Adverse events and discomfort during magnetic resonance imaging in cochlear implant recipients. JAMA Otolaryngol Head Neck Surg 2015;141:45-52.

Kong Sk, et al. The reversed internal magnet of cochlear implant after magnetic resonance imaging. Am J Otolaryngol 2014;35:239-41.

Majdani O, et al. Artifacts caused by cochlear implants with non-removable magnets in 3-T MRI: Phantom and cadaveric studies. Eur Arch Otorhinolaryngol 2009;266:1885-90.

Majdani O, et al. Demagnetization of cochlear implants and temperature changes in 3.0-T MRI environment. Otolaryngol Head Neck Surg 2008;139:833-9.

Ranney DF, Huffaker HH. Magnetic microspheres for the targeted controlled release of drugs and diagnostic agents. Ann NY Acad Sci 1987;507:104-119.

Schneider ML, Walker GB, Dormer KJ. Effects of magnetic resonance imaging on implantable permanent magnets. Am J Otol 1995;16:687-689.

Shellock FG. Magnetic Resonance Procedures: Health Effects and Safety. CRC Press, LLC, Boca Raton, FL, 2001.

Shellock FG. *Ex vivo* assessment of deflection forces and artifacts associated with high-field strength MRI of "mini-magnet" dental prostheses. Magnetic Resonance Imaging 1989;7 (Suppl 1):38.

Young DB, Pawlak AM. An electromagnetically controllable heart valve suitable for chronic implantation. ASAIO Trans 1990;36:M421-M425.

Yuh WTC, et al. Extrusion of an eye socket magnetic implant after MR imaging examination: Potential hazard to a patient with eye prosthesis. J Magn Reson Imag 1991;1:711-713.

Medivance Nasogastric Sump Tube with YSI Series 400 Temperature Sensor

MRI Information. The **Medivance Nasogastric Sump Tube with YSI Series 400 Temperature Sensor**, 18-Fr. (Medivance, Inc., Louisville, CO) was determined to be MR Conditional according to the terminology specified in the American Society for Testing and Materials (ASTM) International, Designation: F2503. Standard Practice for Marking Medical Devices and Other Items for Safety in the Magnetic Resonance Environment.

Non-clinical testing demonstrated that the Medivance Nasogastric Sump Tube with YSI Series 400 Temperature Sensor, 18-Fr. is MR Conditional. A patient with this device can be scanned safely, immediately after placement under the following conditions:

- Static magnetic field of 3-Tesla or less
- Spatial gradient magnetic field of 720-gauss/cm or less
- Maximum MR system reported whole-body-averaged specific absorption rate (SAR) of 3-W/kg for 15 minutes of scanning.

In non-clinical testing, the Medivance Nasogastric Sump Tube with YSI Series 400 Temperature Sensor, 18-Fr. produced a temperature rise of 0.9°C at a maximum MR system-reported whole body averaged specific absorption rate (SAR) of 3-W/kg for 15-minutes of MR scanning in a 3-Tesla MR system using a transmit/receive body coil (Excite, Software G3.0-052B, General Electric Healthcare, Milwaukee, WI).

MR image quality may be compromised if the area of interest is in the exact same area or relatively close to the position of the Medivance Nasogastric Sump Tube with YSI Series 400 Temperature Sensor, 18-Fr. Therefore, optimization of MR imaging parameters to compensate for the presence of this device may be necessary.

Artifact Information

Pulse Sequence	T1-SE	T1-SE	GRE	GRE
Signal Void Size	10,377-mm^2	90-mm^2	3,992-mm^2	75-mm^2
Plane Orientation	Parallel	Perpendicular	Parallel	Perpendicular

IMPORTANT NOTE: To ensure patient safety during MRI, the Medivance Nasogastric Sump Tube with YSI Series 400 Temperature Sensor, 18-Fr. must be labeled to verify that it is positioned exactly as it was for this MRI assessment: straight down the center of the patient, with the remaining tubing/connector going out the back of the MR system. The Medivance Nasogastric Sump Tube with YSI Series 400 Temperature Sensor, 18-Fr. should NOT be connected to a monitor and there should be NO loops or coils present. See additional information below:

1) The Medivance Nasogastric Sump Tube with YSI Series 400 Temperature Sensor, 18-Fr. must disconnected from the monitor prior to the MRI procedure.

2) Remove all electrically conductive material from the bore of the MR system that is not required for the procedure (i.e. unused surface coils, cables, etc.).

3) Keep electrically conductive material that must remain in the bore of the MR system from directly contacting the patient by placing insulation or space between the conductive material and the patient.

4) Position the Medivance Nasogastric Sump Tube with YSI Series 400 Temperature Sensor, 18-Fr. in a straight configuration to prevent cross points, coils, and loops. The remaining portion of this device, along with the connector should be positioned in a straight line out the BACK of the MR system (i.e. NOT along side the inside of the MR system).

5) Ensure that the Medivance Nasogastric Sump Tube with YSI Series 400 Temperature Sensor, 18-Fr. exiting the patient does not touch the patient.

6) Monitor the patient continuously using a verbal means (e.g., intercom). If the patient reports any unusual sensation, discontinue the MRI procedure immediately. Notably, MRI procedures should not be performed in patients that are unable to communicate (e.g., sedated, anesthetized, etc.).

MedStream Programmable Infusion System
Codman

The MedStream Programmable Infusion System (Catalog No. 91-4200US & 91-4201US; Codman) is MR Conditional. Comprehensive labeling information must be reviewed to ensure patient safety.

Carefully review the latest MRI labeling conditions and guidelines at: www.depuysynthes.com/hcp/codman-neuro/products

Important Note to MR Healthcare Professionals: Different MRI guidelines may exist for different countries. Therefore, use the appropriate information for your country.

[MR healthcare professionals are advised to contact the respective manufacturer in order to obtain the latest safety information to ensure patient safety relative to the use of an MR procedure.]

REFERENCE

Depuy Synthes, www.depuysynthes.com
Depuy Synthes, www.depuysynthes.com/hcp/codman-neuro/products

Miscellaneous Implants and Devices

Many miscellaneous implants, materials, devices, and objects have been tested with regard to MR procedures and the MR environment. For example, various types of firearms have been evaluated in the MR environment. These firearms exhibited strong ferromagnetism. In fact, two of the six firearms that underwent testing discharged in a reproducible manner while in the MR system room. Obviously, firearms should remain outside of the MR environment to prevent problems or possible injuries.

MR-guided biopsy, therapeutic, and minimally invasive surgical procedures are important clinical applications that are performed on conventional, open-architecture, or "double-donut" MR systems specially designed for this work. These procedures present challenges for the instruments and devices that are needed to support these interventions. Metallic surgical instruments and other devices potentially pose hazards (e.g., "missile" effects) or other problems (i.e. image artifacts and distortion that can obscure the area of interest) that must be addressed to apply MR-guided techniques effectively. Various manufacturers have used "weakly" ferromagnetic, nonferromagnetic or nonmetallic materials to make special instruments for interventional MR procedures.

Other medical products and devices have been developed with metallic components that are either entirely nonferromagnetic and nonconducting or made from metals that have a low magnetic susceptibility (e.g., titanium, non-magnetic types of stainless steel, etc.) that are acceptable for use in the MR environment.

MRI at 3-Tesla and Miscellaneous Implants and Devices. Many implants and devices have been tested in association with 3-Tesla MR systems. Refer to **The List** to determine information about specific miscellaneous implants and devices assessed at 3-Tesla.

REFERENCES

Audet-Griffin A, Pakbaz S, Shellock FG. Evaluation of MRI issues for a new, liquid embolic device. Journal of Interventional Neuroradiology 2014;6:624-9.

Dula AN, Virostko J, Shellock FG. Assessment of MRI issues at 7-Tesla for 28 implants and other objects. Am J Roentgenol 2014;202:401-405.

Go KG, et al. Interaction of metallic neurosurgical implants with magnetic resonance imaging at 1.5-Tesla as a cause of image distortion and of hazardous movement of the implant. Clin Neurosurg 1989;91:109-115.

Kanal E, Shaibani A. Firearm safety in the MR imaging environment. Radiology 1994;193:875-876.

Lufkin R, Jordan S, Lylyck P, et al. MR imaging with topographic EEG electrodes in place. Am J Neuroradiol 1988;9:953-954.

Planert J, et al. Measurements of magnetism-forces and torque moments affecting medical instruments, implants, and foreign objects during magnetic resonance imaging at all degrees of freedom. Med Physics 1996;23:851-856.

Sammet, CL, Yang X, Wassenaar P, Bourekas EC, Yuh BA, Shellock FG, Sammet S, Knopp MV. MRI heating assessment of passive, extracranial neurosurgical implants at 7-Tesla. Magnetic Resonance Imaging 2013;31:1029-34.

Shellock FG. Biomedical implants and devices: Assessment of magnetic field interactions with a 3.0-Tesla MR system. J Magn Reson Imag 2002;16:721-732.

Shellock FG. MR-compatibility of an endoscope designed for use in interventional MR procedures. Am J Roentgenol 1998;71:1297-1300.

Shellock FG. Magnetic Resonance Procedures: Health Effects and Safety. CRC Press, LLC, Boca Raton, FL, 2001.

Shellock FG. MR safety update 2002: Implants and devices. J Magn Reson Imag 2002;16:485-496.

Shellock FG. Metallic neurosurgical implants: Assessment of magnetic field interactions, heating, and artifacts at 1.5-Tesla. Radiology 2001;218:611.

Shellock FG. Surgical instruments for interventional MRI procedures: Assessment of MR safety. J Magn Reson Imag 2001;13:152-157.

Shellock FG, Audet-Griffin A. Evaluation of magnetic resonance imaging issues for a wirelessly-powered lead used for epidural, spinal cord stimulation. Neuromodulation 2014;17:334-339.

Shellock FG, Shellock VJ. Ceramic surgical instruments: Evaluation of MR-compatibility at 1.5-Tesla. J Magn Reson Imag 1996;6:954-956.

Shellock FG, Shellock VJ. Evaluation of MR compatibility of 38 bioimplants and devices. Radiology 1995;197:174.

Titterington B, Shellock FG. A new vascular coupling device: Assessment of MRI issues at 3-Tesla. Magn Reson Imaging 2014;32:585-9.

Zhang J, et al. Temperature changes in nickel-chromium intracranial depth electrodes during MR scanning. Am J Neuroradiol 1993;14:497-500.

Neurostimulation Systems: General Information

The incidence of patients receiving implanted neurostimulation or neuromodulation systems for treatment of neurological disorders and other conditions continues to increase. Because of the inherent design and intended function of neurostimulation systems, [including those used for deep brain stimulation (DBS), spinal cord stimulation (SCS), vagus nerve stimulation (VNS), and other similar devices], the electromagnetic fields used for MR procedures may produce a variety of problems. For example, altered function of a neurostimulation system that results from exposure to the electromagnetic fields of an MR system may cause discomfort, pain, or serious injuries to patients.

MRI-related heating has been reported to create the greatest concern for various devices used for neuromodulation. Variables that impact heating include, but are not limited to, the following:

- The specific type of neuromodulation system
- The electrical characteristics of the specific neuromodulation system
- The field strength and RF wavelength of the MR system
- The type of transmit RF coil (i.e. transmit head vs transmit body RF coil) used for MRI
- The amount of RF energy delivered (i.e. the RF power level, SAR)
- The technique used to calculate or estimate SAR used by the MR system
- The patient's anatomy undergoing MR imaging
- The landmark position or body part undergoing MRI relative to the transmit RF coil
- The orientation and configuration of the implantable pulse generator (IPG), extension (e.g., the cable connecting the pulse generator (PG) to the implanted lead), and the lead relative to the source of RF energy (i.e. the transmit RF coil)

Importantly, the exact criteria for the particular neurostimulation system with regard to the pulse generator, leads, electrodes, and operational aspects of the device as well as the MR system conditions must be defined by comprehensive testing and carefully followed to ensure patient safety. On-going investigations continue to define the acceptable criteria to permit MR examinations, including those involving 1.5- and 3-Tesla MR systems, to be performed in patients with neurostimulation systems. Importantly, various device manufacturers now have certain neurostimulation systems that have been specially designed to be MR Conditional, which have fewer limitations for MR imaging procedures compared to older devices.

REFERENCES

Aziz TZ. Current and future directions of post-deep brain stimulation implant magnetic resonance imaging scanning. World Neurosurg 2011;76:69-70.

Baker K, Nyenhuis JA, Hridlicka G, Rezai AR, Tkach JA, Sharan A, Shellock FG. Neurostimulator implants: Assessment of magnetic field interactions associated with 1.5- and 3.0-Tesla MR systems. J Magn Reson Imag 2005;21:72-77.

Baker KB, Tkach JA, Nyenhuis JA, Phillips M, Shellock FG, Gonzalez-Martinez J, Rezai AR. Evaluation of specific absorption rate as a dosimeter of MRI-Related implant heating. J Magn Reson Imag 2004;20:315-320.

Baker KB, Tkach J, Hall JD, Nyenhuis JA, Shellock FG, Rezai AR. Reduction of MRI-related heating in deep brain stimulation leads using a lead management system. Neurosurgery 2005;57:392-397.

Baker KB, et al. Variability in RF-induced heating of a deep brain stimulation implant across MR systems. J Magn Reson Imag 2006;24:1236-42.

Baker KB, et al. Deep brain stimulation for obsessive-compulsive disorder: using functional magnetic resonance imaging and electrophysiological techniques: Technical case report. Neurosurgery 2007;61(5 Suppl 2):E367-8.

Bhidayasiri R, Bronstein JM, Sinha S, Krahl SE, Ahn S, Behnke EJ, Cohen MS, Frysinger R, Shellock FG. Bilateral neurostimulation systems used for deep brain stimulation: *In vitro* study of MRI-related heating at 1.5-Tesla and implications for clinical imaging of the brain. Magnetic Resonance Imaging 2005;23:549-555.

Bosma RL, et al. Spinal cord response to stepwise and block presentation of thermal stimuli: A functional MRI study. J Magn Reson Imaging 2015;41:1318-25.

Bronstein JM, et al. Deep brain stimulation for Parkinson disease: An expert consensus and review of key issues. Arch Neurol 2011;68:165.

Buentjen L, et al. Direct targeting of the thalamic anteroventral nucleus for deep brain stimulation by T1-weighted magnetic resonance imaging at 3T. Stereotact Funct Neurosurg 2014;92:25-30.

Cabot E, et al. Evaluation of the RF heating of a generic deep brain stimulator exposed in 1.5 T magnetic resonance scanners. Bioelectromagnetics 2013;34:104-13.

Carmichael DW, et al. Functional MRI with active, fully implanted, deep brain stimulation systems: Safety and experimental confounds. Neuroimage 2007;37:508.

Chhabra V, Sung E, et al. Safety of magnetic resonance imaging of deep brain stimulator systems: A serial imaging and clinical retrospective study. J Neurosurg 2010;112:497-502.

Cheng CH, et al. 1.5-T versus 3-T MRI for targeting subthalamic nucleus for deep brain stimulation. Br J Neurosurg 2014;28:467-70.

Coffey RJ, et al. Magnetic resonance imaging conditionally safe neurostimulation leads: Investigation of the maximum safe lead tip temperature. Neurosurgery 2014;74:215-24.

De Andres J, Valia JC, et al. Magnetic resonance imaging in patients with spinal neurostimulation systems. Anesthesiology 2007;106:779-86.

De Andres J, et al. MRI-compatible spinal cord stimulator device and related changes in patient safety and imaging artifacts. Pain Med 2014;15:815-9.

de Jonge JC, et al. Safety of a dedicated brain MRI protocol in patients with a vagus nerve stimulator. Epilepsia 2014;55:112-5.

Desai MJ, et al. The rate of magnetic resonance imaging in patients with spinal cord stimulation. Spine 2015;40:E531-7.

Dormont D, et al. Chronic thalamic stimulation with three-dimensional MR stereotactic guidance. Am J Neuroradiol 1997;18:1093-1097.

Elkelini MS, Hassouna MM. Safety of MRI at 1.5-Tesla in patients with implanted sacral nerve neurostimulator. Eur Urol 2006;50:311-6.

Englot DJ, et al. Abnormal T2-weighted MRI signal surrounding leads in a subset of deep brain stimulation patients. Stereotact Funct Neurosurg 2011;89:311-317.

Eryaman Y, et al. Parallel transmit pulse design for patients with deep brain stimulation implants. Magn Reson Med 2015;73:1896-1903.

Finelli DA, Rezai AR, Ruggieri P, Tkach J, Nyenhuis J, Hridlicka G, Sharan A, Stypulkowski PH, Shellock FG. MR-related heating of deep brain stimulation electrodes: An *in vitro* study of clinical imaging sequences. Am J Neuroradiol 2002;23:1795-1802.

Fraix V, et al. Effects of magnetic resonance imaging in patients with implanted deep brain stimulation systems. J Neurosurg 2010;113:1242-5.

Georgi A-C, Stippich C, Tronnier VM, Heiland S. Active deep brain stimulation during MRI: A feasibility study. Magn Reson in Medicine 2003;51:380-388.

Gleason CA, et al. The effect of magnetic resonance imagers on implanted neurostimulators. Pacing Clin Electrophysiol 1992;15:81-94.

Gorny KR, et al. 3 Tesla MRI of patients with a vagus nerve stimulator: Initial experience using a T/R head coil under controlled conditions. J Magn Reson Imag 2010;31:475-81.

Gupte AA, et al. MRI-related heating near deep brain stimulation electrodes: More data are needed. Stereotact Funct Neurosurg 2011;89:131-40.

Henderson J, Tkach J, Phillips M, Baker K, Shellock FG, Rezai A. Permanent neurological deficit related to magnetic resonance imaging in a patient with implanted deep brain stimulation electrodes for Parkinson's disease: Case report. Neurosurgery 2005;57:E1063.

Kerl HU, et al. The subthalamic nucleus at 7.0 Tesla: Evaluation of sequence and orientation for deep-brain stimulation. Acta Neurochir (Wien) 2012;154:2051-62.

Kovacs N, Nagy F, Kover F, et al. Implanted deep brain stimulator and 1.0-Tesla magnetic resonance imaging. J Magn Reson Imag 2006;24:1409-12.

Larson PS, et al. Magnetic resonance imaging of implanted deep brain stimulators: Experience in a large series. Stereotact Funct Neurosurg 2008;86:92-100.

Liem LA, van Dongen VC. Magnetic resonance imaging and spinal cord stimulation systems. Pain 1997;70:95-97.

Maldonado IL, et al. Magnetic resonance-based deep brain stimulation technique: A series of 478 consecutive implanted electrodes with no perioperative intracerebral hemorrhage. Neurosurgery 2009;65(6 Suppl):196-201.

Moens M, et al. Spinal cord stimulation modulates cerebral function: An fMRI study. Neuroradiology 2012;54:1399-407.

Moeschler SM, et al. Spinal cord stimulator explanation for magnetic resonance imaging: A case series. Neuromodulation 2015;18:285-8; discussion 288.

Mogilner AY, Rezai AR. Brain stimulation: History, current clinical application, and future prospects. Acta Neurochir Suppl 2003;87:115-120.

Mohsin SA, Sheikh NM, Saeed U. MRI-induced heating of deep brain stimulation leads. Phys Med Biol 2008;53:5745-56.

Nazzaro JM, Lyons KE, Wetzel LH, Pahwa R. Use of brain MRI after deep brain stimulation hardware implantation. Int J Neurosci 2010;120:176-83.

Nazzaro JM, et al. Deep brain stimulation lead-contact heating during 3T MRI: Single- versus dual channel pulse generator configurations. Int J Neurosci 2014;124:166-74.

Nolte IS, et al. Visualization of the internal globus pallidus: Sequence and orientation for deep brain stimulation using a standard installation protocol at 3.0 Tesla. Acta Neurochir (Wien) 2012;154:481-94.

Nowinski WL, et al. Simulation and assessment of cerebrovascular damage in deep brain stimulation using a stereotactic atlas of vasculature and structure derived from multiple 3- and 7-Tesla scans. J Neurosurg 2010;113:1234-41

Ostrem JL, et al. Clinical outcomes of PD patients having bilateral STN DBS using high-field interventional MR-imaging for lead placement. Clin Neurol Neurosurg 2013;115:708-12.

Phillips MD, et al. Parkinson disease: Pattern of functional MR imaging activation during deep brain stimulation of subthalamic nucleus--initial experience. Radiology 2006;239:209-16.

Rezai AR, et al. Thalamic stimulation and functional magnetic resonance imaging: Localization of cortical and subcortical activation with implanted electrodes. J Neurosurg 1999;90:583-590.

Rezai AR, Baker K, Tkach J, Phillips M, Hrdlicka G, Sharan A, Nyenhuis J, Ruggieri P, Henderson J, Shellock FG. Is magnetic resonance imaging safe for patients with neurostimulation systems used for deep brain stimulation (DBS)? Neurosurgery 2005;57:1056-1062.

Rezai AR, Finelli D, Ruggieri P, Tkach J, Nyenhuis JA, Shellock FG. Neurostimulators: Potential for excessive heating of deep brain stimulation electrodes during MR imaging. J Magn Reson Imag 2001;14:488-489.

Rezai AR, Finelli D, Nyenhuis JA, Hrdlick G, Tkach J, Ruggieri P, Stypulkowski PH, Sharan A, Shellock FG. Neurostimulator for deep brain stimulation: *Ex vivo* evaluation of MRI-related heating at 1.5-Tesla. J Magn Reson Imag 2002;15:241-250.

Rezai AR, Phillips M, Baker K, Sharan AD, Nyenhuis J, Tkach J, Henderson J, Shellock FG. Neurostimulation system used for deep brain stimulation (DBS): MR safety issues and implications of failing to follow guidelines. Investigative Radiology 2004;39:300-303.

Rise MT. Instrumentation for neuromodulation. Archives Of Medical Research 2000;31:237-247.

Ryu SI, et al. Asymptomatic transient MRI signal changes after unilateral deep brain stimulation electrode implantation for movement disorder. Stereotact Funct Neurosurg 2004;82:65-9.

Sankar T, Lozano AM. Magnetic resonance imaging and deep brain stimulation: Questions of safety. World Neurosurg 2011;76:71-3.

Sarkar SN, et al. Low-power inversion recovery MRI preserves brain tissue contrast for patients with Parkinson disease with deep brain stimulators. AJNR Am J Neuroradiol 2014;35:1325-9.

Sarkar SN, et al. Utilizing fast spin echo MRI to reduce image artifacts and improve implant/tissue interface detection in refractory Parkinson's patients with deep brain stimulators. Parkinsons Dis 2014;2014:508576].

Sarkar SN, et al. Three-dimensional brain MRI for DBS patients within ultra-low radiofrequency power limits. Mov Disord 2014;29:546-9.

Shrivastava D, et al. Heating induced near deep brain stimulation lead electrodes during magnetic resonance imaging with a 3T transceive volume head coil. Phys Med Biol 2012;57:5651-65.

Shellock FG. MRI Safety and Neuromodulation Systems. In: Neuromodulation. Krames ES, Peckham PH, Rezai, AR, Editors. Academic Press/Elsevier, New York, 2009.

Shellock FG. MR imaging and electronically-activated devices. Radiology 219:294-295, 2001.

Shellock FG, Audet-Griffin A. Evaluation of magnetic resonance imaging issues for a wirelessly-powered lead used for epidural, spinal cord, stimulation. Neuromodulation 2014;17:334-339.

Shellock FG. Begnaud J, Inman DM. VNS Therapy System: In vitro evaluation of MRI-related heating and function at 1.5- and 3-Tesla. Neuromodulation 2006;9:204-213.

Shellock FG, et al. Implantable microstimulator: Magnetic resonance safety at 1.5-Tesla. Investigative Radiology 2004;39:591-594.

Shrivastava D, et al. Effect of the extracranial deep brain stimulation lead on radiofrequency heating at 9.4 Tesla (400.2 MHz). J Magn Reson Imag 2010;32:600-7.

Smith CD, et al. Chapter 16. Health effects of induced electrical currents: Implications for implants. In: Magnetic Resonance: Health Effects and Safety, FG Shellock, Editor, CRC Press, Boca Raton, FL, 2001; pp. 393-413.

Spiegel J, et al. Transient dystonia following magnetic resonance imaging in a patient with deep brain stimulation electrodes for the treatment of Parkinson disease. J Neurosurgery 2003;99:772-774.

Tagliati M, et al. and the National Parkinson Foundation DBS Working Group. Safety of MRI in patients with implanted deep brain stimulation devices. Neuroimage 2009;47 Suppl 2:T53-7.

Thani NB, et al. Accuracy of postoperative computed tomography and magnetic resonance image fusion for assessing deep brain stimulation electrodes. Neurosurgery 2011;69:207-14.

Thornton JS. Technical challenges and safety of magnetic resonance imaging with in situ neuromodulation from spine to brain. Eur J Paediatr Neurol 2017;21:232-241.

Tronnier VM, et al. Magnetic resonance imaging with implanted neurostimulation systems: An *in vitro* and *in vivo* study. Neurosurgery 1999;44:118-25.

Tronnier HT, et al. Risk assessment of magnetic resonance imaging in chronically implanted paddle electrodes for cortical stimulation. Stereotact Funct Neurosurg 2015;93:182-9.

Ullman M, et al. A pilot study of human brain tissue post-magnetic resonance imaging: Information from the National Deep Brain Stimulation Brain Tissue Network (DBS-BTN). Neuroimage 2011;54 Suppl 1:S233-

Utti RJ, Tsuboi Y, et al. Magnetic resonance imaging and deep brain stimulation. Neurosurgery 2002;51:1423-1431.

Walsh KM, et al. Spinal cord stimulation: A review of the safety literature and proposal for perioperative evaluation and management. Spine J 2015;15:1864-9.

Weise LM, et al. Postoperative MRI examinations in patients treated by deep brain stimulation using a non-standard protocol. Acta Neurochir (Wien) 2010;152:2021-7.

Zekaj E, et al. Does magnetic resonance imaging induce tissue damage due to DBS lead heating? Acta Neurochir 2013;155:1677-8.

Zonenshayn M, Mogilner AY, Rezai AR. Neurostimulation and functional brain stimulation. Neurological Research 2000;22:318-325.

Zrinzo L, et al. Clinical safety of brain magnetic resonance imaging with implanted deep brain stimulation hardware: Large case series and review of the literature. World Neurosurg 2011;76:164-72.

Neurostimulation Systems: Deep Brain Stimulation
Medtronic Inc.

MRI Guidelines for Medtronic Deep Brain Stimulation Systems

Models include:
Kinetra: 7428
Soletra: 7426
Itrel II: 7424
Activa PC Deep Brain Neurostimulator (Model 37601)
Activa RC Deep Brain Neurostimulator (Model 37612)
Activa SC Deep Brain Neurostimulator (Model 37602)
Activa SC Deep Brain Neurostimulator (Model 37603)

Various deep brain stimulation devices from Medtronics, Inc. are MR Conditional. Certain devices have strict limitations for MRI procedures, while others that utilize SureScan MRI technology are less restrictive and referred to as "full-body eligible". Comprehensive labeling information must be reviewed to ensure patient safety.

Carefully review the latest MRI labeling conditions and guidelines at: www.medtronic.com/mri

Note to MR Healthcare Professionals: Different MRI guidelines exist for different countries. Therefore, use the appropriate information for your country.

[MR healthcare professionals are advised to contact the respective manufacturer in order to obtain the latest safety information to ensure patient safety relative to the use of an MR procedure.]

REFERENCES

Medtronic, Inc., www.medtronic.com
Medtronic, Inc., www.medtronic.com/mri

Neurostimulation System: EndoStim Lower Esophagus Stimulation (LES) Stimulation System
EndoStim BV

The EndoStim Lower Esophagus Stimulation (LES) Stimulation System (EndoStim BV, The Hague, Netherlands) is MR Conditional and designed to allow patients to be safely undergo MRI procedures under highly specific conditions and guidelines.

The **EndoStim LES Stimulation System (Gen 1 Model 1002 – SN <999, with lead Model 1003)** has received CE Marking for use with magnetic resonance imaging (MRI) under the following conditions:

- Head and extremities (limbs) imaging with local transmit/receive coil only in 1.5T/64MHz machines.
- The device must be switched off prior to the MRI scan and switched back on afterwards.

The **EndoStim II LES Stimulation System (Gen 2 Model 1006 – SN 1000+, with lead Model 1003)** has received CE Marking for use with magnetic resonance imaging (MRI) under the following conditions:

- Full body MRI scans using 3.0-T/128MHz systems.
- Head and extremities (limbs) MRI scans with local transmit/receive coil in 1.5T/64MHz or 3.0T/128MHz machines.
- The device must be switched off prior to the MRI scan and switched back on afterwards.

The EndoStim Programmer System is considered MR Unsafe, meaning that it cannot be present and/or used in the same room as the MR system.

For full MRI labeling information, visit: www.endostim.com

Important Note to MR Healthcare Professionals: Different MRI guidelines may exist for different countries. Therefore, use the appropriate information for your country.

[MR healthcare professionals are advised to contact the respective manufacturer in order to obtain the latest safety information to ensure patient safety relative to the use of an MR procedure.]

REFERENCE

EndoStim BV, www.endostim.com

Neurostimulation System: Enterra Therapy, Gastric Electrical Stimulation (GES)
Medtronic, Inc.

The Enterra Therapy, Gastric Electrical Stimulation (GES) System (Medtronic, Inc.), is a neurostimulation system indicated for treatment of patients with chronic, intractable (drug refractory) nausea and vomiting secondary to gastroparesis of diabetic or idiopathic etiology.

The Enterra Therapy, Gastric Electrical Stimulation System (Enterra Models: Enterra Model 3116, Enterra II Model 37800) is MR Unsafe.

Magnetic Resonance Imaging (MRI) – Patients with an implanted device should not be exposed to the electromagnetic fields produced by magnetic resonance imaging (MRI). Use of MRI may potentially result in system failure, dislodgement, heating, or induced voltages in the neurostimulator and/or lead. An induced voltage through the neurostimulator or lead may cause uncomfortable, "jolting," or "shocking" levels of stimulation. Clinicians should carefully weigh the decision to use MRI in patients with an implanted neurostimulation system, and note the following:

- Magnetic and radio-frequency (RF) fields produced by MRI may change the neurostimulator settings and injure the patient.

[MR healthcare professionals are advised to contact the respective manufacturer in order to obtain the latest safety information to ensure patient safety relative to the use of an MR procedure.]

REFERENCE

Medtronic, Inc., www.medtronic.com/mri

Neurostimulation System: InterStim Therapy - Sacral Nerve Stimulation (SNS) for Urinary Control
Medtronic, Inc.

InterStim Therapy - Sacral Nerve Stimulation (SNS) for Urinary Control (Medtronic, Inc.) is a treatment for urinary urge incontinence, non-obstructive urinary retention, and significant symptoms of urgency-frequency in patients who have failed or could not tolerate more conservative treatments.

InterStim Therapy - Sacral Nerve Stimulation (SNS) for Urinary Control (Medtronic, Inc.) is MR Conditional (information applies to Interstim and Interstim II, Models 3058 and 3023). Comprehensive labeling information must be reviewed to ensure patient safety.

Carefully review the latest MRI labeling conditions and guidelines at: www.medtronic.com/mri

[MR healthcare professionals are advised to contact the respective manufacturer in order to obtain the latest safety information to ensure patient safety relative to the use of an MR procedure.]

REFERENCE

Medtronic, Inc., www.medtronic.com/mri

Neurostimulation System: Pulsante SPG (Sphenopalatine Ganglion) Microstimulator
Autonomic Technologies, Inc.

Autonomic Technologies, Inc. developed the Pulsante SPG (Sphenopalatine Ganglion) Microstimulator System (also known as the ATI Neurostimulation System) to provide on-demand SPG stimulation therapy with the intention to relieve the debilitating pain of cluster headache. The Pulsante SPG System is a minimally-invasive, rechargeable, multi-channel, peripheral nerve stimulation system. The System includes:

The Insert. Pulsante SPG Microstimulator (ATI Neurostimulator), a microstimulator with an integral lead designed to fit the facial anatomy. The microstimulator is available in four sizes to accommodate a range of facial anatomies. The insert has CE-marked MR Conditional labeling for whole-body MRI.

The Remote Controller. A hand-held device with simple therapy controls that provides on-demand patient-controlled SPG therapy. Therapy settings are individualized and can be adjusted quickly by physicians using a programmer laptop.

Magnetic Resonance Imaging (MRI)

The ATI Neurostimulator is MR Conditional. It poses no known hazards in *specified* MRI environment with *specified* conditions of use.

Non-clinical testing has demonstrated the ATI Neurostimulator is MR Conditional. It can be scanned safely under the following conditions:

- Static magnetic field of 3.0 Tesla
- Spatial gradient field of 8 Tesla/meter
- Maximum whole body averaged specific absorption rate (SAR) of 2 W/kg for 15 minutes of scanning.

In non-clinical testing in a 3.0 Tesla MR scanner, the ATI Neurostimulator produced a temperature rise of less than 5.0°C at a maximum whole body averaged specific absorption rate (SAR) of 2 W/kg, as assessed by calorimetry for 15 minutes of MR scanning.

The image artifact extends approximately 40 mm from the device, including the lead, when scanned using the spin and gradient echo pulse sequence.

Refer to the ATI Neurostimulation System manuals for additional warnings and information for the use of the ATI Neurostimulation System.

The ATI Remote Controller is MR Unsafe. It is hazardous in all MRI environments.

Important Note to MR Healthcare Professionals: Different MRI guidelines may exist for different countries. Therefore, use the appropriate information for your country.

[MR healthcare professionals are advised to contact the respective manufacturer in order to obtain the latest safety information to ensure patient safety relative to the use of an MR procedure.]

REFERENCE

Autonomic Technologies, Inc., www.ati-spg.com

Neurostimulation System: Senza Spinal Cord Stimulation System
Nevro Corporation

The implanted Senza Spinal Cord Stimulation (SCS) System (Nevro Corporation) is MR Conditional and has been demonstrated to present no known hazards in a specified MRI environment when following specific guidelines as described in the 1.5-T and 3-T Magnetic Resonance Imaging (MRI) Guidelines for the Senza system.

Important Note to MR Healthcare Professionals: Different MRI guidelines may exist for different countries. Therefore, use the appropriate information for your country.

[MR healthcare professionals are advised to contact the respective manufacturer in order to obtain the latest safety information to ensure patient safety relative to the use of an MR procedure.]

REFERENCE

Nevro Corporation, www.nevrocorp.com

Neurostimulation System: RNS System
Neuropace

The responsive neurostimulation device or RNS system (Neuropace) is designed for the treatment of medically refractory partial epilepsy and includes implantable and external products. The RNS System is an adjunctive therapy in reducing the frequency of seizures in individuals 18 years of age or older with partial onset seizures from no more than two foci that are refractory to two or more antiepileptic medications.

Magnetic Resonance Imaging. MRI is contraindicated for patients with an implanted RNS System. Do not perform an MRI on a patient with any implanted RNS Neurostimulator or Lead (or any portion of a Lead). The RNS System is MR Unsafe. Testing has not been performed to define conditions of use to ensure safety of the RNS System in an MR environment.

[MR healthcare professionals are advised to contact the respective manufacturer in order to obtain the latest safety information to ensure patient safety relative to the use of an MR procedure.]

REFERENCE

Neuropace, www.neuropace.com

Neurostimulation Systems: Spinal Cord Stimulation
Boston Scientific

Precision Spectra Spinal Cord Stimulator (SCS) System

The Precision Spectra Spinal Cord Stimulator (SCS) System is MR Conditional. Comprehensive labeling information must be reviewed to ensure patient safety.

Carefully review the latest MRI labeling conditions and guidelines at: www.bostonscientific.com

Precision Montage MRI Spinal Cord Stimulation (SCS) System

The Precision Montage MRI Spinal Cord Stimulation (SCS) System (Boston Scientific) is MR Conditional. Comprehensive labeling information must be reviewed to ensure patient safety.

Carefully review the latest MRI labeling conditions and guidelines at: www.bostonscientific.com

Spectra WaveWriter Spinal Cord Stimulation (SCS) System

The Spectra WaveWriter Spinal Cord Stimulation (SCS) System is MR Conditional. Comprehensive labeling information must be reviewed to ensure patient safety.

Carefully review the latest MRI labeling conditions and guidelines at: www.bostonscientific.com/manuals/manuals/landing-page.html

Important Note to MR Healthcare Professionals: Different MRI guidelines may exist for different countries. Therefore, use the appropriate information for your country.

[MR healthcare professionals are advised to contact the respective manufacturer in order to obtain the latest safety information to ensure patient safety relative to the use of an MR procedure.]

REFERENCE

Boston Scientific, www.bostonscientific.com

Neurostimulation Systems: Spinal Cord Stimulation
St. Jude Medical

Genesis, GenesisXP, GenesisRC, Eon, Eon C, Eon Mini, and Renew

The Genesis, GenesisXP, GenesisRC, Eon, EonC, Eon Mini, and Renew neuromodulation devices (St. Jude Medical) used for spinal cord stimulation are indicated as aids in the management of chronic intractable pain of the trunk and/or limbs including unilateral or bilateral pain associated with any of the following: failed back surgery syndrome, intractable low back and leg pain, as well as for the treatment of other conditions.

MRI Information. The labeling information for these afore-mentioned products states:

"Warnings/Precautions: Diathermy therapy, cardioverter defibrillators, magnetic resonance imaging (MRI), explosive or flammable gases, theft detectors and metal screening devices, lead movement, operation of machinery and equipment, postural changes, pediatric use, pregnancy, and case damage. Patients who are poor surgical risks, with multiple illnesses, or with active general infections should not be implanted."

In addition, the following information is stated:

Magnetic resonance imaging (MRI). Patients with implanted neurostimulation systems should not be subjected to MRI. The electromagnetic field generated by an MRI may forcefully dislodge implanted components, damage the device electronics, and induce voltage through the lead that could jolt or shock the patient."

Therefore, these devices are contraindicated (i.e. MR Unsafe) for patients referred for MR procedures.

Protégé MRI Spinal Cord Stimulation System, St. Jude Medical

The Protégé MRI Spinal Cord Stimulation System (St. Jude Medical) is MR Conditional. This MR Conditional neurostimulation system must be used in conjunction with the proper leads from St. Jude Medical and used in accordance with MR Conditional labeling requirements.

Carefully review the latest MRI labeling conditions and guidelines at: www.sjm.com.

Important note to MR Healthcare Professionals: Different MRI guidelines may exist for different countries. As such, use the appropriate information for your country.

[MR healthcare professionals are advised to contact the respective manufacturer in order to obtain the latest safety information to ensure patient safety relative to the use of an MR procedure.]

REFERENCE

St. Jude Medical, www.sjm.com

Neurostimulation Systems: Spinal Cord Stimulation
Medtronic, Inc.

Models include:
PrimeAdvanced Spinal Cord Neurostimulator
(PrimeAdvanced, Model 37702)
RestoreAdvanced Spinal Cord Neurostimulator
(RestoreAdvanced, Model 37713)
RestoreUltra Spinal Cord Neurostimulator
(RestoreUltra, Model 37712)
Itrel 3: 7425
Restore: 37711
Synergy: 7427
SynergyPlus: 7479
Synergy Versitrel: 7427V
SynergyCompact: 7479B

PrimeAdvanced SureScan MRI, Model 97702
RestoreUltra SureScan MRI, Model 91112
RestoreAdvanced SureScan MRI, Model 97713
RestoreSensor SureScan MRI, Model 97714

Various spinal cord stimulation (SCS devices from Medtronics, Inc. are MR Conditional. Certain devices have strict limitations for MRI procedures, while others that utilize SureScan MRI technology are less restrictive and referred to as "full-body eligible". Comprehensive labeling information must be reviewed to ensure patient safety.

Carefully review the latest MRI labeling conditions and guidelines at: www.medtronic.com/mri

Note to MR Healthcare Professionals: Different MRI guidelines exist for different countries. Therefore, use the appropriate information for your country.

[MR healthcare professionals are advised to contact the respective manufacturer in order to obtain the latest safety information to ensure patient safety relative to the use of an MR procedure.]

REFERENCES

Medtronic, Inc., www.medtronic.com
Medtronic, Inc., www.medtronic.com/mri

Neurostimulation System: Spinal Cord Stimulation
Stimwave Technologies, Inc.

Freedom Spinal Cord Stimulator (SCS) System

Models: FRT4-A001, FRE4-A001

The Freedom Spinal Cord Stimulator (SCS) System (spinal cord stimulation system) (Stimwave Technologies, Inc.) is intended as the sole mitigating agent, or as an adjunct to other modes of therapy used in a multidisciplinary approach for chronic, intractable pain of the trunk and/or lower limbs, including unilateral or bilateral pain. The Freedom SCS System features leads that are MR Conditional for full body MR procedures at 1.5- and 3-T.

Magnetic Resonance Imaging (MRI) – An MRI examination may be safely performed under specific conditions. Refer to the Product Safety Guide for specific MRI guidelines, www.stimwave.com

Additional devices from Stimwave Technologies, Inc. are also labeled MR Conditonal. For a full listing of the other MR Conditional neuromodulation systems, visit www.stimwave.com.

[MR healthcare professionals are advised to contact the respective manufacturer in order to obtain the latest safety information to ensure patient safety relative to the use of an MR procedure.]

REFERENCES

Shellock FG, Audet-Griffin A. Evaluation of magnetic resonance imaging issues for a wirelessly-powered lead used for epidural, spinal cord stimulation. Neuromodulation 2014;17:334-339.

Stimwave, www.stimwave.com

Neurostimulation System: Vagus Nerve Stimulation
Cyberonics/LivaNova

Vagus Nerve Stimulation, Vagal Nerve Stimulator, VNS Therapy, NeuroCybernetic Prosthesis (NCP) System

Current MRI information for the Vagus Nerve Stimulator, VNS Therapy, NeuroCybernetic Prosthesis (NCP) System may be found by visiting:

https://us.livanova.cyberonics.com/healthcare-professionals/prescribing-information

Performing MRI in Patients with Cut Lead. Labeling information exists to perform MRI examinations in patients with cut VNS leads. Carefully review the latest MRI labeling conditions and guidelines at: **www.livanova.cyberonics.com**

Note to MR Healthcare Professionals: Different MRI guidelines exist for different countries. Therefore, use the appropriate information for your country.

[MR healthcare professionals are advised to contact the respective manufacturer in order to obtain the latest safety information to ensure patient safety relative to the use of an MR procedure.]

REFERENCES

Cyberonics/Livanova, www.livanova.cyberonics.com

https://us.livanova.cyberonics.com/healthcare-professionals/prescribing-information

Ocular Implants, Lens Implants, and Devices

Of the different ocular implants, lens implants, and devices that have undergone MRI testing, the Fatio eyelid spring, the retinal tack made from martensitic (i.e. ferromagnetic) stainless steel (Western European), the Troutman magnetic ocular implant, and the Unitek round wire eyelid spring demonstrated positive magnetic field interactions in association with 1.5-Tesla MR systems. By comparison, many lens implants pose no hazard to the patient during an MRI procedure since they are not made from metallic or conducting materials (see **The List**).

A patient with a Fatio eyelid spring or round wire eyelid spring may experience discomfort but would probably not be injured as a result of exposure to an MR system. In fact, patients have undergone MR examinations with eyelid wires after having a protective plastic covering placed around the globe along with a firmly applied eye patch as a precaution.

The retinal tack made from martensitic stainless steel and Troutman magnetic ocular implant may injure a patient undergoing an MR procedure, although no such case has ever been reported.

Interestingly, Tokue, et al. (2013) reported that certain color contact lenses (which are a type of cosmetic contact lens) may contain iron oxide or other metals, which is problematic for MRI due to the associated imaging artifacts.

[For additional information pertaining to ocular-related prostheses, see **Glaucoma Drainage Implants (Shunt Tubes)**, **Magnetically-Activated Implants and Devices**, and **Scleral Buckle (Scleral Buckling) Procedure**.]

REFERENCES

Albert DW, Olson KR, Parel JM, et al. Magnetic resonance imaging and retinal tacks. Arch Ophthalmol 1990;108:320-321.

Allemann R, et al. Ultra high-field magnetic resonance imaging of a glaucoma microstent. Curr Eye Res 2011;36:719-26.

de Keizer RJ, Te Strake L. Intraocular lens implants (pseudophakoi) and steelwire sutures: A contraindication for MRI? Doc Ophthalmol 1984;61:281-284.

Joondeph BC, Peyman GA, Mafee MF, et al. Magnetic resonance imaging and retinal tacks [Letter]. Arch Ophthalmol 1987;105:1479-1480.

Marra S, et al. Effect of magnetic resonance imaging on implantable eyelid weights. Ann Otol Rhinol Laryngol 1995;104:448-452.

Roberts CW, Haik BG, Cahill P. Magnetic resonance imaging of metal loop intraocular lenses. Arch Ophthalmol 1990;108:320-321.

Seiff SR, et al. Eyelid palpebral springs in patients undergoing magnetic resonance imaging: An area of possible concern [Letter]. Arch Ophthalmol 1991;109:319.

Shellock FG. Magnetic Resonance Procedures: Health Effects and Safety. CRC Press, LLC, Boca Raton, FL, 2001.

Shellock FG, Kanal E. Magnetic Resonance: Bioeffects, Safety, and Patient Management. Second Edition, Lippincott-Raven Press, New York, 1996.

Shellock FG, Myers SM, Schatz CJ. *Ex vivo* evaluation of ferromagnetism determined for metallic scleral "buckles" exposed to a 1.5-T MR scanner. Radiology 1992;185:288-289.

Tokue H, et al. Incidental discovery of circle contact lens by MRI: You can't scan my poker face, circle contact lens as a potential MRI hazard. BMC Med Imaging 2013;13:11.

van Rijn GA, et al. Magnetic resonance compatibility of intraocular lenses measured at 7 Tesla. Invest Ophthalmol Vis Sci 2012;53:3449-3453.

Orthopedic Implants, Materials, and Devices

Most of the orthopedic implants, materials, and devices evaluated for MRI issues (i.e. magnetic field interactions, heating, and artifacts) are made from nonferromagnetic materials and, therefore, are safe or "MR Conditional" according to the conditions specified for patients undergoing MR procedures. However, due to the length of the implant or the formation of a conductive loop, MRI-related heating may be a problem for some orthopedic implants, especially cervical fixation devices and internal or external fixation systems (see below).

The Perfix interference screw used for reconstruction of the anterior cruciate ligament is highly ferromagnetic, as reported by Shellock, et al. (1992). Because this interference screw is firmly imbedded in bone for its specific application, it is held in place with sufficient retentive force to prevent movement or dislodgment in association with MRI. Patients with Perfix interference screws have safely undergone MR procedures using MR systems operating at 1.5-Tesla.

Patients with the "MR Safe" or "MR Conditional" orthopedic implants, materials, and devices indicated in **The List** have undergone MR procedures using MR systems operating at 3-Tesla or less without incident by following specific conditions defined by MRI proper testing.

External Fixation Systems. External fixation systems comprise specially designed frames, clamps, rods, rod-to-rod couplings, pins, posts, fasteners, wire fixations, fixation bolts, washers, nuts, hinges, sockets, connecting bars, screws and other components used in orthopedic and reconstructive surgery. Indications for external fixation systems are varied and include the following treatment applications:

- Open and closed fracture fixation;
- Correction of pseudoarthroses of long bones (both congenital and acquired);
- Limb lengthening by metaphyseal or epiphyseal distraction;
- Correction of bony or soft tissue defects; and
- Correction of bony or soft tissue deformities.

The assessment of MRI issues for external fixation systems is particularly challenging because of the myriad of possible components (many of which are made from conductive materials) and configurations used for these devices. The primary concern is MRI-related heating which is dependent on particular aspects (e.g., the lengths of the component parts) of the external fixation system. Importantly, the MRI conditions (strength of the static magnetic field, frequency of the RF field, type of RF transmit coil, pulse sequence, body part imaged, position of the fixation device relative to the transmit RF coil, etc.) used greatly impacts the safety aspects of scanning patients with external fixation systems.

To ensure patient safety, guidelines are typically applied on a case by case basis and, therefore, MR professionals are referred to product labeling approved by the U.S. Food and Drug Administration or other noitifed body for a given external fixation system. Notably, the acceptable MRI conditions typically apply to the specific configuration(s) used in the evaluation of a given fixation device, only. Other configurations may be unsafe for the patient in association with MRI.

There are several external fixation systems with MR Conditional labeling that are deemed acceptable for scanning patients as long as the frame is not in the bore of the MR system (i.e. within the transmit RF body coil). For example, the Large External Fixator, External Fixation System (Depuy Synthes, www.depuysynthes.com) has the following MR Conditional labeling:

Large External Fixator (external fixation system) devices used in a typical construct include clamps, rods and various attachments. A patient with a Synthes Large External Fixator frame (Depuy Synthes, www.depuysynthes.com) may be scanned safely after placement of the frame under the following conditions:

- Static magnetic field of 1.5 Tesla or 3.0 Tesla when the fixator frame is positioned outside the MRI Bore at Normal Operator or in First Level Control Mode
- Highest spatial gradient magnetic field of 720 Gauss/cm or less
- Maximum MR system reported whole body averaged specific absorption rate (SAR) of 2 W/kg for the Normal Operating Mode and 4 W/kg for the First Level Controlled Mode for 15 minutes of scanning
- Use only whole body RF transmit coil, no other transmit coils are allowed, local receive only coils are allowed

- Specialty coils, such as knee or head coils, should not be used as they have not been evaluated for RF heating and may result in higher localized heating
- Do not place any radio frequency (RF) transmit coils over the Large External Fixator frame

Note: In nonclinical testing, the Large External Fixator frame was tested in several different configurations. This testing was conducted with the construct position 7 cm within the outside edge of the MRI bore. The results showed a maximum observed heating for a pelvic frame of less than 1°C for 1.5 T and 3.0 T with a machine reported whole body averaged SAR of 2 W/kg.

Importantly, certain external fixation systems are labeled, MR Unsafe, such as the Hybrid Ring Fixator, External Fixation Recon System: The "Hybrid Ring Fixator" is MR Unsafe. Do not use this device in any MR environment. This device is known to pose hazards in all MR environments.

Vibration Associated With MR Procedures. Graf, et al. (2006) reported that torque acting on 'relatively large metallic implants due to eddy-current induction in associated with MR imaging can be considerable. Larger implants (such as fixation devices) made from conducting materials are especially affected. Gradient switching has been shown to produce fast alternating torque. Significant vibrations at off-center positions of the metal parts may explain why some patients with metallic implants sometimes report feeling heating sensations during MR examinations.

MRI Simulations and Orthopedic Implants. Because orthopedic implants tend to have a variety of sizes and shapes, it is particularly challenging to assess MRI-related heating for these devices. An efficient means of addressing this issue is to conduct MRI simulations to determine the worst-case of MRI-induced heating for a given orthopedic implant of different sizes under 1.5-T/64-MHz and 3-T/128-MHz conditions and then to apply an experimental test to validate the numerical results for worst-case heating, as described by Liu, et al. (2013).

MRI at 3-Tesla and Orthopedic Implants, Materials, and Devices. A variety of orthopedic implants have been evaluated for magnetic field interactions at 3-Tesla (see **The List**). Many are considered to be acceptable for patients undergoing MRI examinations based on findings for magnetic field interactions and MRI-related heating. Excessive temperature rises may be a concern for some orthopedic implants, especially cervical fixation devices and internal or external fixation systems.

[MR healthcare professionals are advised to contact the respective manufacturer in order to obtain the latest safety information to ensure patient safety relative to the use of an MR procedure.]

REFERENCES

Bagheri MH, et al. Metallic artifact in MRI after removal of orthopedic implants. Eur J Radiol 2012;81:584-90.

Depuy Synthes, www.depuysynthes.com

Elsissy P, et al. MRI evaluation of the knee with non-ferromagnetic external fixators,. Eur J Orthop Surg Traumatol 2015;25:933-9.

Farrelly C, et al. Imaging of soft tissues adjacent to orthopedic hardware: Comparison of 3-T and 1.5-T MRI. Am J Roentgenol 2010;194:W60-4.

Graf H, et al. Eddy-current induction in extended metallic parts as a source of considerable torsional moment. J Magn Reson Imag 2006;23:585-590.

Jungmann PM, et al. Advances in MRI around metal. J Magn Reson Imaging 2017;46:972-991.

Knott PT, et al. A comparison of magnetic and radiographic imaging artifact after using three types of metal rods: Stainless steel, titanium, and vitallium. Spine J 2010;10:789-94.

Koch KM, et al. Magnetic resonance imaging near metal implants. J Magn Reson Imag 2010;32:773-87.

Liu Y, et al. Numerical investigations of MRI RF field induced heating for external fixation devices. Biomed Eng Online 2013;12:12.

Liu Y, et al. Effect of insulating layer material on RF-induced heating for external fixation system in 1.5T MRI system. Electromagn Biol Med 2014;33:223-7.

Liu Y, Chen J, Shellock FG, Kainz W. Computational and experimental studies of an orthopedic implant: MRI-related heating at 1.5-Tesla/64-MHz and 3-Tesla/128-MHz. J Magn Reson Imaging 2013;37:491-497.

Luechinger R, Boesiger P, Disegi JA. Safety evaluation of large external fixation clamps and frames in a magnetic resonance environment. J Biomed Mater Res B Appl Biomater 2007;82:17-22.

Lyons CJ, et al. The effect of magnetic resonance imaging on metal spine implants. Spine 1989;14:670-672.

McComb C, Allan D, Condon B. Evaluation of the translational and rotational forces acting on a highly ferromagnetic orthopedic spinal implant in magnetic resonance imaging. J Magn Reson Imag 2009;29:449-53.

Mechlin M, et al. Magnetic resonance imaging of postoperative patients with metallic implants. Am J Roentgenol 1984;143:1281-1284.

Mesgarzadeh M, et al. The effect on medical metal implants by magnetic fields of magnetic resonance imaging. Skeletal Radiol 1985;14:205-206.

Muranaka H, et al. Evaluation of RF heating on hip joint implant in phantom during MRI examinations. Nippon Hoshasen Gijutsu Gakkai Zasshi 2010;66:725-33.

Powell J, et al. Numerical simulation of SAR induced around Co-Cr-Mo hip prostheses *in situ* exposed to RF fields associated with 1.5 and 3 T MRI body coils. Magn Reson Med 2012;68:960-8.

Shellock FG, Crues JV, Editors. MRI Bioeffects, Safety, and Patient Management. Biomedical Research Publishing Group, Los Angeles, CA, 2014.

Shellock FG. Biomedical implants and devices: Assessment of magnetic field interactions with a 3.0-Tesla MR system. J Magn Reson Imag 2002;16:721-732.

Shellock FG, Kanal E. Magnetic Resonance: Bioeffects, Safety, and Patient Management. Second Edition, Lippincott-Raven Press, New York, 1996.

Shellock FG, Mink JH, Curtin S, et al. MRI and orthopedic implants used for anterior cruciate ligament reconstruction: Assessment of ferromagnetism and artifacts. J Magn Reson Imag 1992;2:225-228.

Shellock FG, Morisoli S, Kanal E. MR procedures and biomedical implants, materials, and devices: 1993 update. Radiology 1993;189:587-599.

Stradiotti P, et al. Metal-related artifacts in instrumented spine. Techniques for reducing artifacts in CT and MRI: State of the art. Eur Spine J 2009;18 Suppl 1:102-8.

Talbot BS, Weinberg EP. MR imaging with metal-suppression sequences for evaluation of total joint arthroplasty. Radiographics 2016;36:209-25.

Tsukimura I, et al. Assessment of magnetic field interactions and radiofrequency-radiation-induced heating of metallic spinal implants in 7 T field. J Orthop Res 2017;35:1831-1837.

.Yang CW, et al. Magnetic resonance imaging of artificial lumbar disks: Safety and metal artifacts. Chin Med J (Engl) 2009;20;122:911-6.

Zou YF, et al. Evaluation of MR issues for the latest standard brands of orthopedic metal implants: Plates and screws. Eur J Radiol 2015;84:450-7.

Otologic Implants

Of the otologic implants evaluated for the presence of magnetic field interactions (note, MRI-related heating is not considered to be an issue for these relatively small implants), the McGee stapedectomy piston prosthesis, made from platinum and chromium-nickel alloy stainless steel, is ferromagnetic. The manufacturer recalled this otologic implant. Patients who received this device were issued warnings to avoid MR procedures. The specific item and lot numbers of the McGee implants recalled and regarded as a contraindication for MR procedures are as follows (Personal Communication, Winston Geer, Smith & Nephew Richards Inc., Barlett, TN, 1995):

Item No.	Lot Number
14-0330	1W91100, 4UO9690
14-0331	4U09700
14-0332	1W91110, 4U58540, 4U86300
14-0333	4U09710, 1W34390, 2WR4073
14-0334	4U09720, 1W34390, 2WR4073
14-0335	1W34400, 4U09730
14-0336	3U18350, 3U50470, 4UR2889
14-0337	3U18370, 4UR2889
14-0338	3U18390, 4U02900, 4UR1453
14-0339	3U18400, 3U50500
14-0340	3U18410, 3U50500
14-0341	3U41200, 4UR2889

MR Unsafe Otologic Implants. Besides the above information, there are several other MR Unsafe otologic implants that exist including, the following:

- Tuebingen Type Ventilation Tubes with Wire, Gold-Platinum, Stainless Steel
- Tuebingen Type Ventilation Tubes with Wire, Gilded Silver, Stainless steel
- Tuebingen Type Ventilation Tubes with Wire, Pure Titanium, Stainless Steel
- Minimal Type Ventilation Tube, Gold-coated, Stainless Steel (Kurz, www.kurzmed.de/en/products/mri-safety/)

368 Otologic Implants

MRI at 3-Tesla and Otologic Implants. Many otologic implants have been evaluated for magnetic field interactions at 3-Tesla (see **The List**). In consideration of the relatively small sizes of these items, MRI-related heating is not a concern. For the ones tested, all are considered to be acceptable for patients based on findings for translational attraction, torque, and according to the intended *in vivo* uses of these specific devices. Azadarmaki R, et al. (2014) has reviewed the current MRI information for otologic implants. For MRI information on other otologic implants, please refer to **The List.**

Otologic Implants, Micromedics, Inc. (Eagan, MN). MRI testing at 3-Tesla was conducted on the following products from Micromedics, Inc:

Stainless Steel Vent Tube & Stainless Steel Wire

Because of the size of the metallic mass associated with these particular products, the MRI test findings (MR Conditional 6, 3-Tesla or less) apply to all of the product families listed below (Micromedics, Inc., Eagan, MN):

VT-0205-, Fluoroplastic with stainless steel wire
VT-0702-, Silicone with stainless steel wire
VT-1402-, Stainless steel with stainless steel wire
VT-1412-, Titanium with stainless steel wire
VT-1505-, Polyethylene with stainless steel wire

Otologic Implants, Grace Medical (Memphis, TN). The otologic device families from Grace Medical (www.gracemedical.com) listed below are **MR Safe** because these items are made from nonmetallic and nonconducting materials:

Device Family	Family Product Number(s)	Device Material(s)
Stapes Prostheses-Pistons	401-XXX, 402-XXX, 403-XXX, 404-XXX, 405-XXX, 406-XXX, 408-XXX	Fluoroplastic
Partial and Total Prostheses	1XX, 190-XXX, 749-XXX	Hydroxyapatite
Partial and Total Prostheses	2XX, 193	Hydroxyapatite, Silicone

(XX = 00 through 99) (XXX = 000 through 999, i.e. Product number 190-XXX means all products ranging from 190-000 through 190-999)

The Otologic device families listed below are **MR Conditional** according to MRI tests conducted on selected implants that represented worst case with regard to materials and mass.

Device Family	Family Product Number(s)	Device Material(s)
ALTO Partial and Total Prostheses	6XX, 612-001L, 612-002R	Titanium, Silicone, Hydroxyapatite
K-Helix Prostheses	756-XXX, 757-XXX	Titanium
Strasnick Prostheses	220-XXX, 270-XXX	Titanium, Silicone
Precise Prostheses and Other Ossicular Prostheses	602-XXX, 652-XXX, 700-XXX, 705-XXX, 706-XXX, 707-XXX, 720-XXX, 750-XXX, 751-XXX, 765-XXX, 770-XXX	Titanium, Hydroxyapatite
Stapes Prostheses-Piston	409-XXX, 410-XXX, 411-XXX, 412-XXX, 413-XXX, 415-XXX, 417-XXX, 418-XXX, 419-XXX, 452-XXX, 453-XXX, 465-XXX, 466-XXX, 467-XXX, 468-XXX, 469-XXX	Titanium, Platinum, Stainless Steel, Nitinol, Fluoroplastic
Stapes Prostheses-Buckets	409-XXX, 410-XXX, 411-XXX, 412-XXX, 413-XXX, 415-XXX, 416-XXX, 417-XXX, 418-XXX, 419-XXX, 440-XXX, 442-XXX, 450-XXX, 451-XXX, 452-XXX, 453-XXX, 456-XXX, 460-XXX, 461-XXX, 462-XXX, 464-XXX, 465-XXX, 466-XXX, 467-XXX, 468-XXX, 469-XXX, 470-XXX, 471-XXX	Titanium, Nitinol
Stapes Prostheses-Buckets	420-XXX, 421-XXX, 422-XXX, 423-XXX, 424-XXX, 425-XXX, 426-XXX, 427-XXX, 428-XXX, 429-XXX, 430-XXX, 431-XXX, 432-XXX	Titanium, Nitinol
Foot Shoes	636-XXX	Titanium
Incudo Stapedial Joint, ISJ	755	Nitinol

(XX = 00 through 99) (XXX = 000 through 999, i.e. Product number 190-XXX means all products ranging from 190-000 through 190-999)

The **MRI Information** for these otologic implants is, as follows: Non-clinical testing has demonstrated that patients with these specific Grace Medical ossicular implants can undergo MRI safely, immediately after implantation under the following conditions:

- Static magnetic field of 3-Tesla or less
- Maximum spatial gradient magnetic field of 20,000-gauss/cm (extrapolated) or less
- Maximum MR system reported, whole body averaged specific absorption rate (SAR) of 4-W/kg for 15 minutes of scanning (i.e.

per pulse sequence) in the First Level Controlled Operating Mode of operation for the MR system

REFERENCES

Applebaum EL, Valvassori GE. Effects of magnetic resonance imaging fields on stapedectomy prostheses. Arch Otolaryngol 1985;11:820-821.

Applebaum EL, Valvassori GE. Further studies on the effects of magnetic resonance fields on middle ear implants. Ann Otol Rhinol Laryngol 1990;99:801-804.

Azadarmaki R, et al. MRI information for commonly used otologic implants: review and update. Otolaryngol Head Neck Surg 2014;150:512-9.

Bauknecht HC, et al. Behaviour of titanium middle ear implants at 1.5 and 3 Tesla field strength in magnetic resonance imaging. Laryngorhinootologie 2009;88:236-40.

Fritsch MH. MRI scanners and the stapes prosthesis. Otol Neurotol 2007;28:733-738.

Fritsch MH, Mosier KM. MRI compatibility issues in otology. Curr Opin Otolaryngol Head Neck Surg 2007;15:335-340.

Fritsch MH, Gutt JJ. Ferromagnetic movements of middle ear implants and stapes prostheses in a 3-T magnetic resonance field. Otol Neurotol 2005;26:225-230.

Leon JA, Gabriele OF. Middle ear prothesis: Significance in magnetic resonance imaging. Magnetic Resonance Imaging 1987;5:405-406.

Martin AD, et al. Safety evaluation of titanium middle ear prostheses at 3.0 Tesla. Otolaryngol Head Neck Surg 2005;132:537-42.

Nogueira M, Shellock FG. Otologic bioimplants: *Ex vivo* assessment of ferromagnetism and artifacts at 1.5-Tesla. Am J Roentgenol 1995;163:1472-1473.

Shellock FG, Crues JV, Editors. MRI Bioeffects, Safety, and Patient Management. Biomedical Research Publishing Group, Los Angeles, CA, 2014.

Shellock FG, et al. *In vitro* magnetic resonance imaging evaluation of ossicular implants at 3-T. Otol Neurotol 2012;33:871-7

Shellock FG, Morisoli S, Kanal E. MR procedures and biomedical implants, materials, and devices: 1993 update. Radiology 1993;189:587-599.

White DW. Interaction between magnetic fields and metallic ossicular prostheses. Am J Otol 1987;8:290-292.

Wild DC, Head K, Hall DA. Safe magnetic resonance scanning of patients with metallic middle ear implants. Clin Otolaryngol 2006;31:508-510.

www.gracemedical.com

www.kurzmed.com/en/products/

Oxygen Tanks and Gas Cylinders

According to Chaljub, et al. (2001), accidents related to ferromagnetic oxygen tanks and other gas cylinders that can become projectiles may be increasing. In fact, missile-related accidents for these objects as well as other items have resulted in at least one fatality, several injuries, damage to MR systems, and down-time (i.e. loss of revenue) for many MRI centers.

Therefore, MRI facilities must implement a policy for safe administration of oxygen to patients undergoing MR procedures. In lieu of utilizing pipes to directly deliver gases to patients, the use of non-magnetic (usually aluminum) gas cylinders is one means of preventing "missile effect" hazards in the MR environment. Non-magnetic oxygen tanks and cylinders for other gases are commercially available from various vendors.

MRI centers should have a sufficient number of nonmagnetic oxygen tanks and strict policies in place to prevent staff members from introducing ferromagnetic objects into the MR environment. Notably, some hospital-based MRI facilities have nonmagnetic oxygen tanks used throughout their buildings to prevent projectile accidents.

Nonmagnetic tanks must be prominently labeled and/or color-coded to avoid confusion with magnetic cylinders. Additionally, only regulators tested and demonstrated to be acceptable for use in a high magnetic field environment should be used with the nonmagnetic cylinders. Furthermore, all healthcare workers that work in the MR environment must be informed regarding the fact that only nonmagnetic oxygen and other gas cylinders are allowed into the MR system room.

Nonmagnetic or weakly magnetic (i.e. MR Conditional) oxygen regulators, flow meters, cylinder carts, cylinder stands, cylinder holders for wheelchairs, and suction devices are also commercially available to provide safe respiratory support and management of patients in the MR environment.

REFERENCES

Chaljub G, et al. Projectile cylinder accidents resulting from the presence of ferromagnetic nitrous oxide or oxygen tanks in the MR suite. Am J Roentgenol 2001;177:27-30.

Colletti PM. Size "H" oxygen cylinder: Accidental MR projectile at 1.5-Tesla. J Magn Reson Imag 2004;19:141-143.

ECRI Institute. Patient Death Illustrates the Importance of Adhering to Safety Precautions in Magnetic Resonance Environments. ECRI Institute, Plymouth Meeting, PA, Aug. 6, 2001.

Jolesz FA, et al. Compatible instrumentation for intraoperative MRI: Expanding resources. J Magn Reson Imag 1998;8:8-11.

Keeler EK, et al. Accessory equipment considerations with respect to MRI compatibility. J Magn Reson Imag 1998;8:12-18.

Shellock FG, Crues JV, Editors. MRI Bioeffects, Safety, and Patient Management. Biomedical Research Publishing Group, Los Angeles, CA, 2014.

Palatal System Implant Assembly

The **Palatal System Implant Assembly** (Pavad Medical, Inc., Fremont, CA) is designed to treat sleep disordered breathing.

MRI Information

The Palatal System Implant Assembly was determined to be MR Conditional according to the terminology specified in the ASTM International, Designation: F2503. Standard Practice for Marking Medical Devices and Other Items for Safety in the Magnetic Resonance Environment.

Non-clinical testing demonstrated that the Palatal System Implant Assembly is MR Conditional. A patient with this implant can be scanned safely, immediately after placement under the following conditions:

- Static magnetic field of 1.5-Tesla
- Maximum spatial gradient magnetic field of 250-gauss/cm
- Maximum MR system reported whole-body-averaged specific absorption rate (SAR) of 3.5-W/kg for 15 minutes of scanning (per pulse sequence)

In non-clinical testing, the Palatal System Implant Assembly produced a temperature rise of 0.8 degrees C at a maximum MR system-reported whole body averaged specific absorption rate (SAR) of 3.5-W/kg for 15-minutes of MR scanning in a 1.5-Tesla MR system using a transmit/receive body coil (1.5-Tesla, Magnetom, Software Numaris/4, Version Syngo MR 2002B DHHS, Siemens Medical Solutions, Malvern, PA).

MR image quality may be compromised if the area of interest is in the exact same area or relatively close to the position of the Palatal System Implant Assembly. Therefore, optimization of MR imaging parameters to compensate for the presence of this implant may be necessary. The following chart provides artifact information for the Palatal System Implant Assembly in relation to different pulse sequences at 1.5-Tesla:

Pulse sequence	Signal Void
T1-weighted spin echo, long axis orientation	2.7-cm^2
T1-weighted spin echo, short axis orientation	2.7-cm^2
Gradient echo, long axis orientation	8.8-cm^2
Gradient echo, short axis orientation	9.6-cm^2

MRI Procedures and Function of the Palatal System Implant Assembly

The effects of MRI procedures on the functional aspects of Palatal System Implant Assembly devices were assessed. *In-vitro* testing was performed on a phantom with six Palatal System Implant Assembly devices placed in various orientations relative to the MR system. MRI was conducted using 1.5-Tesla/64 MHz MR system (transmit/receive RF body coil) to perform 8 different MR imaging pulse sequences, as follows: T1-weighted spin echo, T1-weighted fast spin echo, T2-weighted spin echo, T2- weighted fast spin echo, three dimensional fast gradient echo, turbo/fast gradient echo, turbo/fast spoiled gradient echo, echo planar imaging.

The findings indicated that there was no apparent damage or alteration in the function of the Palatal System Implant Assembly. Thus, the Palatal System Implant Assembly was demonstrated to maintain full functionality after exposure to the MRI conditions indicated above.

Additional guidelines for the Palatal System Implant Assembly include:

- Do not use MR systems other than 1.5 Tesla MR systems.
- Continuously monitor the patients using visual and audio means (i.e. intercom system) throughout the MR procedure.
- Instruct the patient to alert the MR system operator of any unusual sensations or problems so the MR system operator can terminate the MRI procedure, if needed.
- Provide the patient with a means to alert the MR system operator of any unusual sensations or problems that may be experienced during the MRI procedure.

Patent Ductus Arteriosus (PDA) Occluders, Atrial Septal Defect (ASD) Occluders, Ventricular Septal Defect (VSD) Occluders, and Patent Foramen Ovale (PFO) Closure Devices

Cardiac occluders and closure devices are implants used to treat patients with patent ductus arteriosus (PDA), atrial septal defect (ASD), ventricular septal defect (VSD), or patent foramen ovale (PFO) heart conditions. For implants that have been evaluated relative to the use of 1.5-Tesla MR systems, as long as the proper size occluder or closure device is used, the amount of retention provided by the folded-back, hinged arms of the implant is sufficient to keep it in place immediately after implantation. Eventually, tissue growth covers the cardiac occluder or closure device and facilitates retention.

Certain metallic PDA, ASD, VSD occluders and PFO closure devices tested for magnetic qualities were made from either 304V stainless steel or MP35N. Occluders made from 304V stainless steel were found to be "weakly" ferromagnetic, whereas those made from MP35N were nonferromagnetic in association with a 1.5-Tesla MR system.

Patients with cardiac occluders made from MP35N (i.e. a nonferromagnetic alloy) may undergo MR procedures at 1.5-Tesla or less any time after placement of these implants. However, patients with cardiac occluders made from 304V stainless steel (i.e. a "weakly ferromagnetic" material) are advised to wait a minimum of six weeks after implantation before undergoing MR procedures. This wait period permits tissue ingrowth to provide additional retentive forces for the occluders made from weakly ferromagnetic materials.

If there is any question about the integrity of the retention aspects of a metallic cardiac occluder made from a ferromagnetic material, the individual or patient should not be allowed into the MR environment or to undergo an MR procedure.

MRI at 3-Tesla and PDA, ASD, VSD Occluders and PFO Closure Devices. Various PDA, ASD, VSD occluders and PFO closure devices have been evaluated at 3-Tesla (see **The List**). All of these implants tested to date are considered acceptable for patients referred for MR examinations based on findings for deflection angles, torque, MRI-related heating and the intended *in vivo* uses of these specific devices.

REFERENCES

Shellock FG, Crues JV, Editors. MRI Bioeffects, Safety, and Patient Management. Biomedical Research Publishing Group, Los Angeles, CA, 2014.

Shellock FG, Morisoli SM. *Ex vivo* evaluation of ferromagnetism and artifacts for cardiac occluders exposed to a 1.5-Tesla MR system. J Magn Reson Imag 1994;4:213-215.

Shellock FG, Valencerina S. Septal repair implants: Evaluation of MRI safety at 3-Tesla. Magnetic Resonance Imaging 2005;23:1021-1025.

Pellets, Bullets, and Shrapnel

The majority of pellets and bullets tested in the MR environment were found to be composed of nonferromagnetic materials, however, these items are often "contaminated" by ferromagnetic metals. Ammunition that proved to be ferromagnetic tended to be manufactured in foreign countries and/or used for military applications. Shrapnel typically contains steel and, therefore, presents a potential hazard for patients undergoing MR procedures.

Because pellets, bullets, and shrapnel are frequently contaminated with ferromagnetic materials, the risk versus benefit of performing an MR procedure should be carefully considered. Additional consideration must be given to whether the metallic object is located near or in a vital anatomic structure, with the assumption that the object is likely to be ferromagnetic and can potentially move.

In an effort to reduce lead poisoning in "puddling" type ducks, the federal government requires many of the eastern United States to use steel shotgun pellets instead of lead. The presence of steel shotgun pellets presents a potential hazard to patients undergoing MR procedures and causes substantial imaging artifacts at the immediate position of these metallic objects.

In one case, a small metallic BB located in a subcutaneous site caused painful symptoms in a patient exposed to an MR system, although no serious injury occurred. Accordingly, MR healthcare professionals should exercise caution when deciding to perform MR procedures in patients with pellets, bullets, shrapnel or other similar ballistic objects.

Smugar, et al. (1999) conducted an investigation to determine whether neurological problems developed in patients with intraspinal bullets or bullet fragments in association with MR imaging performed at 1.5-Tesla. Patients were queried during scanning for symptoms of discomfort, pain, or changes in neurological status. Additionally, detailed neurological examinations were performed prior to MRI, post MRI, and at the patients' discharge. Based on these findings, Smugar, et al. concluded that a patient with a complete spinal cord injury may undergo MR imaging with an intraspinal bullet or fragment without concern for affects on the physical or neurological status. Thus, metallic fragments in the spinal canals of paralyzed patients are believed to represent only a relative contraindication to MR procedures.

Eshed, et al. (2010) conducted a retrospective investigation of the potential hazards for patients undergoing MRI at 1.5-Tesla with retained metal fragments from combat and terrorist attacks. Metallic fragments in 17 patients were in ranged in size between one and 10-mm. One patient reported a superficial migration of a 10-mm fragment after MRI. No other adverse reaction was reported. The authors concluded that 1.5-Tesla MRI examinations are safe in patients with retained metallic fragments from combat and terrorist attacks not in the vicinity of vital organs. However, caution is advised as well as an assessment of risk versus benefit for the patient.

Dedini, et al. (2013) studied bullets and shotgun pellets that were a representative sample of ballistic objects commonly encountered in association with criminal trauma using 1.5-, 3- and 7-Tesla MR systems. The findings indicated that non-steel containing bullets and pellets did not exhibit substantial magnetic field interactions at 1.5-, 3-, and 7-Tesla, and that both steel-containing and non-steel-containing bullets did not significantly heat, even under extreme MRI conditions at 3-Tesla. Steel-containing bullets were potentially unsafe for patients referred for MRI due to their potential to move *in vivo*, although this recommendation must be interpreted on a case-by-case basis with respect to the restraining effect of the specific tissue environment, time *in situ*, proximity of vital or delicate structures, and with careful consideration given to the risk versus benefit for the patient.

REFERENCES

Bolliger SA, et al. Movement of steel-jacketed projectiles in biological tissue in the magnetic field of a 3-T magnetic resonance unit. Int J Legal Med 2017 (In press).

Dedini RD, Karacozoff AM, Shellock FG, et al. MRI issues for ballistic objects: Information obtained at 1.5-, 3-, and 7-Tesla. Spine Journal 2013;13:815-22.

Diallo I, et al. Magnetic field interactions of military and law enforcement bullets at 1.5 and 3 Tesla. Mil Med 2016;181:710-3.

Eggert S, et al. Fairly direct hit! Advances in imaging of shotgun projectiles in MRI. Eur Radiol 2015;25:2745-53.

Eggert S, et al. The influence of 1.5 and 3 T magnetic resonance unit magnetic fields on the movement of steel-jacketed projectiles in ordnance gelatin. Forensic Sci Med Pathol 2015;11:544-51.

Eshed I, et al. Is magnetic resonance imaging safe for patients with retained metal fragments from combat and terrorist attacks? Acta Radiol 2010;51:170-4.

Genç A, et al. When the bullet moves! Surgical caveats from a migrant intraspinal bullet. Neurol Neurochir Pol 2016;50:387-391.

Karacozoff AM, Pekmezci M, Shellock FG. Armor-piercing bullet: 3-Tesla MRI findings and identification by a ferromagnetic detection system. Military Medicine 2013;178:e380-e385.

Martinez-del-Campo E, et al. Magnetic resonance imaging in lumbar gunshot wounds: An absolute contraindication? Neurosurg Focus 2014;37:E13.

Shellock FG, Kanal E. Magnetic Resonance: Bioeffects, Safety, and Patient Management. Second Edition, Lippincott-Raven Press, New York, 1996.

Smugar SS, Schweitzer ME, Hume E. MRI in patients with intraspinal bullets. J Magn Reson Imag 1999;9:151-153.

Teitelbaum GP. Metallic ballistic fragments: MR imaging safety and artifacts [Letter]. Radiology 1990;177:883.

Teitelbaum GP, et al. Metallic ballistic fragments: MR imaging safety and artifacts. Radiology 1990;175:855-859.

Winklhofer S, et al. Added value of dual-energy computed tomography versus single-energy computed tomography in assessing ferromagnetic properties of ballistic projectiles: Implications for magnetic resonance imaging of gunshot victims. Invest Radiol 2014;49:431-7.

Penile Implants

Several types of penile implants and prostheses have been evaluated for magnetic field interactions associated with MR systems. Of these, two (i.e. the Duraphase and Omniphase models) demonstrated substantial ferromagnetic qualities when exposed to a 1.5-Tesla MR system. Fortunately, it is unlikely for a penile implant to severely injure a patient undergoing an MR procedure because of the degree of magnetic field interactions associated with a 1.5-Tesla MR system. This is especially true when one considers the manner in which this device is utilized. Nevertheless, it would be uncomfortable for a patient with a ferromagnetic penile implant to undergo an MR examination. For this reason, subjecting a patient with the Duraphase or Omniphase penile implant to the MR environment or an MR procedure is inadvisable.

MRI at 3-Tesla and Penile Implants. Several different penile implants have been tested for magnetic field interactions and MRI-related heating in association with 3-Tesla MR systems. Findings for these specific penile implants indicated that they either exhibited no magnetic field interactions or relatively minor or "weak" magnetic field interactions. Accordingly, these specific penile implants are considered acceptable for patients undergoing MR procedures using MR systems operating at 3-Tesla or less and according to the MR Conditional labeling (see **The List**).

REFERENCES

Lowe G, et al. A catalog of magnetic resonance imaging compatibility of penile prostheses. J Sex Med 2012;9:1482-1487.

Shellock FG, Crues JV, Editors. MRI Bioeffects, Safety, and Patient Management. Biomedical Research Publishing Group, Los Angeles, CA, 2014.

Shellock FG, Crues JV, Sacks SA. High-field magnetic resonance imaging of penile prostheses: *In vitro* evaluation of deflection forces and imaging artifacts [Abstract]. In: Book of Abstracts, Society of Magnetic Resonance in Medicine. Berkeley, CA: Society of Magnetic Resonance in Medicine, 1987;3:915.

Shellock FG, Kanal E. Magnetic Resonance: Bioeffects, Safety, and Patient Management. Second Edition, Lippincott-Raven Press, New York, 1996.

Pessaries

A pessary is a relatively small medical device that is inserted into the vagina or rectum and held in place by the pelvic floor musculature. In some instances, a pessary may contain metal to permit forming it into a shape to facilitate proper fit and retention. Typically, the pessary is a firm ring or similar structure that presses against the wall of the vagina and urethra to help decrease urinary leakage or other condition. Indications for the pessary include pelvic support defects, such as uterine prolapse and vaginal prolapse, as well as stress urinary incontinence.

MRI Information. A wide variety of pessary styles exist, including those made entirely from nonmetallic, nonconducting materials (e.g., plastic, silicone, or latex) as well as those that have metallic components. Pessaries made from nonmetallic, nonconducting materials pose no problems for patients undergoing MR procedures. However, pessaries that have metallic components may cause substantial artifacts and/or may pose risks to patients undergoing MR examinations. As such, a patient with a pessary that contains metal should be given additional consideration prior to the MR examination. To date, there is no report of injury or other significant problem related to performing MR examinations in patients with these devices.

REFERENCES

Brubacker L. The vaginal pessary. In: Friedman AJ, Editor. American Urogynecologic Society Quarterly Report 1991.

Davila GW. Vaginal prolapse: Management with nonsurgical techniques. Postgrad Med 1996;99:171-176.

Deger RB, Menzin AW, Mikuta JJ. The vaginal pessary: Past and present. Postgrad Obstet Gynecol 1993;13:1-8.

Komesu YM, et al. Restoration of continence by pessaries: Magnetic resonance imaging assessment of mechanism of action. Am J Obstet Gynecol 2008;198:563.e1-6.

Miller DS. Contemporary use of the pessary. In: Sciarra JJ, Editor. Gynecology and obstetrics. Philadelphia: Lippencott-Raven, 1997:1-12.

Zeitlin MP, Lebherz TB. Pessaries in the geriatric patient. J Am Geriatr Soc 1992;40:635-9.

PillCam Capsule Endoscopy Devices

The PillCam Capsule Endoscopy Devices include the following versions: Pillcam M2A, PillCam SB, PillCam SB2, PillCam ESO, PillCam ESO2, PillCam COLON 2, and PillCam Patency (Given Imaging, Inc.). These devices are ingestible devices utilized in the gastrointestinal (GI) tract. Peristalsis moves the PillCam Capsule smoothly and painlessly throughout the gastrointestinal tract, transmitting color video images or these products are used to assess other aspects GI function. The procedure allows patients to continue daily activities during the examination.

The PillCam Capsule Endoscopy Device has been utilized to diagnose diseases of the small intestine including Crohn's Disease, celiac disease and other malabsorption disorders, benign and malignant tumors of the small intestine, vascular disorders and medication related small bowel injuries.

MRI Information

The User Manual for the PillCam Capsule Endoscopy Device states:

"Undergoing an MRI while the capsule is inside the patient's body may result in serious damage to his/her intestinal tract or abdominal cavity. If the patient did not positively verify the excretion of the PillCam Capsule from his/her body, he/she should contact the physician for evaluation and possible abdominal X-ray before undergoing an MRI examination."

This information applies to all versions/models of the PillCam devices.

REFERENCE

Given Imaging, www.givenimaging.com

Prometra Programmable Pumps

There are two different versions of the Prometra Programmable Pumps (Flowonix Medical, Inc.):

Prometra Programmable Pump, Model # 11827

Prometra II Programmable Pump, Model # 13827

Carefully review the latest MRI labeling conditions and guidelines to ensure patient safety.

Important Note to MR Healthcare Professionals: Different MRI guidelines may exist for different countries. Therefore, use the appropriate information for your country.

[MR healthcare professionals are advised to contact the respective manufacturer in order to obtain the latest safety information to ensure patient safety relative to the use of an MR procedure.]

REFERENCE

Flowonix Medical, www.flowonix.com

Reveal Plus Insertable Loop Recorder
Medtronic, Inc.

The 9526 Reveal Plus Insertable Loop Recorder (Medtronic, Inc.) is MR Conditional. Comprehensive labeling information must be reviewed to ensure patient safety.

Carefully review the latest MRI labeling conditions and guidelines at: www.medtronic/mri

Important Note to MR Healthcare Professionals: Different MRI guidelines may exist for different countries. Therefore, use the appropriate information for your country.

[MR healthcare professionals are advised to contact the respective manufacturer in order to obtain the latest safety information to ensure patient safety relative to the use of an MR procedure.]

REFERENCES

Gimbel JR, Wilkoff BL. Artefact mimicking tachycardia during magnetic resonance imaging in a patient with an implantable loop recorder. Heart 2003;89:e10.

Gimbel JR. Magnetic resonance imaging of implantable cardiac rhythm devices at 3.0 Tesla. Pacing Clin Electrophysiol 2008;31:795-801.

Krahn A, et al. Final results from a pilot study with an implantable loop recorder to determine the etiology of syncope in patients with negative non-invasive and invasive testing. American Journal of Cardiology 1998;82:117-119.

Medtroni, Inc., www.medtronic.com/mri

Shellock FG, et al. Cardiac pacemakers, ICDs, and loop recorder: Evaluation of translational attraction using conventional ("long-bore") and "short-bore" MR systems at 1.5- and 3-Tesla. Journal of Cardiovascular Magnetic Resonance 2003;5:387-397.

Shellock FG. MR Safety and the Reveal Insertable Loop Recorder. Signals, No. 49, Issue 3, pp. 8, 2004.

Wong JA, et al. Feasibility of magnetic resonance imaging in patients with an implantable loop recorder. Pacing Clin Electrophysiol 2008;31:333-7.

Reveal DX 9528 and Reveal XT 9529, Insertable Cardiac Monitors
Medtronic, Inc.

The Reveal DX 9528 Insertable Cardiac Monitor and the Reveal XT 9529 Insertable Cardiac Monitor (Medtronic, Inc.) are MR Conditional. Comprehensive labeling information must be reviewed to ensure patient safety.

Carefully review the latest MRI labeling conditions and guidelines at: www.medtronic.com/mri

Important Note to MR Healthcare Professionals: Different MRI guidelines may exist for different countries. Therefore, use the appropriate information for your country.

[MR healthcare professionals are advised to contact the respective manufacturer in order to obtain the latest safety information to ensure patient safety relative to the use of an MR procedure.]

REFERENCE

Medtroni, Inc., www.medtronic.com/mri

Reveal LINQ Model LNQ11 Insertable Cardiac Monitor
Medtronic, Inc.

The Reveal LINQ Model LNQ11 Insertable Cardiac Monitor (Medtronic, Inc.) is MR Conditional.

Comprehensive labeling information must be reviewed to ensure patient safety. Carefully review the latest MRI labeling conditions and guidelines at: www.medtronic/mri.

Important note to MR Healthcare Professionals: Different MRI guidelines may exist for different countries. As such, use the appropriate information for your country.

[MR healthcare professionals are advised to contact the respective manufacturer in order to obtain the latest safety information to ensure patient safety relative to the use of an MR procedure.]

REFERENCE

Medtroni, Inc., www.medtronic.com/mri

St. Jude Medical (SJM) Confirm, Implantable Cardiac Monitor
St. Jude Medical

The SJM Confirm, Implantable Cardiac Monitor, Models DM2100, DM2102, Implantable Cardiac Monitor (St. Jude Medical) are MR Conditional. Comprehensive labeling information must be reviewed to ensure patient safety.

Carefully review the latest MRI labeling conditions and guidelines at: www.sjm.com.

Important Note to MR Healthcare Professionals: Different MRI guidelines may exist for different countries. Therefore, use the appropriate information for your country.

[MR healthcare professionals are advised to contact the respective manufacturer in order to obtain the latest safety information to ensure patient safety relative to the use of an MR procedure.]

REFERENCE

St. Jude Medical, www.sjm.com

SAM Sling

The SAM Sling (SAM Medical Products) is a force-controlled circumferential pelvic belt designed to provide safe and effective reduction and stabilization of open-book pelvic fractures. Pelvic ring fractures are devastating injuries, accompanied by extensive internal bleeding that can often be fatal. Since the mid-nineteenth century, the standard first-aid protocol has been to wrap a bedsheet or belt around the victim's hips, cinch it tight, and hope for the best. This technique works, even for the worst type of pelvic fractures, known as open-book fractures because the pelvic ring has sprung open, like the pages of a book. Compression "closes the book," reduces pain, slows bleeding, and promotes clot formation as the patient is transported to an emergency department.

Researchers determined that the optimum safe pressure for closing unstable open-book fractures falls in a range centered on approximately 150 Newtons, or 33 pounds. That finding allowed the creation of the SAM Sling's patented "autostop" buckle, which has spring-loaded prongs that lock the buckle in place when the right amount of force is applied.

MRI Information. Based on *in vitro* testing, the SAM Sling will not present a hazard or risk to a patient undergoing an MRI procedure using an MR system operating at 3-Tesla or less. The SAM Sling contains ferromagnetic springs in the buckle. Therefore, it is important to ensure that the SAM Sling is firmly applied to the patient prior to entry into the MRI environment (as stated in the labeling for this device). Accordingly, there will be no hazard or risk to a patient undergoing an MRI procedure. The SAM Sling should not be removed from the patient while in the MR system or in the MR system room. This product is not recommended for use on children.

REFERENCE

SAM Medical Products, www.sammedical.com

Scaffolds

Bioresorbable (the terms "bioresorbable", "biodegradeable" and "bioabsorbable" refers to the complete breakdown and removal of a material over time) scaffolds are designed to provide the same benefits as metallic drug-eluting or bare metal stents. Because these scaffolds are made from nonmetallic, non-conducting materials, these implants are MR Safe.

Scaffolds utilized for the coronary arteries and other vascular areas, include:

- Absorb Bioresorbable Vascular Scaffold (BVS) System, Abbott Vascular
- Absorb GT1 Bioresorbable Vascular Scaffold (BVS) System, Abbott Vascular
- DESolve Scaffold System, Elixir Medical
- Fantom Bioresorbable Scaffold, Reva Medical
- Fortitude Bioresorbable Drug-Eluting Coronary Scaffold, Amaranth Medical
- Igaki-Tamai Biodegradable Coronary Artery Scaffold, Kyoto Medical Planning
- Magmaris Bioresorbable Scaffold, Biotronic
- Mirage Microfiber Scaffold, ManLi

Scleral Buckle
(Scleral Buckling Procedure)

The application of a scleral buckle (note, this is a procedure not an implant) or "scleral buckling" is a surgical technique used to repair retinal detachments and was first used experimentally by ophthalmic surgeons in 1937. By the early 1960s, scleral buckling became the method of choice when the development of new materials, particularly silicone, offered surgeons better opportunities to improve patient care.

The buckling element is usually left in place permanently. The element pushes in, or "buckles," the sclera toward the middle of the eye. This buckling effect on the sclera relieves the traction on the retina, allowing the retinal tear to settle against the wall of the eye. The buckle effect may cover only the area behind the detachment or it may encircle the eyeball like a ring. This procedure effectively holds the retina against the sclera until scarring seals the tear and prevents fluid leakage, which could cause further retinal detachment. Scleral buckles come in many shapes and sizes. The encircling band is usually a thin silicone band sewn around the circumference of the sclera of the eye. In rare instances, a metallic clip may be used. Some metallic clips may pose a risk to patients undergoing MRI procedures.

Tantalum Clips
Tantalum clips are less bulky than sutures, allowing the surgeon to adjust the tension of the circling band for the scleral buckle. These clips do not cause tissue reaction and do not harbor infection. Because tantalum is a nonmagnetic metal, these clips are considered to be acceptable for patients undergoing MRI procedures.

REFERENCES

Bakshandeh H, Shellock FG, Schatz CJ, Morisoli SM. Metallic clips used for scleral buckling: *Ex vivo* evaluation of ferromagnetism at 1.5 T. J Magn Reson Imag 1993;3:559.

Lincoff H. Radial buckling in the repair of retinal detachment. Int Ophthalmol Clin. 1976;16:127-34.

Michels RG. Scleral buckling methods for rhegmatogenous retinal detachment. Retina 1986;6:1-49.

Sophono Alpha Magnetic Implant

MRI labeling information for the Sophono Alpha Magnetic Implant (also referred to as the Alpha (M) Bone Conduction Hearing System) (Sophono/Medtronic, Inc. www.sophono.com) is, as follows:

WARNING

Do not perform Magnetic Resonance Imaging (MRI) on a patient wearing an Otomag Alpha Sound Processor, Magnetic Spacer, Headband or Softband. The external portions of the device must be removed prior to entering the MR environment. Severe injury may result if the external portions of the device are not removed prior to entering the MR environment.

- The Alpha (M) Magnetic Implant can be scanned safely using MRI only under certain conditions.

MR Unsafe: The Alpha Sound Processor, Magnetic Spacer, Headband or Softband must be removed before entering the MR environment

MRI Information

Non-clinical testing demonstrated the Alpha (M) Magnetic Implant is MR Conditional and can be scanned safely using MRI only under the following conditions:

- Remove all external components including the Otomag Alpha Sound Processor, Magnetic Spacer, Headband or Softband before entering the MR environment
- Static magnetic field of 3 Tesla or less,
- Spatial gradient field of 720 gauss/cm or less,
- Maximum whole-body averaged specific absorption rate (SAR) of 4 W/kg in the First Level Controlled Mode for a maximum scan time of 15 minutes of continuous scanning.

In non-clinical testing the Alpha (M) Magnetic Implant produced a maximum temperature rise less than 3.2°C during 15 minutes of continuous MR scanning in the First Level Controlled Mode at a maximum whole-body averaged SAR of 4 W/kg. The computed implant temperature increase in response to the worst-case, time-averaged gradient field (94.7-Tesla/sec) for the 15 minute possible exposure for a series of clinical MRI scans is less than 2.6°C.

Image Artifact

The maximum image artifact size extends approximately 5-cm relative to the size and shape of the implant when scanned in nonclinical testing using the Gradient echo (GRE) pulse sequence in a 3 Tesla/128-MH, Excite, Software 14X.M5, General Electric Healthcare, Milwaukee, WI; active-shielded, horizontal field MR system with a send receive RF coil. Artifacts were less with the T1-weighted, spin echo pulse sequence.

Implant Function Following MR Scanning

In non-clinical testing, when positioned parallel to the patient table, the Alpha (M) Magnetic Implant maintained over 95% of its original magnetic strength after 10 insertions into a static MRI field and over 10 minutes of pulse sequence in a 3 Tesla Siemens Tri Clinical MRI Scanner (MRC20587). To minimize demagnetization of the internal magnets, Sophono recommends that the patient's head is positioned along the long axis of the MRI scanner and that the patient is instructed to avoid head movement while lying on the patient table. If the head is tilted at an angle to the long axis of the patient table during a scan, the internal magnets may be demagnetized and a stronger external magnet may be needed to keep the device in place.

Caution

After MRI exposure the Magnetic Spacer Strength should be adjusted as necessary following the instructions "Instructions for Placement / Sizing of the Magnetic Spacers and Alpha Sound Processor" included in the manual for this product (www.sophono.com).

[MR healthcare professionals are advised to contact the manufacturer to ensure that the latest safety information is obtained and carefully followed in order to ensure patient safety relative to the use of an MR procedure.]

REFERENCE

Sophono/Medtronic, Inc., www.sophono.com

Surgical Instruments and Devices

Interventional magnetic resonance (MR) techniques have evolved into clinically viable surgical and therapeutic applications. This has resulted in the development and performance of innovative procedures that include percutaneous biopsy (e.g., breast, bone, brain, abdominal, etc.), endoscopic surgery of the abdomen, spine, and sinuses, neurosurgical procedures, and MR-guided monitoring of thermal therapies (i.e. laser-induced, RF-induced, and cryomediated procedures).

Surgical instruments and devices are an important necessity for interventional MR. Besides the typical MRI issues, there are possible hazards in the interventional MR setting related to the surgical instruments and devices that must be addressed to ensure the safety of healthcare practitioners and patients. Many of the conventional instruments and devices are made from metallic materials and/or conductive materials that can create substantial problems in association with interventional MR.

The interventional MR safety issues that exist for surgical instruments and devices include unwanted movement caused by magnetic field interactions (e.g., the "missile effect", translational attraction, torque), issues related to eddy currents, and excessive temperatures generated by RF-induced heating. Furthermore, the operational aspects of various instruments may be adversely impacted by the electromagnetic fields used for MR procedures. Artifacts associated with the use of a metallic surgical instrument or device can be particularly problematic if in the imaging area of interest during its intended use. Additionally, the operation of certain devices may cause spurious electromagnetic noise, resulting in substantial artifacts. To address these problems, various surgical instruments and devices have been developed that do not present an additional risk or problem to the patient or MR healthcare practitioner in the interventional MR environment.

REFERENCES

Hinks RS, et al. MR systems for image-guided therapy. J Magnetic Resonance Imaging 1998;8:19-25.

Jolesz FA. Interventional and intraoperative MRI: A general overview of the field. J Magn Reson Imag 1998;8:3-7.

Jolesz FA. Image-guided procedures and the operating room of the future. Radiology 1997;204:601-612.

Jolesz FA, et al. Compatible instrumentation for intraoperative MRI: Expanding resources. J Magnetic Resonance Imaging 1998;8:8-11.

Maldonado IL, et al. Magnetic resonance-based deep brain stimulation technique: A series of 478 consecutive implanted electrodes with no perioperative intracerebral hemorrhage. Neurosurgery 2009;65(6 Suppl):196-201.

Shellock FG. Compatibility of an endoscope designed for use in interventional MR imaging procedures. Amer J Roentgenol 1998;171:1297-1300.

Shellock FG. Metallic surgical instruments for interventional MRI procedures: Evaluation of MR safety. J Magn Reson Imag 2001;13:152-157.

Shellock FG. MRI safety of instruments designed for interventional MRI: Assessment of ferromagnetism, heating, and artifacts. Workshop on New Insights into Safety and Compatibility Issues Affecting *In Vivo* MR, Syllabus, International Society of Magnetic Resonance in Medicine, Berkeley, 1998; pp. 39.

Shellock FG, Shellock VJ. Ceramic surgical instruments: Evaluation of MR-compatibility at 1.5 Tesla. J Magn Reson Imag 1996;6:954-956.

Thomas C, et al. Carbon fibre and nitinol needles for MRI-guided interventions: First *in vitro* and *in vivo* application. Eur J Radiol 2011;79:353-358.

Sutures

Sutures are made from a variety of materials, including those that are nonmetallic and metallic. Various sutures *with the needles removed* (i.e. the needles are typically made from ferromagnetic materials) have been testing at 1.5- and 3-Tesla. For the different sutures evaluated at 1.5-Tesla, all were shown to be acceptable for patients.

MRI at 3-Tesla and Sutures. At 3-Tesla, most of the sutures evaluated displayed no magnetic field interactions, while two (Flexon suture and Steel suture, United States Surgical, North Haven, CT) showed minor deflection angles and torque. For these two sutures, the *in situ* application of these materials provides sufficient counter-forces to prevent movement or dislodgment. Therefore, in consideration of their intended *in vivo* use, all of the sutures with the needles removed tested to date are acceptable at 3-Tesla. Additional sutures acceptable for patients undergoing MRI examinations at 3-Tesla may be found on **The List**.

REFERENCE

Shellock FG. Biomedical implants and devices: Assessment of magnetic field interactions with a 3.0-Tesla MR system. J Magn Reson Imag 2002;16:721-732.

SynchroMed, SynchroMed EL, and SynchroMed II Drug Infusion Systems
Medtronic, Inc.

The following drug infusion systems/programmable infusion pumps (Medtronic, Inc.) are MR Conditional:

SynchroMed Pump Models: 8615, 8616, 8617 and 8618

SynchroMed EL Pump Models: All models beginning with 8626, 8627

SynchroMed II Pump, Models: All models beginning with 8637

Comprehensive labeling information must be reviewed to ensure patient safety.

Carefully review the latest MRI labeling conditions and guidelines at: www.medtronic.com/mri

[MR healthcare professionals are advised to contact the respective manufacturer in order to obtain the latest safety information to ensure patient safety relative to the use of an MR procedure.]

REFERENCE

Medtronic, Inc., www.medtronic.com/mri

TheraSeed Radioactive Seed Implant

The TheraSeed radioactive seed implant (Theragenics Corporation; now owned by Bard Medical) is used to deliver low-level radiation to the prostate to treat cancer. The TheraSeed radioactive seed is a relatively small implant comprised of a titanium tube with two graphite pellets and a lead marker inside. The outside dimensions of tube are approximately 0.177-inches in length with a diameter of 0.032-inches.

Palladium-103 is the isotope contained in the TheraSeed implant. Because the radiation is so low and the seeds are placed so precisely, virtually all the radiation is absorbed by the prostate. Treatments with the TheraSeed implant may involve placement of from 80 to 120 of these devices within the prostate. These "seeds" are implanted with "spacers" between them and placed according to treatment plans, so that they do not contact one another during their intended "*in vivo*" use.

Magnetic resonance tests (magnetic field interactions, heating, and artifacts) conducted on the TheraSeed revealed that this implant is acceptable for patients undergoing MR procedures at 3-Tesla or less.

REFERENCES

Bard Medical, www.bardmedical.com
Theragenics, www.theraseed.com

Transdermal Medication Patches and Other Drug Delivery Patches

A transdermal patch allows continuous and prolonged drug delivery that may be more effective and safer than oral medication. In addition, patches offer the potential to deliver medications that would otherwise require injections. Future advances in technology will expand the utilization of drug patches. For example, researchers are currently working on various technologies to "force" larger molecules through the skin. These so-called "active patches" may permit the delivery of insulin to diabetics, as well as the administration of red-cell stimulating erythropoietin for treatment of anemic patients without injections.

Several anecdotal reports have indicated that transdermal medication patches that contain aluminum foil or other similar metallic component may cause excessive heating or a burn in a patient undergoing an MR procedure. For example, the Deponit (nitroglycerin transdermal delivery system) patch that contains an aluminum foil component was worn by a patient during MR imaging. This patient received a second-degree burn during the examination that was performed using conventional pulse sequences and standard imaging procedures (Personal communication, Robert E. Mucha, Schwarz Pharma, Milwaukee, WI; 1995). This injury was likely due to MRI-related heating of the metallic foil associated with this transdermal patch.

The U.S. Food and Drug Administration is aware of at least two other adverse events in which patients wearing nicotine transdermal patches during MRI examinations experienced burns. In one case, the patient was wearing a nicotine (Habitrol) transdermal patch. When the patient was removed from the scanner at the completion of the MRI procedure, he stated that his arm was "burning". Upon examination, his upper left arm appeared to be mildly erythematous and there was a small blister where the patch was located. In another case, a patient underwent a brief MRI examination of the lumbar spine while wearing a nicotine transdermal patch. Later, the patient complained of burn lines on his upper arms that were associated with this patch.

Therefore, a patient wearing a transdermal patch that has a metallic component must be identified prior to undergoing an MR procedure. The patient's physician should be contacted to determine if it is possible to temporarily remove the medication patch to prevent excessive heating and burns. After the MR examination, a new patch should be applied following the directions of the prescribing physician (Personal communication, Robert E. Mucha, Schwarz Pharma, Milwaukee, WI). Importantly, this procedure should be conducted in consultation with the physician responsible for prescribing the transdermal patch or otherwise responsible for the management of the patient.

The Institute for Safe Medical Practices has stated that medication patches such as ANDRODERM, TRANSDERM-NITRO, DEPONIT, NICODERM, NICOTROL, CATAPRES-TTS, and possibly others should be removed prior to an MR examination. In addition, other patches to be aware of include the nicotine patch marketed as Habitrol and its "private label" equivalents and Scopolamine\Hyoscine HydroBromide, marketed as TransDerm Scop (Personal Communication, Crispin C. Fernandez, M.D. Medical Affairs, Novartis Consumer Health, Inc. Parsippany, NJ).

Notably, not all transdermal medication patches contain a metallic component and, therefore, these patches do not need to be removed from the patient in preparation for the MRI examination. Furthermore, if the body part with the patch is not within the transmit RF coil (e.g., performing MRI of the brain using a transmit/receive head coil in a patient with a transdermal medication patch applied to the torso), there is no risk to the patient.

ActiPatch
ActiPatch (BioElectronics, Frederick, MD) is a medical, drug-free device that delivers pulsed electromagnetic frequency therapies to accelerate healing of soft tissue injuries. The ActiPatch has an embedded battery-operated microchip that delivers continuous pulsed therapy to reduce pain and swelling.

ActiPatch and MRI. The ActiPatch must be removed prior to performing an MRI procedure to prevent possible damage to this device and the potential risk of excessive heating. Thus, this device is considered MR Unsafe.

Patches with Magnets

It should be noted that some patches contain small magnets, such as the AcuMed Advanced Pain Patch (Acumed, www.acumedpatches.com). Because of the risks and problems associated with strong magnetic field interactions and artifacts, these patches should be removed from the patient prior to MRI.

REFERENCES

Institute for Safe Medical Practices, Medication Safety Alert! Burns in MRI patients wearing transdermal patches. Vol. 9, Issue 7, April 8, 2004. http://www.ismp.org/msaarticles/burnsprint.htm

Kanal E, Barkovich AJ, Bell C, et al. ACR guidance document for safe MR practices: 2007. Am J Roentgenol 2007;188:1447-1474.

Kuehn BM. FDA warning: remove drug patches before MRI to prevent burns to skin. JAMA. 2009;301:1328.

www.bielcorp.com

FDA Public Health Advisory: Risk of Burns during MRI Scans from Transdermal Drug Patches with Metallic Backings
[Reprinted with permission.]

The FDA has been made aware of information about certain transdermal patches (medicated patches applied to the skin) that contain aluminum or other metals in the backing of the patches. Patches that contain metal can overheat during an MRI scan and cause skin burns in the immediate area of the patch.

Transdermal patches slowly deliver medicines through the skin. Some patches contain metal in the layer of the patch that is not in contact with the skin (the backing). The metal in the backing of these patches may not be visible. The labeling for most of the medicated patches that contain metal in the backing provides a warning to patients about the risk of burns if the patch is not removed before an MRI scan. However, not all transdermal patches that contain metal have this warning for patients in the labeling.

The FDA is in the process of reviewing the labeling and composition of all medicated patches to ensure that those made with materials containing metal provide a warning about the risk of burns to patients who wear the patches during an MRI scan.

Until this review is complete, FDA recommends that healthcare professionals referring patients to have an MRI scan identify those patients who are wearing a patch before the patients have the MRI scan. The healthcare professional should advise these patients about the procedures for removing and disposing of the patch before the MRI scan, and replacing the patch after the MRI scan. MRI facilities should follow published safe practice recommendations concerning patients who are wearing patches (1, 2).

Until this safety issue is resolved, FDA recommends that patients who use medicated patches (including nicotine patches) do the following:

- Tell the doctor referring you for an MRI scan that you are using a patch and why you are using it (such as, for pain, smoking cessation, hormones).
- Ask your doctor for guidance about removing and disposing of the patch before having an MRI scan and replacing it after the procedure.
- Tell the MRI facility that you are using a patch. You should do this when making your appointment and during the health history questions you are asked when you arrive for your appointment.

The FDA urges health care professionals and patients to report possible cases of skin burns while wearing patches during an MRI to the FDA through the MedWatch program by phone (1-800-FDA-1088) or by the Internet at http://www.fda.gov/medwatch/index.html.

(1) Kanal, et. al, ACR Guidance Document for Safe MR Practices: 2007. Amer J Roentgenol 2007;188:1–27.

(2) Guidelines for Screening Patients For MR Procedures and Individuals for the MR Environment, Institute for Magnetic Resonance Safety, Education, and Research, www.imrser.org.

FDA Update (03/09/2009). The FDA evaluated the composition of available patches to determine which of them contain metal components and to assure that this information is included in their labeling. Based on current information from this evaluation, the FDA is working with the manufacturers of the following patches to update the labeling to include adequate warnings to patients about the risk of burns to the skin if the patch is worn during an MRI scan. It should be noted that some of the drugs listed may have a generic equivalent and more than one size and strength of patch. The FDA will update this posting as information becomes available.

Proprietary Name Generic/Established Name

Catapres TTS/Clonidine, Neupro / Rotigotine, Lidopel/Lidocaine HCl and Epinephrine, Synera/Lidocaine/Tetracaine, Transderm-Scop Scopolamine, Prostep/Nicotine Transdermal System, Habitrol/Nicotine Transdermal System, Nicotrol TD/Nicotine transdermal system, Androderm/Testosterone Transdermal System, Fentanyl/Fentanyl, Salonpas Power Plus / Methyl Salicylate/Menthol

Vascular Access Ports, Infusion Pumps, and Catheters

Vascular access ports, infusion pumps, and catheters are implants and devices commonly used to provide long-term vascular administration of chemotherapeutic agents, antibiotics, analgesics and other medications (also, see information pertaining to other similar devices including **Ambulatory Infusion Pumps, Insulin Pumps,** the **IsoMed Implantable Constant-Flow Infusion Pump, Prometra Programmable Pumps,** the **SynchroMed, SynchroMED EL,** and **SynchroMed II Drug Infusion Systems**).

Vascular access ports are usually implanted in a subcutaneous pocket over the upper chest wall with the catheters inserted in the jugular, subclavian, or cephalic vein. Vascular access ports have a variety of similar features (e.g., a reservoir, central septum, and catheter) and may be constructed from different materials including stainless steel, titanium, silicone, and plastic. Because of the widespread use of vascular access ports and associated catheters and the high probability that patients with these devices may require MR procedures, it has been important to characterize the MRI issues for these implants.

Three of the implantable vascular access ports and catheters evaluated for safety with MR procedures showed measurable magnetic field interactions during exposure to the MR systems (typically 1.5-Tesla) used for testing, but the interactions were minor relative to the *in vivo* applications of these implants. Therefore, an MR procedure is acceptable at 1.5-Tesla or less in a patient that has one of the vascular access ports or catheters shown in **The List**.

With respect to MR imaging and artifacts, in general, vascular access ports that produce the least amount of artifact are made entirely from nonmetallic materials. The ones that produce the largest artifacts are composed of metal(s) or have metal in an unusual shape (e.g., the OmegaPort Access Devices).

MRI at 3-Tesla and Vascular Access Ports and Catheters. For the vascular access ports and catheters assessed for magnetic field interactions at 3-Tesla, these items did not exhibit substantial magnetic field interactions and, therefore, will not move or dislodge in this MR environment. Because of the design aspects typically used for vascular access ports, excessive MRI-related heating causing an injury in a patient is not an issue. However, for certain catheters, MRI-related heating can be substantial and pose possible problems for patients referred for MRI examinations, as reported by Owen, et al. (2014).

For the accessories, some (e.g., Huber needle) showed measurable magnetic field interactions (see **The List**). However, during the *intended uses* of these accessories, it is unlikely that they will present a problem in 3-Tesla or less MR environments considering that the simple application of adhesive tape or other appropriate means of retention effectively counterbalances the magnetic qualities of these devices (Unpublished Observations, F.G. Shellock).

REFERENCES

Owens S, et al. Evaluation of epidural and peripheral nerve catheter heating during magnetic resonance imaging. Reg Anesth Pain Med 2014;39:534-9.

Shellock FG. Biomedical implants and devices: Assessment of magnetic field interactions with a 3.0-Tesla MR system. J Magn Reson Imag 2002;16:721-732.

Shellock FG, Nogueira M, Morisoli S. MR imaging and vascular access ports: *Ex vivo* evaluation of ferromagnetism, heating, and artifacts at 1.5-T. J Magn Reson Imag 1995;4:481-484.

Shellock FG, Shellock VJ. Vascular access ports and catheters tested for ferromagnetism, heating, and artifacts associated with MR imaging. Magnetic Resonance Imaging 1996;14:443-447.

Titterington B, Shellock FG. Evaluation of MRI issues for an access port with a radiofrequency identification (RFID) tag. Magnetic Resonance Imaging 2013;31:1439-44.

VeriChip Microtransponder

The VeriChip Microtransponder is a miniaturized, implantable radio frequency identification device (RFID). This is a passive device that contains an electronic circuit that is activated externally by a low-power electro-magnetic field emitted by a battery powered scanner. The Microtransponder is implanted subcutaneously.

With regard to MRI procedures, the labeling for this device is, as follows: Patients with the VeriChip Microtransponder may safely undergo MRI diagnostics in up to 7-Tesla cylindrical systems. See section below.

INSTRUCTIONS FOR PATIENTS UNDERGOING MRI

- The patient should be monitored continuously throughout the MRI procedure using visual and audio means (e.g., intercom system).
- Instruct the patient to alert the MR system operator of any unusual sensations or problems so that, if necessary, the MR system operator can immediately terminate the procedure.
- Provide the patient with a means to alert the MR system operator of any unusual sensations or problems.
- Do not perform MRI if the patient is sedated, anesthetized, confused or otherwise unable to communicate with the MR system operator.

VOCARE Bladder System, Implantable Functional Neuromuscular Stimulator

The NeuroControl VOCARE Bladder System (also referred to as the FineTech-Brindley Bladder System, Finetech Medical, Ltd.) is a radiofrequency (RF) powered motor control neurostimulation system that consists of both implanted and external components. The VOCARE Bladder System delivers low levels of electrical stimulation to a spinal cord injured patient's intact sacral spinal nerve roots to elicit functional contraction of the muscles innervated by them. The VOCARE Bladder System consists of the following subsystems:

- The **Implanted Components** include the Implantable Receiver-Stimulator and Extradural Electrodes.
- The **External Components** include the External Controller, External Transmitter, External Cable, Transmitter Tester, Battery Charger and Power Cord.
- The **Surgical Components** include the Surgical Stimulator, Intradural Surgical Probe, Extradural Surgical Probe, Surgical Test Cable, and Silicone Adhesive.

PRECAUTIONS

- **X-rays, Diagnostic Ultrasound**: X-ray imaging, and diagnostic ultrasound have not been reported to affect the function of the Implantable Receiver-Stimulator or Extradural Electrodes. However, the implantable components may obscure the view of other anatomic structures.
- **MRI**: Testing of the VOCARE Bladder System in a 1.5-Tesla scanner with a maximum spatial gradient of 450 gauss/cm or less, exposed to an average Specific Absorption Rate (SAR) of 1.1 W/kg, for a 30 minute duration resulted in localized temperature rises up to 5.5 degrees C in a gel phantom (without blood flow) and translational force less than that of a 12 gram mass and torque of 0.47 N-cm (less than that produced by the weight of the device). A patient with a VOCARE Bladder System may undergo an MR procedure using a shielded or

unshielded MR system with a static magnetic field of 1.5-Tesla <u>only</u> and a maximum spatial gradient of 450 gauss/cm or less. The implantable components may obscure the view of other nearby anatomic structures. Artifact size is dependent on variety of factors including the type of pulse sequence used for imaging (e.g., larger for gradient echo pulse sequences and smaller for spin echo and fast spin echo pulse sequences), the direction of the frequency encoding, and the size of the field of view used for imaging. The use of non-standard scanning modes to minimize image artifact or improve visibility should be applied with caution and with the Specific Absorption Rate (SAR) not to exceed an average of 1.1-W/kg and gradient magnetic fields no greater than 20 Tesla/sec. The use of Transmit RF Coils other than the scanner's Body RF Coil or a Head RF Coil is prohibited. Testing of the function of each electrode should be conducted prior to MRI scanning to ensure no leads are broken. Do not expose patients to MRI if any lead is broken or if integrity cannot be established as excessive heating may result in a broken lead. Patients should be advised to empty their bladder or bowel prior to MRI scanning as a precaution. The external components of the VOCARE Bladder System must be removed prior to MRI scanning. Patients must be continuously observed during the MRI procedure and instructed to report any unusual sensations (e.g., warming, burning, or neuromuscular stimulation). Scanning must be discontinued immediately if any unusual sensation occurs.

Note to MR Healthcare Professionals: Different MRI guidelines exist for different countries. Therefore, use the appropriate information for your country.

[MR healthcare professionals are advised to contact the respective manufacturer in order to obtain the latest safety information to ensure patient safety relative to the use of an MR procedure.]

REFERENCE

Finetech Medical, www.finetech-medical.co.uk

The List – Information and Terminology

The List contains information for thousands of implants, devices, materials, and other products. The objects in **The List** are divided into general categories to facilitate access and review of pertinent information.

To properly utilize **The List**, particular attention must be given to the information indicated for the highest static magnetic **Field Strength** used for testing and the **Status** information indicated for a given **Object.** The "default" **Field Strength** indicated for an *MR Safe* implant is typically 1.5-Tesla. However, in some cases "3-Tesla" or "1.5- and 3-Tesla" is indicated if MRI testing was conducted.

Note: These specific terms correspond to the column headings for information compiled in **The List**. In addition, for certain objects (e.g., those designated as *Conditional 5)*, it may be necessary to refer to specific recommendations or guidelines in **SECTION II** of this textbook or to contact the manufacturer of the implant or device for the latest MRI labeling information, particularly if the implant/device is an "active" implant. Frequently, specific MRI information may be found on the implant/device company's website. See **Appendix III** for a list of websites for device manufacturers. It should be noted that, in some cases, the MRI labeling information is different in the United States (U.S.) versus outside of the United States.

The relevant terminology for **The List** is, as follows:

Object: This is the implant, device, material, or product that underwent evaluation relative to an MR procedure or the MR environment. Information is provided for the material(s) used to make the object and the manufacturer of the object, if known. The term "SS" refers to stainless steel. Note that there are magnetic and nonmagnetic forms of stainless steel.

Status: This information pertains to the results of the tests conducted on the object. Testing typically included an assessment of magnetic field interactions (i.e. deflection and/or torque) and MRI-related heating, as needed. In some cases, medical products were assessed for induced electrical currents and the impact of an MR procedure or the MR environment on the functional or operational aspects of the object.

Information for each object has been specifically categorized using a **Status** designation, which indicates the object to be **Safe, Conditional,** or **Unsafe**, as follows (***IMPORTANT NOTE***: Please see the section entitled *Terminology Applied to Implants and Devices):

Safe – The object is considered to be safe for the patient undergoing an MR procedure or an individual in the MR environment, with special reference to the highest static magnetic field strength that was used for the evaluation. The object has undergone testing to demonstrate that it is safe or it is made from material(s) considered to be safe (e.g., nonmetallic, nonconducting materials such as plastic, silicone, glass, etc.) with regard to the MR environment or an MR procedure. Refer to additional information for the particular object indicated in the text of **SECTION II** of this textbook (please see the **Table of Contents**).

Terminology from the American Society for Testing and Materials (ASTM) International and utilized by the Food and Drug Administration as well as other notified bodies refers to MR Safe as an item that poses no known hazards in all MRI environments. Using the current terminology, MR Safe items include nonconducting, nonmetallic, items such as a plastic Petri dish.

Conditional – The object may or may not be safe for the patient undergoing an MR procedure or an individual in the MR environment, depending on the specific conditions that are present.

Current terminology from the American Society for Testing and Materials (ASTM) International and utilized by the Food and Drug Administration refers to MR Conditional as an item that has been demonstrated to pose no known hazards in a specified MRI environment with specified conditions of use. Field conditions that define the MRI environment include static magnetic field strength, highest spatial gradient of the magnetic field*, dB/dt (time varying magnetic fields), radio frequency (RF) fields, and specific absorption rate (SAR). Additional conditions, including specific configurations of the item (e.g., the routing of leads used for a neurostimulation system), may be required.

*[Please review: Commentary - Regarding the Value Reported for the Term "Spatial Gradient Magnetic Field" and How This Information Is Applied to Labeling of Medical Implants and

Devices*, Shellock FG, Kanal E, Gilk TB. Am J Roentgenol, 2011;196:142-145. To obtain this article, visit **www.IMRSER.org**.]

IMPORTANT NOTE: Recently, the Food and Drug Administration has approved MRI labeling pertaining to spatial gradient magnetic field values that have been calculated (or extrapolated) to higher values for implants and devices based on information for the measured deflection angles. Note that there may or may not be an indication in the MRI labeling that the higher spatial gradient magnetic field value was calculated (or extrapolated) for a given implant or device.

MR Conditional information has been sub-categorized to indicate specific recommendations for the particular object, as follows:

Conditional 1 – The object is acceptable for the patient or individual in the MR environment, despite the fact that it showed positive findings for magnetic field interactions during testing. Notably, the object is considered to be "weakly" ferromagnetic, *only*.

In general, the object is safe because the magnetic field interactions were characterized as "mild" or "weak" relative to the *in vivo* forces or counter-forces present for the object. For example, certain prosthetic heart valve prostheses and annuloplasty rings showed measurable magnetic field interactions during exposure to the MR systems used for testing, but the magnetic field interactions were less than the forces exerted on the implants by the beating heart.

Additionally, there may be substantial "retentive" or counter-forces provided by the presence of sutures or other means of fixation (e.g., screws, cement, etc.), tissue ingrowth, scarring, or granulation that serve to prevent the object from presenting a risk or hazard to the patient undergoing an MR procedure or an individual in the MR environment.

For a device or product that is used for an MR-guided procedure, there may be minor magnetic field interactions in association with the MR system. Eddy currents may also be present. However, the device or product is considered to be acceptable if it is used in its "intended" manner, as specified by the manufacturer. Special attention should be given to the strength of the static magnetic field and RF frequency used for testing the device or product. Functional or operational aspects may need to be considered.

Additionally, specific recommendations for the use of the device or product in the MR environment or during an MR procedure (i.e.

typically presented in the *Product Insert* or *Instructions for Use*) should be followed carefully.

Conditional 2 – Certain "weakly" ferromagnetic objects – including coils, filters, stents, clips, cardiac occluders, or other implants - typically become firmly incorporated into the tissue six weeks following placement. Therefore, it is unlikely that these objects will be moved or dislodged by interactions with the magnetic fields of MR systems operating at the static magnetic field strength used for testing. Furthermore, to date, there has been no report of an injury to a patient or individual in association with an MR procedure for these coils, stents, filters, cardiac occluders or other similar implants designated as "**Conditional 2**".

Of note is that if the implant is made from a nonmagnetic material (e.g., Phynox, Elgiloy, Titanium, Titanium alloy, MP35N, Nitinol, etc.), it is *not* necessary to wait a period of time before performing an MR procedure using an MR system operating at 1.5-Tesla or less. In some cases, this may also apply to 3-Tesla.

Special Note: If there is any concern regarding the implant or the integrity of the tissue with regard to its ability to retain the object in place during an MR procedure or during exposure to the MR environment, the patient or individual should not be allowed into the MR environment.

Conditional 3 – Certain transdermal patches with metallic foil (e.g., Deponit, nitroglycerin transdermal delivery system) or other metallic components, although not attracted to an MR system, have been reported to heat excessively during MR procedures if located within the area of the transmit RF coil. This excessive heating may produce discomfort or burn a patient or individual wearing a transdermal patch with a metallic component. Therefore, it is recommended that the patch with a metallic component be removed prior to the MR procedure. A new patch should be applied immediately after the examination. This procedure should only be done in consultation with the patient's personal physician responsible for prescribing the transdermal medication patch.

Conditional 4 - This particular halo vest or cervical fixation device may have ferromagnetic component parts, however, the magnetic field interactions have not been determined or they are not excessive. Nevertheless, there has been no report of patient injury in association with the presence of this device in the MR environment at the static magnetic field strength used for MR safety testing. Issues may still be present with regard to MRI-related heating. As such, guidelines provided in the *Product Insert* or *Instructions for Use* for a given halo vest or cervical fixation device should be carefully followed. Halo vests and cervical fixation devices made from conducting metals may heat excessively during an MR procedure, resulting in serious patient injury. Contact the manufacturer for further information. Also, refer to the latest information for cervical fixation devices and note that several products have been evaluated at 3-Tesla.

Conditional 5 - This object is acceptable for a patient undergoing an MR procedure or an individual in the MR environment *only* if specific guidelines or recommendations are followed. See specific information for a given object in **SECTION II** and contact the manufacturer for further information, as needed. Please refer to the specific criteria for performing the MR procedure by reviewing the information for the object in this textbook. Consult the manufacturer of the particular device for the latest safety information. Frequently, this information may be found at the company's website. *A list of biomedical company websites is provided in **Appendix III**.*

Conditional 6 - This implant/device was determined to be MR Conditional according to the terminology specified in the American Society for Testing and Materials (ASTM) International, Designation: F2503. Standard Practice for Marking Medical Devices and Other Items for Safety in the Magnetic Resonance Environment.

Non-clinical testing demonstrated that the implant/device is MR Conditional. A patient with this implant/device can be scanned safely immediately after placement under the following conditions:

- Static magnetic field of 3-Tesla or less
- Maximum spatial gradient magnetic field of 720-gauss/cm (a higher spatial gradient magnetic field value may apply if properly calculated)
- Maximum MR system reported whole-body-averaged specific absorption rate (SAR) of 2-W/kg for 15 minutes of scanning (per pulse sequence).

MRI-Related Heating

In non-clinical testing, the implant/device produced a temperature rise of less than or equal to 6.0 degrees C using an MR system reported, whole body averaged specific absorption rate (SAR) of 2-

W/kg for 15-minutes (per pulse sequence) of scanning in a 3-Tesla MR system.

Artifact
MR image quality may be compromised if the area of interest is in the exact same area or relatively close to the position of the implant/device. In some cases, the artifact size relative to the size of the implant or device may be indicated.

Attention: Contact the manufacturer of this implant/device for further information, as needed.

Conditional 7 - *Important Note:* This device is not intended for use inside of the MR system during the operation of the scanner for an MR procedure. That is, this device should not be *inside of the bore* of the MR system, exposing this device to the time-varying and RF fields that are present during an MR procedure.

Attention: Contact the manufacturer of this implant/device for further information.

Conditional 8 – Note: This information pertains to an implant/device that has MRI labeling at 1.5-Tesla and 3-Tesla, only. In some cases, it may pertain to a single and two-overlapped version of a stent. In other cases, Conditional 8 may apply to other implants or devices.

The implant/device was determined to be MR Conditional according to the terminology specified in the American Society for Testing and Materials (ASTM) International, Designation: F2503. Standard Practice for Marking Medical Devices and Other Items for Safety in the Magnetic Resonance Environment.

Non-clinical testing demonstrated that the implant/device is MR Conditional. A patient with this implant/device can be scanned safely immediately after placement under the following conditions:

- Static magnetic field of 1.5-Tesla and 3-Tesla only
- Maximum spatial gradient magnetic field of 720-gauss/cm (a higher spatial gradient magnetic field value may apply if properly calculated)
- Maximum MR system reported whole-body-averaged specific absorption rate (SAR) of 2-W/kg for 15 minutes of scanning (per pulse sequence)

MRI-Related Heating

In non-clinical testing, the implant/device produced the following temperature rises during MRI performed for 15-minutes (i.e. per pulse sequence) in 1.5-Tesla and 3-Tesla MR systems, using an MR system reported, whole body averaged SAR of 2-W/kg or less, as follows:

Highest temperature changes

Less than or equal to 6.0 degrees C at 1.5-T/64-MHz

Less than or equal to 6.0 degrees C at 3-T/128-MHz

Artifact
MR image quality may be compromised if the area of interest is in the exact same area or relatively close to the position of the implant/device. In some cases, the artifact size relative to the size of the implant or device may be indicated.

Attention: Contact the manufacturer of this implant/device for further information.

Terminology from the American Society for Testing and Materials (ASTM) International and utilized by the Food and Drug Administration refers to <u>MR Unsafe</u> as an item that is known to pose hazards in all MRI environments. MR Unsafe items include magnetic items such as a pair of ferromagnetic scissors.

Unsafe 1 – The object is considered to pose a potential or realistic risk or hazard to a patient or individual in the MR environment primarily as the result of movement or dislodgment of the object. Other risks or a different hazard may also exist. Therefore, in general, the presence of this object is considered to be a contraindication for an MR procedure and/or for an individual to enter the MR environment depending on the nature of the object or item.

Note that the "default" static magnetic field strength for an *MR Unsafe* implant or device is typically 1.5-Tesla.

Unsafe 2 – This object may display only minor magnetic field interactions which, in consideration of the *in vivo* application of this object, is unlikely to pose a hazard or risk in association with movement or dislodgment. Nevertheless, the presence of this object is considered to be a contraindication for an MR procedure or for an individual in the MR environment. Potential risks of performing an MR procedure in a patient or individual with this object include possible induced currents, excessive heating, or other potentially hazardous conditions. Therefore, it is inadvisable to perform an MR procedure in a patient or individual with this object.

For example, although certain cardiovascular catheters and accessories typically do not exhibit magnetic field interactions, there are other mechanisms whereby these devices may pose a hazard to the patient or individual in the MR environment (e.g., excessive MRI-related heating).

The Swan-Ganz thermodilution catheter (and other similar catheters) displays no attraction to the MR system. However, there has been a report of a Swan-Ganz catheter that "melted" in a patient during an MR procedure. Therefore, the presence of this cardiovascular catheter and/or other similar device is considered to be a contraindication for a patient undergoing an MR procedure.

Note that the "default" static magnetic field strength for an *MR Unsafe* implant or device is typically 1.5-Tesla.

Field Strength – This is the highest strength of the static magnetic field of the MR system that was used for the evaluation of the object. In many cases, a 1.5-Tesla MR system was used for testing. However, there are some objects that were tested at field strengths lower (e.g., 0.15-Tesla) or higher (e.g., 3-Tesla, 7-Tesla, etc.) than 1.5-Tesla.

Note that the "default" field strength for an MR Unsafe implant or device is typically 1.5-Tesla.

Important Note: An object that exhibits only "mild" or "weak" magnetic field interactions in association with exposure to a 1.5-Tesla MR system may be attracted with sufficient force by a higher field strength scanner (e.g., 3-Tesla), potentially posing a risk to a patient or individual. Therefore, careful consideration must be given to each object relative to the static magnetic field strength of the MR system used for testing as well as the conditions that are present for the patient or individual under consideration prior to exposure to the MR environment.

Furthermore, for implants and devices that have an elongated shape or form a loop of a certain diameter, MRI-related heating may be of concern.

Reference – This is the peer-reviewed publication or other documentation used for the MRI safety information indicated for a particular object.

*Terminology Applied to Implants and Devices

IMPORTANT NOTE: See the section, **Terminology Applied to Implants and Devices,** for a full explanation of the proper terms used for MRI labeling.

Also, for a comprehensive explanation, see Shellock FG, Woods TO, Crues JV. MRI labeling information for implants and devices: Explanation of terminology. Radiology 2009;253:26-30 (available as a PDF file on *www.IMRSER.org*).

Use of Terminology

The current MRI labeling terminology is intended to help elucidate matters related to biomedical implants and devices to ensure the safe use of MRI technology. Notably, this terminology (i.e. MR Safe, MR Conditional, and MR Unsafe) has not been applied *retrospectively* to implants and devices that previously received U.S. Food and Drug Administration (FDA) approved labeling using the older terms "MR Safe" or "MR Compatible" (i.e. this applies to those objects tested prior to 2005). Accordingly, this should be understood to avoid undue confusion regarding the matter of MRI-related labeling for "older" vs. "newer" implants.

REFERENCES

American Society for Testing and Materials (ASTM) International, Designation: F2503. Standard Practice for Marking Medical Devices and Other Items for Safety in the Magnetic Resonance Environment. ASTM International, West Conshohocken, PA.

Shellock FG, Kanal E, Gilk T. Regarding the value reported for the term "spatial gradient magnetic field" and how this information is applied to labeling of medical implants and devices. Am J Roentgenol 2011;196:142-145.

Shellock FG, Woods TO, Crues JV. MRI labeling information for implants and devices: Explanation of terminology. Radiology 2009;253:26-30.

Woods TO. Standards for medical devices in MRI: Present and future. J Magn Reson Imag 2007;26:1186-9.

Woods TO. Guidance for Industry and FDA Staff - Establishing Safety and Compatibility of Passive Implants in the Magnetic Resonance (MR) Environment. Document issued on: August 21, 2008; http://www.fda.gov/cdrh/osel/guidance/1685.html

Object	Status	Field Strength (T)	Reference

Aneurysm Clips

Object	Status	Field Strength (T)	Reference
Aesculap Aneurysm Clip Device Family *Yasargil Clip Family Product Numbers* *FE5xxK, FE6xxK, FE7xxK, FE8xxK, FE9xxK, Phynox* *Aesculap, Inc., www.Aesculap.com*	Conditional 5	1.5, 3	
Aesculap Aneurysm Clip Device Family *Yasargil Clip, Family Product Numbers* *FT0xxT, FT1xxT, FT2xxT, FT3xxT, FT5xxT,* *FT6xxT, FT7xxT, FT7xxD, FT8xxT, FT9xxT, Titanium* *Aesculap, Inc., www.Aesculap.com*	Conditional 5	1.5, 3	
Aesculap AVM Clip, Curved, Phynox *Aesculap, Inc., www.aesculapusa.com*	Safe	1.5, 3	
Aesculap AVM Clip, Straight, Phynox *Aesculap, Inc., www.aesculapusa.com*	Safe	1.5, 3	
Codman AVM Micro Clip *Codman, www.depuysynthes.com*	Conditional 6	3	116
Codman Slim-Line Aneurysm Clip *Codman, www.depuysynthes.com*	Conditional 6	3	116
Codman Slim-Line Aneurysm Clip Graft *Codman, www.depuysynthes.com*	Conditional 6	3	116
Codman Slim-Line Mini Aneurysm Clip *Codman, www.depuysynthes.com*	Conditional 6	3	116
Codman Slim-Line Temporary Vessel Aneurysm Clip *Codman, www.depuysynthes.com*	Conditional 6	3	116
Downs Multi-Positional, Aneurysm Clip *17-7PH*	Unsafe 1	1.44	1
Drake (DR 14, DR 21), Aneurysm Clip *Edward Weck, Triangle Park, NJ*	Unsafe 1	1.44	1
Drake (DR 16), Aneurysm Clip *Edward Weck, Triangle Park, NJ*	Unsafe 1	0.147	1
Drake Aneurysm Clip, 301 SS *Edward Weck, Triangle Park, NJ*	Unsafe 1	1.5	
GIANT L-Aneurysm Clip, Titanium Permanent *Aneurysm Clip, 40-mm Straight Blade* *Peter Lazic Microsurgical, www.lazic.de/en/*	Conditional 6	3	
Heifetz Aneurysm Clip, 17-7PH *Edward Weck, Triangle Park, NJ*	Unsafe 1	1.5	
Heifetz Aneurysm Clip, Elgiloy *Edward Weck, Triangle Park, NJ*	Safe	1.5	
Housepian Aneurysm Clip	Unsafe 1	0.147	1
Kapp Aneurysm Clip, 405 SS *V. Mueller*	Unsafe 1	1.5	

Object	Status	Field Strength (T)	Reference
Kapp, Curved Aneurysm Clip, 404 SS *V. Mueller*	Unsafe 1	1.44	1
Kapp, Straight Aneurysm Clip, 404 SS *V. Mueller*	Unsafe 1	1.44	1
Kopitnik AVM Microclips, All FE Models *Aesculap, Inc., www.aesculapusa.com*	Safe	3	
Kopitnik AVM Microclip, Aneurysm Clip *Peter Lazic Microsurgical, www.lazic.de/en/*	Safe	1.5	
L-Aneurysm Clip System, Titanium *Peter Lazic GmbH* *www.lazic.de/en/*	Safe	3	
L-Aneurysm Clip *20 degree Angle, 5-mm, 7.5-mm, 10-mm, Titanium* *Peter Lazic Microsurgical, www.lazic.de/en/*	Conditional 6	3	
L-Aneurysm Clip *45 degree Angle, 5-mm, 7.5-mm, 10-mm, Titanium* *Peter Lazic Microsurgical, www.lazic.de/en/*	Conditional 6	3	
L-Aneurysm Clip *90 degree Angle, 5-mm, 7.5-mm, 10-mm, Titanium* *Peter Lazic Microsurgical, www.lazic.de/en/*	Conditional 6	3	
L-Aneurysm Clip *Angle with radius, 7.5-mm, 10-mm, Titanium* *Peter Lazic Microsurgical, www.lazic.de/en/*	Conditional 6	3	
L-Aneurysm Clip *Bayonet, 7-mm, 10-mm, 12-mm, Titanium* *Peter Lazic Microsurgical, www.lazic.de/en/*	Conditional 6	3	
L-Aneurysm Clip, Curved *7-mm, 9-mm, 12-mm, 15-mm, Titanium* *Peter Lazic Microsurgical, www.lazic.de/en/*	Conditional 6	3	
L-Aneurysm Clip, Fenestrated *3.5-mm 45 degree Angle, 5-mm, 7.5-mm, 10-mm,* *Titanium* *Peter Lazic Microsurgical, www.lazic.de/en/*	Conditional 6	3	
L-Aneurysm Clip, Fenestrated *3.5-mm 90 degree Angle, 5-mm, 7.5-mm, 10-mm,* *Titanium* *Peter Lazic Microsurgical, www.lazic.de/en/*	Conditional 6	3	
L-Aneurysm Clip, Fenestrated *3.5-mm Straight* *4-mm, 6-mm, 9-mm, Titanium* *Peter Lazic Microsurgical, www.lazic.de/en/*	Conditional 6	3	

Object	Status	Field Strength (T)	Reference
L-Aneurysm Clip, Fenestrated *5-mm 45 degree Angle* *5-mm, 7.5-mm, 10-mm, Titanium* *Peter Lazic Microsurgical, www.lazic.de/en/*	Conditional 6	3	
L-Aneurysm Clip, Fenestrated *5-mm 90 degree Angle* *5-mm, 7.5-mm, 10-mm, Titanium* *Peter Lazic Microsurgical, www.lazic.de/en/*	Conditional 6	3	
L-Aneurysm Clip, Fenestrated *5-mm Straight* *4-mm, 6-mm, 9-mm, 12-mm, Titanium* *Peter Lazic Microsurgical, www.lazic.de/en/*	Conditional 6	3	
L-Aneurysm Clip, Giant Aneurysm Clip Bayonet, *21-mm, Titanium* *Peter Lazic Microsurgical, www.lazic.de/en/*	Conditional 6	3	
L-Aneurysm Clip, Giant Aneurysm Clip Straight *21-mm, 25-mm, 30-mm, 35-mm, 40-mm, Titanium* *Peter Lazic Microsurgical, www.lazic.de/en/*	Conditional 6	3	
L-Aneurysm Clip, J Curved *7-mm, 9-mm, 11-mm, Titanium* *Peter Lazic Microsurgical, www.lazic.de/en/*	Conditional 6	3	
L-Aneurysm Clip, Mini Clip Angle and Curved *5-mm, Titanium* *Peter Lazic Microsurgical, www.lazic.de/en/*	Conditional 6	3	
L-Aneurysm Clip, Mini Clip Angle *7-mm, Titanium* *Peter Lazic Microsurgical, www.lazic.de/en/*	Conditional 6	3	
L-Aneurysm Clip, Mini Clip Bayonet *4-mm, 7-mm, Titanium* *Peter Lazic Microsurgical, www.lazic.de/en/*	Conditional 6	3	
L-Aneurysm Clip, Mini Clip Curved Narrow Jaw *4-mm, Titanium* *Peter Lazic Microsurgical, www.lazic.de/en/*	Conditional 6	3	
L-Aneurysm Clip, Mini Clip Curved *4-mm, 5-mm, Titanium* *Peter Lazic Microsurgical, www.lazic.de/en/*	Conditional 6	3	
L-Aneurysm Clip, Mini Clip Sideward Angle *5-mm, Titanium* *Peter Lazic Microsurgical, www.lazic.de/en/*	Conditional 6	3	
L-Aneurysm Clip, Mini Clip Sideward Curved *6-mm, Titanium* *Peter Lazic Microsurgical, www.lazic.de/en/*	Conditional 6	3	

Object	Status	Field Strength (T)	Reference
L-Aneurysm Clip, Mini Clip *Slightly Curved Narrow Jaw* *3-mm, 4-mm, Titanium* *Peter Lazic Microsurgical, www.lazic.de/en/*	Conditional 6	3	
L-Aneurysm Clip, Mini Clip Slightly Curved *4-mm, 5-mm, 7-mm, Titanium* *Peter Lazic Microsurgical, www.lazic.de/en/*	Conditional 6	3	
L-Aneurysm Clip, Mini Clip Straight Narrow Jaw *3-mm, 5-mm, Titanium* *Peter Lazic Microsurgical, www.lazic.de/en/*	Conditional 6	3	
L-Aneurysm Clip, Mini Clip Straight *3-mm, 5-mm, 7-mm, Titanium* *Peter Lazic Microsurgical, www.lazic.de/en/*	Conditional 6	3	
L-Aneurysm Clip, Sideward Angle *8-mm, 12-mm, Titanium* *Peter Lazic Microsurgical, www.lazic.de/en/*	Conditional 6	3	
L-Aneurysm Clip, Sideward Curved *9-mm, Titanium* *Peter Lazic Microsurgical, www.lazic.de/en/*	Conditional 6	3	
L-Aneurysm Clip, Slightly Curved *7-mm, 9-mm, 12-mm, 15-mm, 18-mm, Titanium* *Peter Lazic Microsurgical, www.lazic.de/en/*	Conditional 6	3	
L-Aneurysm Clip, Straight *7-mm, 9-mm, 12-mm, 15-mm, 18-mm, Titanium* *Peter Lazic Microsurgical, www.lazic.de/en/*	Conditional 6	3	
Lazic D-Aneurysm Clip, PEEK *Peter Lazic Microsurgical Innovations, www.lazic.de/en*	Conditional 8	1.5, 3	
Lazic L-Aneurysm Clip, Titanium *Peter Lazic Microsurgical Innovations, www.lazic.de/en*	Conditional 8	1.5, 3	
Mayfield Aneurysm Clip, 301 SS *Codman, www.depuysynthes.com*	Unsafe 1	1.5	3
Mayfield Aneurysm Clip, 304 SS *Codman, www.depuysynthes.com*	Unsafe 1	1.5	5
McFadden Aneurysm Clip, 301 SS *Codman, www.depuysynthes.com*	Unsafe 1	1.5	
McFadden Vari-Angle, Aneurysm Clip *Micro Clip, fenestrated, 9-mm straight blade, MP35N* *Codman, www.depuysynthes.com*	Safe	1.5	
McFadden Vari-Angle, Aneurysm Clip *Micro Clip, 9-mm straight blade, MP35N* *Codman, www.depuysynthes.com*	Safe	1.5	
Olivercrona *Aneurysm Clip*	Safe	1.44	1

Object	Status	Field Strength (T)	Reference
Perneczky Aneurysm Clip *curved, 9-mm* *Zeppelin Chirurgische Instrumente, Germany*	Safe	1.5	
Perneczky Aneurysm Clip *curved, 20-mm* *Zeppelin Chirurgische Instrumente, Germany*	Safe	1.5	
Perneczky Aneurysm Clip *straight, 2-mm blade* *Zeppelin Chirurgische Instrumente, Germany*	Safe	1.5, 3	82
Perneczky Aneurysm Clip *straight, 3-mm* *Zeppelin Chirurgische Instrumente, Germany*	Safe	1.5	
Perneczky Aneurysm Clip *straight, 6-mm blade* *Zeppelin Chirurgische Instrumente, Germany*	Safe	1.5, 3	82
Perneczky Aneurysm Clip *straight, 7-mm blade* *Zeppelin Chirurgische Instrumente, Germany*	Safe	1.5, 3	82
Perneczky Aneurysm Clip *straight, 9-mm* *Zeppelin Chirurgische Instrumente, Germany*	Safe	1.5	
Pivot Aneurysm Clip *17-7PH*	Unsafe 1	1.5	
R. Spetzler Titanium Aneurysm Clip *for Permanent Occlusion, 5-mm Fenestrated Bayonet* *11-mm blade length (M-9248), Titanium alloy* *Allegiance Healthcare Corporation, V. Mueller* *Neuro/Spine, San Carlos, CA*	Safe	1.5, 3	
R. Spetzler Titanium Aneurysm Clip *for Permanent Occlusion, 5-mm Fenestrated Straight* *12-mm blade length (M-9227), Titanium alloy* *Allegiance Healthcare Corporation, V. Mueller* *Neuro/Spine, San Carlos, CA*	Safe	1.5, 3	
R. Spetzler Titanium Aneurysm Clip for *Permanent Occlusion* *Mini 40 degree Side* *5-mm blade length (M-9450), Titanium alloy* *Allegiance Healthcare Corporation, V. Mueller* *Neuro/Spine, San Carlos, CA*	Safe	1.5, 3	
R. Spetzler Titanium Aneurysm Clip for *Permanent Occlusion* *Standard Bayonet* *12-mm blade length (M-9152), Titanium alloy* *Allegiance Healthcare Corporation, V. Mueller* *Neuro/Spine, San Carlos, CA*	Safe	1.5, 3	

Object	Status	Field Strength (T)	Reference
R. Spetzler Titanium Aneurysm Clip *for Permanent Occlusion* *Standard Straight* *15-mm blade length (M-9113), Titanium alloy* *Allegiance Healthcare Corporation, V. Mueller* *Neuro/Spine, San Carlos, CA*	Safe	1.5, 3	
Scoville Aneurysm Clip, EN58J *Downs Surgical, Inc., Decatur, GA*	Safe	1.5	
Slim-Line Aneurysm Clip *Fenestrated Straight, 4-mm opening* *6-mm blade, MP35N* *Codman, www.depuysynthes.com*	Safe	1.5, 3	
Spetzler Pure Titanium Aneurysm Clip *Model C-2200, straight, 5-mm blade* *C.P. Titanium* *NMT Neurosciences, Duluth, Georgia*	Safe	1.5, 3	82
Spetzler Pure Titanium Aneurysm Clip *Model C-2203, straight, 11-mm blade* *C.P. Titanium* *NMT Neurosciences, Duluth, Georgia*	Safe	1.5, 3	82
Spetzler Pure Titanium Aneurysm Clip *Model C-2212, curved, 7-mm blade* *C.P. Titanium* *NMT Neurosciences, Duluth, Georgia*	Safe	1.5, 3	82
Spetzler Pure Titanium Aneurysm Clip *Model C-2214, curved, 11-mm blade* *C.P. Titanium* *NMT Neurosciences, Duluth, Georgia*	Safe	1.5, 3	82
Spetzler Pure Titanium Aneurysm Clip *Model C-2224, straight, 11-mm/3.5-mm fenestrated blade* *C.P. Titanium* *NMT Neurosciences, Duluth, Georgia*	Safe	1.5, 3	82
Spetzler Pure Titanium Aneurysm Clip *Model C-2526, straight, 11-mm blade* *C.P. Titanium* *NMT Neurosciences, Duluth, Georgia*	Safe	1.5, 3	82
Spetzler Pure Titanium Aneurysm Clip *straight, 9-mm blade* *C. P. Titanium* *Elekta Instruments, Atlanta, GA*	Safe	1.5, 3	82
Spetzler Titanium Aneurysm Clip *straight, 13-mm blade, double turn* *C.P. Titanium* *Elekta Instruments, Inc., Atlanta, GA*	Safe	1.5	68

Object	Status	Field Strength (T)	Reference
Spetzler Titanium Aneurysm Clip *straight, 13-mm blade, single turn* *C.P. Titanium* *Elekta Instruments, Inc., Atlanta, GA*	Safe	1.5, 3	68, 82
Spetzler Titanium Aneurysm Clip *straight, 9-mm blade, double turn* *C.P. Titanium* *Elekta Instruments, Inc., Atlanta, GA*	Safe	1.5	68
Spetzler Titanium Aneurysm Clip *straight, 9-mm blade, single turn* *C.P. Titanium* *Elekta Instruments, Inc., Atlanta, GA*	Safe	1.5, 3	68, 82
Stevens Aneurysm Clip, silver alloy	Safe	0.15	6
Sugita Aneurysm Clip, Elgiloy *Downs Surgical, Inc., Decatur, GA*	Safe	1.5	
Sugita Aneurysm Clip, Elgiloy, Fenestrated *Mizuho America, Inc., www.mizuho.com*	Safe	1.5, 3	82
Sugita Aneurysm Clip *for Permanent Occlusion* *Mizuho America Inc., www.mizuho.com*	Conditional 8	1.5, 3	
Sugita Titanium Aneurysm Clip *mini temporary* *angled, 5-mm blade, Titanium alloy* *Mizuho America, Inc., www.mizuho.com*	Safe	1.5	
Sugita Titanium Aneurysm Clip *mini temporary* *straight large, 6-mm blade, Titanium alloy* *Mizuho America, Inc., www.mizuho.com*	Safe	1.5	
Sugita Titanium Aneurysm Clip *mini temporary* *straight slim, 6-mm blade, Titanium alloy* *Mizuho America, Inc., www.mizuho.com*	Safe	1.5	
Sugita Titanium Aneurysm Clip *mini, angled, 5-mm blade, Titanium alloy* *Mizuho America, Inc., www.mizuho.com*	Safe	1.5	
Sugita Titanium Aneurysm Clip *mini, angled, 7-mm blade, Titanium alloy* *Mizuho America, Inc., www.mizuho.com*	Safe	1.5	
Sugita Titanium Aneurysm Clip *mini, bayonet, 5-mm blade, Titanium alloy* *Mizuho America, Inc., www.mizuho.com*	Safe	1.5	
Sugita Titanium Aneurysm Clip *mini, curved slim, 5.2-mm blade, Titanium alloy* *Mizuho America, Inc., www.mizuho.com*	Safe	1.5	

Object	Status	Field Strength (T)	Reference
Sugita Titanium Aneurysm Clip *mini, curved slim, 6.7-mm blade, Titanium alloy* *Mizuho America, Inc., www.mizuho.com*	Safe	1.5	
Sugita Titanium Aneurysm Clip *mini, curved slim, 8.2-mm blade, Titanium alloy* *Mizuho America, Inc., www.mizuho.com*	Safe	1.5	
Sugita Titanium Aneurysm Clip *mini, curved, 4.5-mm blade* *Titanium alloy* *Mizuho America, Inc., www.mizuho.com*	Safe	1.5	
Sugita Titanium Aneurysm Clip *mini, curved, 5.5-mm blade* *Titanium alloy* *Mizuho America, Inc., www.mizuho.com*	Safe	1.5	
Sugita Titanium Aneurysm Clip *mini, curved, 5-mm blade, Titanium alloy* *Mizuho America, Inc., www.mizuho.com*	Safe	1.5	
Sugita Titanium Aneurysm Clip *mini, side curved, 7-mm blade, Titanium alloy* *Mizuho America, Inc., www.mizuho.com*	Safe	1.5	
Sugita Titanium Aneurysm Clip *mini, straight large, 6-mm blade, Titanium alloy* *Mizuho America, Inc., www.mizuho.com*	Safe	1.5	
Sugita Titanium Aneurysm Clip *mini, straight slim, 4-mm blade, Titanium alloy* *Mizuho America, Inc., www.mizuho.com*	Safe	1.5	
Sugita Titanium Aneurysm Clip *mini, straight slim, 6-mm blade, Titanium alloy* *Mizuho America, Inc., www.mizuho.com*	Safe	1.5	
Sugita Titanium Aneurysm Clip *mini, straight small, 4-mm blade, Titanium alloy* *Mizuho America, Inc., www.mizuho.com*	Safe	1.5	
Sugita Titanium Aneurysm Clip *standard* *1/4 curved, 11-mm blade, Titanium alloy* *Mizuho America, Inc., www.mizuho.com*	Safe	1.5	
Sugita Titanium Aneurysm Clip *standard* *1/4 curved, large, 8.6-mm blade, Titanium alloy* *Mizuho America, Inc., www.mizuho.com*	Safe	1.5	
Sugita Titanium Aneurysm Clip *standard* *1/4 curved, small, 7.6-mm blade, Titanium alloy* *Mizuho America, Inc., www.mizuho.com*	Safe	1.5	

Object	Status	Field Strength (T)	Reference
Sugita Titanium Aneurysm Clip *standard* *45 degree curved, large, 10-mm blade, Titanium alloy* *Mizuho America, Inc., www.mizuho.com*	Safe	1.5	
Sugita Titanium Aneurysm Clip *standard* *45 degree curved, medium, 7.5-mm blade, Titanium alloy* *Mizuho America, Inc., www.mizuho.com*	Safe	1.5	
Sugita Titanium Aneurysm Clip *standard* *45 degree curved, small, 5-mm blade, Titanium alloy* *Mizuho America, Inc., www.mizuho.com*	Safe	1.5	
Sugita Titanium Aneurysm Clip *standard* *angled, 12-mm blade, Titanium alloy* *Mizuho America, Inc., www.mizuho.com*	Safe	1.5	
Sugita Titanium Aneurysm Clip *standard* *angled, 8-mm blade, Titanium alloy* *Mizuho America, Inc., www.mizuho.com*	Safe	1.5	
Sugita Titanium Aneurysm Clip *standard* *bayonet large, 12-mm blade, Titanium alloy* *Mizuho America, Inc., www.mizuho.com*	Safe	1.5	
Sugita Titanium Aneurysm Clip *standard* *bayonet small, 10-mm blade, Titanium alloy* *Mizuho America, Inc., www.mizuho.com*	Safe	1.5	
Sugita Titanium Aneurysm Clip *standard* *bayonet, 7-mm blade, Titanium alloy* *Mizuho America, Inc., www.mizuho.com*	Safe	1.5	
Sugita Titanium Aneurysm Clip *standard* *curved (155 g), 9-mm blade, Titanium alloy* *Mizuho America, Inc., www.mizuho.com*	Safe	1.5	
Sugita Titanium Aneurysm Clip *standard* *curved (160 g), 9-mm blade, Titanium alloy* *Mizuho America, Inc., www.mizuho.com*	Safe	1.5	
Sugita Titanium Aneurysm Clip *standard* *for permanent occlusion* *45 degree angled, 19-mm* *serrated blade, Titanium alloy* *Mizuho America, Inc., www.mizuho.com*	Safe	1.5, 3	82

Object	Status	Field Strength (T)	Reference
Sugita Titanium Aneurysm Clip *standard* *J-angled, large, 9-mm blade, Titanium alloy* *Mizuho America, Inc., www.mizuho.com*	Safe	1.5	
Sugita Titanium Aneurysm Clip *standard* *J-angled, medium, 7.5-mm blade, Titanium alloy* *Mizuho America, Inc., www.mizuho.com*	Safe	1.5	
Sugita Titanium Aneurysm Clip *standard* *J-angled, small, 6-mm blade, Titanium alloy* *Mizuho America, Inc., www.mizuho.com*	Safe	1.5	
Sugita Titanium Aneurysm Clip *standard* *L-angled, large, 10-mm blade, Titanium alloy* *Mizuho America, Inc., www.mizuho.com*	Safe	1.5	
Sugita Titanium Aneurysm Clip *standard* *L-angled, medium, 7.5-mm blade, Titanium alloy* *Mizuho America, Inc., www.mizuho.com*	Safe	1.5	
Sugita Titanium Aneurysm Clip *standard* *L-angled, small, 5-mm blade, Titanium alloy* *Mizuho America, Inc., www.mizuho.com*	Safe	1.5	
Sugita Titanium Aneurysm Clip *standard* *L-curved, large, 10-mm blade, Titanium alloy* *Mizuho America, Inc., www.mizuho.com*	Safe	1.5	
Sugita Titanium Aneurysm Clip *standard* *L-curved, small, 7.5-mm blade, Titanium alloy* *Mizuho America, Inc., www.mizuho.com*	Safe	1.5	
Sugita Titanium Aneurysm Clip *standard* *side angled, 12-mm blade, Titanium alloy* *Mizuho America, Inc., www.mizuho.com*	Safe	1.5	
Sugita Titanium Aneurysm Clip *standard* *side angled, 8-mm blade, Titanium alloy* *Mizuho America, Inc., www.mizuho.com*	Safe	1.5	
Sugita Titanium Aneurysm Clip *standard* *side curved bayonet, 8.5-mm blade, Titanium alloy* *Mizuho America, Inc., www.mizuho.com*	Safe	1.5	

Object	Status	Field Strength (T)	Reference
Sugita Titanium Aneurysm Clip *standard* *side curved, 9-mm blade, Titanium alloy* *Mizuho America, Inc., www.mizuho.com*	Safe	1.5	
Sugita Titanium Aneurysm Clip *standard* *slight curved bayonet, 12-mm blade, Titanium alloy* *Mizuho America, Inc., www.mizuho.com*	Safe	1.5	
Sugita Titanium Aneurysm Clip *standard* *slightly angled, 8-mm blade, Titanium alloy* *Mizuho America, Inc., www.mizuho.com*	Safe	1.5	
Sugita Titanium Aneurysm Clip *standard* *slightly curved (165), 11-mm blade, Titanium alloy* *Mizuho America, Inc., www.mizuho.com*	Safe	1.5	
Sugita Titanium Aneurysm Clip *standard* *slightly curved (170), 11-mm blade, Titanium alloy* *Mizuho America, Inc., www.mizuho.com*	Safe	1.5	
Sugita Titanium Aneurysm Clip *standard* *slightly curved, 18-mm blade, Titanium alloy* *Mizuho America, Inc., www.mizuho.com*	Safe	1.5	
Sugita Titanium Aneurysm Clip *standard* *slightly curved, 9-mm blade, Titanium alloy* *Mizuho America, Inc., www.mizuho.com*	Safe	1.5	
Sugita Titanium Aneurysm Clip *standard* *slightly curved, small, 14-mm blade, Titanium alloy* *Mizuho America, Inc., www.mizuho.com*	Safe	1.5	
Sugita Titanium Aneurysm Clip *standard* *small curved, 9-mm blade, Titanium alloy* *Mizuho America, Inc., www.mizuho.com*	Safe	1.5	
Sugita Titanium Aneurysm Clip *standard* *staight (small), 12-mm blade, Titanium alloy* *Mizuho America, Inc., www.mizuho.com*	Safe	1.5	
Sugita Titanium Aneurysm Clip *standard* *straight large, 18-mm blade, Titanium alloy* *Mizuho America, Inc., www.mizuho.com*	Safe	1.5	

Object	Status	Field Strength (T)	Reference
Sugita Titanium Aneurysm Clip *standard* *straight medium, 15-mm blade, Titanium alloy* *Mizuho America, Inc., www.mizuho.com*	Safe	1.5	
Sugita Titanium Aneurysm Clip *standard* *straight, large, 10-mm blade, Titanium alloy* *Mizuho America, Inc., www.mizuho.com*	Safe	1.5	
Sugita Titanium Aneurysm Clip *standard* *straight, small, 7-mm blade, Titanium alloy* *Mizuho America, Inc., www.mizuho.com*	Safe	1.5	
Sugita Titanium Aneurysm Clip *temporary* *bayonet, 7-mm blade, Titanium alloy* *Mizuho America, Inc., www.mizuho.com*	Safe	1.5	
Sugita Titanium Aneurysm Clip *temporary* *curved, 8-mm blade, Titanium alloy* *Mizuho America, Inc., www.mizuho.com*	Safe	1.5	
Sugita Titanium Aneurysm Clip *temporary* *slightly curved, 11-mm blade, Titanium alloy* *Mizuho America, Inc., www.mizuho.com*	Safe	1.5	
Sugita Titanium Aneurysm Clip *temporary* *straight large, 10-mm blade, Titanium alloy* *Mizuho America, Inc., www.mizuho.com*	Safe	1.5	
Sugita Titanium Aneurysm Clip *temporary* *straight small, 7-mm blade, Titanium alloy* *Mizuho America, Inc., www.mizuho.com*	Safe	1.5	
Sugita Titanium Aneurysm Clip II *for Permanent Occlusion* *Mizuho America Inc., www.mizuho.com*	Conditional 8	1.5, 3	
Sugita, AVM Micro Clip *Aneurysm Clip, Elgiloy* *Mizuho America, Inc., www.mizuho.com*	Safe	1.5	
Sugita, Bent, Mini Aneurysm Clip *for temporary occlusion, Elgiloy* *Mizuho America, Inc., www.mizuho.com*	Safe	1.5	
Sugita, Bent, Standard Aneurysm Clip *for temporary occlusion, Elgiloy* *Mizuho America, Inc., www.mizuho.com*	Safe	1.5	

Object	Status	Field Strength (T)	Reference
Sugita, Sideward CVD Bayonet, standard *Aneurysm Clip for permanent occlusion* *Mizuho America, Inc., www.mizuho.com*	Safe	1.5	
Sugita, Straight, Large *Aneurysm Clip for permanent occlusion, Elgiloy* *Mizuho America, Inc., www.mizuho.com*	Safe	1.5	
Sugita *Fenestrated Large Fujita* *Blade Deflected Type* *Aneurysm Clip for permanent occlusion* *angled, 10-mm serrated blade, Elgiloy* *Mizuho America, Inc., www.mizuho.com*	Safe	1.5, 3	82
Sugita *Fenestrated large, bent* *Aneurysm Clip* *for permanent occlusion, Elgiloy* *Mizuho America, Inc., www.mizuho.com*	Safe	1.5	
Sugita *Large Aneurysm Clip for* *permanent occlusion* *straight, 21-mm serrated blade, Elgiloy* *Mizuho America, Inc., www.mizuho.com*	Safe	1.5, 3	82
Sugita *Long Aneurysm Clip for permanent occlusion* *straight, 19-mm nonserration blade, Elgiloy* *Mizuho America, Inc., www.mizuho.com*	Safe	1.5, 3	82
Sugita *Standard bent Aneurysm Clip* *8-mm blade, Elgiloy* *Mizuho America, Inc., www.mizuho.com*	Safe	1.5, 3	82
Sugita *Standard curved Aneurysm Clip* *6-mm blade, Elgiloy* *Mizuho America, Inc., www.mizuho.com*	Safe	1.5, 3	82
Sugita *Temporary Mini Aneurysm Clip* *bent, 7-mm blade, Elgiloy* *Mizuho America, Inc., www.mizuho.com*	Safe	1.5, 3	82
Sugita *Temporary standard straight* *Aneurysm Clip, 7-mm blade, Elgiloy* *Mizuho America, Inc., www.mizuho.com*	Safe	1.5, 3	82
Sundt AVM Micro Aneurysm Clip System *MP35N* *Codman, www.depuysynthes.com*	Conditional 6	3	

Object	Status	Field Strength (T)	Reference
Sundt AVM Micro CLIP *# 3, MP35N* *Codman, www.depuysynthes.com*	Safe	1.5, 3	
Sundt AVM Micro CLIP *# 4, MP35N* *Codman, www.depuysynthes.com*	Safe	1.5, 3	
Sundt AVM Micro CLIP *# 5, MP35N* *Codman, www.depuysynthes.com*	Safe	1.5, 3	
Sundt AVM, Micro Clip *Aneurysm Clip, MP35N* *Codman, www.depuysynthes.com*	Safe	1.5	
Sundt Slim-Line Aneurysm Clip *# 6, Bayonet, MP35N* *Codman, www.depuysynthes.com*	Safe	1.5, 3	
Sundt Slim-Line Aneurysm Clip *# 6, Forward Angle, MP35N* *Codman, www.depuysynthes.com*	Safe	1.5, 3	
Sundt Slim-Line Aneurysm Clip *Fenestrated Bayonet* *Straight, 6-mm opening* *15-mm blade, MP35N* *Codman, www.depuysynthes.com*	Safe	1.5, 3	
Sundt Slim-Line Aneurysm Clip *Fenestrated Straight* *4-mm opening, 24-mm blade, MP35N* *Codman, www.depuysynthes.com*	Safe	1.5, 3	
Sundt Slim-Line Aneurysm Clip *Sharp Right Angle* *12-mm blade, MP35N* *Codman, www.depuysynthes.com*	Safe	1.5, 3	
Sundt Slim-Line Mini Aneurysm Clip *# 6, Right Angle, MP35N* *Codman, www.depuysynthes.com*	Safe	1.5, 3	
Sundt Slim-Line Mini Aneurysm Clip *# 6, Straight, MP35N* *Codman, www.depuysynthes.com*	Safe	1.5, 3	
Sundt Slim-Line Mini Aneurysm Clip *# 7, Right Angle, MP35N* *Codman, www.depuysynthes.com*	Safe	1.5, 3	
Sundt Slim-Line Mini Aneurysm Clip *also known as Slimline, MP35N* *Codman, www.depuysynthes.com*	Conditional 6	3	

Object	Status	Field Strength (T)	Reference
Sundt Slim-Line Temporary Vessel Aneurysm Clip *also known as Slimline, MP35N* *Codman, www.depuysynthes.com*	Conditional 6	3	
Sundt Slim-Line, Graft Clip *Aneurysm Clip, MP35N* *Codman, www.depuysynthes.com*	Safe	1.5	
Sundt Slim-Line, Temporary Aneurysm Clip *10-mm blade, MP35N* *Codman, www.depuysynthes.com*	Safe	1.5	
Sundt-Kees Multi-Angle *Aneurysm Clip, 17-7PH* *Downs Surgical, Inc., Decatur, GA*	Unsafe 1	1.5	
Sundt-Kees Slim-Line Aneurysm Clip *also known as Slimline* *30 Degree Forward Angle, MP35N* *Codman, www.depuysynthes.com*	Conditional 6	3	
Sundt-Kees Slim-Line Aneurysm Clip *also known as Slimline* *30 Degree Forward Curve, MP35N* *Codman, www.depuysynthes.com*	Conditional 6	3	
Sundt-Kees Slim-Line Aneurysm Clip *also known as Slimline* *Bayonet, 30 Degree Curved Forward-Left, MP35N* *Codman, www.depuysynthes.com*	Conditional 6	3	
Sundt-Kees Slim-Line Aneurysm Clip *also known as Slimline* *Bayonet, 30 Degree Curved Forward-Right, MP35N* *Codman, www.depuysynthes.com*	Conditional 6	3	
Sundt-Kees Slim-Line Aneurysm Clip *also known as Slimline* *Bayonet, Straight, MP35N* *Codman, www.depuysynthes.com*	Conditional 6	3	
Sundt-Kees Slim-Line Aneurysm Clip *also known as Slimline* *Curved, MP35N* *Codman, www.depuysynthes.com*	Conditional 6	3	
Sundt-Kees Slim-Line Aneurysm Clip *also known as Slimline* *Fenestrated 45 Degree Angle, 6-mm Opening, MP35N* *Codman, www.depuysynthes.com*	Conditional 6	3	
Sundt-Kees Slim-Line Aneurysm Clip *also known as Slimline* *Fenestrated 45 Degree Angle* *4-mm Opening, 30 Degree, MP35N* *Codman, www.depuysynthes.com*	Conditional 6	3	

Object	Status	Field Strength (T)	Reference
Sundt-Kees Slim-Line Aneurysm Clip *also known as Slimline* *Fenestrated 90 Degree Angle, 4-mm Opening, MP35N* *Codman, www.depuysynthes.com*	Conditional 6	3	
Sundt-Kees Slim-Line Aneurysm Clip *also known as Slimline* *Fenestrated 90 Degree Angle, 6-mm Opening, MP35N* *Codman, www.depuysynthes.com*	Conditional 6	3	
Sundt-Kees Slim-Line Aneurysm Clip *also known as Slimline* *Fenestrated Bayonet Straight, 6-mm Opening, MP35N* *Codman, www.depuysynthes.com*	Conditional 6	3	
Sundt-Kees Slim-Line Aneurysm Clip *also known as Slimline* *Fenestrated Straight, 3-mm Extended Tandem, 6-mm,* *MP35N* *Codman, www.depuysynthes.com*	Conditional 6	3	
Sundt-Kees Slim-Line Aneurysm Clip *also known as Slimline* *Fenestrated Straight, 4-mm Opening, MP35N* *Codman, www.depuysynthes.com*	Conditional 6	3	
Sundt-Kees Slim-Line Aneurysm Clip *also known as Slimline* *Fenestrated Straight, 5-mm Extended Tandem, 6-mm,* *MP35N* *Codman, www.depuysynthes.com*	Conditional 6	3	
Sundt-Kees Slim-Line Aneurysm Clip *also known as Slimline* *Fenestrated Straight, 6-mm Opening, MP35N* *Codman, www.depuysynthes.com*	Conditional 6	3	
Sundt-Kees Slim-Line Aneurysm Clip *also known as Slimline* *Graft, 4-mm Diameter, MP35N* *Codman, www.depuysynthes.com*	Conditional 6	3	
Sundt-Kees Slim-Line Aneurysm Clip *also known as Slimline* *Reinforcing 30 Degree Angle, 6-mm Wide, MP35N* *Codman, www.depuysynthes.com*	Conditional 6	3	
Sundt-Kees Slim-Line Aneurysm Clip *also known as Slimline* *Reinforcing 60 Degree Angle, 6-mm Wide, MP35N* *Codman, www.depuysynthes.com*	Conditional 6	3	
Sundt-Kees Slim-Line Aneurysm Clip *also known as Slimline* *Reinforcing Zero Degree Angle, 6-mm Wide, MP35N* *Codman, www.depuysynthes.com*	Conditional 6	3	

Object	Status	Field Strength (T)	Reference
Sundt-Kees Slim-Line Aneurysm Clip *also known as Slimline* *Right Angle, MP35N* *Codman, www.depuysynthes.com*	Conditional 6	3	
Sundt-Kees Slim-Line Aneurysm Clip *also known as Slimline* *Sharp Right Angle, MP35N* *Codman, www.depuysynthes.com*	Conditional 6	3	
Sundt-Kees Slim-Line Aneurysm Clip *also known as Slimline* *Sideward Angle, MP35N* *Codman, www.depuysynthes.com*	Conditional 6	3	
Sundt-Kees Slim-Line Aneurysm Clip *also known as Slimline* *Slightly curved, MP35N* *Codman, www.depuysynthes.com*	Conditional 6	3	
Sundt-Kees Slim-Line Aneurysm Clip *also known as Slimline* *Straight, MP35N* *Codman, www.depuysynthes.com*	Conditional 6	3	
Sundt-Kees Slim-Line Aneurysm Clip *also known as Slimline* *Super Bayonet, MP35N* *Codman, www.depuysynthes.com*	Conditional 6	3	
Sundt-Kees Slim-Line *Fenestrated, Aneurysm Clip* *9-mm blade, MP35N* *Codman, www.depuysynthes.com*	Safe	1.5	
Sundt-Kees, Slim-Line *9-mm blade MP35N, Aneurysm Clip* *Codman, www.depuysynthes.com*	Safe	1.5	
Vari-Angle Aneurysm Clip, 17-7PH *Codman, www.depuysynthes.com*	Unsafe 1	1.5	
Vari-Angle McFadden Aneurysm Clip *MP35N* *Codman, www.depuysynthes.com*	Safe	1.5	
Vari-Angle Micro Aneurysm Clip, 17-7PH *Codman, www.depuysynthes.com*	Unsafe 1	1.5	
Vari-Angle Spring Aneurysm Clip, 17-7PH *Codman, www.depuysynthes.com*	Unsafe 1	1.5	
Yasargil Aneurysm Clip *All "FD" Models, per the manufacturer* *Aesculap, Inc., www.aesculapusa.com*	Unsafe 1	1.5	

Object	Status	Field Strength (T)	Reference
Yasargil Aneurysm Clip *All "FE" Models per the manufacturer* *Aesculap, Inc., www.aesculapusa.com*	Safe	3	
Yasargil Aneurysm Clip *All "FT" Models, per the manufacturer* *Aesculap, Inc., www.aesculapusa.com*	Safe	3	
Yasargil Aneurysm Clip, 316L SS *Aesculap, Inc., www.aesculapusa.com*	Safe	1.5	
Yasargil Aneurysm Clip, Model FD *Aesculap, Inc., www.aesculapusa.com*	Unsafe 1	1.5	
Yasargil Aneurysm Clip, Model FE 720T *mini, permanent, 7-mm blade, Titanium alloy* *Aesculap, Inc., www.aesculapusa.com*	Safe	1.5	
Yasargil Aneurysm Clip, Model FE 740T *standard, permanent, 7-mm blade, Titanium alloy* *Aesculap, Inc., www.aesculapusa.com*	Safe	1.5	
Yasargil Aneurysm Clip, Model FE 748 *standard, 9-mm blade, bayonet* *Phynox* *Aesculap, Inc., www.aesculapusa.com*	Safe	1.5	
Yasargil Aneurysm Clip, Model FE 750 *9-mm blade, straight* *Phynox* *Aesculap, Inc., www.aesculapusa.com*	Safe	1.5	
Yasargil Aneurysm Clip, Model FE 750T *standard, permanent, 9-mm blade* *Titanium alloy* *Aesculap, Inc., www.aesculapusa.com*	Safe	1.5	
Yasargil Aneurysm Clip, Model FE *Aesculap, Inc., www.aesculapusa.com*	Safe	1.5	
Yasargil Aneurysm Clip, Standard Clip, Permanent *FT790D, Titanium, blade length 20-mm* *Aesculap, Inc., www.Aesculap.com*	Conditional 5	3	
Yasargil Mini Clip, Titanium *Aneurysm Clip, Model FT728T* *bayonet, 7-mm blade, Titanium alloy* *Aesculap, Inc., www.aesculapusa.com*	Safe	1.5, 3	82
Yasargil Phynox Aneurysm Clip *All FE Models* *Aesculap, Inc., www.aesculapusa.com*	Safe	3	
Yasargil Phynox Aneurysm Clip, Long Clip *Permanent, FE863K, blade length 40-mm* *Aesculap, Inc., www.Aesculap.com*	Conditional 5	3	

Object	Status	Field Strength (T)	Reference
Yasargil Phynox Aneurysm Clip *Long Clip, Permanent, FE863K* *Aesculap, Inc., www.Aesculap.com*	Conditional 6	3	
Yasargil, Standard Aneurysm Clip Titanium *Model FT740T, straight, 7-mm blade* *Titanium alloy* *Aesculap, Inc., www.aesculapusa.com*	Safe	1.5, 3	82
Yasargil, Standard Aneurysm Clip Titanium *Model FT758T, bayonet, 12-mm blade* *Titanium alloy* *Aesculap, Inc., www.aesculapusa.com*	Safe	1.5, 3	82
Yasargil, Standard Aneurysm Clip Titanium *Model FT760T, 11-mm blade* *Titanium alloy* *Aesculap, Inc., www.aesculapusa.com*	Safe	1.5, 3	82
Yasargil, Standard Aneurysm Clip Titanium *Model FT790T, straight, 20-mm blade* *Titanium alloy* *Aesculap, Inc., www.aesculapusa.com*	Safe	1.5, 3	82
Yasargil, Standard Aneurysm Clip, Permanent *Model FE660K* *straight, 12-mm blade* *Phynox, SN FYA21* *Aesculap, Inc., www.aesculapusa.com*	Safe	3	
Yasargil, Standard Aneurysm Clip, Permanent *Model FE660K* *straight, 12-mm blade* *Phynox, SN FYA46* *Aesculap, Inc., www.aesculapusa.com*	Safe	3	
Yasargil, Standard Aneurysm Clip, Permanent *Model FE662K* *angled, 10-mm blade* *Phynox, SN FKJ41* *Aesculap, Inc., www.aesculapusa.com*	Safe	3	
Yasargil, Standard Aneurysm Clip, Permanent *Model FE662K* *angled, 10-mm blade* *Phynox, SN FUJ53* *Aesculap, Inc., www.aesculapusa.com*	Safe	3	
Yasargil, Standard Aneurysm Clip, Permanent *Model FE840K* *straight, 25-mm blade* *Phynox, SN FYR65* *Aesculap, Inc., www.aesculapusa.com*	Safe	3	

Object	Status	Field Strength (T)	Reference
Yasargil, Standard Aneurysm Clip, Permanent *Model FE840K* *straight, 25-mm blade* *Phynox, SN FYS01* *Aesculap, Inc., www.aesculapusa.com*	Safe	3	
Yasargil, Standard Aneurysm Clip, Permanent *Model FT650T* *straight, 9-mm blade* *Titanium alloy, SN CQY63* *Aesculap, Inc., www.aesculapusa.com*	Safe	3	
Yasargil, Standard Aneurysm Clip, Permanent *Model FT650T* *straight, 9-mm blade* *Titanium alloy, SN CQY83* *Aesculap, Inc., www.aesculapusa.com*	Safe	3	
Yasargil, Standard Aneurysm Clip, Permanent *Model FT662T* *angled, 10-mm blade* *Titanium alloy, SN CLU37* *Aesculap, Inc., www.aesculapusa.com*	Safe	3	
Yasargil, Standard Aneurysm Clip, Permanent *Model FT662T* *angled, 10-mm blade* *Titanium alloy, SN CLU54* *Aesculap, Inc., www.aesculapusa.com*	Safe	3	
Yasargil, Standard Aneurysm Clip, Permanent *Model FTD790D* *straight, 20-mm blade* *Titanium alloy, SN CTW58* *Aesculap, Inc., www.aesculapusa.com*	Safe	3	
Yasargil, Standard Aneurysm Clip, Permanent *Model FTD790D* *straight, 20-mm blade* *Titanium alloy, SN CTW73* *Aesculap, Inc., www.aesculapusa.com*	Safe	3	
Yasargil, Standard Aneurysm Clip *Model FE750* *straight, 9-mm blade, Phynox* *Aesculap, Inc., www.aesculapusa.com*	Safe	1.5, 3	82
Yasargil, Standard Aneurysm Clip *Model FE780* *straight, 14-mm blade, Phynox* *Aesculap, Inc., www.aesculapusa.com*	Safe	1.5, 3	82

Object	Status	Field Strength (T)	Reference
Yasargil, Standard Aneurysm Clip *Model FE786* *curved, 15.3-mm blade, Phynox* *Aesculap, Inc., www.aesculapusa.com*	Safe	1.5, 3	82
Yasargil, Standard Aneurysm Clip *Model FE790K* *straight, 20-mm blade, Phynox* *Aesculap, Inc., www.aesculapusa.com*	Safe	1.5, 3	82
Yasargil, Standard Aneurysm Clip *Model FE798* *Bayonet, 20-mm blade, Phynox* *Aesculap, Inc., www.aesculapusa.com*	Safe	1.5, 3	82
Yasargil, Standard Aneurysm Clip *Model FE798* *Bayonet, 20-mm blade, Phynox* *Aesculap, Inc., www.aesculapusa.com*	Safe	1.5, 3	82
Yasargil, Standard Aneurysm Clip *Model FE887* *7-mm blade, Phynox* *Aesculap, Inc., www.aesculapusa.com*	Safe	1.5, 3	82
Yasargil Clip Standard Permanent *Aneurysm Clip, Phynox* *25-mm straight blade* *Peter Lazic Microsurgical, www.lazic.de/en/*	Conditional 6	3	
Yasargil Clip Standard Permanent *Aneurysm Clip, Phynox* *90 degree Angle* *5-mm, 7-mm, 10-mm* *Peter Lazic Microsurgical, www.lazic.de/en/*	Conditional 6	3	
Yasargil Clip Standard Permanent *Aneurysm Clip, Phynox* *Angle with Radius* *8-mm, 10-mm* *Peter Lazic Microsurgical, www.lazic.de/en/*	Conditional 6	3	
Yasargil Clip Standard Permanent *Aneurysm Clip, Phynox* *Bayonet 45 degree Angle* *5-mm, 7-mm, 9-mm, 11-mm* *Peter Lazic Microsurgical, www.lazic.de/en/*	Conditional 6	3	
Yasargil Clip Standard Permanent *Aneurysm Clip, Phynox* *Bayonet Angle, 5-mm* *2.5-mm, 3.5-mm, 4.5-mm* *Peter Lazic Microsurgical, www.lazic.de/en/*	Conditional 6	3	

Object	Status	Field Strength (T)	Reference
Yasargil Clip Standard Permanent *Aneurysm Clip, Phynox* *Bayonet Angle* *5-mm* *Peter Lazic Microsurgical, www.lazic.de/en/*	Conditional 6	3	
Yasargil Clip Standard Permanent *Aneurysm Clip, Phynox* *Bayonet* *7-mm, 10-mm, 12-mm, 17-mm, 20-mm* *Peter Lazic Microsurgical, www.lazic.de/en/*	Conditional 6	3	
Yasargil Clip Standard Permanent *Aneurysm Clip, Phynox* *Curved and Angle, 8-mm* *Peter Lazic Microsurgical, www.lazic.de/en/*	Conditional 6	3	
Yasargil Clip Standard Permanent *Aneurysm Clip, Phynox* *Curved, 7-mm, 9-mm, 11-mm, 15-mm, 17-mm* *Peter Lazic Microsurgical, www.lazic.de/en/*	Conditional 6	3	
Yasargil Clip Standard Permanent *Aneurysm Clip, Phynox* *Fenestrated 3.5-mm 45 degree Angle* *5-mm, 7-mm, 11-mm* *Peter Lazic Microsurgical, www.lazic.de/en/*	Conditional 6	3	
Yasargil Clip Standard Permanent *Aneurysm Clip, Phynox* *Fenestrated 3.5-mm 90 degree Angle* *5-mm, 7-mm, 11-mm* *Peter Lazic Microsurgical, www.lazic.de/en/*	Conditional 6	3	
Yasargil Clip Standard Permanent *Aneurysm Clip, Phynox* *Fenestrated 3.5-mm Straight* *3-mm, 4-mm, 5-mm, 7-mm, 9-mm, 12-mm* *Peter Lazic Microsurgical, www.lazic.de/en/*	Conditional 6	3	
Yasargil Clip Standard Permanent *Aneurysm Clip, Phynox* *Fenestrated 5-mm 45 degree Angle Opening Sideward* *Left, 5-mm, 7-mm* *Peter Lazic Microsurgical, www.lazic.de/en/*	Conditional 6	3	
Yasargil Clip Standard Permanent *Aneurysm Clip, Phynox* *Fenestrated 5-mm 45 degree Angle Opening Sideward* *Right, 5-mm, 7-mm* *Peter Lazic Microsurgical, www.lazic.de/en/*	Conditional 6	3	

Object	Status	Field Strength (T)	Reference
Yasargil Clip Standard Permanent *Aneurysm Clip, Phynox* *Fenestrated 5-mm 45 degree Angle* *5-mm, 7-mm, 11-mm* *Peter Lazic Microsurgical, www.lazic.de/en/*	Conditional 6	3	
Yasargil Clip Standard Permanent *Aneurysm Clip, Phynox* *Fenestrated 5-mm 90 degree Angle Jaw Curved Left* *5-mm, 7-mm, 10-mm* *Peter Lazic Microsurgical, www.lazic.de/en/*	Conditional 6	3	
Yasargil Clip Standard Permanent *Aneurysm Clip, Phynox* *Fenestrated 5-mm 90 degree Angle Jaw Curved Right* *5-mm, 7-mm, 10-mm* *Peter Lazic Microsurgical, www.lazic.de/en/*	Conditional 6	3	
Yasargil Clip Standard Permanent *Aneurysm Clip, Phynox* *Fenestrated 5-mm 90 degree Angle Opening Sideward Left* *5-mm, 7-mm* *Peter Lazic Microsurgical, www.lazic.de/en/*	Conditional 6	3	
Yasargil Clip Standard Permanent *Aneurysm Clip, Phynox* *Fenestrated 5-mm 90 degree Angle Opening Sideward Right* *5-mm, 7-mm* *Peter Lazic Microsurgical, www.lazic.de/en/*	Conditional 6	3	
Yasargil Clip Standard Permanent *Aneurysm Clip, Phynox* *Fenestrated 5-mm 90 degree Angle* *5-mm, 7-mm, 11-mm* *Peter Lazic Microsurgical, www.lazic.de/en/*	Conditional 6	3	
Yasargil Clip Standard Permanent *Aneurysm Clip, Phynox* *Fenestrated 5-mm Bayonet* *5-mm, 7-mm, 11-mm* *Peter Lazic Microsurgical, www.lazic.de/en/*	Conditional 6	3	
Yasargil Clip Standard Permanent *Aneurysm Clip, Phynox* *Fenestrated 5-mm Straight Opening Sideward Right* *5-mm, 7-mm, 10-mm* *Peter Lazic Microsurgical, www.lazic.de/en/*	Conditional 6	3	

Object	Status	Field Strength (T)	Reference
Yasargil Clip Standard Permanent *Aneurysm Clip, Phynox* *Fenestrated 5-mm Straight* *3-mm, 4-mm, 5-mm, 7-mm, 9-mm, 12-mm* *Peter Lazic Microsurgical, www.lazic.de/en/*	Conditional 6	3	
Yasargil Clip Standard Permanent *Aneurysm Clip, Phynox* *J Curved, 7-mm, 9-mm, 11-mm* *Peter Lazic Microsurgical, www.lazic.de/en/*	Conditional 6	3	
Yasargil Clip Standard Permanent *Aneurysm Clip, Phynox* *Mini Clip Angle and Curved* *5-mm* *Peter Lazic Microsurgical, www.lazic.de/en/*	Conditional 6	3	
Yasargil Clip Standard Permanent *Aneurysm Clip, Phynox* *Mini Clip Angle, 7-mm* *Peter Lazic Microsurgical, www.lazic.de/en/*	Conditional 6	3	
Yasargil Clip Standard Permanent *Aneurysm Clip, Phynox* *Mini Clip Bayonet, 4-mm, 7-mm* *Peter Lazic Microsurgical, www.lazic.de/en/*	Conditional 6	3	
Yasargil Clip Standard Permanent *Aneurysm Clip, Phynox* *Mini Clip Curved Narrow Jaw, 4-mm* *Peter Lazic Microsurgical, www.lazic.de/en/*	Conditional 6	3	
Yasargil Clip Standard Permanent *Aneurysm Clip, Phynox* *Mini Clip Curved, 4-mm, 5-mm* *Peter Lazic Microsurgical, www.lazic.de/en/*	Conditional 6	3	
Yasargil Clip Standard Permanent *Aneurysm Clip, Phynox* *Mini Clip Sideward Angle* *5-mm* *Peter Lazic Microsurgical, www.lazic.de/en/*	Conditional 6	3	
Yasargil Clip Standard Permanent *Aneurysm Clip, Phynox* *Mini Clip Sideward Curved* *6-mm* *Peter Lazic Microsurgical, www.lazic.de/en/*	Conditional 6	3	
Yasargil Clip Standard Permanent *Aneurysm Clip, Phynox* *Mini Clip Slightly Curved Narrow Jaw* *3-mm, 4-mm* *Peter Lazic Microsurgical, www.lazic.de/en/*	Conditional 6	3	

Object	Status	Field Strength (T)	Reference
Yasargil Clip Standard Permanent *Aneurysm Clip, Phynox* *Mini Clip Slightly Curved* *4-mm, 5-mm, 7-mm* *Peter Lazic Microsurgical, www.lazic.de/en/*	Conditional 6	3	
Yasargil Clip Standard Permanent *Aneurysm Clip, Phynox* *Mini Clip Straight Narrow Jaw* *3-mm, 5-mm* *Peter Lazic Microsurgical, www.lazic.de/en/*	Conditional 6	3	
Yasargil Clip Standard Permanent *Aneurysm Clip, Phynox* *Mini Clip Straight, 3-mm, 5-mm, 7-mm* *Peter Lazic Microsurgical, www.lazic.de/en/*	Conditional 6	3	
Yasargil Clip Standard Permanent *Aneurysm Clip, Phynox* *Sideward Angle, 7-mm, 11-mm* *Peter Lazic Microsurgical, www.lazic.de/en/*	Conditional 6	3	
Yasargil Clip Standard Permanent *Aneurysm Clip, Phynox* *Sideward Curved, 9-mm* *Peter Lazic Microsurgical, www.lazic.de/en/*	Conditional 6	3	
Yasargil Clip Standard Permanent *Aneurysm Clip, Phynox* *Slightly Curved* *7-mm, 9-mm, 11-mm, 15-mm, 17-mm, 20-mm* *Peter Lazic Microsurgical, www.lazic.de/en/*	Conditional 6	3	
Yasargil Clip Standard Permanent *Aneurysm Clip, Phynox* *Straight with Radius* *9-mm, 10-mm* *Peter Lazic Microsurgical, www.lazic.de*	Conditional 6	3	
Yasargil Clip Standard Permanent *Aneurysm Clip, Phynox* *Straight* *7-mm, 8-mm, 11-mm, 15-mm, 17-mm, 20-mm, 25-mm* *Peter Lazic Microsurgical, www.lazic.de/en/*	Conditional 6	3	
Yasargil Clip Standard Permanent *Aneurysm Clip, Phynox* *Tangential Angle* *13-mm* *Peter Lazic Microsurgical, www.lazic.de/en/*	Conditional 6	3	

Object	Status	Field Strength (T)	Reference
Yasargil T-Bar Aneurysm Clip *Permanent* *Model FE853K* *45 degree angle, 9-mm blade* *Phynox* *Aesculap, Inc., www.aesculapusa.com*	Safe	3	
Yasargil T-Bar Aneurysm Clip *Permanent* *Model FE856K* *90 degree angle, 13-mm blade* *Phynox* *Aesculap, Inc., www.aesculapusa.com*	Safe	3	
Yasargil T-Bar Aneurysm Clip *Permanent* *Model FT853T* *45 degree angle, 9-mm blade* *Titanium* *Aesculap, Inc., www.aesculapusa.com*	Safe	3	
Yasargil T-Bar Aneurysm Clip *Permanent* *Model FT856T* *90 degree angle, 13-mm blade* *Titanium* *Aesculap, Inc., www.aesculapusa.com*	Safe	3	
Yasargil Titanclip *Standard Permanent* *Aneurysm Clip, Titanium* *25-mm straight blade* *Peter Lazic Microsurgical, www.lazic.de/en/*	Conditional 6	3	
Yasargil Titanclip *Standard Permanent* *Aneurysm Clip, Titanium* *45 degree Angle* *5-mm, 7-mm, 9-mm, 11-mm* *Peter Lazic Microsurgical, www.lazic.de/en/*	Conditional 6	3	
Yasargil Titanclip *Standard Permanent* *Aneurysm Clip, Titanium* *90 degree Angle* *5-mm, 7-mm, 10-mm* *Peter Lazic Microsurgical, www.lazic.de/en/*	Conditional 6	3	
Yasargil Titanclip *Standard Permanent* *Aneurysm Clip, Titanium* *Angle with Radius* *8-mm, 10-mm* *Peter Lazic Microsurgical, www.lazic.de/en/*	Conditional 6	3	

Object	Status	Field Strength (T)	Reference
Yasargil Titanclip *Standard Permanent* *Aneurysm Clip, Titanium* *Bayonet Angle* *2.5-mm, 3.5-mm, 4.5-mm* *Peter Lazic Microsurgical, www.lazic.de/en/*	Conditional 6	3	
Yasargil Titanclip *Standard Permanent* *Aneurysm Clip, Titanium* *Bayonet Angle* *5-mm* *Peter Lazic Microsurgical, www.lazic.de/en/*	Conditional 6	3	
Yasargil Titanclip *Standard Permanent* *Aneurysm Clip, Titanium* *Bayonet* *7-mm, 10-mm, 12-mm, 17-mm, 20-mm* *Peter Lazic Microsurgical, www.lazic.de/en/*	Conditional 6	3	
Yasargil Titanclip *Standard Permanent* *Aneurysm Clip, Titanium* *Curved and Sideward Angle* *8-mm* *Peter Lazic Microsurgical, www.lazic.de/en/*	Conditional 6	3	
Yasargil Titanclip *Standard Permanent* *Aneurysm Clip, Titanium* *Curved* *7-mm, 9-mm, 11-mm, 15-mm, 17-mm* *Peter Lazic Microsurgical, www.lazic.de/en/*	Conditional 6	3	
Yasargil Titanclip *Standard Permanent* *Aneurysm Clip, Titanium* *Fenestrated 3.5-mm 45 degree Angle* *5-mm, 7-mm, 11-mm* *Peter Lazic Microsurgical, www.lazic.de/en/*	Conditional 6	3	
Yasargil Titanclip *Standard Permanent* *Aneurysm Clip, Titanium* *Fenestrated 3.5-mm 90 degree Angle* *5-mm, 7-mm, 11-mm* *Peter Lazic Microsurgical, www.lazic.de/en/*	Conditional 6	3	

Object	Status	Field Strength (T)	Reference
Yasargil Titanclip *Standard Permanent* *Aneurysm Clip, Titanium* *Fenestrated 3.5-mm Straight* *3-mm, 4-mm, 5-mm, 7-mm, 9-mm, 12-mm* *Peter Lazic Microsurgical, www.lazic.de/en/*	Conditional 6	3	
Yasargil Titanclip *Standard Permanent* *Aneurysm Clip, Titanium* *Fenestrated 45 degree Opening Sideward Left* *5-mm, 7-mm* *Peter Lazic Microsurgical, www.lazic.de/en/*	Conditional 6	3	
Yasargil Titanclip *Standard Permanent* *Aneurysm Clip, Titanium* *Fenestrated 45 degree Opening Sideward Right* *5-mm, 7-mm* *Peter Lazic Microsurgical, www.lazic.de/en/*	Conditional 6	3	
Yasargil Titanclip *Standard Permanent* *Aneurysm Clip, Titanium* *Fenestrated 5-mm 45 degree Angle* *5-mm, 7-mm, 11-mm* *Peter Lazic Microsurgical, www.lazic.de/en/*	Conditional 6	3	
Yasargil Titanclip *Standard Permanent* *Aneurysm Clip, Titanium* *Fenestrated 5-mm 90 degree Angle Jaw Curved Left* *5-mm, 7-mm, 10-mm* *Peter Lazic Microsurgical, www.lazic.de/en/*	Conditional 6	3	
Yasargil Titanclip *Standard Permanent* *Aneurysm Clip, Titanium* *Fenestrated 5-mm 90 degree Angle Jaw Curved Right* *5-mm, 7-mm, 10-mm* *Peter Lazic Microsurgical, www.lazic.de/en/*	Conditional 6	3	
Yasargil Titanclip *Standard Permanent* *Aneurysm Clip, Titanium* *Fenestrated 5-mm 90 degree Angle* *5-mm, 7-mm, 11-mm* *Peter Lazic Microsurgical, www.lazic.de/en/*	Conditional 6	3	

Object	Status	Field Strength (T)	Reference
Yasargil Titanclip *Standard Permanent* *Aneurysm Clip, Titanium* *Fenestrated 5-mm Bayonet* *5-mm, 7-mm, 11-mm* *Peter Lazic Microsurgical, www.lazic.de/en/*	Conditional 6	3	
Yasargil Titanclip *Standard Permanent* *Aneurysm Clip, Titanium* *Fenestrated 5-mm Straight Opening Sideward Right* *5-mm, 7-mm, 10-mm* *Peter Lazic Microsurgical, www.lazic.de/en/*	Conditional 6	3	
Yasargil Titanclip *Standard Permanent* *Aneurysm Clip, Titanium* *Fenestrated 5-mm Straight* *3-mm, 4-mm, 5-mm, 7-mm, 9-mm, 12-mm* *Peter Lazic Microsurgical, www.lazic.de/en/*	Conditional 6	3	
Yasargil Titanclip *Standard Permanent* *Aneurysm Clip, Titanium* *Fenestrated 90 degree Opening Sideward* *Left, 5-mm, 7-mm* *Peter Lazic Microsurgical, www.lazic.de/en/*	Conditional 6	3	
Yasargil Titanclip *Standard Permanent* *Aneurysm Clip, Titanium* *Fenestrated 90 degree Opening Sideward* *Right, 5-mm, 7-mm* *Peter Lazic Microsurgical, www.lazic.de/en/*	Conditional 6	3	
Yasargil Titanclip *Standard Permanent* *Aneurysm Clip, Titanium* *J Curved* *7-mm, 9-mm, 11-mm* *Peter Lazic Microsurgical, www.lazic.de/en/*	Conditional 6	3	
Yasargil Titanclip *Standard Permanent* *Aneurysm Clip, Titanium* *Mini Clip Angle and Curved, 5-mm* *Peter Lazic Microsurgical, www.lazic.de/en/*	Conditional 6	3	
Yasargil Titanclip *Standard Permanent* *Aneurysm Clip, Titanium* *Mini Clip Angle, 7-mm* *Peter Lazic Microsurgical, www.lazic.de/en/*	Conditional 6	3	

Object	Status	Field Strength (T)	Reference
Yasargil Titanclip *Standard Permanent* *Aneurysm Clip, Titanium* *Mini Clip Bayonet, 4-mm, 7-mm* *Peter Lazic Microsurgical, www.lazic.de/en/*	Conditional 6	3	
Yasargil Titanclip *Standard Permanent* *Aneurysm Clip, Titanium* *Mini Clip Curved Narrow Jaw, 4-mm* *Peter Lazic Microsurgical, www.lazic.de/en/*	Conditional 6	3	
Yasargil Titanclip *Standard Permanent* *Aneurysm Clip, Titanium* *Mini Clip Curved, 4-mm, 5-mm* *Peter Lazic Microsurgical, www.lazic.de/en/*	Conditional 6	3	
Yasargil Titanclip *Standard Permanent* *Aneurysm Clip, Titanium* *Mini Clip Sideward Angle, 5-mm* *Peter Lazic Microsurgical, www.lazic.de/en/*	Conditional 6	3	
Yasargil Titanclip *Standard Permanent* *Aneurysm Clip, Titanium* *Mini Clip Sideward Curved, 6-mm* *Peter Lazic Microsurgical, www.lazic.de/en/*	Conditional 6	3	
Yasargil Titanclip *Standard Permanent* *Aneurysm Clip, Titanium* *Mini Clip Slightly Curved Narrow Jaw, 3-mm, 4-mm* *Peter Lazic Microsurgical, www.lazic.de/en/*	Conditional 6	3	
Yasargil Titanclip *Standard Permanent* *Aneurysm Clip, Titanium* *Mini Clip Slightly Curved, 4-mm, 5-mm, 7-mm* *Peter Lazic Microsurgical, www.lazic.de/en/*	Conditional 6	3	
Yasargil Titanclip *Standard Permanent* *Aneurysm Clip, Titanium* *Mini Clip Straight Narrow Jaw, 3-mm, 5-mm* *Peter Lazic Microsurgical, www.lazic.de/en/*	Conditional 6	3	
Yasargil Titanclip *Standard Permanent* *Aneurysm Clip, Titanium* *Mini Clip Straight, 3-mm, 5-mm, 7-mm* *Peter Lazic Microsurgical, www.lazic.de/en/*	Conditional 6	3	

Object	Status	Field Strength (T)	Reference
Yasargil Titanclip *Standard Permanent* *Aneurysm Clip, Titanium* *Sideward Angle, 7-mm, 11-mm* *Peter Lazic Microsurgical, www.lazic.de/en/*	Conditional 6	3	
Yasargil Titanclip *Standard Permanent* *Aneurysm Clip, Titanium* *Sideward Curved, 9-mm* *Peter Lazic Microsurgical, www.lazic.de/en/*	Conditional 6	3	
Yasargil Titanclip *Standard Permanent* *Aneurysm Clip, Titanium* *Slightly Curved, 7-mm, 9-mm, 11-mm, 15-mm, 17-mm, 20-mm* *Peter Lazic Microsurgical, www.lazic.de/en/*	Conditional 6	3	
Yasargil Titanclip *Standard Permanent* *Aneurysm Clip, Titanium* *Straight with Radius, 9-mm, 11-mm* *Peter Lazic Microsurgical, www.lazic.de/en/*	Conditional 6	3	
Yasargil Titanclip *Standard Permanent* *Aneurysm Clip, Titanium* *Straight, 7-mm, 9-mm, 11-mm, 15-mm, 17-mm, 20-mm, 25-mm* *Peter Lazic Microsurgical, www.lazic.de/en/*	Conditional 6	3	
Yasargil Titanclip *Standard Permanent* *Aneurysm Clip, Titanium* *Tangential Angle, 13-mm* *Peter Lazic Microsurgical, www.lazic.de/en/*	Conditional 6	3	
Yasargil Titanium Aneurysm Clips *All FT Models* *Aesculap, Inc., www.aesculapusa.com*	Safe	3	

Biopsy Needles, Markers, and Devices

Object	Status	Field Strength (T)	Reference
Achieve Marker *CareFusion, www.carefusion.com*	Conditional 6	3	128
Adjustable, Automated Aspiration Biopsy Gun *10, 15, and 20-mm* *MD Tech, Watertown, MA*	Unsafe 1	1.5	7
Adjustable, Automated Biopsy Gun *6, 13, and 19-mm* *MD Tech, Watertown, MA*	Unsafe 1	1.5	7

Object	Status	Field Strength (T)	Reference
AOS Marker Seed *Alpha-Omega Services, Inc., Bellflower, CA*	Conditional 6	3	
ASAP 16, Automatic 16 G Core Biopsy System *19-cm length, 304 SS*	Unsafe 1	1.5	7
Aspiration Needle MRI *MRI Devices Corporation, Waukesha, WI*	Safe	1.5	
ATEK TriMark, Biopsy Marker *Hologic, www.hologic.com*	Conditional 5	3	
Automatic Cutting Needle with Depth Markings *14 G, 10-cm length* *Biopsy Needle* *Manan, Northbrook, IL*	Unsafe 1	1.5	7
Automatic Cutting Needle with Ultrasound Tip *& Depth Markings 18 G, 16-cm length* *Biopsy Needle* *Manan, Northbrook, IL*	Unsafe 1	1.5	7
Automatic Cutting Needle with Ultrasound Tip *& Depth Markings* *18 G, 20-cm length* *Biopsy Needle* *Manan, Northbrook, IL*	Unsafe 1	1.5	7
Basic II Hookwire Breast Localization Needle *MD Tech, Watertown, MA*	Unsafe 1	1.5	7
Beaded Breast Localization Wire Set *19 G, 3-1/2 inch needle with 7-7/8 inch wire* *Inrad, Grand Rapids, MI*	Unsafe 1	1.5	7
Beaded Breast Localization Wire Set *20 G, 2 inch needle with 5-7/8 inch wire* *Inrad, Grand Rapids, MI*	Unsafe 1	1.5	7
Biopsy Gun, 13-mm, Biopsy Needle *Meadox, Oakland, NJ*	Unsafe 1	1.5	7
Biopsy Gun, 25-mm, Biopsy Needle *Meadox, Oakland, NJ*	Unsafe 1	1.5	7
Biopsy Needle, 17 G, 10-cm length *Meadox, Oakland, NJ*	Unsafe 1	1.5	7
Biopsy Needle, 20 G, 15-cm length *Meadox, Oakland, NJ*	Unsafe 1	1.5	7
Biopsy Needle, 22 G, 15-cm length *Cook Medical, Inc., www.cookmedical.com*	Unsafe 1	1.5	7
Biopsy Needle, 22 G, 15-cm length *Meadox, Oakland, NJ*	Unsafe 1	1.5	7
Biopty-Cut Biopsy Needle, 14 G, 10-cm length *Bard Medical, www.bardmedical.com*	Unsafe 1	1.5	7

Object	Status	Field Strength (T)	Reference
Biopty-Cut Biopsy Needle, 16 G, 16-cm length *Bard Medical, www.bardmedical.com*	Unsafe 1	1.5	7
Biopty-Cut Biopsy Needle, 18 G, 18-cm length *Bard Medical, www.bardmedical.com*	Unsafe 1	1.5	7
Biopty-Cut Biopsy Needle, 18 G, 20-cm length *Bard Medical, www.bardmedical.com*	Unsafe 1	1.5	7
BioZorb Tissue Marker *Focal Therapeutics, www.focaltherapeutics.com*	Conditional 5	3	
BoneBiopsy Set MRI *manual version, includes trocar,* *stylet, drill and ejector* *MRI Devices Corporation, Waukesha, WI*	Safe	1.5	
Breast Localization Needle, 20 G, 5-cm length *Manan, Northbrook, IL*	Unsafe 1	1.5	7
Breast Localization Needle, 20 G, 7-cm length *Manan, Northbrook, IL*	Unsafe 1	1.5	7
CeleroMark, Biopsy Marker *Hologic, www.hologic.com*	Conditional 5	3	
Chiba Needle and HiLiter *Ultrasound Enhancement* *22 G, 3-7/8 inch Biopsy Needle* *Inrad, Grand Rapids, MI*	Unsafe 1	1.5	7
Cianna Tissue Marker *Cianna Medical, Inc., wwwcianna.com*	Conditional 6	3	
Coaxial Needle Set Chiba-type *22 G, 5-7/8 inch Biopsy Needle* *Inrad, Grand Rapids, MI*	Unsafe 1	1.5	7
Coaxial Needle Set Introducer *19G, 2-15/16 inch Biopsy Needle* *Inrad, Grand Rapids, MI*	Unsafe 1	1.5	7
CoaxNeedle MRI *MRI Devices Corporation, Waukesha, WI*	Safe	1.5	
CorMARK, Biopsy Marker *Hologic, www.hologic.com*	Conditional 5	3	
CorMark Tissue Marker *Ethicon, www.ethicon.com*	Safe	3	
Cutting Needle & Gun *18 G, 155-mm length, Biopsy Needle* *Meadox, Oakland, NJ*	Unsafe 1	1.5	7
Cutting Needle, 14 G, 9-cm length *Biopsy Needle* *West Coast Medical, Laguna Beach, CA*	Unsafe 1	1.5	7

Object	Status	Field Strength (T)	Reference
Cutting Needle, 16 G, 17-mm length *Biopsy Needle* *BIP USA, Inc.* *Niagara Falls, NY*	Unsafe 1	1.5	7
Cutting Needle, 16 G, 19-mm length *Biopsy Needle* *BIP USA, Inc.* *Niagara Falls, NY*	Unsafe 1	1.5	7
Cutting Needle, 18 G, 100-mm length *Biopsy Needle* *Meadox, Oakland, NJ*	Unsafe 1	1.5	7
Cutting Needle, 18 G, 15-cm length *Biopsy Needle* *West Coast Medical, Laguna Beach, CA*	Unsafe 1	1.5	7
Cutting Needle, 18 G, 150-mm length *Biopsy Needle* *Meadox, Oakland, NJ*	Unsafe 1	1.5	7
Cutting Needle, 18 G, 9-cm length *Biopsy Needle* *West Coast Medical, Laguna Beach, CA*	Unsafe 1	1.5	7
Cutting Needle, 19 G, 15-cm length *Biopsy Needle* *West Coast Medical, Laguna Beach, CA*	Unsafe 1	1.5	7
Cutting Needle, 19 G, 6-cm length *Biopsy Needle* *West Coast Medical, Laguna Beach, CA*	Unsafe 1	1.5	7
Cutting Needle, 19 G, 9-cm length *Biopsy Needle* *West Coast Medical, Laguna Beach, CA*	Unsafe 1	1.5	7
Cutting Needle, 20 G, 15-cm length *Biopsy Needle* *West Coast Medical, Laguna Beach, CA*	Unsafe 1	1.5	7
Cutting Needle, 20 G, 20-cm length *Biopsy Needle* *West Coast Medical, Laguna Beach, CA*	Unsafe 1	1.5	7
Cutting Needle, 20 G, 9-cm length *Biopsy Needle* *West Coast Medical, Laguna Beach, CA*	Unsafe 1	1.5	7
Disposable Biopsy Needle, MDBN-08-28 *Ad-Tech Medical, www.adtechmedical.com*	Conditional 8	1.5, 3	
DUALOK Breast Lesion Localization Wire *Bard Biopsy, www.bardbiopsy.com*	Unsafe 1	1.5	
Echotip Ultra Fiducial Marker *Cook Medical, www.cookmedical.com*	Conditional 6	3	

Object	Status	Field Strength (T)	Reference
EnCor MRI Directional Vacuum-Assisted Biopsy Device and Driver *Bard Biopsy, www.bardbiopsy.com*	Conditional 5	1.5, 3	
EnCor Ultra Breast Biopsy System *Bard Biopsy, www.bardbiopsy.com*	Unsafe 1	1.5	
FINESSE ULTRA Breast Biopsy System, Biopsy Driver *Bard Biopsy, www.bardbiopsy.com*	Unsafe 1	1.5	
Fully Automatic BiopsyGun MRI *MRI Devices Corporation, Waukesha, WI*	Safe	1.5	
Hawkins Blunt Needle, Biopsy Needle *MD Tech, Watertown, MA*	Unsafe 1	1.5	7
Hawkins III Breast Localization Needle *MD Tech, Watertown, MA*	Unsafe 1	1.5	7
Heart Breast Tissue Marker *Bard Peripheral Vascular, www.bardbiopsy.com*	Conditional 6	3	
HydroMARK, Biopsy Marker *Hologic, www.hologic.com*	Conditional 5	3	
Gold Anchor *Naslund Medical AB, www.fineneedlemarker.com*	Conditional 8	1.5, 3	
Gold Seed Fiducial *Covidien, www.covidien.com*	Conditional 5	3	
KMD-Mark1Marker *Kent Medical Devices, Inc., Minneapolis, MN*	Conditional 6	3	
Kopans Breast Lesion Localization Needle *Cook Medical Inc., www.cookmedical.com*	Unsafe 1	1.5	
LeLoc MRI Tumor Localizer *MRI Devices Corporation, Waukesha, WI*	Safe	1.5	
LOCalizer RFID Breast Lesion Localization System *Health Beacons, www.healthbeacons.com*	Conditional 8	1.5, 3	
Lufkin Aspiration Cytology Needle *20 G, 5-cm length, Biopsy Needle* *E-Z-Em, Inc., Westbury, NY*	Safe	1.5	9
Lufkin Biopsy Needle *18 G, 15-cm length* *E-Z-Em, Inc., Westbury, NY*	Safe	1.5	8
Lufkin Biopsy Needle *18 G, 5-cm length* *E-Z-Em, Inc., Westbury, NY*	Safe	1.5	8
Lufkin Biopsy Needle *22 G, 10-cm length* *E-Z-Em, Inc., Westbury, NY*	Safe	1.5	8

Object	Status	Field Strength (T)	Reference
Lufkin Biopsy Needle *22 G, 15-cm length* *E-Z-Em, Inc., Westbury, NY*	Safe	1.5	8
Lufkin Biopsy Needle *22 G, 5-cm length* *E-Z-Em, Inc., Westbury, NY*	Safe	1.5	8
Magseed Magnetic Marker System *Endomagnetics Ltd., www.endomag.com*	Conditional 5	1.5, 3	
MammoMARK, Biopsy Marker *Hologic, www.hologic.com*	Conditional 5	3	
MammoMark Tissue Marker *Ethicon, www.ethicon.com*	Safe	3	
MammoMark Tissue Marker Deployment Device *Ethicon, www.ethicon.com*	Safe	3	
MammoMark Tissue Marker *Ethicon, www.ethicon.com*	Safe	3	
MammoMark Tissue Marker Deployment Device *Ethicon, www.ethicon.com*	Safe	3	
MammoMark II Tissue Marker *Ethicon, www.ethicon.com*	Safe	3	
MammoMark II Tissue Marker Deployment Device *Ethicon, www.ethicon.com*	Safe	3	
MammoMARK, Biopsy Marker *Hologic, www.hologic.com*	Conditional 5	3	
Micromark Clip, Marking Clip *Biopsys Medical, Irvine, CA*	Safe	1.5	61
MicroMark II Clip, 316L SS *Ethicon, www.ethicon.com*	Safe	1.5, 3	
MReye Biopsy and Special Purpose Needles *Cook Medical Inc., www.cookmedical.com*	Conditional 5	1.5	
MReye Chiba Biopsy Needle *Cook Medical Inc., www cookmedical.com*	Safe	1.5	
MReye Franseen Lung Biopsy Needle *Cook Medical Inc., www cookmedical.com*	Conditional 5	1.5	
MReye Interventional Needle, Biopsy Needle *Cook Medical Inc., www.cookmedical.com*	Conditional 5	1.5	
MReye Kopans Breast Lesion Localization Needle *Reference Part Numbers beginning with IDKBL* *Cook Medical Inc., www.cookmedical.com*	Conditional 5	1.5	
MR Ghiatas Beaded Breast Localization Wire Set *Inrad Inc., Kentwood, MI*	Conditional 6	3	
MR Ghiatas Breast Localization Wire Set *C. R. Bard, Inc., Murray Hill, NJ*	Conditional 6	3	

Object	Status	Field Strength (T)	Reference
MR Ghiatas Beaded Localization Wire *MR GHIATAS Localization Wire* *Bard Biopsy, www.bardbiopsy.com*	Conditional 6	3	
MRI BioGun, 18 G, 10-cm length, Biopsy Needle *E-Z-Em, Inc., Westbury, NY*	Safe	1.5	8
MRI BiopsyKit *MRI Devices Corporation, Waukesha, WI*	Safe	1.5	
MRI Histology Needle, 18 G, 15-cm length *Biopsy Needle* *E-Z-Em, Inc., Westbury, NY*	Safe	1.5	7
MRI Histology Needle, 18 G, 5-cm length *Biopsy Needle* *E-Z-Em, Inc., Westbury, NY*	Safe	1.5	8
MRI Histology Needle, 20 G, 10-cm length *Biopsy Needle* *E-Z-Em, Inc., Westbury, NY*	Safe	1.5	8
MRI Histology Needle, 20 G, 15-cm length *Biopsy Needle* *E-Z-Em, Inc., Westbury, NY*	Safe	1.5	8
MRI Histology Needle, 20 G, 5-cm length *Biopsy Needle* *E-Z-Em, Inc., Westbury, NY*	Safe	1.5	7
MRI Histology Needle, 20 G, 7.5-cm length *Biopsy Needle* *E-Z-Em, Inc., Westbury, NY*	Safe	1.5	8
MRI Lesion Marking System, 20 G, 7.5-cm length *E-Z-Em, Inc., Westbury, NY*	Safe	1.5	8
MRI Needle, 20-gauge, 9-cm *QSUM Biopsy Disposables LLC, www.qsum.net*	Conditional 7	3	
MRI Needle, Biopsy Needle *Cook Medical, Inc., www.cookmedical.com*	Safe	1.5	7
mrt Biopsy Needle, All Sizes *Daum Medical*	Safe	1.5	
NeuroCut Needle MRI *MRI Devices Corporation, Waukesha, WI*	Safe	1.5	
NeuroGate Set MRI *MRI Devices Corporation, Waukesha, WI*	Safe	1.5	
NeuroPunctureNeedle MRI *MRI Devices Corporation, Waukesha, WI*	Safe	1.5	
Percucut Biopsy Needle and Stylet *19.5 gauge x 10-cm* *E-Z-Em, Inc., Westbury, NY*	Unsafe 1	1.5	7

Object	Status	Field Strength (T)	Reference
Percucut Biopsy Needle and Stylet *21 gauge x 10-cm* *E-Z-Em, Inc., Westbury, NY*	Unsafe 1	1.5	7
PunctureNeedle MRI *MRI Devices Corporation, Waukesha, WI*	Safe	1.5	
Sadowsky Breast Marking System *20 G, 5-cm length needle and 7 inch hook wire* *Ranfac Corporation, Avon, MA*	Unsafe 1	1.5	7
SecureMark, Biopsy Marker *Hologic, www.hologic.com*	Conditional 5	3	
Semi-Automatic BiopsyGun MRI *MRI Devices Corporation, Waukesha, WI*	Safe	1.5	
SenoMark UltraCor MRI, SS *M shaped breast biopsy marker clip* *SenoRx, Aliso Viejo, CA*	Conditional 6	3	
SenoMark UltraCor MRI, Titanium *X shaped breast biopsy marker clip* *SenoRx, Aliso Viejo, CA*	Conditional 6	3	
Single Loop Titanium Marker *Tissue Marker, Titanium alloy* *RUBICOR Medical Inc., Redwood City, CA*	Conditional 6	3	
Sirius MRI Marker NS *C4 Imaging, www.c4imagining.com*	Conditional 5	1.5, 3	
SmartGuide CT/MRI *MRI Devices Corporation, Waukesha, WI*	Safe	1.5	
Soft Tissue Biopsy Needle Gun & Biopsy Needle *Anchor Procducts Co., Addison, IL*	Unsafe 1	1.5	7
Spirotome Single Use 10 Standard *Biopsy Device* *MEDINVENTS, Belgium*	Conditional 5	3	
superLock Cobra, Marker *SuperDimension, www.superdimension.com*	Conditional 6	3	120
Surgical Mesh with X-Ray Marker *NuVasive, Inc., San Diego, CA*	Conditional 6	3	
Tantalum Marker *Altomed Limited, www.altomed.com*	Conditional 6	3	
TargoGrid positioning grid for *biopsies and punctures* *MRI Devices Corporation, Waukesha, WI*	Safe	1.5	
TriMark, Biopsy Marker *Hologic, www.hologic.com*	Conditional 5	3	
Trocar Needle, Biopsy Needle *BIP USA, Inc., Niagara Falls, NY*	Unsafe 1	1.5	7

Object	Status	Field Strength (T)	Reference
Trocar Needle, Disposable Biopsy Needle *Cook Medical, Inc., www.cookmedical.com*	Unsafe 1	1.5	7
TumoLoc MRI, Tumor Localizer *MRI Devices Corporation, Waukesha, WI*	Safe	1.5	
UltraClip II, MR Tissue Marker Device *Inrad Inc., Kentwood, MI*	Conditional 6	3	
UltraClip II, MR Tissue Marker Device *C. R. Bard, Inc., Murray Hill, NJ*	Conditional 6	3	
UltraClip II, Tissue Marker, Clip Only *Bard Peripheral Vascular, www.bardbiopsy.com*	Conditional 6	3	
UltraClip II, Tissue Marker, Coil *Bard Peripheral Vascular, www.bardbiopsy.com*	Conditional 6	3	
UltraClip II, Tissue Marker, Ribbon *Bard Peripheral Vascular, www.bardbiopsy.com*	Conditional 6	3	
UltraClip II, Tissue Marker, Wing *Bard Peripheral Vascular, www.bardbiopsy.com*	Conditional 6	3	
Ultra-Core, Biopsy Needle *16 G, 16-cm length*	Unsafe 1	1.5	7
UltraCor Twirl Breast Tissue Marker *Bard Biopsy, www.bardbiopsy.com*	Conditional 5	3	
VACORA Biopsy System *Bard Biopsy, www.bardbiopsy.com*	Conditional 5	3	
Venus Breast Tissue Marker *Bard Peripheral Vascular, www.bardbiopsy.com*	Conditional 6	3	

Breast Tissue Expanders and Implants

Object	Status	Field Strength (T)	Reference
ACCUSPAN Tissue Expander with Magnetic Port *PMT Corporation, www.pmtcorp.com*	Unsafe 1	1.5	
ACX Tissue Expander, Integrated Magnetic *Injection Port (various models)* *Sientra, www.sientra.com*	Unsafe 1	1.5	
Becker Expander/Mammary Mentor H/S *Breast Implant* *Mentor, www.mentorwwllc.com*	Safe	1.5	10
Breast Tissue Expander *Style 133 FV with MAGNA-SITE Injection Site* *Magnetic Port* *McGhan Medical/INAMED Aesthetics, Santa Barbara, CA*	Unsafe 1	1.5	86
Breast Tissue Expander *Style 133 LV with MAGNA-SITE Injection Site* *Magnetic Port* *McGhan Medical/INAMED Aesthetics, Santa Barbara, CA*	Unsafe 1	1.5	86

Object	Status	Field Strength (T)	Reference
Breast Tissue Expander *Style 133 MV with MAGNA-SITE Injection Site* *Magnetic Port* *McGhan Medical/INAMED Aesthetics, Santa Barbara, CA*	Unsafe 1	1.5	86
Breast Tissue Expander *STYLE 133V (133 V) Series, MAGNA-SITE Injection Site* *Allergan, Inc., www.allergan.com*	Unsafe 1	1.5	
Breast Tissue Expander *STYLE 133 FV, MAGNA-SITE Injection Site* *Allergan, Inc., www.allergan.com*	Unsafe 1	1.5	
Breast Tissue Expander *STYLE 133 FX, MAGNA-SITE Injection Site* *Allergan, Inc., www.allergan.com*	Unsafe 1	1.5	
Breast Tissue Expander *STYLE 133 LV, MAGNA-SITE Injection Site* *Allergan, Inc., www.allergan.com*	Unsafe 1	1.5	
Breast Tissue Expander *STYLE 133 MV, MAGNA-SITE Injection Site* *Allergan, Inc., www.allergan.com*	Unsafe 1	1.5	
Breast Tissue Expander *STYLE 133 MX, MAGNA-SITE Injection Site* *Allergan, Inc., www.allergan.com*	Unsafe 1	1.5	
Breast Tissue Expander *STYLE 133 SV, MAGNA-SITE Injection Site* *Allergan, Inc., www.allergan.com*	Unsafe 1	1.5	
Breast Tissue Expander *STYLE 133 SX, MAGNA-SITE Injection Site* *Allergan, Inc., www.allergan.com*	Unsafe 1	1.5	
Breast Tissue Expander *Natrelle 133* *MAGNA-SITE Injection Site* *Allergan, Inc., www.allergan.com*	Unsafe 1	1.5	
CONTOUR PROFILE Tissue Expander *Mentor, www.mentorwwllc.com*	Unsafe 1	1.5	
CONTOUR PROFILE Tissue Expander *With Bufferzone Area* *Mentor, www.mentorwwllc.com*	Unsafe 1	1.5	
CPX2 Tissue Expander *Mentor, www.mentorwwllc.com*	Unsafe 1	1.5	
CPX3 Tissue Expander *Mentor, www.mentorwwllc.com*	Unsafe 1	1.5	
Double Chamber Breast Tissue Expander *Model 20739-400* *SILIMED, Inc., Dallas, TX*	Unsafe 1	1.5	

Object	Status	Field Strength (T)	Reference
Infall, Breast Implant with Magnetic Port *Heyerschultzz*	Unsafe 1	1.5	
Integra Breast Tissue Expander with Magnetic Port *PMT Corporation, www.pmtcorp.com*	Unsafe 1	1.5	125
Integra Tissue Expander with Magnetic Port *PMT Corporation, www.pmtcorp.com*	Unsafe 1	1.5	
MemoryGel Breast Implant *Mentor, www.mentorwwllc.com*	Safe	1.5, 3	
MemoryGel SILTEX Breast Implant *Mentor, www.mentorwwllc.com*	Safe	1.5, 3	
Motiva Implant, Ergonomix Round SILKSURFACE *Corse' with Qid* *Establishment Labs S.A., www.establishmentlabs.com*	Conditional 8	1.5, 3	
Motiva Implant, Round VELVETSURFACE PLUS *Corse' with Qid* *Establishment Labs S.A., www.establishmentlabs.com*	Conditional 8	1.5, 3	
Motiva Implant, Round SILKSURFACE *Corse' with Qid* *Establishment Labs S.A., www.establishmentlabs.com*	Conditional 8	1.5, 3	
NanoSkin Surfact Breast Implant, All Sizes *Groupe SEBBIN SAS, www.sebbin.com/en/*	Safe	1.5, 3	
Radovan Tissue Expander, 316L SS *Mentor, www.mentorwwllc.com*	Safe	1.5	10
Sillmed Breast Tissue Expander(s) *with Magnetic Port(s)* *Sillmed, www.silimed.com.br*	Unsafe 1	1.5	
SILTEX CONTOUR PROFILE *Breast Implant, Adjustable* *Mentor, www.mentorwwllc.com*	Safe	1.5, 3	
SILTEX CONTOUR PROFILE *Saline Breast Implant* *Mentor, www.mentorwwllc.com*	Safe	1.5, 3	
SILTEX CONTOUR PROFILE Tissue Expander *Mentor, www.mentorwwllc.com*	Unsafe 1	1.5	
SILTEX Low, Medium, *and Tall Height Tissue Expander, Style 6100* *Mentor, www.mentorwwllc.com*	Unsafe 1	1.5	
SILTEX Round Saline Breast Implant *Mentor, www.mentorwwllc.com*	Safe	1.5, 3	
SILTEX SPECTRUM *Breast Implant, Adjustable* *Mentor, www.mentorwwllc.com*	Safe	1.5, 3	

Object	Status	Field Strength (T)	Reference
Siltex Spectrum Post-Operatively *Adjustable Saline-Filled Mammary Prosthesis, 316L SS* *Mentor, www.mentorwwllc.com*	Safe	1.5	10
SPECTRUM Breast Implant, Adjustable *Mentor, www.mentorwwllc.com*	Safe	1.5, 3	
Tissue Expander with Magnetic Port, Breast Implant *McGhan Medical Corporation, Santa Barbara, CA*	Unsafe 1	1.5	

Cardiac Pacemakers, ICDs, and Cardiac Monitors

Object	Status	Field Strength (T)	Reference
Abbott and St. Jude Medical, Cardiac Pacemaker *List of MR Conditional Versions* *Abbott and St. Jude Medical, Inc.,* *www.sjm.com/mriready*	Conditional 5	1.5	
Abbott and St. Jude Medical, Cardiac Pacemaker *List of MR Conditional Versions* *Abbott and St. Jude Medical, Inc.,* *www.sjm.com/mriready*	Conditional 5	1.5, 3	
Abbott and St. Jude Medical, Implantable *Cardioverter Defibrillator (ICD)* *List of MR Conditional Versions* *Abbott and St. Jude Medical, Inc.,* *www.sjm.com/mriready*	Conditional 5	1.5	
Abbott and St. Jude Medical, Implantable *Cardioverter Defibrillator (ICD)* *List of MR Conditional Versions* *Abbott and St. Jude Medical, Inc.,* *www.sjm.com/mriready*	Conditional 5	1.5, 3	
Accent MRI and Accent ST MRI Cardiac *Pacemaker Systems* *Models PM1224, PM2224, PM1226,* *PM2226, PM1124 PM2124* *St. Jude Medical, www.sjm.com/mriready*	Conditional 5	1.5	
Adapta Cardiac Pacemaker *Medtronic, Inc., www.medtronic.com/mri*	Unsafe 2	1.5	
ADVANTIO MRI Pacemaker, Cardiac Pacemaker *Boston Scientific, www.bostonscientific.com*	Conditional 5	1.5	
Advisa DR MRI SureScan Pacing System *Medtronic, Inc., www.medtronic.com/mri*	Conditional 5	1.5, 3	
Advisa SR MRI SureScan Pacing System *Medtronic, Inc., www.medtronic.com/mri*	Conditional 5	1.5, 3	
Amplia MRI Quad CRT-D *Cardiac Resynchronization Therapy Defibrillator (CRT-D)* *Medtronic, Inc., www.medtronic.com/mri*	Conditional 5	1.5	
AngelMed Guardian, Implantable Cardiac Monitor *Angel Medical Systems, Shrewsbury, NJ*	Unsafe 1	1.5	

Object	Status	Field Strength (T)	Reference
Assurity MRI Cardiac Pacemaker System *Models PM1272, PM2272* *St. Jude Medical, Inc.* *St. Jude Medical, Inc., www.sjm.com/mriready*	Conditional 5	1.5	
Biotronik Cardiac Pacemaker *List of MR Conditional Versions* *Biotronik, www.biotronikusa.com/manuals/index.cfm*	Conditional 5	1.5	
Biotronik Cardiac Pacemaker *List of MR Conditional Versions* *Biotronik, www.biotronikusa.com/manuals/index.cfm*	Conditional 5	1.5, 3	
Biotronik Cardiac Implantable Cardioverter *Defibrillator (ICD)* *List of MR Conditional Versions* *Biotronik, www.biotronikusa.com/manuals/index.cfm*	Conditional 5	1.5	
Biotronik Cardiac Implantable Cardioverter *Defibrillator (ICD)* *List of MR Conditional Versions* *Biotronik, www.biotronikusa.com/manuals/index.cfmá*	Conditional 5	1.5, 3	
Boston Scientific Cardiac Pacemaker *List of MR Conditional Versions* *Boston Scientific, www.bostonscientific.com*	Conditional 5	1.5	
Boston Scientific Cardiac Pacemaker *List of MR Conditional Versions* *Boston Scientific, www.bostonscientific.com*	Conditional 5	1.5, 3	
Boston Scientific Implantable Cardioverter *Defibrillator (ICD)* *List of MR Conditional Versions* *Boston Scientific, www.bostonscientific.com*	Conditional 5	1.5	
Boston Scientific Implantable Cardioverter *Defibrillator (ICD)* *List of MR Conditional Versions* *Boston Scientific, www.bostonscientific.com*	Conditional 5	1.5, 3	
Compia MRI Quad CRT-D *Cardiac Resynchronization Therapy Defibrillator (CRT-D)* *Medtronic, Inc., www.medtronic.com/mri*	Conditional 5	1.5	
Concerto II Cardiac Resynchronization Therapy, CRT *Medtronic, Inc., www.medtronic.com/mri*	Unsafe 2	1.5	
Consulta CRT-D Cardiac Resynchronization Therapy, CRT *Medtronic, Inc., www.medtronic.com/mri*	Unsafe 2	1.5	
Consulta CRT-P Cardiac Resynchronization Therapy, CRT *Medtronic, Inc., www.medtronic.com/mri*	Unsafe 2	1.5	
Cosmos, Model 283-01, Pacemaker *Intermedics, Inc., Freeport, TX*	Unsafe 1	3	85

Object	Status	Field Strength (T)	Reference
Cosmos II, Model 283-03, Pacemaker *Intermedics, Inc., Freeport, TX*	Unsafe 2	3	85
Cosmos II, Model 284-05, Pacemaker *Intermedics, Inc., Freeport, TX*	Unsafe 1	3	85
Delta TRS, Type DDD, Model 0937 Pacemaker *Cardiac Pacemakers, Inc., St. Paul, MN*	Unsafe 1	3	85
Endurity Cardiac Pacemaker System *Models PM1162, PM2162* *St. Jude Medical, Inc.* *St. Jude Medical, Inc., www.sjm.com/mriready*	Conditional 5	1.5	
Endurity MRI Cardiac Pacemaker System *Models PM1172, PM2172* *St. Jude Medical, Inc.* *St. Jude Medical, Inc., www.sjm.com/mriready*	Conditional 5	1.5	
EnRhythm MRI SureScan Pacing System *Medtronic, Inc., www.medtronic.com/mri*	Conditional 5	1.5	
Ensura DR MRI SureScan Pacing System *Medtronic, Inc., www.medtronic.com/mri*	Conditional 5	1.5, 3	
Evera MRI SureScan Defibrillation System *Implantable Cardioverter Defibrillator, ICD* *Medtronic, Inc., www.medtronic.com,* *www.medtronic.com/mri*	Conditional 5	1.5, 3	
Evera MRI SureScan Defibrillation System *Implantable Cardioverter Defibrillator, ICD* *XT DR, XT VR, S DR* *Medtronic, Inc., www.medtronic.com,* *www.medtronic.com/mri*	Conditional 5	1.5, 3	
GEM DR 7271, Dual Chamber Implantable *Cardioverter Defibrillator* *Medtronic, Inc., www.medtronic.com/mri*	Unsafe 1	3	85
GEM II DR 7273, Dual Chamber Implantable *Cardioverter Defibrillator* *Medtronic, Inc., www.medtronic.com/mri*	Unsafe 1	3	85
Implantable Cardioverter Defibrillator (ICD), *ProMRI Lumax 740 Series, VR-T, DR-T, HF-T* *Biotronik, US: www.biotronikusa.com/promri Outside US:* *www.biotronik.com/promri*	Conditional 5	1.5	
INGENIO MRI Pacemaker (Cardiac Pacemaker) *Boston Scientific, www.bostonscientific.com*	Conditional 5	1.5	
InSync Maximo II Cardiac Resynchronization *Therapy, CRT* *Medtronic, Inc., www.medtronic.com/mri*	Unsafe 2	1.5	

Object	Status	Field Strength (T)	Reference
KAPPA DR403, Dual Chamber Rate Responsive *Pacemaker* *Medtronic, Inc., www.medtronic.com/mri*	Unsafe 2	3	85
KAPPA DR706, Dual Chamber Rate Responsive *Pacemaker* *Medtronic, Inc., www.medtronic.com/mri*	Unsafe 1	3	85
KORA (various models) Cardiac Pacemaker *Sorin, www.sorin.com*	Conditional 5	1.5	
LivaNova and Sorin Cardiac Pacemaker *List of MR Conditional Versions* *LivaNova and Sorin, www.livanova.sorin.com*	Conditional 5	1.5	
LivaNova and Sorin Cardiac Pacemaker *List of MR Conditional Versions* *LivaNova and Sorin, www.livanova.sorin.com*	Conditional 5	1.5, 3	
LivaNova and Sorin Implantable Cardioverter *Defibrillator (ICD)* *List of MR Conditional Versions* *LivaNova and Sorin, www.livanova.sorin.com*	Conditional 5	1.5	
LivaNova and Sorin Implantable Cardioverter *Defibrillator (ICD)* *List of MR Conditional Versions* *LivaNova and Sorin, www.livanova.sorin.com*	Conditional 5	1.5, 3	
MARQUIS DR 7274 Implantable Cardioverter *Defibrillator* *Medtronic, Inc., www.medtronic.com/mri*	Unsafe 1	3	85
Maximo II Implantable Cardioverter Defibrillator *Medtronic, Inc., www.medtronic.com/mri*	Unsafe 2	1.5	
Medtronic Cardiac Pacemaker *List of MR Conditional Versions* *Medtronic, Inc., www.medtronic.com/MRI*	Conditional 5	1.5	
Medtronic Cardiac Pacemaker *List of MR Conditional Versions* *Medtronic, Inc., www.medtronic.com/MRI*	Conditional 5	1.5, 3	
Medtronic Implantable Cardioverter Defibrillator *(ICD)* *List of MR Conditional Versions* *Medtronic, Inc., www.medtronic.com/MRI*	Conditional 5	1.5	
Medtronic Implantable Cardioverter Defibrillator *(ICD)* *List of MR Conditional Versions* *Medtronic, Inc., www.medtronic.com/MRI*	Conditional 5	1.5, 3	
Micra Transcather Pacing System (TPS) *Medtronic, Inc., www.medtronic.com/mri*	Conditional 5	1.5, 3	

Object	Status	Field Strength (T)	Reference
MICRO JEWEL II 7223CX Implantable Cardioverter *Defibrillator* *Medtronic, Inc., www.medtronic.com/mri*	Unsafe 1	3	85
Nanostim Leadless Pacemaker *St. Jude Medical, www.sjm.com*	Conditional 5	1.5	
Nova Model 281-01Pacemaker *Intermedics, Inc., Freeport, TX*	Unsafe 1	3	85
Nova II, Model 281-05, Pacemaker *Intermedics, Inc., Freeport, TX*	Unsafe 2	3	85
Nova II, Model 282-04, Pacemaker *Intermedics, Inc., Freeport, TX*	Unsafe 2	3	85
ProMRI Cardiac Pacemaker Systems (Biotronik): *Exclusion Zone MRI at 1.5-T/64-MHz* *Information applies various components.* *Must follow highly specific conditions and guidelines* *Biotronik, US: www.biotronikusa.com/promri* *Outside US: www.biotronik.com/promri*	Conditional 5	1.5	
ProMRI Cardiac Pacemaker Systems (Biotronik): *Full Body MRI at 1.5-T/64-MHz* *Information applies various components.* *Must follow highly specific conditions and guidelines* *Biotronik, US: www.biotronikusa.com/promri* *Outside US: www.biotronik.com/promri*	Conditional 5	1.5	
ProMRI Cardiac Resynchronization Systems (CRT), *Cardiac Pacemaker Systems (Biotronik):* *Exclusion Zone MRI at 1.5-T/64-MHz* *Information applies various components.* *Must follow highly specific conditions and guidelines* *Biotronik, US: www.biotronikusa.com/promri* *Outside US: www.biotronik.com/promri*	Conditional 5	1.5	
ProMRI Cardiac Resynchronization Systems (CRT), *Implantable Cardioverter Defibrillator Systems (ICDs)* *(Biotronik): Exclusion Zone MRI at 1.5-T/64-MHz* *Information applies various components.* *Must follow highly specific conditions and guidelines* *Biotronik, US: www.biotronikusa.com/promri* *Outside US: www.biotronik.com/promri*	Conditional 5	1.5	
ProMRI Implantable Cardioverter Defibrillator *Systems (ICDs)(Biotronik):* *Exclusion Zone MRI at 3-T/128 MHz* *Information applies various components.* *Must follow highly specific conditions and guidelines* *Biotronik, US: www.biotronikusa.com/promri* *Outside US: www.biotronik.com/promri*	Conditional 5	3	

Object	Status	Field Strength (T)	Reference
ProMRI Implantable Implantable Cardioverter *Defibrillator Systems (ICDs) (Biotronik):* *Full Body MRI at 1.5-T/64-MHz* *Information applies various components.* *Must follow highly specific conditions and guidelines* *Biotronik, US: www.biotronikusa.com/promri* *Outside US: www.biotronik.com/promri*	Conditional 5	1.5	
ProMRI Loop Recorder (Biotronik): *Full Body MRI at 1.5-T/64-MHz* *Loop Recorder: BioMonitor* *Must follow highly specific conditions and guidelines* *Biotronik, US: www.biotronikusa.com/promri* *Outside US: www.biotronik.com/promri*	Conditional 5	1.5	
Protecta CRT-D Cardiac Resynchronization Therapy *Medtronic, Inc., www.medtronic.com/mri*	Unsafe 2	1.5	
Protecta Implantable Cardioverter Defibrillator *Medtronic, Inc., www.medtronic.com/mri*	Unsafe 2	1.5	
Protecta XT CRT-D Cardiac Resynchronization *Therapy* *Medtronic, Inc., www.medtronic.com/mri*	Unsafe 2	1.5	
Protecta XT Implantable Cardioverter Defibrillator *Medtronic, Inc., www.medtronic.com/mri*	Unsafe 2	1.5	
Quantum, Model 253-19, Pacemaker *Intermedics, Inc., Freeport, TX*	Unsafe 1	3	85
Relay, Model 294-03, Pacemaker *Intermedics, Inc., Freeport, TX*	Unsafe 1	3	85
Revo MRI SureScan Pacing System, RVDRO1 *Revo MRI SureScan, RVDR01, CapSureFix MRI* *SureScan, 5086MRI* *Cardiac Pacemaker* *Medtronic, Inc., www.Medtronic.com*	Conditional 5	1.5	
Reveal DX 9528 *Insertable Cardiac Monitor* *Medtronic, Inc., www.medtronic.com/mri*	Conditional 5	1.5, 3	
Reveal LINQ Insertable Cardiac Monitoring *(ICM) System* *Medtronic Reveal LINQ Model LNQ11* *Insertable Cardiac Monitor* *Medtronic, Inc., www.medtronic.com/mri*	Conditional 5	1.5, 3	
Reveal Plus Insertable Loop Recorder (ILR) *9526 Reveal Plus Insertable Loop Recorder* *Medtronic, Inc., www.medtronic.com/mri*	Conditional 5	1.5	90, 91
Reveal XT 9529 Insertable Cardiac Monitor *Medtronic, Inc., www.medtronic.com/mri*	Conditional 5	1.5, 3	

Object	Status	Field Strength (T)	Reference
Res-Q ACE *Model 101-01 Pacemaker* *Intermedics, Inc., Freeport, TX*	Unsafe 1	3	85
S-ICD System, Implantable Cardioverter Defibrillator *Cameron Health, www.cameronhealth.com*	Unsafe 2	1.5	
Secura Implantable Cardioverter Defibrillator *Medtronic, Inc., www.medtronic.com/mri*	Unsafe 2	1.5	
Sensia Cardiac Pacemaker *Medtronic, Inc., www.medtronic.com/mri*	Unsafe 2	1.5	
SIGMA SDR306 Dual Chamber Rate *Responsive Pacemaker* *Medtronic, Inc., www.medtronic.com/mri*	Unsafe 1	3	85
SJM Confirm, Model DM2100 *Implantable Cardiac Monitor* *Note: MRI labeling is different for the United States* *versus Outside of the United States* *St. Jude Medical, www.sjm.com*	Conditional 5	1.5	
SJM Confirm, Model DM2102 *Implantable Cardiac Monitor* *Note: MRI labeling is different for the United States* *versus Outside of the United States* *St. Jude Medical, www.sjm.com*	Conditional 5	1.5	
Syncra CRT-P Cardiac Resynchronization Therapy *Medtronic, Inc., www.medtronic.com/mri*	Unsafe 2	1.5	
THERA VDD 8968I Dual Chambe, Atrial Sensing, *Ventricular Sensing Pacemaker* *Medtronic, Inc., www.medtronic.com/mri*	Unsafe 2	3	85
Versa Cardiac Pacemaker *Medtronic, Inc., www.medtronic.com/mri*	Unsafe 2	1.5	
Virtuoso Implantable Cardioverter Defibrillator *Medtronic, Inc., www.medtronic.com/mri*	Unsafe 2	1.5	
Visia AF MRI SureScan *Implantable Cardioverter Defibrillator, ICD* *Medtronic, Inc., www.medtronic.com,* *www.medtronic.com/mri*	Conditional 5	1.5	
ZIO Patch *iRhythm Technologies, www.irhythmtech.com*	Unsafe 2	1.5	
ZIO XT Patch *iRhythm Technologies, Inc., www.irhythmtech.com*	Unsafe 2	1.5	

Object	Status	Field Strength (T)	Reference

Cardiovascular Catheters and Accessories

Object	Status	Field Strength (T)	Reference
Apollo Micro Catheter, 15-mm Tip *Covidien and ev3 Inc., www.ev3.net*	Conditional 8	1.5, 3	
Apollo Micro Catheter, 70-mm Tip *Covidien and ev3 Inc., www.ev3.net*	Conditional 8	1.5, 3	
Arrow You-Bend Two Lumen Hemodialysis Catheter *Arrow International Inc., Reading, PA*	Conditional 6	3	
AVA 3xi Catheter, All Models *Edwards Lifesciences, www.edwards.com*	Safe	1.5, 3	
AVA 3xi Introducer Valve, All Models *Edwards Lifesciences, www.edwards.com*	Safe	1.5, 3	
AVA HF Catheter, All Models *Edwards Lifesciences, www.edwards.com*	Safe	1.5, 3	
Bactiseal Endoscopic Ventricular Catheter *Codman, www.depuysynthes.com*	Safe	1.5, 3	
Cannon II Plus, Chronic Hemodialysis Catheter (CHDC) *Teleflex Medical, Inc., www.teleflex.com*	Conditional 6	3	
Codman SureStream Intraspinal Catheter *Codman, www.depuysynthes.com*	Conditional 6	3	
CliniCath Catheter *Smiths Medical, www.smiths-medical.com*	Safe	3	
Cool Line Catheter *Zoll Circulation, www.zoll.com*	Safe	1.5, 3	
Chronic Catheter *Covidien, www.covidien.com*	Conditional 6	3	
Dura-Flow Chronic Dialysis Catheter *Angiodynamics, Inc., www.Angiodynamics.com*	Safe	1.5, 3	
DuraMax Chronic Dialysis Catheter *Angiodynamics, Inc., www.Angiodynamics.com*	Safe	1.5, 3	
EVENMORE Chronic Dialysis Catheter *Angiodynamics, Inc., www.Angiodynamics.com*	Safe	1.5, 3	
FlexTip Plus Epidural Catheter *Regional Anesthesia Device* *Teleflex Medical, www.teleflex.com*	Conditional 5	1.5, 3	
IntroFlex Catheter, All Models *Edwards Lifesciences, www.edwards.com*	Safe	1.5, 3	
LifeJet VP VascPak *Angiodynamics, Inc., www.Angiodynamics.com*	Safe	1.5, 3	
Morpheus Smart PICC *Angiodynamics, Inc., www.Angiodynamics.com*	Safe	1.5, 3	
MultiMed CVC Catheter, All Models *Edwards Lifesciences, www.edwards.com*	Safe	1.5, 3	

Object	Status	Field Strength (T)	Reference
NeoStar Triple Lumen Catheter *Angiodynamics, Inc., www.Angiodynamics.com*	Safe	1.5, 3	
NextStep Retrograde Catheter *Arrow International, www.arrowintl.com*	Conditional 5	3	
ON-Q SilverSoaker Catheter *I-Flow, LLC, www.iflo.com*	Safe	1.5, 3	
Opticath Catheter, Model U400 *Abbott Laboratories, www.abbott.com*	Unsafe 2	1.5	60
Opticath PA Catheter with extra port *Abbott Laboratories, www.abbott.com*	Unsafe 2	1.5	60
Opticath PA Catheter with RV Pacing Port *Abbott Laboratories, www.abbott.com*	Unsafe 2	1.5	60
Opti-Q SvO2/CCO *Catheter* *Abbott Laboratories, www.abbott.com*	Unsafe 2	1.5	60
Oximetric 3, SO2 *Optical Module* *Abbott Laboratories, www.abbott.com*	Unsafe 2	1.5	60
Palindrome Sapphire HD Catheter *Covidien, www.covidien.com*	Conditional 6	3	
PediaSat Oximetry Catheter, All Models *Edwards Lifesciences, www.edwards.com*	Safe	1.5, 3	
PICC Catheter *Angiodynamics, Inc., www.Angiodynamics.com*	Safe	1.5, 3	
PolyFlow Peripherally Inserted Catheter *Smiths Medical, www.smiths-medical.com*	Safe	3	
PreSep OLIGON Oximeter Catheter *XA3820HCDCNL* *Edwards Lifesciences, www.edwards.com*	Conditional 5	3	
PreSep Oximetry Catheter, All Models *Edwards Lifesciences, www.edwards.com*	Safe	1.5, 3	
Quadrathane Cannon II Plus Catheter *Arrow International, www.arrowintl.com*	Conditional 6	3	
Quadrathane NextStep Retrograde Catheter *Arrow International, www.arrowintl.com*	Conditional 6	3	
Quattro Catheter *Zoll Circulation, www.zoll.com*	Safe	1.5	
RV Pacing Lead *Abbott Laboratories, www.abbott.com*	Unsafe 2	1.5	60
SCHON Chronic Hemodialysis Catheter *Angiodynamics, Inc., www.Angiodynamics.com*	Safe	1.5, 3	
SCHON XL Acute Hemodialysis Catheter *Angiodynamics, Inc., www.Angiodynamics.com*	Safe	1.5, 3	

Object	Status	Field Strength (T)	Reference
SecurACath, PICC Catheter with Nitinol Securement *Interrad Medical, Inc., St. Paul, MN*	Conditional 5	3	
StimuCath Continuous Peripheral *Nerve Block (CPNB) Catheter* *Regional Anesthesia Device* *Teleflex Medical, www.teleflex.com*	Conditional 5	1.5, 3	
Swan-Ganz Flow Directed Catheter, *Models 111F7, 115F7* *Edwards Lifesciences, www.edwards.com*	Safe	1.5, 3	
Swan-Ganz Pediatric Catheter, *Oximetry without Thermistor,* *Models 040F4, 040HF4, 015F4, 015HF4* *Edwards Lifesciences, www.edwards.com*	Safe	1.5, 3	
Swan-Ganz Thermodilution Catheter *American Edwards Laboratories, Irvine, CA*	Unsafe 2	1.5	57
Swan-Ganz Triple-lumen Thermodilution Catheter *American Edwards Laboratories, Irvine, CA*	Unsafe 2	1.5	60
TD Thermodilution Catheter *Flow-directed thermodilution pulmonary artery catheter* *Abbott Laboratories, www.abbott.com*	Unsafe 2	1.5	60
TDQ CCO Catheter *Flow-directed thermodilution continuous* *cardiac output pulmonary artery catheter* *Abbott Laboratories, www.abbott.com*	Unsafe 2	1.5	60
Torque-Line Flow-directed *thermodilution pulmonary artery catheter* *Abbott Laboratories, www.abbott.com*	Unsafe 2	1.5	60
Total Abscession Drainage Catheter *Angiodynamics, Inc., www.Angiodynamics.com*	Safe	1.5, 3	
Transpac IV *Abbott Laboratories, www.abbott.com*	Safe	1.5	60
TruFlow Hemodialysis Catheter *Smiths Medical, www.smiths-medical.com*	Safe	3	
VAMP, All Models *Edwards Lifesciences, www.edwards.com*	Safe	3	
VAMP Flex, All Models *Edwards Lifesciences, www.edwards.com*	Safe	3	
VAMP Jr., All Models *Edwards Lifesciences, www.edwards.com*	Safe	3	
Vantex CVC Catheter, All Models *Edwards Lifesciences, www.edwards.com*	Safe	3	
VENTRA Percutaneous Intravenous Catheter *Smiths Medical, www.smiths-medical.com*	Safe	3	

Object	Status	Field Strength (T)	Reference
VolumeView Catheter, VLVF *Edwards Lifesciences, www.edwards.com*	Conditional 8	1.5, 3	
VolumeView Femoral Catheter *Edwards Lifesciences, www.edwards.com*	Conditional 8	1.5, 3	
VolumeView Thermistor Manifold *Edwards Lifesciences, www.edwards.com*	Conditional 7	3	
VolumeView Venous Injectate Kit *Edwards Lifesciences, www.edwards.com*	Conditional 7	1.5, 3	
VP1, VAMP Plus *Edwards Lifesciences, www.edwards.com*	Conditional 7	3	

Carotid Artery Vascular Clamps

Object	Status	Field Strength (T)	Reference
Crutchfield, Carotid Artery Vascular Clamp *Codman, www.depuysynthes.com*	Conditional 5	1.5	11
Kindt, Carotid Artery Vascular Clamp *V. Mueller*	Conditional 5	1.5	11
Poppen-Blaylock, Carotid Artery Vascular Clamp *Codman, www.depuysynthes.com*	Unsafe 1	1.5	11
Salibi, Carotid Artery Vascular Clamp *Codman, www.depuysynthes.com*	Conditional 5	1.5	11
Selverstone, Carotid Artery Vascular Clamp *Codman, www.depuysynthes.com*	Conditional 5	1.5	11

Cerebrospinal Fluid (CSF) Shunt Valves and Accessories

Object	Status	Field Strength (T)	Reference
AccuDrain External CSF Drainage System *Integra NeuroSciences, www.integralife.com*	Safe	3	
ACCU FLO Connector *Right Angle, 316L SS* *Codman, www.depuysynthes.com*	Conditional 6	3	
ACCU FLO Connector *Right Angle, Plastic* *Codman, www.depuysynthes.com*	Safe	3	
ACCU-FLO Connector *Straight, 316L SS* *Codman, www.depuysynthes.com*	Conditional 6	3	
ACCU-FLO Connector *Straight, Plastic* *Codman, www.depuysynthes.com*	Safe	3	
ACCU-FLO Connector *Three Way, 316L SS* *Codman, www.depuysynthes.com*	Conditional 6	3	

Object	Status	Field Strength (T)	Reference
ACCU-FLO Connector *Three Way, Plastic* *Codman, www.depuysynthes.com*	Safe	3	
Accura II *Adult Integral Shunt System* *Phoenix Biomedical Corporation, Valley Forge, PA*	Safe	1.5	103
Accura II *Pediatric Integral Shunt System* *Phoenix Biomedical Corporation, Valley Forge, PA*	Safe	1.5	102
Anti-Siphon Device *Integra NeuroSciences, www.integralife.com*	Safe	3	
Anti-Siphon Device, NL8501415 *Integra NeuroSciences, www.integralife.com*	Safe	3	
Burr Hole Valve System(s) *15527, 15539, 12837, 15530, 12834,* *12838, 15533, 12835, 12839, 15536, 12836* *Integra NeuroSciences, www.integralife.com*	Safe	3	
BUS Device *Ventriculo-peritoneal shunt* *Codman, www.depuysynthes.com*	Conditional 6	3	
Catheter(s), Integra *NL8501200, NL8501376, NL8501328, NL8501201,* *NL8501380, NL8501515, NL8501202, NL8501381,* *NL8501517, NL8501220, NL8501382, NL8501519,* *NL8501221, NL8501228, NL8501390, NL8501222,* *NL8501504, NL8501391, NL8501375, NL8501229,* *NL8501392, NL8501415* *Integra NeuroSciences, www.integralife.com*	Safe	3	
Cerebral Ventricular Shunt Tube Connector, *Accu-flow right angle* *Codman, www.depuysynthes.com*	Safe	1.5	3, 94, 95
Cerebral Ventricular Shunt Tube Connector, *Accu-Flow, straight* *Codman, www.depuysynthes.com*	Safe	1.5	3, 94, 95
Cerebral Ventricular Shunt Tube Connector, *Accu-flow, T-connector* *Codman, www.depuysynthes.com*	Safe	1.5	3, 94, 95
Connector(s), Integra *NL8501902, NL8501911, NL8501913,* *NL8501908, NL8501919* *Integra NeuroSciences, www.integralife.com*	Safe	3	
Connector(s), Integra *991002, 999410, 999412, 999415,* *999411, 999414, 9MZ500* *Integra NeuroSciences, www.integralife.com*	Safe	3	

Object	Status	Field Strength (T)	Reference
Codman ACCU-FLO Straight Connector, 316 SS *Codman, www.depuysynthes.com*	Conditional 6	3	
Codman ACCU-FLO Straight Connector, Plastic *Codman, www.depuysynthes.com*	Safe	1.5, 3	
Codman ACCU-FLO Three Way Connector, Plastic *Codman, www.depuysynthes.com*	Safe	1.5, 3	
Codman ACCU-FLO Three Way Connector, 316 SS *Codman, www.depuysynthes.com*	Conditional 6	3	
Codman ACCU FLO Right Angle Connector *Codman, www.depuysynthes.com*	Conditional 6	3	
Codman Certas Plus Programmable Valve *Programmable CSF Shunt Valve* *Codman, www.depuysynthes.com*	Conditional 5	1.5, 3	
Codman Certas Programmable Valve *Programmable CSF Shunt Valve* *Codman, www.depuysynthes.com*	Conditional 5	1.5, 3	119
Codman EDS CSF External Drainage System *Codman, www.depuysynthes.com*	Safe	1.5, 3	103
Codman HAKIM Precision Pressure Valve *Fixed Pressure CSF Shunt Valve* *Codman, www.depuysynthes.com*	Conditional 6	3	
Codman HAKIM Programmable Valve *Codman, www.depuysynthes.com*	Conditional 5	1.5, 3	110
Codman Holter Cerebral Catheter-Reservoir *LeRoy Design* *Codman, www.depuysynthes.com*	Conditional 6	1.5, 3	
Codman Holter In-Line Shunt Filter, Hoffman Design *Codman, www.depuysynthes.com*	Conditional 6	1.5, 3	
Codman Hydrocephalus Shunt, System Connector *Codman, www.depuysynthes.com*	Conditional 6	1.5, 3	
Codman MEDOS Right Angle Connector *also known as CODMAN Hakim Right Angle Connector* *Codman, www.depuysynthes.com*	Conditional 6	3	
Codman MEDOS Straight Connector *also known as CODMAN Hakim Straight Connector* *Codman, www.depuysynthes.com*	Conditional 6	3	
Contour-Flex Valve System(s) *Integra NeuroSciences, www.integralife.com*	Safe	3	
CRx Universal Shunt *Cerebral Spinal Fluid (CSF) Shunt Valve* *Sophysa, www.sophysa.com*	Safe	1.5, 3	

Object	Status	Field Strength (T)	Reference
CRx Valve *Cerebral Spinal Fluid (CSF) Shunt Valve* *Sophysa, www.sophysa.com*	Safe	1.5, 3	
CSF Flow Control Valve, Fixed Pressure *Medtronic, Inc., www.medtronic.com/mri*	Safe	1.5	
Delta Shunt Assembly *Medtronic, Inc., www.medtronic.com/mri*	Safe	3	96, 103
Delta Valve *Medtronic, Inc., www.medtronic.com/mri*	Safe	1.5	
Diamond valve *Cerebral Spinal Fluid (CSF), Shunt Valve* *Sophysa, www.sophysa.com*	Safe	1.5, 3	
Diamond II model valve *Cerebral Spinal Fluid (CSF), Shunt Valve* *Sophysa, www.sophysa.com*	Safe	1.5, 3	
EDM Ventricular Catheter *External CSF Drainage Product* *Medtronic, Inc., www.medtronic.com/mri*	Safe	3	103
EDS 2 CSF External Drainage System *Codman, www.depuysynthes.com*	Safe	3	103
EDS 3 CSF External Drainage System *Codman, www.depuysynthes.com*	Safe	3	103
Edwards-Barbaro Shunt *Integra NeuroSciences, www.integralife.com*	Safe	3	
Equi-Flow Valve System *Integra NeuroSciences* *www.integralife.co*	Safe	3	
GAV 2.0, Gravitational Valve (GV) *Miethke GmbH & Co. KG, www.miethke.com*	Conditional 8	1.5, 3	
HOLTER Cerebral Catheter-Reservoir *LeRoy Design* *Codman, www.depuysynthes.com*	Conditional 6	3	
HOLTER In Line Shunt Filter *Codman, www.depuysynthes.com*	Conditional 5	3	
HOLTER In Line Shunt Filter *Hoffman Design* *Codman, www.depuysynthes.com*	Conditional 6	3	
HOLTER Reservoir, 316L SS *Codman, www.depuysynthes.com*	Conditional 6	3	
HOLTER Rickham Reservoir, 316L SS *Codman, www.depuysynthes.com*	Conditional 6	3	
HOLTER Rickham Reservoir, Plastic *Codman, www.depuysynthes.com*	Safe	3	

Object	Status	Field Strength (T)	Reference
HOLTER Salmon-Rickham, Ventriculostomy *Reservoir, 316L SS* *Codman, www.depuysynthes.com*	Conditional 6	3	
HOLTER Salmon-Rickham, Ventriculostomy *Reservoir, Plastic* *Codman, www.depuysynthes.com*	Safe	3	
HOLTER Selker Ventriculostomy Reservoir, Plastic *Codman, www.depuysynthes.com*	Safe	3	
HOLTER Type A Connector *Codman, www.depuysynthes.com*	Conditional 6	3	
HOLTER Type B Connector *Codman, www.depuysynthes.com*	Conditional 6	3	
HOLTER Ventricular Catheter *Codman, www.depuysynthes.com*	Conditional 6	3	
HOLTER, Selker Valve, 316L SS *Codman, www.depuysynthes.com*	Conditional 6	3	
Horizontal-Vertical (H-V) Lumbar Valve System *Integra NeuroSciences, www.integralife.com*	Conditional 5	3	
Integra Flow Regulating Valve *Low Flow Lumbar* *Integra NeuroSciences, www.integralife.com*	Conditional 5	3	
Integra Flow Regulating Valve *Low Flow Mini* *Integra NeuroSciences, www.integralife.com*	Conditional 5	3	
Integra Flow Regulating Valve *Low Flow Standard* *Integra NeuroSciences, www.integralife.com*	Conditional 5	3	
Integra NPH Valve System(s) *909500, 909507, 909515, 909501,* *909507S, 909518, 909502, 909508,* *909520, 909503, 909508S, 909521,* *909504, 909512, 90S512, 909505,* *909513, 90S521, 909506, 909514,* *90S5211* *Integra NeuroSciences, www.integralife.com*	Safe	3	
LP Shunt *Medtronic, Inc., www.medtronic.com/mri*	Safe	1.5	
LPVII Valve System(s) *NL8509810, NL8509830, NL8509850, NL8509811,* *NL8509831,* *NL8509851, NL8509820, NL8509840, NL8509860,* *NL8509821 NL8509841 NL8509861* *Integra NeuroSciences, www.integralife.com*	Safe	3	

Object	Status	Field Strength (T)	Reference
Miethke proGAV Programmable Shunt System *B. Braun, www.bbraun.com*	Conditional 5	1.5, 3	
Miethke proGAV Shunt System *B. Braun, www.bbraun.com*	Conditional 5	3	
Miethke proSA Shunt System *B. Braun, www.bbraun.com*	Conditional 5	3	
Mishler Valve System(s) *NL8500311, NL8500313, NL8500315, NL8500312,* *NL8500314* *Integra NeuroSciences, www.integralife.com*	Safe	3	
Multi Purpose On-Off Valve System(s) *NL8500108 NL8500125 NL8500128* *Integra NeuroSciences, www.integralife.com*	Safe	3	
Novus Valve System(s) *NL8509010, NL8509021, NL8509610, NL8509011,* *NL8509311 NL8509620, NL8509020, NL8509321* *Integra NeuroSciences, www.integralife.com*	Safe	3	
One Piece Shunt Valve System(s) *NL8506102, NL8506302, NL8506403, NL8506201* *NL8506401, NL8506501, NL8506202, NL8506402* *Integra NeuroSciences, www.integralife.com*	Safe	3	
OSV II Low Flow Lumbar Valve System(s) *Integra NeuroSciences, www.integralife.com*	Safe	3	
OSV II Low Pro Valve System(s) *Integra NeuroSciences, www.integralife.com*	Safe	3	
OSV II Lumbar Valve System(s) *Integra NeuroSciences, www.integralife.com*	Safe	3	
OSV II Smart Valve *Integra NeuroSciences, www.integralife.com*	Safe	3	
OSV II Valve System(s) *Integra NeuroSciences, www.integralife.com*	Safe	3	
POLARIS Adjustable Pressure Valve *Sophysa, www.sophysa.com*	Conditional 5	3	97, 103
proGAV Adjustable Valve *Aesculap, Inc., www.aesculapusa.com*	Conditional 5	3	104
proGAV 2.0 (proGAV II) Hydrocephalus Shunt Valve *Christoph Miethke GmbH & Co., www.miethke.com*	Conditional 5	3	
PS Medical CSF-Flow Control Valve *Medtronic, Inc., www.medtronic.com/mri*	Safe	1.5	96
PS Medical CSF-Ventricular Access Port *Medtronic, Inc., www.medtronic.com/mri*	Safe	1.5	96
PS Medical CSF-Ventricular Reservoir *Medtronic, Inc., www.medtronic.com/mri*	Safe	1.5	96

Object	Status	Field Strength (T)	Reference
PS Medical CSF-Ventriculostomy Reservoir *Medtronic, Inc., www.medtronic.com/mri*	Safe	1.5	96
PS Medical Strata Burr Hole Valve *Medtronic, Inc., www.medtronic.com/mri*	Conditional 5	3	
PS Medical Strata II Valve *Medtronic, Inc., www.medtronic.com/mri*	Conditional 5	3	
PS Medical Strata NSC Burr Hole Valve *Medtronic, Inc., www.medtronic.com/mri*	Conditional 5	3	
PS Medical Strata NSC Lumboperitoneal *Shunt System* *Medtronic, Inc., www.medtronic.com/mri*	Conditional 5	3	
PS Medical Strata NSC Lumboperitoneal Valve *Medtronic, Inc., www.medtronic.com/mri*	Conditional 5	3	
PS Medical Strata NSC Valve *Medtronic, Inc., www.medtronic.com/mri*	Conditional 5	3	
PS Medical Strata Valve(s), Small and Regular *Medtronic, Inc., www.medtronic.com/mri*	Conditional 5	3	
PS Medical Strata Valve *Adjustable Cerebral Spinal Fluid Valve* *Medtronic, Inc., www.medtronic.com/mri*	Conditional 5	1.5	96
Pudenz Valve System(s) *NL8501330, NL8501358, NL8501411, NL8501331,* *NL8501359, NL8501412, NL8501356, NL8501410,* *NL8501413, NL8501357 NL8501414* *Integra NeuroSciences, www.integralife.com*	Safe	3	
Pulsar Valve *Sophysa, www.sophysa.com*	Safe	1.5	97
Reservoir(s), Integra *NL8501210, NL8501214, NL8501121, NL8501211,* *NL8501215 NL8501132, NL8501212, NL8500150,* *NL8501192, NL8501213, NL8500155 NL8501195* *Integra NeuroSciences, www.integralife.com*	Safe	3	
Reservoir(s), Integra *999015, 999112, 999303, 999016, 999113,* *999304, 999017, 999301, 951305, 999110,* *999302, 951307, 999111* *Integra NeuroSciences, www.integralife.com*	Safe	3	
Rickham Reservoir, 316L SS *Codman, www.depuysynthes.com*	Conditional 6	3	
Right Angle Connector, Nylon *Codman, www.depuysynthes.com*	Safe	3	
Selker Valve, 316L SS *Codman, www.depuysynthes.com*	Conditional 6	3	

Object	Status	Field Strength (T)	Reference
Selker Valve, Nylon *Codman, www.depuysynthes.com*	Safe	3	
Shunt Valve, Holter-Hausner Type *Holter-Hausner, Inc., Bridgeport, PA*	Safe	1.5	55
Shunt Valve, Holtertype *The Holter Co., Bridgeport, PA*	Unsafe 1	1.5	55
Single Valve, Cerebral Spinal Fluid (CSF) *Shunt Valve* *Sophysa, www.sophysa.com*	Safe	1.5, 3	
Sophy Adjustable Pressure Valve, Model SP3 *Sophysa, www.sophysa.com*	Conditional 5	1.5	97
Sophy Adjustable Pressure Valve, Model SU8 *Sophysa, www.sophysa.com*	Conditional 5	1.5	97
Sophy Adjustable Pressure Valve, *Sophysa, www.sophysa.com*	Conditional 5	1.5	97
Sophy Mini Monopressure Valve *Sophysa, www.sophysa.com*	Safe	1.5	97
Straight Connector, Nylon *Codman, www.depuysynthes.com*	Safe	3	
Strata II Programmable CSF Shunt Valve *Medtronic, Inc., www.medtronic.com/mri*	Conditional 5	3	
StrataMR Programmable Valves and Shunts *Medtronic, Inc., www.Medtronic.com/MRI*	Conditional 8	1.5, 3	
Strata NSC Programmable CSF Shunt Valve *Medtronic, Inc., www.medtronic.com/mri*	Conditional 5	3	
Strata Programmable CSF Shunt Valve *Medtronic, Inc., www.medtronic.com/mri*	Conditional 5	3	
Suture Tubing Clamp(s), Integra *999004, 999005, 999007* *Integra NeuroSciences, www.integralife.com*	Safe	3	
Three Way Connector, Silicone, Nylon *Codman, www.depuysynthes.com*	Safe	3	
UltraVS Valve System(s) *NL8501109, NL8501115, NL8501127, NL8501110,* *NL8501123, NL8501128, NL8501111, NL8501124,* *NL8501129, NL8501113, NL8501125, NL8501130,* *NL8501114, NL8501126, NL8501131* *Integra NeuroSciences, www.integralife.com*	Safe	3	

Object	Status	Field Strength (T)	Reference
Ventricular Catheter(s), Peritoneal Catheter(s), *Atrial Catheter(s) 953100, 951102A, 9MZ207, 9MZ100, 9MD1022, 9MZ208, 953101, 9MD102A, 9MZ209, 9MZ101, 9MD102B, 9MZ210, 9MZ1011, 9MZ203, 9MZ211, PC1, 9MZ204, VC1, 951101, 9MZ205, 999013, 951101A, 9MZ206, 999014, 951102* *Integra NeuroSciences, www.integralife.com*	Safe	3	

Coils, Stents, Filters, and Grafts

Object	Status	Field Strength (T)	Reference
2D Helical, 35 Fibered Platinum Coil *Boston Scientific, www.bostonscientific.com*	Conditional 5	1.5, 3	
AAA Endograft *TriVascular2, Inc., Santa Rosa, CA*	Conditional 6	3	
Abre Stent *Medtronic, Inc., www.Medtronic.com/MRI*	Conditional 8	1.5, 3	
Absolute Biliary Stent *Abbott Vascular, www.abbottvascular.com*	Conditional 5	3	
Absolute .035 Biliary Self-Expanding Stent *Abbott Vascular, www.abbottvascular.com*	Conditional 5	3	
Absolute Pro .035 Biliary Self-Expanding Stent *Abbott Vascular, www.abbottvascular.com*	Conditional 5	3	
Absolute Pro Stent *Nickel Titanium with Nickel Titanium Platinum markers* *8-mm x 120-mm* *single version* *Abbott Vascular, www.abbottvascular.com*	Conditional 6	3	
Absolute Pro Stent *Nickel Titanium with Nickel Titanium Platinum markers* *8-mm x 348-mm* *three overlapped version* *Abbott Vascular, www.abbottvascular.com*	Conditional 6	3	
Absolute Pro Peripheral Stent *Abbott Vascular, www.abbottvascular.com*	Conditional 5	3	
Absorb Bioresorbable Vascular Scaffold *(BVS) System* *Abbott Vascular, www.abbottvascular.com*	Safe	1.5, 3	
Absorb GT1 Bioresorbable Vascular Scaffold *(BVS) System* *Abbott Vascular, www.abbottvascular.com*	Safe	1.5, 3	
Acculink Carotid Stent *Abbott Vascular, www.abbottvascular.com*	Conditional 5	3	
ACS Multi-Link Coronary Stent *Abbott Vascular, www.abbottvascular.com*	Conditional 5	3	

Object	Status	Field Strength (T)	Reference
ACS Multi-Link RX Duet *Stent, 316L SS* *Abbott Vascular, www.abbottvascular.com*	Safe	1.5	72
ACS Multi-Link DUET Coronary Stent *Abbott Vascular, www.abbottvascular.com*	Conditional 5	3	
ACS Multi-Link TRISTAR Coronary Stent *Abbott Vascular, www.abbottvascular.com*	Conditional 5	3	
ACS Multi-Link ULTRA Coronary Stent *Abbott Vascular, www.abbottvascular.com*	Conditional 5	3	
ACS RX Multi-Link *15 x 3.0-mm, Stent, 316L SS* *Abbott Vascular, www.abbottvascular.com*	Safe	1.5	72
ACS RX Multi-Link *15 x 4.0-mm, Stent, 316L SS* *Abbott Vascular, www.abbottvascular.com*	Safe	1.5	72
ACS RX Multi-Link *25 x 3.0-mm, Stent, 316L SS* *Abbott Vascular, www.abbottvascular.com*	Safe	1.5	72
ACS Stent, 316L SS *Abbott Vascular, www.abbottvascular.com*	Safe	1.5	
ACURATE Stent *Symetis SA, Switzerland*	Conditional 6	3	
Adapt Carotid Stent *Carotid Artery Stent* *Endotex Interventional Systems, Inc., Cupertino, CA*	Conditional 6	3	
Advanta SST Aortic Repair Graft *Atrium Medical Corporation, www.atriummed.com and* *Maquet Cardiovascular LLC, www.maquet.com/vascular*	Safe	1.5, 3	
Advanta SST PTFE Vascular Graft *Atrium Medical Corporation, www.atriummed.com and* *Maquet Cardiovascular LLC, www.maquet.com/vascular*	Safe	1.5, 3	
Advanta VS PTFE Vascular Graft *Atrium Medical Corporation, www.atriummed.com and* *Maquet Cardiovascular LLC, www.maquet.com/vascular*	Safe	1.5, 3	
Advanta VST PTFE Vascular Graft *Atrium Medical Corporation, www.atriummed.com and* *Maquet Cardiovascular LLC, www.maquet.com/vascular*	Safe	1.5, 3	
Advanta V12 Stent *Atrium Medical Corporation, Hudson, New Hampshire*	Conditional 6	3	
AEROmini Stent *Merit Medical, www.merit.com*	Conditional 8	1.5, 3	
AEROmini Tracheobronchial Stent *Merit Medical, www.meritmedical.com*	Conditional 8	1.5, 3	

Object	Status	Field Strength (T)	Reference
AERO Tracheobronchial Stent *Merit Endotek, Merit Medical, www.merit.com*	Conditional 6	3	
Aero Tracheal Stent *Alveolus, Inc., Charlotte, NC*	Conditional 6	3	
Aero Tracheal Stent *Nitinol with Polyurethane Cover* *Alveolus, Inc., Charlotte, NC*	Conditional 6	3	
ALIMAXX-B Biliary Stent *Uncovered Biliary Stent* *Merit Endotek* *Merit Medical, www.merit.com*	Conditional 6	3	
ALIMAXX-B Covered Biliary Stent *Alveolus, Inc., Charlotte, NC*	Conditional 6	3	
ALIMAXX-B Uncovered Biliary Stent *Alveolus, Inc. Charlotte, NC*	Conditional 6	3	
ALIMAXX-ES Stent *Merit Medical, www.merit.com*	Conditional 8	1.5, 3	
ALIMAXX-ES Esophageal Stent *Merit Endotek* *Merit Medical, www.merit.com*	Conditional 6	3	
ALN Vena Cava Filter, 316L SS *ALN Implants Chirurgicaux, www.aln2b.com*	Conditional 6	3	
ALN Vena Cava Filter, 12 Legs *ALN Implants Chirurgicaux, www.aln2b.com*	Conditional 8	1.5, 3	
ALN Vena Cava Filter, 12 Legs with Hook *ALN Implants Chirurgicaux, www.aln2b.com*	Conditional 8	1.5, 3	
AmM Fortitude Bioresorbable Drug-Eluting *Coronary Scaffold* *Amaranth Medical, www.amaranthmedical.com*	Safe	1.5, 3	
Amplatzer Vascular Graft (AVG) *AGA Medical Corporation, www.sjm.com/aga-medical*	Conditional 8	1.5, 3	
Amplatz IVC Filter *Cook Medical, Inc., www.cookmedical.com*	Safe	4.7	21
Anaconda Endovascular Device *Vascutek Ltd.*	Conditional 6	3	
ANCURE Endograft Sten *Guidant Corporation*	Safe	1.5	
AneuRx AAA Stent Grafts System *Medtronic, Inc., www.medtronic.com/mri*	Conditional 6	3	
AneuRx AAAdvantage Stent Grafts System *Medtronic, Inc., www.medtronic.com/mri*	Safe	3	
AneuRx II Bifurcation Stent Graft *Medtronic, Inc., www.medtronic.com/mri*	Safe	3	

Object	Status	Field Strength (T)	Reference
Angiomed Memotherm Femoral Stent *4-mm x 120-mm, Nitinol* *C.R. Bard, Inc., www.crbard.com*	Safe	1.5	
Angiomed Memotherm Femoral Stent *5-mm x 20-mm, Nitinol* *C.R. Bard, Inc., www.crbard.com*	Safe	1.5	
Angiomed Memotherm Iliac Stent *12-mm x 110-mm, Nitinol* *C.R. Bard, Inc., www.crbard.com*	Safe	1.5	
Angiomed Memotherm Iliac Stent *8-mm x 20-mm, Nitinol* *C.R. Bard, Inc., www.crbard.com*	Safe	1.5	
AngioStent Stent, 15-mm *Platinum, Iridium* *Angiodynamics* *Queensbury, NY*	Safe	1.5	
Aorfix Bifurcated Stent Graft system *Lombard Medical, www.LombardMedical.com*	Conditional 5	3	
Apollo Cerebral Stent, 316LVM SS *MicroPort Medical, www.microport.com.cn/english*	Conditional 6	3	
Apollo Intracranial Stent *MicroPort Medical, www.microport.com.cn/english*	Conditional 8	1.5, 3	
ArchStent *Ostial Corporation, www.ostialcorp.com*	Conditional 6	3	
aSpire Covered Stent *100 x 14-mm* *Vascular Architects, Portola, CA*	Safe	1.5	
aSpire II Stent *Nitinol with an ePTFE covering* *Vascular Architects, Inc., San Jose, CA*	Safe	3	
Assurant Cobalt Iliac Stent *single and two overlapped versions* *Medtronic, Inc., www.medtronic.com/mri*	Conditional 8	1.5, 3	
Astron Stent, Nitinol, gold markers *Biotronik, www.Biotronik.com*	Conditional 6	3	
Athena Embolization Coil *Medina Medical, www.medina-medical.com*	Conditional 8	1.5, 3	
Atrioventricular Valved Stent (AVS) *Navigate Cardiac Structures, Inc., www.navigatecsi.com*	Conditional 8	1.5, 3	
AVE GFX Stent, 316L SS *Arterial Vascular Engineering, Santa Rosa, CA*	Safe	1.5	69
AVE Micro I Stent, 316L SS *Arterial Vascular Engineering, Santa Rosa, CA*	Safe	1.5	69

Object	Status	Field Strength (T)	Reference
AVE Micro II Stent, 316L SS *Arterial Vascular Engineering, Santa Rosa, CA*	Safe	1.5	69
AXIOS Stent *Xlumena, Inc., www.xlumena.com*	Conditional 8	1.5, 3	
Axium Detachable Coil, Embolization Coil *Covidien and ev3, Inc., www.ev3.net*	Conditional 6	3	
Axium Detachable Implant for *Neurovascular Malformation* *Embolization coil* *Covidien and ev3, Inc., www.ev3.net*	Conditional 6	3	
Axium Embolization Coil *All Sizes* *Medtronic, www.medtronic.com*	Conditional 8	1.5, 3	
Axxess Biolimus A9 Eluting Bifurcation Stent *Coronary Artery Stent* *Nitinol* *Devax, Inc., Irvine, CA*	Conditional 6	3	
Axxess Stent, Coronary Artery Stent *Devax, Inc., Irvine, CA*	Safe	3	
Azur Peripheral Endovascular *Embolization Coil System* *Azur Detachable* *MicroVention, Inc., Tustin, CA*	Conditional 6	3	
Babygraft - Cardiovascular Arterial Graft L-Hydro *Labcor Laboratorios Ltda., www.labcor.com*	Safe	1.5, 3	
BARD CONFORMEXX, Biliary Stent *C. R. Bard & Angiomed GmbH & Co. Medizintechnik KG,* *Germany*	Safe	1.5, 3	83
Bard DeBakey Woven Graft *Bard Peripheral Vascular, www.bardpv.com*	Safe	3	
Bard E-LUMINEXX (ELUMINEXX) Biliary Stent *Bard Peripheral Vascular, www.bardpv.com*	Conditional 6	3	
Bard E-LUMINEXX (ELUMINEXX) Vascular Stent *Bard Peripheral Vascular, www.bardpv.com*	Conditional 6	3	
Bard LifeStent FlexStar XL Stent *Bard Peripheral Vascular, www.bardpv.com*	Conditional 5	1.5, 3	
Bard Low Porosity PTFE Felt *Bard Peripheral Vascular, www.bardpv.com*	Safe	1.5, 3	
Bard LUMINEXX 3 Biliary and Vascular Stent *C. R. Bard & Angiomed GmbH & Co.* *Medizintechnik KG, Germany*	Safe	1.5, 3	

Object	Status	Field Strength (T)	Reference
BARD LUMINEXX *Biliary and Vascular Stent* *C. R. Bard & Angiomed GmbH & Co.* *Medizintechnik KG, Germany*	Safe	1.5, 3	83
Bard Polyester Felt *Bard Peripheral Vascular, www.bardpv.com*	Safe	1.5, 3	
Bard PTFE Felt *Bard Peripheral Vascular, www.bardpv.com*	Safe	1.5, 3	
Bard PTFE Felt Pledget *Bard Peripheral Vascular, www.bardpv.com*	Safe	1.5, 3	
Bard Stent, Bifurcated *36 x 20-mm, Nitinol* *Bard Peripheral Vascular, www.bardpv.com*	Safe	1.5	70
Bard ViVEXX Carotid Stent *Nitinol* *C. R. Bard & Angiomed GmbH & Co. Medizintechnik KG,* *Germany*	Safe	3	
Bard XT Stent *15 x 3.0-mm, 316 LVM* *Bard Interventional Products, Billerica, MA*	Safe	1.5	72
Bard XT Stent *316 LVM* *Bard Limited, Ireland*	Safe	1.5	69
Berenstein Hydroflex Embolization Coil *MicroVention, Inc., www.microvention.com*	Conditional 6	3	
BeStent, 15 x 3.0-mm *Medtronic, Inc., www.medtronic.com/mri*	Safe	1.5	72
BeStent, 25 x 3.0-mm *Medtronic, Inc., www.medtronic.com/mri*	Safe	1.5	72
BeStent, MR Safe SS *Medtronic, Inc., www.medtronic.com/mri*	Safe	1.5	69
Bifurcated EXCLUDER Endoprosthesis *Nitinol* *Stent* *W.L. Gore and Associates, Inc., www.goremedical.com*	Safe	1.5	
Biliary Amsterdam Stent *Hobbs Medical, www.hobbsmedical.com*	Safe	1.5	
Biliary Pigtail Stent *Hobbs Medical, www.hobbsmedical.com*	Safe	1.5	
BIOFLEX Stent, Coronary Artery Stent *316L SS* *Biosensors International, La Jolla, CA*	Safe	3	
BioFreedom Drug Coated Stent (DCS) *Biosensors International, www.biosensors.com*	Conditional 8	1.5, 3	

Object	Status	Field Strength (T)	Reference
BioMatrix Flex Stent *Biosensors International, La Jolla, CA*	Conditional 8	1.5, 3	
BioMatrix Flex BTK Stent *Biosensors Research USA, Inc.,* *www.biosensors.com/usa/*	Conditional 8	1.5, 3	
BioNIR Stent *Medinol Ltd., www.medinol.com*	Conditional 8	1.5, 3	
Biosoft duo Multilength Hydro-coated *Double Loop Ureteral Stent* *Coloplast, www.coloplast.com*	Safe	1.5, 3	
Black Silicone Filiform Double Pigtail Ureteral Stent *Cook Medical, www.cookmedical.com*	Conditional 6	3	
Blazer Stent *OrbusNeich, www.orbusneich.com*	Conditional 6	3	
Blockade Medical Barricade Coil System *Embolization Coil* *Blockade Medical, blockademedical.com*	Conditional 6	3	
Bovine Pericardium Heterological Graft *Labcor Laboratorios Ltda., www.labcor.com*	Safe	1.5, 3	
BRAVO Flow Diverter *Codman Neurovascular, www.depuysynthes.com*	Conditional 5	1.5, 3	
Bridge Constant Stent *Medtronic, Inc., www.medtronic.com/mri*	Safe	3	
Bronchial Stent *Hood Laboratories, www.hoodlabs.com*	Safe	1.5, 3	
Bulbar Urethral Stent *Allium Medical Solutions Ltd., www.allium-medical.com*	Conditional 8	1.5, 3	
BX Stent *316L SS* *Cordis, Miami Lakes, FL*	Safe	1.5	69
BX Velocity Balloon-Expander *Intracranial Intravascular Stent, 4.0-mm x 8-mm* *Cordis, www.depuysynthes.com*	Safe	1.5, 3	83
Cappella Sideguard Coronary Sidebranch Stent *Sideguard Stent (Side Guard Stent)* *Capella Medical Devices, Ltd., www.cappella-med.com*	Conditional 5	1.5, 3	
CarboStent Isthmus Iliac Stent *CID, cidvascular.com*	Conditional 8	1.5, 3	
CARDIOROOT Aortic Graft *Atrium Medical Corporation, www.atriummed.com and* *Maquet Cardiovascular LLC, www.maquet.com/vascular*	Safe	1.5, 3	
Carotid Stent (RD11-014) *Microvention, Inc., www.microvention.com*	Conditional 5	3	

Object	Status	Field Strength (T)	Reference
Carotid WALLSTENT Endoprosthesis *Boston Scientific, www.bostonscientific.com*	Conditional 5	3	
CASHMERE Microcoil *Embolization Coil* *Micrus Endovascular, www.micrusendovascular.com*	Conditional 5	3	
Castor Branched Aortic Stent Graft *MicroPort Medical, www.microport.com.cn/english*	Conditional 8	1.5, 3	
Celect Vena Cava Filter *Cook Medical, Inc., www.cookmedical.com*	Conditional 5	3	
Celosia Covered Stent *InSitu Technologies, Inc., www.insitu-tech.com*	Conditional 5	1.5, 3	
CenterFlex Vascular Graft *Carbon-impregnated ePTFE* *Bard Peripheral Vascular, www.bardpv.com*	Safe	1.5, 3	
CGuard Carotid Stent, All Sizes *InspireMD Ltd., www.inspiremd.com*	Conditional 8	1.5, 3	
ChampioNIR Stent, All Sizes *Medinol Ltd., www.medinol.com*	Conditional 8	1.5, 3	
CHOOSTENT *M.I. Tech Co., Ltd., www.mitech.co.kr*	Conditional 8	1.5, 3	
CHOOSTENT Covered Esophagus Stent *M.I. Tech, www.mitech.co.kr*	Conditional 8	1.5, 3	
Chromaxx BX Stent *Cobalt Chromium Alloy* *Angiomed GmbH & Co., Germany*	Conditional 6	3	
Chromium Coronary Stent *Biocore Biotecnologia S.A., Canoas, Brazil*	Conditional 8	1.5, 3	
Cinatra Cobalt-Chromium *Coronary Artery Stent* *Atrium Medical Corporation, Hudson, NH*	Conditional 8	1.5, 3	
Cobra BMS, Bare Metal Stent *Medlogics Device Corporation, Santa Rosa, CA*	Conditional 6	3	
COBRA PzF Coronary Stent *CeloNova BioSciences, Inc., www.celonova.com*	Conditional 8	1.5, 3	
Cobra Stent *MEDLOGICS Device Corporation, Santa Rosa, CA*	Conditional 6	3	
Coherex FlatStent EF *Coherex Medical, Salt Lake City, UT*	Conditional 6	3	
Complete SE Stent *Medtronic, Inc., www.medtronic.com/mri*	Conditional 8	1.5, 3	
Complex Helical 18 Coil *Boston Scientific, www.bostonscientific.com*	Conditional 5	1.5, 3	

Object	Status	Field Strength (T)	Reference
CONCERTO Detachable Coil, Embolization Coil *Covidien and ev3 Inc., www.ev3.net*	Conditional 5	3	
ConvertX Nephroureteral Stent *BrightWater Medical, www.brightwatermed.com*	Conditional 8	1.5, 3	
Cook Celect Vena Cava Filter *Cook Medical, Inc., www.cookmedical.com*	Conditional 5	3	
Cook Occluding Spring Embolization Coil *MWCE- 338-5-10* *Cook Medical, Inc., www.cookmedical.com*	Conditional 5	1.5	
Cook-Z Stent, Gianturco-Rosch Biliary Design *Cook Medical, Inc., www.cookmedical.com*	Conditional 5	1.5	
Cook-Z Stent, Gianturco-Rosch Tracheobronchial *Design* *Cook Medical, Inc., www.cookmedical.com*	Conditional 5	1.5	
Cook-Z Stent Gianturco Self-Expandable *Vena Cava and Venous Design* *Cook Medical Inc., www.cookmedical.com*	Conditional 5	1.5, 3	
CORDIS ENTERPRISE Vascular Reconstruction *Device* *Cordis, www.depuysynthes.com*	Conditional 5	3	
Corograft Arterial Graft L-Hydro *Labcor Laboratorios Ltda., www.labcor.com*	Safe	1.5, 3	
CoRectCoil, Nitinol *Intratherapeutics, Inc., St. Paul, MN*	Safe	1.5	
Corvita Endoluminal Graft *for Abdominal Aortic Aneurysm* *Schneider (USA) Inc.,* *Pfizer Medical Technology Group, Minneapolis, MN*	Safe	1.5	64
CoStar Coronary Stent *Cobalt Chromium* *Conor Medsystems, Menlo Park, CA*	Safe	3	
CoStar Paclitaxel-Eluting Coronary Stent *Conor Medsystems, Menlo Park, CA*	Safe	3	
Covered UltraFlex Esophageal Stent *Nitinol Stent with polyurethane covering* *Boston Scientific, www.bostonscientific.com*	Safe	1.5	
Covered WallFlex Biliary RX Stent *Boston Scientific, www.bostonscientific.com*	Conditional 6	3	
cPAX Embolization Material *NeuroVASx, Inc., Maple Grove, MN*	Safe	1.5, 3	

Object	Status	Field Strength (T)	Reference
Cragg Nitinol Spiral Filter	Safe	4.7	21
Cristallo Ideale Carotid Self-Expanding Stent *Conical version* *Invatec Technology Center GmbH,* *Thurgau, Switzerland*	Conditional 6	3	
Cristallo Ideale Carotid Self-Expanding Stent *Cylindrical version* *Invatec Technology Center GmbH,* *Thurgau, Switzerland*	Conditional 6	3	
Crossflex Stent, 316L SS *Cordis, www.depuysynthes.com*	Safe	1.5	69
Crown Stent, 316L SS *Cordis, www.depuysynthes.com*	Safe	1.5	69
Crux Filter Vena Cava Filter *Crux Biomedical, Inc., Portola Valley, CA*	Conditional 6	3	
Cypher Select, Sirolimus-Eluting Stent *Cordis, www.depuysynthes.com*	Conditional 5	1.5, 3	
Cypher Sirolimus-eluting Coronary Stent *Cordis, www.cordis.com*	Conditional 5	1.5, 3	
DELTAFILL Microcoil, Embolization Coil *Codman Neurovascular and Depuy Synthes,* *www.depuysynthes.com*	Conditional 6	3	
DELTAMAXX Microcoil, Embolization Coil *Codman Neurovascular and Depuy Synthes,* *www.depuysynthes.com*	Conditional 6	3	
DELTAPAQ Microcoil, Embolization Coil *Codman Neurovascular and Depuy Synthes,* *www.depuysynthes.com*	Conditional 6	3	
DELTAPLUSH Microcoil, Embolization Coil *Codman Neurovascular and Depuy Synthes,* *www.depuysynthes.com*	Conditional 6	3	
DELTASFT Microcoil, Embolization Coil *Codman Neurovascular and Depuy Synthes,* *www.depuysynthes.com*	Conditional 6	3	
Denali Vena Cava Filter *Bard Peripheral Vascular, www.bardpv.com*	Conditional 6	3	
DESolve Scaffold System *Elixir Medical, www.elixirmedical.com*	Safe	1.5, 3	
Detachable Microcoil System (DMC) *INCUMEDx, www.incumedx.net*	Conditional 8	1.5, 3	
Detach Embolization Coil System *Cook Medical, Inc., www.cookmedical.com*	Conditional 6	3	

Object	Status	Field Strength (T)	Reference
Diamond Colonic Stent *26-mm diameter x 10-cm length* *Boston Scientific, www.bostonscientific.com*	Safe	1.5	
Distaflo Bypass Graft *Carbon-impregnated ePTFE* *Bard Peripheral Vascular, www.bardpv.com*	Safe	3	
DISTAFLO Bypass Graft *Carbon-impregnated ePTFE* *Bard Peripheral Vascular, www.bardpv.com*	Safe	3	
Diverter Stent *8-mm x 32-mm* *Elgiloy (Conichrome), Tantalum* *MindGuard, Ltd., Israel*	Safe	1.5	
Double-J Closed Tip Ureteral Stent *Gyrus ACMI (Olympus Medical),* *www.medical.olympusamerica.com*	Safe	3	
Double-J II Closed Tip Ureteral Stent *Gyrus ACMI (Olympus Medical),* *www.medical.olympusamerica.com*	Safe	3	
Double Pigtail Ureteral Stent *Gyrus ACMI (Olympus Medical),* *www.medical.olympusamerica.com*	Safe	3	
Double Pigtail Ureteral Stent *Polyurethane* *Gyrus ACMI (Olympus Medical),* *www.medical.olympusamerica.com*	Safe	3	
Driver Sprint Stent *Medtronic, Inc., www.medtronic.com/mri*	Conditional 5	3	
Driver Stent, Including Driver RX, Driver MXII *MicroDriver, MicroDriver MXII* *MicroDriver RX Coronary Stent* *Medtronic, Inc., www.medtronic.com/mri*	Conditional 5	3	
Duraflex Coronary Artery Stent *Goodman Co., LTD., www.goodmankk.com/english/*	Conditional 8	1.5, 3	
Duraflex SE Stent *Flexible Stenting Solutions, Inc., Eatontown, NJ*	Conditional 8	1.5, 3	
DuNing Bioabsorbable Stent *DuNing, Inc., Irvine, CA*	Conditional 6	3	
Dynaflo Bypass Graft *Bard Peripheral Vascular, www.bardpv.com*	Safe	1.5	
Dynalink Biliary Stent *Abbott Vascular, www.abbottvascular.com*	Conditional 5	3	

Object	Status	Field Strength (T)	Reference
Dynalink Stent *10-mm x 100-mm, Nickel/Titanium* *Abbott Vascular, www.abbottvascular.com*	Safe	1.5, 3	
Dynalink Stent *5-mm x 100-mm, Nickel/Titanium* *Abbott Vascular, www.abbottvascular.com*	Safe	1.5, 3	
Dynalink Stent, 5 to 10-mm (OTW), Nitinol *Abbott Vascular, www.abbottvascular.com*	Safe	1.5	
Dynalink E Stent, Drug Eluting Stent *Abbott Vascular, www.abbottvascular.com*	Conditional 6	3	
Dynamic Stent *Biotronik, www.Biotronik.com*	Conditional 6	3	
Dynamic Renal Stent *Biotronik, www.Biotronik.com*	Conditional 6	3	
Eclipse Filter, Vena Cava Filter *Bard Peripheral Vascular, www.bardpv.com*	Conditional 5	3	
Eliachar Laryngeal Stent *Hood Laboratories, www.hoodlabs.com*	Safe	1.5, 3	
EluNIR Stent *Medinol Ltd., www.medinol.com*	Conditional 8	1.5, 3	
Embolization Coil, IMWCE-38-15-15, Inconel *Cook Medical, Inc., www.cookmedical.com*	Conditional 5	3	
Embolization Coil, IMWCE-38-20-15, Inconel *Cook Medical, Inc., www.cookmedical.com*	Conditional 5	3	
Embolization Coil, MWCE-38-14-12 NESTER *Platinum, Inconel* *Cook Medical, Inc., www.cookmedical.com*	Conditional 5	3	
Embolization Coil, Stainless Steel *Cook Medical, Inc., www.cookmedical.com*	Conditional 5	3	
Endeavor Drug Eluting Stent *Medtronic, Inc., www.medtronic.com/mri*	Conditional 5	3	88
Endeavor Resolute Zotarolimus-Eluting *Coronary Stent* *Medtronic, Inc., www.medtronic.com/mri*	Conditional 5	3	
Endeavor Stent, Including Endeavor Sprint *Endeavor MXII* *Endeavor Zotarolimus Eluting Coronary Stent* *Medtronic, Inc., www.medtronic.com/mri*	Conditional 5	3	
EndoCoil Stent *Intratherapeutics, Inc., St. Paul, MN*	Safe	1.5	
EndoCoil-T Stent *Intratherapeutics, Inc., St. Paul, MN*	Safe	1.5	

Object	Status	Field Strength (T)	Reference
EndoFit Endoluminal Stent Graft, Cuff(C) *ENDOMED, Inc., Phoenix, AZ*	Safe	1.5	
EndoFit Endoluminal Stent Graft, Extender (E) *ENDOMED, Inc., Phoenix, AZ*	Safe	1.5	
EndoFit Endoluminal Stent Graft, Occluder (O) *ENDOMED, Inc., Phoenix, AZ*	Safe	1.5	
EndoFit Endoluminal Stent Graft, *Tapered Aortomonoiliac (A)* *ENDOMED, Inc., Phoenix, AZ*	Safe	1.5	
EndoFit Endoluminal Stent Graft, Thoracic (T) *ENDOMED, Inc., Phoenix, AZ*	Safe	1.5	
EndoMAXX Stent *Merit Medical, www.merit.com*	Conditional 8	1.5, 3	
Endurant II Stent Graft *Medtronic, Inc., www.medtronic.com/mri*	Conditional 5	1.5, 3	
Endurant IIs Stent Graft *Medtronic, Inc., www.medtronic.com/mri*	Conditional 5	1.5, 3	
Endurant Stent Graft *Medtronic, Inc., www.medtronic.com/mri*	Conditional 5	1.5, 3	
Enforcer Stent *Cardiovascular Dynamics, Inc.*	Safe	1.5	
Enovus AAA Bifurcated Stent Graft *TriVascular, Inc., Santa Rosa, CA*	Safe	3	
Enovus Iliac Stent Graft *Boston Scientific, www.bostonscientific.com*	Conditional 6	3	
ENROUTE Carotid Artery Stent *Silk Road Medical, www.silkroadmedical.com*	Conditional 8	1.5, 3	
Enterprise Stent *Nitinol with Tantalum Markers* *Cordis, www.depuysynthes.com*	Safe	3	
Enterprise 2 Stent *Codman Neurovascular, Inc.,* *www.depuysynthes.com/Codman*	Conditional 8	1.5, 3	
EOS (Endoluminal Occlusion System) Implant *Medical Murray, Inc., medicalmurray.com*	Conditional 5	1.5, 3	
Epic Stent *Boston Scientific, www.bostonscientific.com*	Conditional 5	1.5, 3	
EsophaCoil-S Stent *Intratherapeutics, Inc., St. Paul, MN*	Safe	1.5	
Esophageal Stent *Hood Laboratories, www.hoodlabs.com*	Safe	1.5, 3	
Esophageal Stent, Niti-S & Comvi Model E2423 *TaeWoong Medical Co., Ltd., www.Stent.net*	Conditional 8	1.5, 3	

Object	Status	Field Strength (T)	Reference
Esophageal TTS Stent *TaeWoong Medical Co., Ltd., www.stent.net*	Conditional 8	1.5, 3	
Esophagus Full-Covered Stent *CG BIO CO., LTD. www.cgbio.co.kr/en/*	Conditional 8	1.5, 3	
Esophagus Stent, For Benign/Malignant Strictures *M.I. Tech, www.mitech.co.kr*	Conditional 8	1.5, 3	
Eta-2 TA Stent *Angiomed GmbH & Co., Germany*	Conditional 6	3	
Evolution Biliary Stent *Cook Medical, Inc., www.cookmedical.com*	Conditional 8	1.5, 3	
Evolution Colonic Stent *Cook Medical, Inc., www.cookmedical.com*	Conditional 8	1.5, 3	
Evolution Colonic Stent *Nitinol wire, Tantalum marker bands* *Cook Medical, www.cookmedical.com*	Conditional 6	3	
Evolution Duodenal Stent *Cook Medical, Inc., www.cookmedical.com*	Conditional 8	1.5, 3	
Evolution Esophageal Stent *Cook Medical, Inc., www.cookmedical.com*	Conditional 8	1.5, 3	
Evolution Colonic Uncovered *Controlled-Release Stent* *Cook Medical, www.cookmedical.com*	Conditional 8	1.5, 3	
EXXCEL Soft Vascular Graft *Atrium Medical Corporation, www.atriummed.com and* *Maquet Cardiovascular LLC, www.maquet.com/vascular*	Safe	1.5, 3	
EXCLUDER Bifurcated Endoprosthesis, Stent Graft *W.L. Gore and Associates, www.goremedical.com*	Conditional 8	1.5, 3	
Exhale Drug Eluting Stent *Broncus Technologies, Inc., Mountain View, CA*	Conditional 6	3	
Exponent Carotid Stent *Medtronic, Inc., www.medtronic.com/mri*	Safe	3	
Express Biliary SD Stent *Boston Scientific, www.bostonscientific.com*	Conditional 5	3	
Express LD Stent *Boston Scientific, www.bostonscientific.com*	Conditional 5	3	
Express SD Stent *Boston Scientific, www.bostonscientific.com*	Conditional 5	3	
Express2 Coronary Stent *Boston Scientific, www.bostonscientific.com*	Conditional 5	3	
Fanelli Laparoscopic Endobiliary Stent *Cook Medical, www.cookmedical.com*	Safe	1.5	
Fantom Bioresorbable Scaffold *Reva Medical, www.revamedical.com*	Safe	1.5, 3	

Object	Status	Field Strength (T)	Reference
Filiform Double Pigtail, Silicone Stent	Safe	1.5	
Cook Medical, www.cookmedical.com			
Figure 8 18 Coil	Conditional 5	1.5, 3	
Boston Scientific, www.bostonscientific.com			
Firebird2 Coronary Artery Stent	Conditional 8	1.5, 3	
MicroPort Medical, www.microport.com.cn/english			
FLAIR Endovascular Stent Graft	Conditional 5	1.5, 3	
Bard Peripheral Vascular, www.bardpv.com			
Flamingo WallStent Esophageal Endoprosthesis	Safe	1.5	
Schneider GmbH, Bulach, Switzerland			
FlexStent, Stent	Conditional 8	1.5, 3	
Flexible Stenting Solutions, www.flexibleStent.com			
FLIXENE IFG (Intraluminal Flow Guard)	Conditional 8	1.5, 3	
with Assisted Delivery Vascular Graft			
Atrium Medical Corporation, www.atriummed.com and			
Maquet Cardiovascular LLC, www.maquet.com/vascular			
FLIXENE IFG Vascular Graft	Safe	1.5, 3	
Atrium Medical Corporation, www.atriummed.com and			
Maquet Cardiovascular LLC, www.maquet.com/vascular			
FLIXENE Vascular Graft	Safe	1.5, 3	
Atrium Medical Corporation, www.atriummed.com and			
Maquet Cardiovascular LLC, www.maquet.com/vascular			
SAFE			
Flower Embolization Microcoil, Platinum	Safe	1.5	22
Target Therapeutics, San Jose, CA			
Flowise Cerebral Flow Diverter Stent	Conditional 5	1.5, 3	
TaeWoong Medical Co., Ltd, www.stent.net			
FLUENCY Plus Endovascular Stent Graft	Conditional 8	1.5, 3	
Bard Peripheral, Vascular, www.bardpv.com			
FLUENCY Plus Tracheobronchial Stent Graft	Conditional 6	3	
Bard Peripheral Vascular, www.bardpv.com			
FLUENCY Plus Vascular Stent Graft	Conditional 6	3	
Bard Peripheral Vascular, www.bardpv.com			
FLUENCY Vascular and	Conditional 6	3	
Tracheobronchial Stent Graft			
Bard Peripheral Vascular, www.bardpv.com			
Formula Stent Including Formula Renal Stent	Conditional 8	1.5, 3	
and Formula 414 Rx Renal Stent			
Cook Medical, Inc., www.cookmedical.com			
Formula 418 Biliary Balloon Expandable Stent	Conditional 5	3	
Cook Medical, Inc., www.cookmedical.com			
Formula 535 Vascular Stent	Conditional 8	1.5, 3	
Cook Medical, www.cookmedical.com			

Object	Status	Field Strength (T)	Reference
Fortitude Bioresorbable Drug-Eluting *Coronary Scaffold* *Amaranth Medical, www.amaranthmedical.com*	Safe	1.5, 3	
Freeman-Aliperti Straight Pancreatic Stent *Hobbs Medical, www.hobbsmedical.com*	Safe	1.5, 3	
Freeman Pancreatic Flexi-Stent *Hobbs Medical, www.hobbsmedical.com*	Safe	1.5, 3	
Fusion Zilver Biliary Stent System *Cook Medical, www.cookmedical.com*	Conditional 5	3	
G2 Express Vena Cava Filter *Bard Peripheral Vascular, www.bardpv.com*	Conditional 6	3	
G2 Filter Vena Cava Filter *Femoral Vein* *Bard Peripheral Vascular, www.bardpv.com*	Conditional 5	1.5	
G2 X Vena Cava Filter *Bard Peripheral Vascular, www.bardpv.com*	Conditional 5	3	
G2 X Filter Vena Cava Filter, Femoral Vein *Bard Peripheral Vascular, www.bardpv.com*	Conditional 5	3	
G2 X Filter Vena Cava Filter, Jugular Vein *Bard Peripheral Vascular, www.bardpv.com*	Conditional 5	3	
GDC 3D Coil, All Shape and Sizes *Stryker Neurovascular, www.stryker.com*	Conditional 5	1.5, 3	
GDC 360 Degree Coil *Stryker Neurovascular, www.stryker.com*	Conditional 5	1.5, 3	
GDC Detachable Coil, GDC 10-3D, 3-D Shape *Platinum alloy* *Stryker Neurovascular, www.stryker.com*	Conditional 5	1.5, 3	
GDC Detachable Coil, GDC 10-Soft *Stryker Neurovascular, www.stryker.com*	Conditional 5	1.5, 3	
GDC Detachable Coil, GDC 10-Standard *Stryker Neurovascular, www.stryker.com*	Conditional 5	1.5, 3	
GDC Detachable Coil, GDC 18-2D, 2 Diameter *Stryker Neurovascular, www.stryker.com*	Conditional 5	1.5, 3	
GDC Detachable Coil, GDC 18-3D, 3-D Shape *Stryker Neurovascular, www.stryker.com*	Conditional 5	1.5, 3	
GDC Detachable Coil, GDC 18-Soft *Stryker Neurovascular, www.stryker.com*	Conditional 5	1.5, 3	
GDC Detachable Coil, GDC 18-Standard *Stryker Neurovascular, www.stryker.com*	Conditional 5	1.5, 3	
GDC Detachable Coil, GDC 2D, 2 Diameter *Stryker Neurovascular, www.stryker.com*	Conditional 5	1.5, 3	

Object	Status	Field Strength (T)	Reference
GDC SR Coil Stretch Resistant, Various sizes *Embolization Coil* *Boston Scientific/Target and Stryker Neurovascular,* *www.stryker.com*	Conditional 5	1.5, 3	
GDC TriSpan Coil, 14-mm *Stryker Neurovascular, www.stryker.com*	Conditional 5	1.5, 3	
GDC TriSpan Coil, 16-mm *Stryker Neurovascular, www.stryker.com*	Conditional 5	1.5, 3	
GDC TriSpan, Various sizes *Boston Scientific/Target and Stryker Neurovascular,* *www.stryker.com*	Conditional 5	1.5, 3	
GDC 18-Fibered VortX Detachable Coil *Stryker Neurovascular, www.stryker.com*	Conditional 5	1.5, 3	
GDC Stretch Resistant Detachable Coil *GDC 10-Soft 2D SR* *Stryker Neurovascular, www.stryker.com*	Conditional 5	1.5, 3	
GDC Stretch Resistant Detachable Coil *GDC 10-Soft SR* *Stryker Neurovascular, www.stryker.com*	Conditional 5	1.5, 3	
GDC Stretch Resistant Detachable Coil *GDC 10-UltraSoft SR* *Stryker Neurovascular, www.stryker.com*	Conditional 5	1.5, 3	
GDC TriSpan Coil *Stryker Neurovascular, www.stryker.com*	Conditional 5	1.5, 3	
GFS Stent *Medtronic, Inc., www.medtronic.com/mri*	Conditional 5	3	
GFX (DOW, DGFW, DFW) Stent *Medtronic, Inc., www.medtronic.com/mri*	Conditional 5	3	
Genous Bio-Engineered R Stent, 316L SS *OrbusNeich Medical, Inc., Fort Lauderdale, FL*	Conditional 6	3	
Genous Bio-engineered R Stent *Coronary Artery Stent* *OrbusNeich Medical, Inc., Fort Lauderdale, FL*	Conditional 6	3	
Gianturco Bird's Nest IVC Filter *Cook Medical, Inc., www.cookmedical.com*	Conditional 5	1.5	21
Gianturco Zig-Zag Stent *Cook Medical, Inc., www.cookmedical.com*	Conditional 5	1.5	21
Gianturco-Roehm Bird's Nest Vena Cava Filter *Cook Medical, Inc., www.cookmedical.com*	Conditional 6	3	
Gianturco-Roubin II *20 x 3.0-mm Stent, 316L SS* *Cook Medical, Inc., www.cookmedical.com*	Safe	1.5	72

Object	Status	Field Strength (T)	Reference
Gianturco-Roubin Flex Stent *Cook Medical, Inc., www.cookmedical.com*	Conditional 5	3	
Gianturco-Roubin Stent, 316L SS *Cook Medical, www.cookmedical.com*	Safe	1.5	69
GODIVER Covered Stent, Bare Metal Stent (BMS) *Goodman Co., Ltd., www.goodmankk.com/english/*	Conditional 8	1.5, 3	
Goldvalve Detachable Balloon *Coils, Filters, Stents* *NFocus Neuromedical, Palo Alto, CA*	Conditional 6	3	
GORE Carotid Stent *W.L. Gore and Associates, www.goremedical.com*	Conditional 8	1.5, 3	
GORE Conformable EXCLUDER (cEXC) *W.L. Gore, and Associates, www.gore.com*	Conditional 8	1.5, 3	
GORE EXCLUDER AAA Endoprosthesis *Stent Graft* *W.L. Gore and Associates, Inc., www.goremedical.com*	Conditional 8	1.5, 3	
GORE Intering Vascular Graft *W.L. Gore & Associates, www.goremedical.com*	Safe	1.5	
GORE MYCROMESH Biomaterial *W.L. Gore & Associates, www.goremedical.com*	Safe	1.5	
GORE MYCROMESH PLUS Biomaterial *W.L. Gore & Associates, www.goremedical.com*	Safe	1.5	
GORE PRECLUDE Pericardial Membrane *W.L. Gore & Associates, www.goremedical.com*	Safe	1.5	
GORE PROPATEN Vascular Graft *W.L. Gore & Associates, www.goremedical.com*	Safe	1.5	
Gore TAG Thoracic Endoprosthesis *W. L. Gore & Associates, Inc., www.goremedical.com*	Conditional 8	1.5, 3	
GORE-TEX Stretch Vascular Graft *W.L. Gore & Associates, www.goremedical.com*	Safe	1.5	
GORE-TEX Vascular Graft *W.L. Gore & Associates, www.goremedical.com*	Safe	1.5	
GORE TIGRIS Vascular Stent, All Sizes *W.L. Gore and Associates, www.goremedical.com*	Conditional 8	1.5, 3	
GORE TIPS Endoprosthesis *W. L. Gore & Associates, Inc., www.goremedical.com*	Safe	1.5	
GRAFTMASTER RX Coronary Stent Graft *Abbott Vascular, www.abbottvascular.com*	Conditional 5	1.5, 3	
Greenfield Stainless Steel Femoral, Vena Cava Filter *Boston Scientific, www.bostonscientific.com*	Conditional 5	1.5	
Greenfield Stainless Steel Jugular, Vena Cava Filter *Boston Scientific, www.bostonscientific.com*	Conditional 5	1.5	

Object	Status	Field Strength (T)	Reference
Greenfield Vena Cava Filter *MD Tech, Watertown, MA*	Conditional 5	1.5	21
Greenfield Vena Cava Filter, Titanium alloy *Ormco, Glendora, CA*	Safe	1.5	21
GTX Coronary Artery Stent, CoCr *Global Therapeutics, Broomfield, CO*	Conditional 8	1.5, 3	
Guglielmi Detachable Coil, Platinum *Target Therapeutics, San Jose, CA*	Safe	1.5	25
Gunther IVC Filter *Cook Medical, www.cookmedical.com*	Conditional 5	1.5	21
Gunther Tulip Vena Cava Filter *Cook Medical, Inc., www.cookmedical.com*	Conditional 6	3	
Gunther Tulip Vena Cava Filter, Conichrome *Cook Medical, www.cookmedical.com*	Conditional 5	3	
Gunther Tulip Vena Cava MReye Filter, Conichrome *Cook Medical, www.cookmedical.com*	Conditional 5	3	
HELIPAQ Microcoil, Embolization Coil *Micrus Endovascular, www.micrusendovascular.com*	Conditional 5	3	
HANAROSTENT *M.I. Tech Co., Ltd., www.mitech.co.kr*	Conditional 8	1.5, 3	
HANAROSTENT Esophagus (CCC) *M.I. Tech Co., Ltd, www.mitech.co.kr*	Conditional 8	1.5, 3	
HANAROSTENT Esophagus Valve (CCC) *M.I. Tech, www.mitech.co.kr*	Conditional 8	1.5, 3	
HANAROSTENT Esophagus ST (CCN) *M.I. Tech Co., Ltd., www.mitech.co.kr*	Conditional 8	1.5, 3	
HANAROSTENT Plumber *M.I. Tech, www.mitech.co.kr*	Conditional 8	1.5, 3	
Harrell Y Stent *Hood Laboratories, www.hoodlabs.com*	Safe	1.5, 3	
HEMAGARD Carotid Knitted Vascular Patch *Atrium Medical Corporation, www.atriummed.com and* *Maquet Cardiovascular LLC, www.maquet.com/vascular*	Safe	1.5, 3	
HEMAGARD Carotid Ultra Thin Knitted Vascular Patch *Atrium Medical Corporation, www.atriummed.com and* *Maquet Cardiovascular LLC, www.maquet.com/vascular*	Safe	1.5, 3	
HEMAGARD Knitted Vascular Graft *Atrium Medical Corporation, www.atriummed.com and* *Maquet Cardiovascular LLC, www.maquet.com/vascular*	Safe	1.5, 3	
HEMAGARD Patch Knitted *Atrium Medical Corporation, www.atriummed.com and* *Maquet Cardiovascular LLC, www.maquet.com/vascular*	Safe	1.5, 3	

Object	Status	Field Strength (T)	Reference
HEMAPATCH Woven *Atrium Medical Corporation, www.atriummed.com, Maquet Cardiovascular LLC, www.maquet.com/vascular*	Safe	1.5, 3	
HEMASHIELD Gold Knitted Double Velour *Vascular Graft* *Atrium Medical Corporation, www.atriummed.com and Maquet Cardiovascular LLC, www.maquet.com/vascular*	Safe	1.5, 3	
HEMASHIELD Gold Woven Three Branch *Vascular Graft* *Atrium Medical Corporation, www.atriummed.com and Maquet Cardiovascular LLC, www.maquet.com/vascular*	Safe	1.5, 3	
HEMASHIELD Platinum Woven Double Velour *Vascular Graft* *Atrium Medical Corporation, www.atriummed.com and Maquet Cardiovascular LLC, www.maquet.com/vascular*	Safe	1.5, 3	
Hercules Bifurcated Main Body Stent Graft *MicroPort Medical, www.microport.com.cn/english*	Conditional 8	1.5, 3	
Hercules Tubular Stent Graft *MicroPort Medical, www.microport.com.cn/english*	Conditional 8	1.5, 3	
Herculink Elite Stent *Abbott Vascular, www.abbottvascular.com*	Conditional 5	1.5, 3	
Herculink Elite Biliary Stent *Abbott Vascular, www.abbottvascular.com*	Conditional 5	1.5, 3	
Herculink Plus Biliary Stent *Abbott Vascular, www.abbottvascular.com*	Conditional 5	1.5, 3	
Hilal Embolization Microcoil *Cook Medical, Inc., www.cookmedical.com*	Conditional 5	3	
Horizon Prostatic Stent, Nitinol *Endocare, Irvine, CA*	Safe	1.5	
Hour Glass Stent *Hood Laboratories, www.hoodlabs.com*	Safe	1.5, 3	
HydroCoil Embolic System, Embolization Coil *MicroVention, Inc., www.microvention.com*	Conditional 6	3	
HydroCoil Embolic System (HES) Implant *Microvention, www.microvention.com*	Conditional 6	3	
iCast *Atrium Medical Corporation, www.atriummed.com*	Conditional 8	1.5, 3	
iChrom Stent *IHT Innovation, Barcelona, Spain*	Conditional 8	1.5, 3	
IDC Interlocking Detachable Coil *Boston Scientific, www.bostonscientific.com*	Conditional 5	1.5, 3	

Object	Status	Field Strength (T)	Reference
Igaki-Tamai Biodegradable Coronary Artery Stent *Scaffold* *Kyoto Medical Planning, www.kyoto-mp.co.jp/en/*	Safe	1.5, 3	
Iliac Wallgraft Endoprosthesis *12 x 90* *Schneider (USA) Inc., Pfizer Medical Technology Group,* *Minneapolis, MN*	Safe	1.5	64
Iliac WallStent Endoprosthesis *5 x 80* *Schneider (USA) Inc., Pfizer Medical Technology Group,* *Minneapolis, MN*	Safe	1.5	64
Iliac WallStent Endoprosthesis *6 X 90* *Schneider (USA) Inc., Pfizer Medical Technology Group,* *Minneapolis, MN*	Safe	1.5	64
IMPRA Carboflo Vascular Graft *Carbon-impregnated ePTFE* *Bard Peripheral Vascular, www.bardpv.com*	Safe	1.5, 3	
IMPRA CenterFlex Vascular Graft *Carbon-impregnated ePTFE* *Bard Peripheral Vascular, www.bardpv.com*	Safe	1.5, 3	
Inflow Gold Stent *15 x 3.0-mm, 316L SS, gold* *Inflow Dynamics, Munich, Germany*	Safe	1.5	72
Inflow Gold Stent, 316L SS, gold plated *Inflow Dynamics, Munich, Germany*	Safe	1.5	72
Inflow Stent, 316L SS *Inflow Dynamics, Munich, Germany*	Safe	1.5	69
Inflow Stent, *316L SS* *Inflow Dynamics, Munich, Germany*	Safe	1.5	72
INNOVA Biliary Stent *INNOVA Self-Expanding Nitinol Biliary Stent* *Boston Scientific, www.bostonscientific.com*	Conditional 5	1.5, 3	
Integrity Coronary Stent *Medtronic, Inc., www.medtronic.com/mri*	Conditional 5	3	
INTERGARD Heparin Ultrathin Vascular Graft *Atrium Medical Corporation, www.atriummed.com and* *Maquet Cardiovascular LLC, www.maquet.com/vascular*	Safe	1.5, 3	
INTERGARD Woven Vascular Graft *Atrium Medical Corporation, www.atriummed.com, Maquet* *Cardiovascular LLC, www.maquet.com/vascular*	Safe	1.5, 3	

Object	Status	Field Strength (T)	Reference
Interlock Fibered IDC Occlusion System *Embolization Coil* *Boston Scientific, www.bostonscientific.com*	Conditional 5	1.5, 3	
INTERPAQ Microcoil *Embolization Coil* *Micrus Endovascular, www.micrusendovascular.com*	Conditional 5	3	
IntraCoil Bronchial Endoprosthesis, Stent *Intratherapeutics, Inc., St. Paul, MN*	Safe	1.5	
IntraStent Biliary Endoprosthesis, Stent *Intratherapeutics, Inc., St. Paul, MN*	Safe	1.5	
IntraStent DoubleStrut Biliary Endoprosthesis *Stent* *Intratherapeutics, Inc., St. Paul, MN*	Safe	1.5	
IntraStent LP Biliary Endoprosthesis *Stent* *Intratherapeutics, Inc., St. Paul, MN*	Safe	1.5	
IntraStent Max LD Biliary Stent *Covidien and ev3, Inc., www.ev3.net*	Conditional 5	1.5	
IntraStent Mega LD Biliary Stent *Covidien and ev3, Inc., www.ev3.net*	Conditional 5	1.5	
ION Stent *Ion Paclitaxel-Eluting Platinum Chromium Stent* *Boston Scientific, www.bostonscientific.com*	Conditional 5	1.5, 3	
Isthmus Logic CarboStent *CID, cidvascular.com*	Conditional 8	1.5, 3	
iVENA Patch *Atrium Medical Corporation, www.atriummed.com,* *Maquet Cardiovascular LLC, www.maquet.com/vascular*	Safe	1.5, 3	
JoStent, 316L SS *Jomed, Helsingborg, Sweden*	Safe	1.5	69
K3 Fibered Platinum Embolization Coil *TaeWoong Medical Co., www.Stent.net*	Conditional 6	3	
Kaneka Stent, Model GGH008 *Coronary Artery Stent* *Kaneka Corporation, Japan*	Conditional 6	3	
Kobi Carotid Stent *Silk Road Medical, www.silkroadmedical.com*	Conditional 5	3	
L605 Stent *Promed Medical Tech, China*	Conditional 6	3	
Large Diameter Covered Stent *Atrium Medical Corporation, www.atriummed.com*	Conditional 8	1.5, 3	

Object	Status	Field Strength (T)	Reference
LEO Plus Next Generation Self-Expanding *Intracranial Stent* *BALT, France*	Conditional 5	1.5, 3	
LGM IVC Filter, Phynox *B. Braun Vena Tech, Evanston, IL*	Safe	1.5	26
Liberte (Liberte') Coronary Artery Stent *Boston Scientific, www.bostonscientific.com*	Conditional 5	3	
Liberte (Liberte') Coronary Stent *Liberte (Liberte') Bare-Metal Coronary Stent* *Boston Scientific, www.bostonscientific.com*	Conditional 5	1.5, 3	
LifeStar Biliary Stent *Bard Peripheral Vascular, www.bardpv.com*	Conditional 5	3	
LifeStent FlexStar Stent *Bard Peripheral Vascular, www.bardpv.com*	Conditional 6	3	
LifeStent FlexStar XL Stent *Bard Peripheral Vascular, www.bardpv.com*	Conditional 6	3	
LifeStent SOLO Vascular Stent *Bard Peripheral Vascular, www.bardpv.com*	Conditional 5	1.5, 3	
LifeStent Vascular Stent *Bard Peripheral Vascular, www.bardpv.com*	Conditional 5	1.5, 3	
LifeStent XL Balloon Expandable Stent *Biliary Stent and Peripheral Vascular Stent* *Bard Peripheral Vascular, www.bardpv.com*	Conditional 6	3	
LithoStent Ureteral Stent, Polyurethane *Gyrus ACMI (Olympus Medical),* *www.medical.olympusamerica.com*	Safe	3	
Low Profile Covered Stent *Atrium Medical Corporation, www.atriummed.com*	Conditional 8	1.5, 3	
LPS Stent, bifurcated *36 x 20-mm, Nitinol* *World Medical Manufacturing Corp., Sunrise, FL*	Safe	1.5	70
LPS Thoracic Stent, 46mm, Nitinol *World Medical Manufacturing Corp., Sunrise, FL*	Safe	1.5	70
Lubri-Flex Open Tip Ureteral Stent *Gyrus ACMI (Olympus Medical),* *www.medical.olympusamerica.com*	Safe	3	
LUNA Aneurysm Embolization System *NFOCUS Neuromedical, Inc., Palo Alto, CA*	Conditional 6	3	
Maas Helical Endovascular Stent *Medinvent, Lausanne, Switzerland*	Safe	4.7	21
Maas Helical IVC Filter *Medinvent, Lausanne, Switzerland*	Safe	4.7	21

Object	Status	Field Strength (T)	Reference
MAC-Stent, 17 x 3-mm *316L SS* *AMG, Munich, Germany*	Safe	1.5	72
Magic WallStent *Schneider, Bulach, Switzerland*	Safe	1.5	69
Magic Wallstent Self-Expanding Coronary Stent *Magic Wallstent Coronary Stent* *Boston Scientific, www.bostonscientific.com*	Safe	1.5	
Magmaris Bioresorbable Scaffold *Biotronic, www.biotronik.com*	Safe	1.5, 3	
Mardis Ureteral Stent With *Hydro Plus Coating, Mardis Soft Stent* *Boston Scientific, www.bostonscientific.com*	Safe	1.5, 3	
Matrix[2] Detachable Coil, Embolization Coil *All Shapes and Sizes* *Stryker Neurovascular, www.stryker.com*	Conditional 5	1.5, 3	
Matrix Detachable Coil, Embolization Coil *All Shapes and Sizes* *Stryker Neurovascular, www.stryker.com*	Conditional 5	1.5, 3	
Matrix Detachable Coil *Matrix Extra Firm-2D, Platinum alloy* *Stryker Neurovascular, www.stryker.com*	Conditional 5	1.5, 3	
Matrix Detachable Coil *Matrix Extra Firm-3D, Platinum alloy* *Stryker Neurovascular, www.stryker.com*	Conditional 5	1.5, 3	
Matrix Detachable Coil *Matrix Firm-2D, Platinum alloy* *Stryker Neurovascular, www.stryker.com*	Conditional 5	1.5, 3	
Matrix Detachable Coil *Matrix Firm-3D, Platinum alloy* *Stryker Neurovascular, www.stryker.com*	Conditional 5	1.5, 3	
Matrix Detachable Coil *Matrix Soft Helical, Platinum alloy* *Stryker Neurovascular, www.stryker.com*	Conditional 5	1.5, 3	
Matrix Detachable Coil *Matrix Soft-2D, Platinum alloy* *Stryker Neurovascular, www.stryker.com*	Conditional 5	1.5, 3	
Matrix Detachable Coil *Matrix Standard-2D, Platinum alloy* *Stryker Neurovascular, www.stryker.com*	Conditional 5	1.5, 3	
Matrix Detachable Coil *Matrix Standard-3D, Platinum alloy* *Stryker Neurovascular, www.stryker.com*	Conditional 5	1.5, 3	

Object	Status	Field Strength (T)	Reference
Matrix Stretch Resistant Detachable Coil *Matrix Soft-SR 2D, Platinum alloy* *Stryker Neurovascular, www.stryker.com*	Conditional 5	1.5, 3	
Matrix Stretch Resistant Detachable Coil *Matrix Soft-SR, Platinum alloy* *Stryker Neurovascular, www.stryker.com*	Conditional 5	1.5, 3	
Matrix Stretch Resistant Detachable Coil *Matrix Standard-SR 2D, Platinum alloy* *Stryker Neurovascular, www.stryker.com*	Conditional 5	1.5, 3	
Matrix Stretch Resistant Detachable Coil *Matrix UltraSoft-SR, Platinum alloy* *Stryker Neurovascular, www.stryker.com*	Conditional 5	1.5, 3	
Medtronic AVE Stent, 316L SS, gold *Medtronic, Inc., www.medtronic.com/mri*	Safe	1.5	70
Medinol Polymer Covered Esophageal Stent *Medinol Ltd, www.medinol.com*	Conditional 5	1.5, 3	
Megalink Biliary Stent *Abbott Vascular, www.abbottvascular.com*	Conditional 5	3	
Mercury Carotid Artery Stent, Nitinol *MicroPort Medical Co., Ltd., People's Republic of China*	Conditional 6	3	
Meridian Filter, Vena Cava Filter, *Jugular and Femoral* *Bard Peripheral Vascular, www.bardpv.com*	Conditional 8	1.5, 3	
Merit Wrapsody Endovascular Stent Graft Family *All Sizes* *Merit Medical Systems, Inc., www.merit.com*	Conditional 8	1.5, 3	
Merlin MD Aneurysm Occlusion Device (AOD) *Merlin MD Pte Ltd, Singapore*	Conditional 6	3	
MGuard Prime Coronary Artery Stent *InspireMD Ltd., www.inspiremd.com*	Conditional 6	3	
Micro-Driver Coronary Stent *Medtronic, Inc., www.medtronic.com/mri*	Conditional 5	3	
Micro-Driver Stent *Medtronic, Inc., www.medtronic.com/mri*	Conditional 5	3	
MicroNester, Nester Embolization Microcoil *Cook Medical, Inc., www.cookmedical.com*	Conditional 5	3	
MicroPlex Coil System, Embolization Coil *MicroVention, Inc., www.microvention.com*	Conditional 6	3	
MicroStent II, 316L SS *Medtronic, Inc., www.medtronic.com/mri*	Safe	1.5	72
Microvention Flow Diverter and Coil-Assist Stent *Microvention, www.microvention.com*	Conditional 8	1.5, 3	

Object	Status	Field Strength (T)	Reference
MICRUSFRAME Microcoil, Embolization Coil *Codman Neurovascular and Depuy Synthes,* *www.depuysynthes.com*	Conditional 6	3	
MICRUSHERE Microcoil, Embolization Coil *Codman Neurovascular and Depuy Synthes,* *www.depuysynthes.com*	Conditional 6	3	
MICRUSHERE XL Microcoil, Embolization Coil *Codman Neurovascular and Depuy Synthes,* *www.depuysynthes.com*	Conditional 6	3	
Mini-Crown Stent, 316L SS *Cordis, www.depuysynthes.com*	Safe	1.5	69
Mirage Microfiber Scaffold, Coronary Artery *Scaffold (Stent)* *ManLi, www.manli.com*	Conditional 6	3	123
Misago Stent *Terumo Medical Corporation, www.terumomedical.com*	Conditional 5	1.5, 3	
Misago Peripheral Stent *Terumo Medical Corporation, www.terumomedical.com*	Conditional 5	1.5, 3	
MiStent Drug-Eluting Coronary Stent *Micell Technologies, Inc., www.micell.com*	Conditional 8	1.5, 3	
Mobin-Uddin IVC/umbrella filter *American Edwards, Santa Ana, CA*	Safe	4.7	21
Mobius HD Stent *Vascular Dynamics, Inc., www.vasculardynamics.com*	Conditional 8	1.5, 3	
Mobius O, Type E Stent *Vascular Dynamics, Israel*	Conditional 6	3	
MReye Embolization Coil *Cook Medical, Inc., www.cookmedical.com*	Conditional 8	1.5, 3	
MReye Flipper Detachable Embolization Coil *Cook Medical, Inc., www.cookmedical.com*	Conditional 5	3	
Multi-Flex Open Tip Ureteral Stent *Gyrus ACMI (Olympus Medical),* *www.medical.olympusamerica.com*	Safe	1.5, 3	
Multi-Link 8 Coronary Artery Stent *Abbott Vascular, www.Abbott.com*	Conditional 5	1.5, 3	
Multi-Link 8 LL Coronary Artery Stent *Abbott Vascular, www.Abbott.com*	Conditional 5	1.5, 3	
Multi-Link 8 SV Coronary Artery Stent *Abbott Vascular, www.Abbott.com*	Conditional 5	1.5, 3	
Multi-Link DUET Stent *Abbott Vascular, www.abbottvascular.com*	Conditional 5	3	
Multi-Link MINI VISION Coronary Stent *Abbott Vascular, www.abbottvascular.com*	Conditional 5	3	

Object	Status	Field Strength (T)	Reference
Multi-Link PENTA Coronary Stent *Abbott Vascular, www.abbottvascular.com*	Conditional 5	3	
Multi-Link PIXEL Coronary Stent *Abbott Vascular, www.abbottvascular.com*	Conditional 5	3	
Multi-Link TETRA Coronary Stent *Abbott Vascular, www.abbottvascular.com*	Conditional 5	3	
Multi-Link TRISTAR Stent *Abbott Vascular, www.abbottvascular.com*	Conditional 5	3	
Multi-Link VISION Coronary Stent *Abbott Vascular, www.abbottvascular.com*	Conditional 5	3	
Multi-Link ULTRA Stent *Abbott Vascular, www.abbottvascular.com*	Conditional 5	3	
Multi-Link ZETA Coronary Stent *Abbott Vascular, www.abbottvascular.com*	Conditional 5	3	
Multi-Link Stent, 2.5 to 4.0-mm (RX and OTW) *Abbott Vascular, www.abbottvascular.com*	Conditional 5	3	
Multiloop 18 Coil *Boston Scientific, www.bostonscientific.com*	Conditional 5	1.5, 3	
NEC Hemi Device *NFocus Neuromedical, Palo Alto, CA*	Conditional 6	3	
Nellix AAA Endoprosthesis *Nellix Endovascular, Palo Alto, CA*	Conditional 8	1.5, 3	
Neovasc Reducer Premounted Stent *Neovasc, Inc., www.neovasc.com*	Conditional 5	1.5, 3	
Neqstent *Cerus Endovascular, www.cerusendo.com*	Conditional 8	1.5, 3	
Nester Embolization Coil *Cook Medical, Inc., www.cookmedical.com*	Conditional 6	3	
Neuroform Stent *Stryker Neurovascular, www.stryker.com*	Conditional 5	3	108
Neuroform EZ Stent *Stryker Neurovascular, www.stryker.com*	Conditional 5	1.5, 3	
Neuroguard Carotid Stent, 6-mm x 40-mm *Contego Medical, contegomedical.com*	Conditional 8	1.5, 3	
Neurolink Stent *Abbott Vascular, www.abbottvascular.com*	Conditional 5	1.5	
Neurostring Embolization Coil *Biomerix Corporation, Fremont, CA*	Conditional 6	3	
Neurovascular Stent *BioAlpha, www.bioalpha.com*	Conditional 5	1.5, 3	

Object	Status	Field Strength (T)	Reference
NEVO Sirolimus-eluting *Coronary Artery Stent* *Cordis Corporation, www.depuysynthes.com*	Conditional 8	1.5, 3	
New retrievable IVC filter *Thomas Jefferson University, Philadelphia, PA*	Conditional 5	1.5	21
NexStent Carotid Stent *Nitinol* *EndoTex Interventional Solutions, Cupertino, CA*	Safe	3	
Nexus Detachable Coil *Embolization Coil* *Covidien and ev3, Inc., www.ev3.net*	Conditional 5	3	
Nexus Embolization Coil *Micro Therapeutics, Inc., Irvine, CA*	Conditional 6	3	
NeXsys Neurovascular Embolization System Implant *Cerus Endovascular Limited, Oxford, United Kingdom*	Conditional 5	1.5, 3	
NIR Coronary Stent *Boston Scientific, www.bostonscientific.com*	Conditional 8	1.5, 3	
NIR Royal Advance Stent *Boston Scientific, www.bostonscientific.com*	Conditional 5	1.5, 3	
NIROYAL Coronary Stent *Boston Scientific, www.bostonscientific.com*	Conditional 8	1.5, 3	
Nitinol Braided Neuro Coil Assist Stent *MicroVention, Inc., www.microvention.com*	Conditional 6	3	
Niti-S Biliary Stent (LCD-type) *TaeWoong Medical Co., Ltd., www.stent.net*	Conditional 8	1.5, 3	
Niti-S SPAXUS Stent *TaeWoong Medical Co., Ltd., www.stent.net*	Conditional 5	1.5, 3	
Non-Covered Biliary Stent *M.I. Tech, www.mitech.co.kr*	Conditional 8	1.5, 3	
Non-Covered Duodenum, Pylorus Stent *M.I. Tech, www.mitech.co.kr*	Conditional 8	1.5, 3	
Non-Vascular Stent, Double Spherical, Covered, *38-mm x 200-mm* *Micro-Tech, www.micro-tech.com.cn/en/*	Conditional 8	1.5, 3	
Non-Vascular Stent, Double Spherical, *38-mm x 200-mm* *Micro-Tech, www.micro-tech.com.cn/en/*	Conditional 8	1.5, 3	
Non-Vascular Stent, Straight *Micro-Tech, www.micro-tech.com.cn/en/*	Conditional 8	1.5, 3	
Non-Vascular Stent, Y-shape *Micro-Tech, www.micro-tech.com.cn/en/*	Conditional 8	1.5, 3	
Novate Sentry IVC Filter *Novate, www.novate.biz*	Conditional 5	1.5, 3	

Object	Status	Field Strength (T)	Reference
NOVATECH GSS, Y-Stent Gold Studded Stent *MRI information applies to all stents in product family* *Novatech, www.novatech.fr*	Conditional 6	3	
Nuloy Stent, Coronary Artery Stent *Icon Interventional Systems, Inc., Cleveland, OH*	Conditional 6	3	
NXT Detachable Coil *Embolization Coil* *Covidien and ev3, Inc., www.ev3.net*	Conditional 5	3	
NXT Tetris Detachable Coil *Embolization Coil* *Covidien and ev3, Inc., www.ev3.net*	Conditional 5	3	
Omnilink Elite Peripheral Stent *Abbott Vascular Devices, www.abbottvascular.com*	Conditional 5	1.5, 3	
Omnilink Elite Stent *Abbott Vascular Instruments Deutschland GmbH,* *Germany*	Conditional 8	1.5, 3	
Omnilink Biliary Stent *Abbott Vascular, www.abbottvascular.com*	Conditional 5	3	
OPTEASE Retrievable Vena Cava Filter *Cordis, www.depuysynthes.com*	Conditional 5	3	
Optima Coil System, All Sizes *Blockade Medical, www.blockademedical.com*	Conditional 8	1.5, 3	
Optimized Flair Endovascular Stent Graft *Bard Peripheral Vascular, www.bardpv.com*	Conditional 6	3	
Optimus Stent, All Sizes *AndraTec GmbH, andratec.com*	Conditional 8	1.5, 3	
OptionELITE Retrievable Vena Cava Filter *Argon Medical, www.argonmedical.com*	Conditional 6	3	
Option Vena Cava Filter *Argon Medical, www.argonmedical.com*	Conditional 6	3	
ORBIT GALAXY Detachable Coil *Codman Neurovascular and Depuy Synthes,* *www.depuysynthes.com*	Conditional 6	3	
Orbit Galaxy Embolization Coil *Codman Neurovascular and Depuy Synthes,* *www.depuysynthes.com*	Conditional 6	3	
ORBIT GALAXY Microcoil, Embolization Coil *Codman Neurovascular and Depuy Synthes,* *www.depuysynthes.com*	Conditional 6	3	
ORBIT GALAXY G2 Microcoil, Embolization Coil *Codman Neurovascular and Depuy Synthes,* *www.depuysynthes.com*	Conditional 6	3	

Object	Status	Field Strength (T)	Reference
ORBIT GALAXY G3 Microcoil, Embolization Coil *Codman Neurovascular and Depuy Synthes,* *www.depuysynthes.com*	Conditional 6	3	
Ovation Abdominal Stent Graft *Trivascular, www.Trivascular.com*	Conditional 6	3	
Ovation Thoracic Stent Graft *Trivascular, www.Trivascular.com*	Conditional 6	3	
pBEAST Peripheral Balloon Expandable Covered Stent *W. L. Gore & Associates., www.goremedical.com*	Conditional 5	1.5, 3	
Palmaz Blue Stent *Cordis, www.depuysynthes.com*	Conditional 5	3	
Palmaz Blue Transhepatic Biliary Stent *Cordis, www.depuysynthes.com*	Conditional 5	3	
Palmaz Endovascular Stent *Cordis, www.depuysynthes.com*	Conditional 5	3	
Palmaz Genesis Stent *Cordis, www.depuysynthes.com*	Conditional 5	3	
Palmaz Genesis Peripheral Stent *Cordis, www.depuysynthes.com*	Conditional 5	3	
Palmaz Genesis Transhepatic Biliary Stent *Cordis, www.depuysynthes.com*	Conditional 5	3	
Palmaz-Schatz Stent, 15 x 3.0-mm *Cordis, www.depuysynthes.com*	Safe	1.5	72
Palmaz-Schatz Stent, P-S 153, 316L SS *Cordis, www.depuysynthes.com*	Safe	1.5	69
Palmaz-Schatz Stent, P-S 154, 316L SS *Cordis, www.depuysynthes.com*	Safe	1.5	69
Palmaz-Schatz Balloon-Expandable Stent *Cordis, www.depuysynthes.com*	Conditional 5	1.5	
ParaMount Mini Biliary Stent *Covidien and ev3, Inc., www.ev3.net*	Conditional 5	1.5	
Passager Stent, Tantalum, 10-mm x 30-mm *Meadox Surgimed, Oakland, NJ*	Safe	1.5	
Passager Stent, Tantalum, 4-mm x 30-mm *Meadox Surgimed, Oakland, NJ*	Safe	1.5	
Penumbra Coil, Embolization Coil *Penumbra, Inc., www.penumbrainc.www*	Conditional 8	1.5, 3	
Penumbra Coil 400, Embolization Coil *Penumbra, Inc., www.penumbrainc.com*	Conditional 8	1.5, 3	
Penumbra Occlusion Coil, POD, Embolization Coil *Penumbr, Inc., www.penumbrainc.com*	Conditional 8	1.5, 3	

Object	Status	Field Strength (T)	Reference
Penumbra Smart Coil, Embolization Coil *Penumbra, Inc., www.penumbrainc.com*	Conditional 8	1.5, 3	
Percuflex Plus *Stent Graft with Suprarenal, Ureteral Stent* *4.8 Fr. (1.6-mm x 220-mm)* *Boston Scientific, www.bostonscientific.com*	Safe	1.5, 3	83
Percuflex Plus Ureteral Stent *With Hydro Plus Coating* *Boston Scientific, www.bostonscientific.com*	Safe	1.5, 3	
Percuflex Ureteral Stent *Boston Scientific, www.bostonscientific.com*	Safe	1.5, 3	
Perdenser Embolization Coil *Beijing Taijieweiye Technology Co., Ltd., China*	Conditional 6	3	
Perigraft Vascular Graft L-Hydro *Labcor Laboratorios Ltda., www.labcor.com*	Safe	1.5, 3	
Peripheral Stent *Covidien, www.covidien.com*	Conditional 8	1.5, 3	
PHAROS Stent, Carotid Artery Stent *Biotronik, www.Biotronik.com*	Conditional 6	3	
Philon Stent *Biotronik, www.Biotronik.com*	Conditional 5	1.5	
Pipeline Embolization Device, PED *Covidien and ev3, Inc., www.ev3.net*	Conditional 5	3	
Polaris Loop Ureteral Stent *Boston Scientific, www.bostonscientific.com*	Safe	1.5, 3	
Polaris Ultra *Dual Durometer Ureteral Stent* *Boston Scientific, www.bostonscientific.com*	Safe	1.5, 3	
Polaris Ultra Ureteral Stent *Boston Scientific, www.bostonscientific.com*	Safe	1.5, 3	
Polyflex Airway Stent *Silicone and polyester* *Boston Scientific, www.bostonscientific.com*	Safe	1.5	
Powerlink Suprarenal *Bifurcated Stent Graft* *Model 34-16-175RBL* *Endologix, Irvine, CA*	Conditional 8	1.5, 3	
PowerLink *Endologix, Inc., Irvine, CA*	Safe	1.5	70
PowerWeb, Model 1 *Endologix, Inc., Irvine, CA*	Safe	1.5	70
PowerWeb *Endologix, Inc., Irvine, CA*	Safe	1.5	70

Object	Status	Field Strength (T)	Reference
Precedent Stent *Boston Scientific, www.bostonscientific.com*	Safe	1.5	70
Precise Microvascular Anastomotic Device (MACD) *316L SS*	Safe	1.5	71
Precise Nitinol Stent, Carotid *Cordis, www.depuysynthes.com, www.cordislabeling.com* *com*	Conditional 5	1.5	
Precise Pro RX Nitinol Stent *Cordis, www.depuysynthes.com, www.cordislabeling.com* *com*	Conditional 5	1.5	
Precise RX Nitinol Stent *Cordis, www.depuysynthes.com, www.cordislabeling.com* *com*	Conditional 5	1.5	
PRESIDIO Microcoil, Embolization Coil *Micrus Endovascular, www.micrusendovascular.com*	Conditional 5	3	
Presillion Stent *Medinol, www.medinol.com*	Conditional 8	1.5, 3	
PRIMUS Biliary Stent *Covidien and ev3, Inc., www.ev3.net*	Conditional 5	1.5	
PRO-Kinetic Energy Stent *Biotronik, www.Biotronik.com*	Conditional 6	3	
PRO-Kinetic Stent, Coronary Artery Stent *Biotronik, www.Biotronik.com*	Conditional 6	3	
PROMUS Element Plus Everolimus-Eluting *Platinum Chromium Coronary Stent* *Boston Scientific, www.bostonscientific.com*	Conditional 5	1.5, 3	
PROMUS Everolimus-Eluting Coronary Stent *PROMUS Stent* *Boston Scientific, www.bostonscientific.com*	Conditional 5	1.5, 3	
PROMUS PREMIER Platinum Chromium *Everolimus-Eluting Coronary Stent* *Boston Scientific, www.bostonscientific.com*	Conditional 5	1.5, 3	
ProPass Stent *Vascular Innovations, Inc., Freemont, CA*	Conditional 6	3	
Protege EverFlex Self-Expanding Biliary Stent *Covidien and ev3, Inc., www.ev3.net*	Conditional 5	1.5	
Protege EverFlex Self-Expanding Stent *Covidien and ev3 Inc., www.ev3.net*	Conditional 5	1.5, 3	
Protege GPS Carotid Stent *Covidien and ev3, Inc., www.ev3.net*	Conditional 5	3	
Protege GPS Self-Expanding Stent *Covidien and ev3 Inc., www.ev3.net*	Conditional 8	1.5, 3	

Object	Status	Field Strength (T)	Reference
Protege GPS Self-Expanding Biliary Stent *Covidien and ev3, Inc., www.ev3.net*	Conditional 5	1.5	
Protege RX Carotid Stent *Covidien and ev3, Inc., www.ev3.net*	Conditional 5	3	
ProVena Graft *B. Braun, www.braun.com*	Safe	1.5, 3	
Pyloric, Duodenal Stent *M.I. Tech, www.mitech.co.kr*	Conditional 8	1.5, 3	
Pyloric Duodenal Stent *TaeWoong Medical Co., Ltd., www.stent.net*	Conditional 5	1.5, 3	
Quadra-coil Ureteral Stent *Gyrus ACMI (Olympus Medical),* *www.medical.olympusamerica.com*	Safe	3	
R Stent, 316 LVM SS *Spectranetics Corporation, Colorado Springs, CO*	Safe	1.5	
R Stent, 316L SS *Orbus Medical Technologies, Fort Lauderdale, FL*	Safe	1.5	
Racer Biliary Stent *Medtronic, Inc., www.medtronic.com/mri*	Safe	3	
Radius Stent, 4.0-mm x 31-mm, Nitinol *Boston Scientific, www.bostonscientific.com*	Safe	1.5, 3	
Radius Stent, Nitinol *Boston Scientific, wwww.bostonscientific.com*	Safe	1.5	69
Rebel Platinum Chromium Coronary Stent *Boston Scientific, www.bostonscientific.com*	Conditional 8	1.5, 3	
Recovery G2 Filter, Vena Cava Filter *Femoral Vein* *Bard Peripheral Vascular, www.bardpv.com*	Conditional 5	1.5	
Recovery Nitinol Filter, Nitinol *Bard Peripheral Vascular, www.bardpv.com*	Safe	3	
Relay Plus Stent Graft *Bolton Medical, Inc., www.boltonmedical.com*	Conditional 8	1.5, 3	
Remedy Biodegradable Stent *Kyoto Medical Planning, www.kyoto-mp.co.jp/en*	Safe	1.5, 3	
Resolute Integrity Zotarolimus-Eluting *Coronary Artery Stent* *Medtronic, Inc., www.medtronic.com/mri*	Conditional 5	1.5, 3	
Resolute Onyx Coronary Artery Stent *Medtronic, Inc., www.Medtronic.com/MRI*	Conditional 8	1.5, 3	
Resonance Double Pigtail Ureteral Stent, MP35N *Cook Medical, www.cookmedical.com*	Conditional 6	3	
Resonance Metallic Ureteral Stent *Cook Medical Inc., www cookmedical.com*	Conditional 5	1.5, 3	

Object	Status	Field Strength (T)	Reference
ReZolve2 *Reva Medical, www.revamedical.com*	Safe	1.5, 3	
Rithron Coronary Stent *Biotronik, www.Biotronik.com*	Conditional 5	1.5	
Ruby Coil, Embolization Coil *Penumbra Inc., www.penumbrainc.com*	Conditional 8	1.5, 3	
RX Herculink Elite, Biliary Stent, 316L SS	Conditional 6	3	
S3 Stent, L605 Cobalt-Chrome *Medlogics Device Corporation, Santa Rosa, CA*	Conditional 6	3	
S540 Stent *Medtronic, Inc., www.medtronic.com/mri*	Conditional 5	3	
S660 Stent *Medtronic, Inc., www.medtronic.com/mri*	Conditional 5	3	
S670, 4.0-mm x 30-mm, 316L SS, Stent *Medtronic, Inc., www.medtronic.com/mri*	Safe	3	
S7, 4.0-mm x 30-mm, 316L SS, Stent *Medtronic, Inc., www.medtronic.com/mri*	Safe	3	
SafeFlo IVC Filter, Inferior Vena Cava Filter *Rafael Medical Technologies, Inc., Israel*	Conditional 6	3	
SALVUS Sirolimus Eluting Stent *Koswire Ltd., South Korea*	Conditional 5	1.5, 3	
Sapphire Detachable Coil *Embolization Coil* *Covidien and ev3, Inc., www.ev3.net*	Conditional 5	1.5	
Scuba Stent, Scuba Co-Cr Peripheral Stent *Invatec/Medtronic, www.invatec.com*	Conditional 8	1.5, 3	
Seaquence Stent, 316L SS *Nycomed Amersham, Princeton, NJ*	Safe	1.5	72
Self-expanding Neuroendograft Stent *Surpass Medical Ltd., www.surpass-med.com*	Conditional 6	3	
Self-Expanding Peripheral Stent *CID s.p.A, www.cidvascular.com*	Conditional 8	1.5, 3	
Silhouette Ureteral Patency Device *MRI information applies to all Silhouette Devices* *Applied Medical Resources, Rancho Santa Margarita, CA*	Conditional 8	1.5, 3	
Silk Artery Reconstruction Device *Stent* *BALT, France*	Conditional 8	1.5, 3	
Single-J Urinary *Diversion Specialty Stent, Silicone* *Gyrus ACMI (Olympus Medical),* *www.medical.olympusamerica.com*	Safe	3	

Object	Status	Field Strength (T)	Reference
Simon Nitinol Filter *Vena Cava Filter* *Bard Peripheral Vascular, www.bardpv.com*	Conditional 6	3	
S.M.A.R.T. (SMART) CONTROL Nitinol Stent *Transhepatic Biliary System* *Cordis, www.depuysynthes.com*	Conditional 5	1.5, 3	
S.M.A.R.T. (SMART) Shape Memory Alloy *Recoverable Technology* *Nitinol Stent* *Cordis, www.depuysynthes.com*	Conditional 5	1.5, 3	
S.M.A.R.T. (SMART) Nitinol Stent, *Transhepatic Biliary System* *Cordis, www.depuysynthes.com*	Conditional 5	1.5, 3	
Sof-Curl Ureteral Stent *Gyrus ACMI (Olympus Medical),* *www.medical.olympusamerica.com*	Safe	3	
SOLITAIRE AB Neurovascular Remodeling Device *Covidien and ev3, Inc., www.ev3.net*	Conditional 5	3	
Solitaire Flow Restoration Stent *Nitinol, SS, Platinum* *Covidien and ev3, Inc., www.ev3.net*	Conditional 8	1.5, 3	
Solus Double Pigtail Stent *Cook Medical, Inc., www.cookmedical.com*	Conditional 6	3	
St. Jude Carotid Stent *10-7 x 40-mm taper Stent, two-overlapped version* *St. Jude Medical, www.sjm.com*	Conditional 6	3	
St. Jude Carotid Stent *10-7 x 50-mm taper Stent, single version* *St. Jude Medical, www.sjm.com*	Conditional 6	3	
Standard Embolization Coil, MWCE-52-15-20, *Stainless Steel* *Cook Medical, www.cookmedical.com*	Conditional 5	1.5	
Stentys Bifurcation Stent *Stentys Inc., www.Stentys.com*	Conditional 6	3	
Stentys Coronary Stent *Stentys Inc., www.Stentys.com*	Conditional 8	1.5, 3	
Stoma Stent *Hood Laboratories, www.hoodlabs.com*	Safe	1.5, 3	
Straight 18 Coil *Boston Scientific, www.bostonscientific.com*	Conditional 5	1.5, 3	
Straight Stoma Stent with Window *Hood Laboratories, www.hoodlabs.com*	Safe	1.5, 3	
Strecker Stent, Tantalum *MD Tech, Watertown, MA*	Safe	1.5	27

Object	Status	Field Strength (T)	Reference
Stretch VL Flexima Ureteral Stent *With Hydro Plus Coating* *Boston Scientific, www.bostonscientific.com*	Safe	1.5, 3	
Strider Stent, Biliary artery, Iliac artery *Nitinol with Tantalum markers* *Medtronic, Inc., www.medtronic.com/mri*	Safe	3	
Supera Biliary Stent *IDEV Technologies, Inc., www.idevmd.com and Abbott* *Vascular, www.abbottvascular.com*	Conditional 5	1.5, 3	
Supera Peripheral Stent, Lengths up to 200-mm *Abbott Vascular, ww.abbottvascular.com*	Conditional 5	1.5, 3	
Supera Stent *IDEV Technologies, Inc., www.idevmd.com and Abbott* *Vascular, www.abbottvascular.com*	Conditional 5	1.5, 3	
Surpass Aneurysm Embolization System, *Self-expanding NeuroEndoGraft* *Surpass Medical, www.surpassmedical.com*	Conditional 5	1.5, 3	
Svelte Bare Metal Stent, single and *two overlapped versions* *Svelte Medical Systems, www.sveltemedical.com*	Conditional 8	1.5, 3	
Svelte Drug-Eluting Coronary Artery Stent *Svelte Medical Systems, www.sveltemedical.com*	Conditional 8	1.5, 3	
SX-ELLA Esophageal Stent HV Plus *ELLA-CS, s.r.o., www.ellacs.eu*	Conditional 8	1.5, 3	
SX-ELLA Stent, Esophageal Degradable BD *ELLA-CS, s.r.o., www.ellacs.eu*	Conditional 8	1.5, 3	
Synergy Coronary Artery Stent *Boston Scientific, www.bostonscientific.com*	Conditional 5	1.5, 3	
TAA Endograft *TriVascular2, Inc., Santa Rosa, CA*	Conditional 6	3	
Taarget Stent Graft *LeMaitre Vascular, Burlington, MA*	Conditional 6	3	
Taewoong Niti-S Nagi Stent *TaeWoong Medical Co., Ltd., www.stent.net*	Conditional 8	1.5, 3	
TAG Endoprosthesis *Thoracic Aneurysm Stent graft* *45-mm x 20-cm endoprostheses* *W.L. Gore & Associates, www.goremedical.com*	Conditional 5	3	
Talent Abdominal Stent Graft *Medtronic, Inc., www.medtronic.com/mri*	Conditional 5	1.5, 3	
Talent Converter Stent Graft *Medtronic, Inc., www.medtronic.com/mri*	Conditional 5	1.5, 3	

Object	Status	Field Strength (T)	Reference
Talent Graft Stent *Bare Spring Model, 16 x 8-m* *World Medical Manufacturing Corp., Sunrise, FL*	Safe	1.5	
Talent Graft Stent *Bare Spring Model, 36 x 20-mm* *World Medical Manufacturing Corp., Sunrise, FL*	Safe	1.5	
Talent Graft Stent *Open Web Model, 16 x 8-mm* *World Medical Manufacturing Corp., Sunrise, FL*	Safe	1.5	
Talent Graft Stent *Open Web Model, 36 x 20-mm* *Nitinol* *World Medical Manufacturing Corp., Sunrise, FL*	Safe	1.5	
Talent Thoracic Graft *Medtronic, Inc., www.medtronic.com/mri*	Conditional 5	1.5, 3	
Target Coil 360 SOFT, Embolization Coil *Stryker Neurovascular, www.stryker.com*	Conditional 5	1.5, 3	
Target Coil 360 STANDARD, Embolization Coil *Stryker Neurovascular, www.stryker.com*	Conditional 5	1.5, 3	
Target Coil 360 ULTRA, Embolization Coil *Stryker Neurovascular, www.stryker.com*	Conditional 5	1.5, 3	
Target Coil HELICAL ULTRA, Embolization Coil *Stryker Neurovascular, www.stryker.com*	Conditional 5	1.5, 3	
Target Detachable Coil, Embolization Coil *All Sizes and Shapes* *Stryker Neurovascular, www.stryker.com*	Conditional 5	1.5, 3	
TAXUS Element Stent *Boston Scientific, www.bostonscientific.com*	Conditional 5	1.5, 3	
TAXUS Express Stent, Paclitaxel-Eluting *Coronary Stent* *Boston Scientific, www.bostonscientific.com*	Conditional 5	1.5, 3	
TAXUS Express2 Atom Stent *Boston Scientific, www.bostonscientific.com*	Conditional 5	1.5, 3	
TAXUS Express2 Atom Paclitaxel-Eluting *Coronary Stent* *Boston Scientific, www.bostonscientific.com*	Conditional 5	1.5, 3	
TAXUS Express2 Coronary Stent *Boston Scientific, www.bostonscientific.com*	Conditional 5	1.5, 3	
TAXUS Liberte (Liberte') Paclitaxel-Eluting *Coronary Stent* *316L SS* *Boston Scientific, www.bostonscientific.com*	Conditional 5	1.5, 3	

Object	Status	Field Strength (T)	Reference
TAXUS Liberte (Liberte') Atom Paclitaxel-Eluting *Coronary Stent* *TAXUS Liberte Atom Stent* *Boston Scientific, www.bostonscientific.com*	Conditional 5	1.5, 3	
TAXUS Liberte (Liberte') Long Paclitaxel-Eluting *Coronary Stent* *TAXUS Liberte Long Stent* *Boston Scientific, www.bostonscientific.com*	Conditional 5	1.5, 3	
Terumo Misago Peripheral Self Expanding Stent *Terumo Medical Corporation, www.terumomedical.com*	Conditional 5	1.5, 3	
Terumo Renzan Stent, All Sizes *MicroVention, Inc., www.microvention.com*	Conditional 8	1.5, 3	
Thoraflex Device, Stent Graft *Vascutek Ltd., www.vascutek.com*	Conditional 8	1.5, 3	
Tornado Embolization Coil *Cook Medical, Inc., www.cookmedical.com*	Conditional 5	3	
Tornado Embolization Microcoil *Cook Medical Inc., www cookmedical.com*	Conditional 5	3	
Trachea/Bronchium Stent *M.I. Tech, www.mitech.co.kr*	Conditional 8	1.5, 3	
Tracheal Stent *Hood Laboratories, www.hoodlabs.com*	Safe	1.5, 3	
Tracheobronchial Wall Stent Endoprosthesis *14 x 80-mm, Stent* *Schneider (USA) Inc., Pfizer Medical Technology Group, Minneapolis, MN*	Safe	1.5	64
Tracheobronchial WallStent Endoprosthesis *24 x 70-mm, Stent* *Schneider (USA) Inc., Pfizer Medical Technology Group, Minneapolis, MN*	Safe	1.5	64
TRAPEASE Permanent Vena Cava Filter *Cordis, www.depuysynthes.com*	Conditional 5	3	
Treovance Abdominal Stent Graft *Bolton Medical, Inc., Sunrise, FL*	Conditional 8	1.5, 3	
Triangular Prostatic Stent *Allium Medical Solutions Ltd., www.allium-medical.com*	Conditional 8	1.5, 3	
TriMaxx Coronary Stent *SS-Tantalum composite* *Stent* *Abbott Vascular Devices, Redwood City, CA*	Safe	3	
TRUFILL DCS ORBIT Detachable Coil *Embolization Coil* *Platinum, Tungsten* *Cordis, www.depuysynthes.com*	Safe	3	87

Object	Status	Field Strength (T)	Reference
TRUFILL Pushable Coils *Vascular Occlusion System* *Platinum* *Cordis, www.depuysynthes.com*	Safe	1.5	
Tryton Side Branch Stent *Tryton Medical, www.trytonmedical.com*	Conditional 6	3	
Uncovered WallFlex Biliary RX Stent System *Boston Scientific, www.bostonscientific.com*	Conditional 6	3	
Uro-Guide Open Tip *Ureteral Stent* *Silicone* *Gyrus ACMI (Olympus Medical),* *www.medical.olympusamerica.com*	Safe	3	
ULTIPAQ Microcoil *Embolization Coil* *Micrus Endovascular, www.micrusendovascular.com*	Conditional 5	3	
Ultraflex Stent *Titanium alloy*	Safe	1.5	73
Ultraflex Tracheobronchial Stent *Boston Scientific, www.bostonscientific.com*	Conditional 5	1.5, 3	
Uro-Guide Open Ureteral Stent *Gyrus ACMI (Olympus Medical),* *www.medical.olympusamerica.com*	Conditional 5	1.5	
V4.0 Abdominal Stent Graft System *TriVascular, Inc., www.trivascular.com*	Conditional 8	1.5, 3	
V12 Renal Covered Stent *Atrium Medical Corporation, www.atriummed.com*	Conditional 8	1.5, 3	
Valecor Platinum Stent *Coronary Artery Stent* *Cornova, Inc., Burlington, MA*	Conditional 8	1.5, 3	
Valeo Biliary Stent *Bard Peripheral Vascular, www.bardpv.com*	Conditional 6	3	
Valiant Thoracic Stent Graft *Medtronic, Inc., www.medtronic.com/mri*	Conditional 5	1.5, 3	
Vanguard Stent *Boston Scientific* *Wayne, NJ*	Safe	1.5	70
VascuFlex Stent *B. Braun Medical, www.bbraun.com*	Conditional 8	1.5, 3	
VascuFlex SE Stent *B. Braun, www.bbraunusa.com*	Conditional 5	1.5, 3	
VascuFlex SEC Stent *B. Braun, www.bbraunusa.com*	Conditional 5	1.5, 3	

Object	Status	Field Strength (T)	Reference
VBS Stent (also known as the Verdi Stent) *Synthes GmbH, Switzerland*	Conditional 6	3	
Vectra VAG, Vascular Access Graft *Bard Peripheral Vascular, www.bardpv.com*	Safe	3	
VENAFLO II Vascular Graft *Carbon-impregnated ePTFE* *Bard Peripheral Vascular, www.bardpv.com*	Safe	3	
VENAFLO Vascular Graft *Carbon-impregnated ePTFE* *Bard Peripheral Vascular, www.bardpv.com*	Safe	3	
Vena Reinforced Organic Valved Arterial Graft *Labcor Laboratorios Ltda., www.labcor.com*	Safe	1.5, 3	
VenaTech Convertible, Vena Cava Filter *B. Braun, www.bbraunusa.com*	Conditional 5	3	
VenaTech LGM Vena Cava Filter *B. Braun, www.bbraunusa.com*	Conditional 5	1.5, 3	
VenaTech LP Vena Cava Filter *B. Braun, www.bbraunusa.com*	Conditional 5	1.5, 3	
Veniti Inferior Vena Cava (IVC) Filter *Veniti, Inc., www.venitimedical.com*	Conditional 5	1.5, 3	
Veniti Vici Venous Stent System *All Sizes Up to 230-mm* *Veniti, Inc., www.veniti.com*	Conditional 8	1.5, 3	
VeriFlex Stent, VeriFlex Coronary Stent *Boston Scientific, www.bostonscientific.com*	Conditional 5	1.5, 3	
VEST Stent *Vascular Graft Solutions LTD, www.graftsolutions.com*	Conditional 5	1.5, 3	
VIABAHN Endoprosthesis *13-mm x 10-cm, Nitinol* *W. L. Gore & Associates, Inc., www.goremedical.com*	Conditional 5	1.5, 3	
VIABAHN Endoprosthesis *8-mm x 25-cm, single version* *Nitinol* *W.L. Gore & Associates, www.goremedical.com*	Conditional 5	1.5, 3	
VIABAHN Endoprosthesis *8-mm x 25-cm, two-overlapped version* *Nitinol* *W.L. Gore & Associates, www.goremedical.com*	Conditional 5	1.5, 3	
VIABAHN Endoprosthesis *9-mm x 15-cm, Nitinol* *W. L. Gore & Associates, Inc., www.goremedical.com*	Conditional 5	1.5, 3	
VIABAHN Endoprosthesis *W.L. Gore and Associates, Inc., www.goremedical.com*	Conditional 5	1.5, 3	

Object	Status	Field Strength (T)	Reference
VIABIL Biliary Endoprosthesis *W.L. Gore and Associates, Inc., www.goremedical.com*	Conditional 5	3	
VIATORR Endoprosthesis *Stent* *Nitinol* *W.L. Gore and Associates, Inc., www.goremedical.com*	Conditional 5	1.5	
VIATORR TIPS Endoprosthesis *W.L. Gore and Associates, Inc., www.goremedical.com*	Conditional 5	3	
Vena Tech LP Vascular Filter *B. Braun, www.bbraunusa.com*	Conditional 5	1.5	
Vici Venous Stent *Veniti, Inc., www.venitimedical.com*	Conditional 8	1.5, 3	
Visi-Pro Balloon Expandable Stent *Covidien and ev3 Inc., www.ev3.net*	Conditional 8	1.5, 3	
Visi-Pro Biliary Stent *Covidien and ev3, Inc., www.ev3.net*	Conditional 5	3	
VIVAL Coronary Stent *Avantec Vascular, Sunnyvale, CA*	Conditional 6	3	
Vortek Hydro-Coated Double Loop Ureteral Stent *Coloplast, www.coloplast.com*	Safe	1.5, 3	
VortX 18 Coil *Boston Scientific, www.bostonscientific.com*	Conditional 5	1.5, 3	
VortX 35 Coil *Boston Scientific, www.bostonscientific.com*	Conditional 5	1.5, 3	
VortX Diamond 18 Coil *Boston Scientific, www.bostonscientific.com*	Conditional 5	1.5, 3	
vProtect Luminal Shield Stent *Prescient Medical, Inc., Doylestown, PA*	Conditional 8	1.5, 3	
V-Track Embolization Coil, HydroCoil *MicroVention, Inc., www.microvention.com*	Conditional 6	3	
V-Track Embolization Coil, MultiPlex *MicroVention, Inc., www.microvention.com*	Conditional 6	3	
V-Trak, HydroCoil, MicroCoil, Embolic Coil *Microvention, www.microvention.com*	Conditional 8	1.5, 3	
Wallaby Medical Embolic Coil System *Wallaby Medical, Inc.*	Conditional 8	1.5, 3	
WallFlex Biliary RX Stent *Boston Scientific, www.bostonscientific.com*	Conditional 5	3	
WallFlex Biliary Stent *covered version* *Boston Scientific, www.bostonscientific.com*	Safe	3	

Object	Status	Field Strength (T)	Reference
WallFlex Biliary Stent *uncovered version* *Boston Scientific, www.bostonscientific.com*	Safe	3	
WallFlex Enteral Colonic Stent with *Anchor Lock Delivery System* *Nitinol* *Boston Scientific, www.bostonscientific.com*	Safe	3	
WallFlex Enteral Duodenal Stent with *Anchor Lock Delivery System* *Nitinol* *Boston Scientific, www.bostonscientific.com*	Safe	3	
WallFlex Partially Covered Esophageal Stent *Boston Scientific, www.bostonscientific.com*	Conditional 5	3	
WallGraft *Boston Scientific, www.bostonscientific.com*	Safe	3	
WallStent Biliary Endoprosthesis, Stent *Schneider USA, Plymouth, MN*	Safe	1.5	28
WallStent Endoprosthesis *Boston Scientific, www.bostonscientific.com*	Conditional 5	3	
WallStent Endoprosthesis *Magic WallStent* *3.5 x 25, Stent* *Schneider (USA) Inc., Pfizer Medical Technology Group,* *Minneapolis, MN*	Safe	1.5	64
WallStent Endoprosthesis *With Permalume covering* *8 x 80, Stent* *Schneider (USA) Inc., Pfizer Medical Technology Group,* *Minneapolis, MN*	Safe	1.5	64
WallStent Esophageal II Endoprosthesis *20 x 130, Stent* *Schneider (USA) Inc., Pfizer Medical Technology Group,* *Minneapolis, MN*	Safe	1.5	64
WallStent Carotid Artery Stent *Boston Scientific, www.bostonscientific.com*	Safe	3	
WallStent *Schneider, Bulach, Switzerland*	Safe	1.5	69
WallStent RX Biliary Endoprosthesis *Boston Scientific, www.bostonscientific.com*	Conditional 5	3	
Walvekar Salivary Duct Stent *Hood Laboratories, www.hoodlabs.com*	Safe	1.5, 3	
WEB Aneurysm Embolization Device *Sequent Medical, Inc., Aliso Viejo, CA*	Conditional 6	3	

Object	Status	Field Strength (T)	Reference
Westaby T-Y Stent *Hood Laboratories, www.hoodlabs.com*	Safe	1.5, 3	
Wiktor Coronary Artery Stent *Medtronic, Inc. www.medtronic.com/mri*	Safe	1.5	
Wiktor GX Stent *Medtronic, Inc., www.medtronic.com/mri*	Safe	1.5	72
Willis Stent *MicroPort Medical, www.microport.com.cn/english*	Conditional 8	1.5, 3	
Wilson-Cook Pancreatic Stent *Cook Medical, www.cookmedical.com*	Safe	1.5	
Wilson-Cook Pancreatic Wedge Stent *Cook Medical, www.cookmedical.com*	Safe	1.5	
Wingspan Stent System *Boston Scientific, www.bostonscientific.com and* *Stryker, www.stryker.com*	Conditional 5	3	
Xact Stent, Nitinol *Abbott Vascular, www.abbottvascular.com*	Conditional 5	3	
XactfleX Carotid Stent, Nitinol *Abbott Vascular, www.abbottvascular.com*	Conditional 5	3	
Xceed Biliary Stent *Abbott Vascular, www.abbottvascular.com*	Conditional 5	3	
XIENCE Alpine Stent *Abbott Vascular, www.abbottvascular.com*	Conditional 5	1.5, 3	
XIENCE Nano Everolimus Eluting Coronary Stent *Abbott Vascular, www.Abbott.com*	Conditional 5	1.5, 3	
XIENCE PRIME Stent *Abbott Vascular, www.abbottvascular.com*	Conditional 5	3	
XIENCE V Everolimus Eluting Coronary Stent *Abbott Vascular, www.abbottvascular.com*	Conditional 5	3	
XIENCE V Stent *Abbott Vascular, www.abbottvascular.com*	Conditional 5	3	
XIENCE Xpedition Stent *Abbott Vascular, www.abbottvascular.com*	Conditional 5	1.5, 3	
Xpert Biliary Stent *Abbott Vascular, www.abbottvascular.com*	Conditional 5	3	
Xpert Stent, Nitinol *Abbott Vascular, www.abbottvascular.com*	Conditional 6	3	
X-Suit NIR Biliary Metallic Stent *Olympus and Medinol, www.medinol.com*	Conditional 5	1.5, 3	
X-Suit NIR Covered Biliary Stent *Medinol Ltd., Israel*	Conditional 8	1.5, 3	

Object	Status	Field Strength (T)	Reference
XTENT Customizable Stent, Coronary Artery Stent *XTENT, Inc., Menlo Park, CA*	Conditional 6	3	
XTRASOFT ORBIT GALAXY Detachable Coil *Codman, www.Depuy.com*	Conditional 6	3	
X-Trode, 3 segment, Stent, 316 SS *C.R. Bard, Inc., www.crbard.com*	Safe	1.5	
X-Trode, 9 segment, Stent, 316 SS *C.R. Bard, Inc., www.crbard.com*	Safe	1.5	
Y Stent *Hood Laboratories, www.hoodlabs.com*	Safe	1.5, 3	
Zenith AAA Endovascular Graft *Ancillary Components, Stent* *Cook Medical, www.cookmedical.com*	Conditional 5	1.5, 3	
Zenith AAA Endovascular Grafts, Bifurcated, Stent *Cook Medical, www.cookmedical.com*	Conditional 5	1.5, 3	
Zenith AAA Endovascular Graft *Zenith Flex AAA Stent* *Including starting with prefix TFB, TFFB, TFLE, ELSE,* *ESBE, ESC, ESP, ZIP, AX1, RX1* *Cook Medical, www.cookmedical.com*	Conditional 5	1.5, 3	
Zenith Alpha Thoracic Endovascular Graft *Cook Medical, www.cook.com*	Conditional 5	1.5, 3	
Zenith Fenestrated AAA Endovascular Graft *Cook Medical, www.cook.com*	Conditional 5	1.5, 3	
Zenith Flex AAA Endovascular Graft Bifurcated *Main Body Graft* *Cook Medical Inc., www cookmedical.com*	Conditional 5	1.5, 3	
Zenith Flex AAA Endovascular Graft Converters *Cook Medical Inc., www cookmedical.com*	Conditional 5	1.5, 3	
Zenith Flex AAA Endovascular Graft Iliac Plug *Cook Medical Inc., www cookmedical.com*	Conditional 5	1.5, 3	
Zenith Flex AAA Endovascular Graft Main *Body Extensions* *Cook Medical Inc., www cookmedical.com*	Conditional 5	1.5, 3	
Zenith Renu AAA Ancillary Graft Converter *Cook Medical Inc., www cookmedical.com*	Conditional 5	1.5, 3	
Zenith Renu AAA Ancillary Graft Main *Body Extension* *Cook Medical Inc., www cookmedical.com*	Conditional 5	1.5, 3	
Zenith Renu AAA Ancillary Graft, Stent *Cook Medical, www.cookmedical.com*	Conditional 5	1.5, 3	
Zenith Spiral-Z AAA Iliac Leg Graft, Stent *Cook Medical, Inc., www.cookmedical.com*	Conditional 5	1.5, 3	

Object	Status	Field Strength (T)	Reference
Zenith TX2 Low-Profile TAA Endovascular Graft *Cook Medical, Inc., www.cookmedical.com*	Conditional 5	1.5, 3	
Zenith TX2 TAA Endovascular Graft *Cook Medical, Inc., www.cookmedical.com*	Conditional 5	1.5, 3	
Zenith TX2 TAA Endovascular Graft with Pro-Form *Cook Medical Inc., www cookmedical.com*	Conditional 5	1.5, 3	
Zenith TX2 TAA Endovascular Graft with Pro-Form *Extensions* *Cook Medical Inc., www cookmedical.com*	Conditional 5	1.5, 3	
Zenith TX2 TAA Endovascular Graft with Pro-Form *Proximal Components* *Cook Medical Inc., www cookmedical.com*	Conditional 5	1.5, 3	
Zenith TX2 TAA Endovascular Graft with Pro-Form *Proximal Tapered Components* *Cook Medical Inc., www cookmedical.com*	Conditional 5	1.5, 3	
Zilver Flex Stent *Cook Medical, Inc., www.cookmedical.com*	Conditional 5	1.5, 3	
Zilver Flex 35 Biliary Stent *Cook Medical, Inc., www.cookmedical.com*	Conditional 5	1.5, 3	
Zilver FLEX 35 Vascular Stent *Cook Medical, Inc., www.cookmedical.com*	Conditional 5	1.5, 3	
Zilver 518 Biliary Self Expanding Stent *Cook Medical, Inc., www.cookmedical.com*	Conditional 5	1.5, 3	
Zilver 518 Vascular Self Expanding Stent *Cook Medical, Inc., www.cookmedical.com*	Conditional 5	1.5, 3	
Zilver 635 Biliary Self Expanding Stent *Cook Medical, Inc., www.cookmedical.com*	Conditional 5	3	
Zilver 635 Vascular Self Expanding Stent *Cook Medical, Inc., www.cookmedical.com*	Conditional 5	3	
Zilver PTX Drug Eluting Peripheral Stent *Cook Medical, Inc., www.cookmedical.com*	Conditional 5	1.5, 3	
Zilver Stent, Iliac Artery *Cook Medical, Inc., www.cookmedical.com*	Conditional 5	3	
Zilver Stent, Nitinol, Gold *Cook Medical, Inc., www.cookmedical.com*	Conditional 5	3	
Zilver Self-Expanding Stent *Cook Medical, Inc., www.cookmedical.com*	Conditional 5	3	
Zimmon Pancreatic Stent *Cook Medical, Inc., www.cookmedical.com*	Conditional 5	1.5, 3	

Object	Status	Field Strength (T)	Reference

Dental Implants, Devices, and Materials

Object	Status	Field Strength (T)	Reference
Alignment Rod *BioTex, Inc., biotexmedical.com*	Conditional 5	3	
B & W Dental Implant System *(CIH-500-150 Implant* *UCI-500-500; CIH Implant 5 x 15-mm* *+ Abutment 5 x 5-mm* *B & W SRL, Argentina*	Conditional 6	3	
Bone Anchor *BioTex, Inc., biotexmedical.com*	Conditional 5	3	
Brace Band, SS *American Dental, Missoula, MT*	Conditional 5	1.5	3
Brace Wire, Chrome Alloy *Ormco Corp., San Marcos, CA*	Conditional 5	1.5	3
Castable Alloy *Golden Dental Products, Inc., Golden, CO*	Conditional 5	1.5	12
Cement-In Keeper *Solid State Innovations, Inc., Mt. Airy, NC*	Conditional 5	1.5	12
CoCr (Cobalt-Chromium) Bridge *Nobel Biocare AB, www.nobelbiocare.com*	Conditional 8	1.5, 3	
Dental amalgam	Safe	1.5	
DentureID *CMP Industries LLC, www.cmpindustries.com*	Conditional 8	1.5, 3	
Dental Implants, PEEK Polymer, PMMA *Straumann www.straumann.com*	Safe	1.5, 3	
GDP Direct Keeper, Pre-formed Post *Golden Dental Products, Inc., Golden, CO*	Conditional 5	1.5	12
Gutta Percha Points *Dental device*	Safe	1.5	
Healing Cap Multi-unit BMK Syst WP *Nobel Biocare AB, www.nobelbiocare.com*	Conditional 6	3	
Hemi Mandibular Reconstruction Construct *(ARTISAN and ARCHITEX)* *Medtronic, www.medtronic.com/mri*	Conditional 8	1.5, 3	
Indian Head Real Silver Points, Dental *Union Broach Co., Inc., New York, NY*	Safe	1.5	
Keeper, Pre-formed Post, Dental *Parkell Products, Inc., Farmingdale, NY*	Safe	1.5	
Magna-Dent, Large Indirect Keeper, Dental *Dental Ventures of America, Yorba Linda, CA*	Safe	1.5	

Object	Status	Field Strength (T)	Reference
Palladium Clad Magnet, Dental *Parkell Products, Inc., Farmingdale, NY*	Unsafe 1	1.5	13
Palladium/Palladium Keeper, Dental *Parkell Products, Inc., Farmingdale, NY*	Conditional 5	1.5	13
Palladium/Platinum Casting Alloy, Dental *Parkell Products, Inc., Farmingdale, NY*	Conditional 5	1.5	13
Permanent Crown, Amalgam, Dental *Ormco Corp.*	Safe	1.5	3
Procera Implant Bridge Including Mounted Implants *(Fixtures)* *Nobel Biocare AB, www.nobelbiocare.com*	Conditional 8	1.5, 3	
Procera Implant Bridge Supported by Two *Zygoma Implants and Standard Implants (Fixtures)* *Nobel Biocare AB, www.nobelbiocare.com*	Conditional 8	1.5, 3	
Reconstruction Plate for Mandibular System *Combined with 14 Screws* *Medicon, www.medicon.de*	Conditional 8	1.5, 3	
Silver Point, Dental *Union Broach Co., Inc., New York, NY*	Safe	1.5	3
Socket Preservation Screw *Medtronic, www.medtronic.com/mri*	Conditional 8	1.5, 3	
SPI Spiral Implant, Dental Implant *Alpha-Bio Tec Ltd., www.alpha-bio.net*	Conditional 6	3	
Stainless Steel Clad Magnet, Dental *Parkell Products, Inc., Farmingdale, NY*	Unsafe 1	1.5	13
Stainless Steel Keeper, Dental *Parkell Products, Inc., Farmingdale, NY*	Conditional 5	1.5	13
T4 5014 Implant, T4 6012-30 Angled Abutment, *T0 2000 Metric Screw* *Nucleoss, www.nucleoss.com*	Conditional 8	1.5, 3	
Titanium Clad Magnet, Dental *Parkell Products, Inc., Farmingdale, NY*	Unsafe 1	1.5	13

ECG Electrodes

Object	Status	Field Strength (T)	Reference
Accutac, ECG Electrode *ConMed Corp., Utica, NY*	Safe	1.5	
Accutac, ECG Electrode, Diaphoretic *ConMed Corp., Utica, NY*	Safe	1.5	
Adult Cloth, ECG Electrode *ConMed Corp., Utica, NY*	Safe	1.5	
Adult ECG, ECG Electrode, Electrode 3-Pack *ConMed Corp., Utica, NY*	Safe	1.5	

Object	Status	Field Strength (T)	Reference
Adult Foam, ECG Electrode *ConMed Corp., Utica, NY*	Safe	1.5	
Blue Sensor, Model 2300 *ECG (EKG) Electrode* *Ambu, www.ambu.com*	Conditional 8	1.5, 3	
Cardiac Monitoring ECG Electrode, 2244 *3M, www.3m.com*	Conditional 5	3	
Cardiac Monitoring ECG Electrode, 2570 *3M, www.3m.com*	Conditional 5	3	
Cardiac Monitoring ECG Electrode, 2660 *3M, www.3m.com*	Conditional 5	3	
Cardiac Monitoring ECG Electrode, 2670 *3M, www.3m.com*	Conditional 5	3	
Cleartrace 2, ECG Electrode *ConMed Corp., Utica, NY*	Safe	1.5	
Dyna/Trace Diagnostic, ECG Electrode *ConMed Corp., Utica, NY*	Safe	1.5	
Dyna/Trace Mini, ECG Electrode *ConMed Corp., Utica, NY*	Safe	1.5	
Dyna/Trace Stress, ECG Electrode *ConMed Corp., Utica, NY*	Safe	1.5	
Dyna/Trace, ECG Electrode *ConMed Corp., Utica, NY*	Safe	1.5	
ECG (EKG) Electrode, Model 2268 *3M, www.3m.com*	Conditional 5	1.5, 3	
ECG (EKG) Electrode, Model 2570 *3M, www.3m.com*	Conditional 5	1.5, 3	
ECG (EKG) Electrode, Model 2670 *3M, www.3m.com*	Conditional 5	1.5, 3	
High Demand, ECG Electrode *ConMed Corp., Utica, NY*	Safe	1.5	
Holtrode, ECG Electrode *ConMed Corp., Utica, NY*	Safe	1.5	
HP M2202A Radio-lucent, ECG Electrode *Hewlett-Packard, Andover, MA*	Safe	1.5	
Invisatrace Adult, ECG Electrode *ConMed Corp., Utica, NY*	Safe	1.5	
Monitoring Electrode, REF 2268 ECG *(EKG) Electrode, Red Dot* *3M, www.3m.com*	Conditional 5	3	

Object	Status	Field Strength (T)	Reference
Neonatal Monitoring Electrode *With Pre-Attached Lead Wire,* *REF 2269T ECG (EKG) Electrode, Red Dot* *3M, www.3m.com*	Conditional 5	3	
Pediatric Foam, ECG Electrode *ConMed Corp., Utica, NY*	Safe	1.5	
Plia Cell Diagnostic, ECG Electrode *ConMed Corp., Utica, NY*	Safe	1.5	
Plia-Cell Diaphoretic, ECG Electrode *ConMed Corp., Utica, NY*	Safe	1.5	
Plia-Cell, ECG Electrode *ConMed Corp., Utica, NY*	Safe	1.5	
Quadtrode MRI, ECG Electrode *InVivo Research, Inc., Orlando, FL*	Safe	1.5	
Resting Electrode, REF 2360 ECG (EKG) Electrode, *Red Dot* *3M, www.3m.com*	Conditional 5	3	
Silvon Adult ECG Electrode *ConMed Corp., Utica, NY*	Safe	1.5	
Silvon Diaphoretic, ECG Electrode *ConMed Corp., Utica,NY*	Safe	1.5	
Silvon Stress, ECG Electrode *ConMed Corp., Utica, NY*	Safe	1.5	
Silvon, ECG Electrode *ConMed Corp., Utica, NY*	Safe	1.5	
Snaptrace, ECG Electrode *ConMed Corp., Utica, NY*	Safe	1.5	
SSE Radiotransparent ECG Electrode *ConMed Corp., Utica, NY*	Safe	1.5	
SSE, ECG Electrode *ConMed Corp., Utica, NY*	Safe	1.5	
WhiteSensor, *Models 0215M, 0315M, 0415M, 0615M,* *0715M, WS/RT, 4841P, 7841P, 4530M,* *4540M, 4570M, 40713, 4440M, 4500M* *ECG (EKG) Electrode* *Ambu, www.ambu.com*	Conditional 8	1.5, 3	

Foley Catheters With and Without Temperature Sensors

Object	Status	Field Strength (T)	Reference
Bardex I.C. Foley Catheter *Silver and Hydrogel Coating,16 Fr.* *Bard Medical, www.bardmedical.com*	Conditional 5	1.5	

Object	Status	Field Strength (T)	Reference
Bardex I.C. Temperature Sensing Foley Catheter *with a 6 foot cable, 16 Fr.* *Bard Medical, www.bardmedical.com*	Conditional 5	1.5	
Bardex Latex-Free Temperature Sensing *400-Series Foley Catheter* *Bard Medical, www.bardmedical.com*	Conditional 5	1.5, 3	
Bardex Lubricath Temperature Sensing *Urotrack Plus Foley Catheter with a 6 foot cable, 16 Fr.* *Bard Medical, www.bardmedical.com*	Conditional 5	1.5	
Bardex Pediatric Temperature Sensing 400-Series *Urotrack Foley Catheter with a detachable cable, 12 Fr.* *Bard Medical, www.bardmedical.com*	Conditional 5	1.5	
CoreView Foley Catheter *CV0016, CV1016, CV1016 with connector, CV0016M* *Bard Medical, www.bardmedical.com*	Conditional 5	1.5, 3	
DeRoyal Foley Catheter With Temperature Sensor, *18-Fr* *DeRoyal Industries, www.DeRoyal.com*	Conditional 5	1.5, 3	
Extension Cable for Foley Catheter *with temperature sensor, 10 feet* *RSP Respiratory Support Products, Inc.* *Smiths Industries, Irvine, CA*	Unsafe 2	1.5	
Foley Catheter *Bard Medical, www.bardmedical.com*	Safe	1.5	
Foley Catheter, SilverTouch Catheter *Medline Industries, Inc., Mundelein, IL*	Conditional 6	3	
Foley Catheter with Temperature Sensor, 10 Fr. *RSP Respiratory Support Products, Inc. &* *Smiths Industries, Irvine, CA*	Conditional 5	1.5	
Foley Catheter with Temperature Sensor, 18 Fr. *RSP Respiratory Support Products, Inc. &* *Smiths Industries, Irvine, CA*	Conditional 5	1.5	
Level 1 Foley Catheter with Temperature Sensor *FC400-08, 8FR* *Global Operations Technology, Rockland, MA*	Conditional 5	1.5, 3	
Level 1 Foley Catheter with Temperature Sensor *FC400-14, 14FR* *Global Operations Technology, Rockland, MA*	Conditional 5	1.5, 3	
Lubri-Sil I.C. Foley Catheter *Bard Medical, www.bardmedical.com*	Safe	3	
Lubri-Sil I.C. Foley Catheter, Temperature Sensing *400-Series Foley Catheter* *Bard Medical, www.bardmedical.com*	Conditional 6	1.5, 3	

Object	Status	Field Strength (T)	Reference
Medline's 100% Silicone 400 Series *Temperature Sensing Foley Catheter* *Medline, www.medline.com*	Conditional 5	1.5, 3	

Halo Vests and Cervical Fixation Devices

Object	Status	Field Strength (T)	Reference
Ambulatory Halo System *Halo and Cervical Fixation*	Conditional 4	1.5	14
Bremer 3D Halo Crown System *with Bremer Air Flo Vest and Titanium Skull Pins* *Cervical Fixation Device* *Depuy Synthes, www.depuysynthes.com*	Conditional 6	3	
Bremer Halo Crown System *with Bremer Air Flo Vest and Titanium Skull Pins* *Cervical Fixation Device* *Depuy Synthes, www.depuysynthes.com*	Conditional 6	3	
Closed-back Halo *Halo and Cervical Fixation* *Depuy Synthes, www.depuysynthes.com*	Safe	1.5	16
Closed Back Halo *Ossur, www.ossur.com*	Unsafe 1	1.5	
EXO Adjustable Coller *Halo and Cervical Fixation* *Florida Manufacturing Co., Daytona, FL*	Conditional 4	1.0	15
Generation 80 Halo System *with Generation 80 Halo Vest and Aluminum Ring* *and Generation 80 Titanium Halo Pins* *Ossur, www.ossur.com*	Unsafe 1	3	114
Guilford Cervical Orthosis, Modified *Halo and Cervical Fixation* *Guilford & Son, Ltd., Cleveland, OH*	Safe	1.0	15
Guilford Cervical Orthosis *Halo and Cervical Fixation* *Guilford & Son, Ltd., Cleveland, OH*	Conditional 4	1.0	15
J-Tongs *Ossur, www.ossur.com*	Unsafe 1	1.5	
JTO Cervico-Thoracic Extension *Ossur, www.ossur.com*	Safe	3	
'LiL Angel Pediatric Halo System *with Jerome Halo Vest and Resolve Glass-composite* *Halo Ring and Resolve Ceramic-tipped Skull Pins* *Ossur, www.ossur.com*	Conditional 6	3	114

Object	Status	Field Strength (T)	Reference
'LiL Angel Pediatric Halo System *with Resolve Halo Vest and Resolve Glass-composite Halo Ring* *and Resolve Ceramic-tipped Skull Pins* *Ossur, www.ossur.com*	Conditional 6	3	114
Mark III Halo Vest *Aluminum Superstructure, SS rivets, Titanium bolts* *Depuy Synthes, www.depuysynthes.com*	Safe	1.5	16
Mark IV Halo Vest *Aluminum Superstructure and Titanium Bolts* *Depuy Synthes, www.depuysynthes.com*	Safe	1.5	16
Miami J Cervical Collar *Ossur, www.ossur.com*	Safe	3	
MR-compatible Halo Vest and Cervical Fixation *Lerman & Son Co., Beverly Hills, CA*	Safe	1.5	
NecLoc Extrication Collar *Ossur, www.ossur.com*	Safe	3	
Occian Collar Back *Ossur, www.ossur.com*	Safe	3	
Open-back Halo, Aluminum *Depuy Synthes, www.depuysynthes.com*	Safe	1.5	16
Open-back Halo with Delrin inserts for Skull Pins *Depuy Synthes, www.depuysynthes.com*	Safe	1.5	16
Papoos Infant Spinal Immobilization Device *Ossur, www.ossur.com*	Safe	3	
Patriot Extrication Collar *Ossur, www.ossur.com*	Safe	3	
Philadelphia Cervical Collar *Ossur, www.ossur.com*	Safe	3	
Philadelphia Coller *Philadelphia Collar Co., Westville, NJ*	Safe	1.0	15
PMT Halo Cervical Orthosis *PMT Corp., Chanhassen, MN*	Safe	1.0	15
PMT Halo Cervical Orthosis with Graphite Rods *and Halo Ring* *PMT Corp., Chanhassen, MN*	Safe	1.0	15
PMT Halo System with Carbon Graphite Open Back *Ring and Titanium Skull Pins* *PMT Corp., Chanhassen, MN*	Conditional 5	3	
Resolve Halo System with Jerome Halo Vest *and Resolve Glass-composite Halo Ring* *and Resolve Ceramic-tipped Skull Pins* *Ossur, www.ossur.com*	Conditional 6	3	114

Object	Status	Field Strength (T)	Reference
Resolve Halo System with Resolve Halo Vest *and Resolve Glass-composite Halo Ring and Resolve Ceramic-tipped Skull Pins* Ossur, www.ossur.com	Conditional 6	3	114
S.O.M.I. Cervical Orthosis *U.S. Manufacturing Co., Pasadena, CA*	Conditional 4	1.0	15
Trippi-Wells Tong, Titanium *Depuy Synthes, www.depuysynthes.com*	Safe	1.5	16
V1 Halo System with V1 Halo Vest *and V1 Halo Ring and V1 Titanium Halo Pins* Ossur, www.ossur.com	Conditional 6	3	114
V2 *Ossur, www.ossur.com*	Unsafe 1	1.5	

Heart Valve Prostheses and Annuloplasty Rings

Object	Status	Field Strength (T)	Reference
AAV-2 Heart Valve, Aortic Heart Valve Prosthesis *Arbor Surgical Technologies, Inc., Irvine, CA*	Conditional 6	3	
AccuFit Mitral Valve Replacement Device *Marvel Medical Technologies, Irvine, CA*	Conditional 5	1.5, 3	
ACURATE TF (Transfemoral) Aortic Bioprosthesis *Symetis SA, www.symetis.com*	Conditional 8	1.5, 3	
AHK 7700, Model 7700 Heart Valve *Medtronic, www.medtronic.com/mri*	Conditional 5	3	
AMEND Mitral Annuloplasty Ring, All Sizes *Valcare Medical LTD., www.valcaremedical.com*	Conditional 8	1.5, 3	
Annuloflex Annuloplasty Ring, Size 26-mm *Carbomedics and www.sorin.com*	Safe	1.5, 3	
Annuloflex Annuloplasty Ring, Size 36-mm *Carbomedics and www.sorin.com*	Safe	1.5, 3	
Annuloflo Annuloplasty Ring, Size 26-mm *Carbomedics and www.sorin.com*	Safe	1.5, 3	
Annuloflo Annuloplasty Ring, Size 36-mm *Carbomedics and www.sorin.com*	Safe	1.5, 3	
AnnuloFlo Mitral Annuloplasty Device *Size 36, Model AR-736* *Carbomedics and www.sorin.com*	Safe	1.5, 3	83
Annuloplasty Ring, Models RNG5 and RNG7 *Dynamic Annuloplasty Ring System* *MiCardia, www.micardia.com*	Conditional 6	3	
Annuloplasty ring, Titanium *Sulzer Medica and Sulzer Carbomedics*	Safe	1.5	
AorTech Aortic, Model 3800 Heart Valve *Aortech Ltd., Strathclyde, U.K.*	Conditional 5	1.5	75

Object	Status	Field Strength (T)	Reference
AorTech Mitral, Model 4800 Heart Valve *Aortech Ltd., Strathclyde, U.K.*	Conditional 5	1.5	75
Aortic Mitroflow Synergy PC *Aortic Pericardial Heart Valve* *Size 19-mm* *Carbomedics and www.sorin.com*	Safe	1.5, 3	
Aortic Mitroflow Synergy PC *Aortic Pericardial Heart Valve* *Size 29-mm* *Carbomedics and www.sorin.com*	Safe	1.5, 3	
Aortic SJM Regent Valve Mechanical Heart Valve *Size 27-mm, Rotatable Aortic* *Standard Cuff-Polyester, AGN* *St. Jude Medical, www.sjm.com*	Conditional 5	3	
Aortic Valve, Size 16-mm *Carbomedics and www.sorin.com*	Safe	1.5, 3	
Apical Connector, Model 174A, Heart Valve *Medtronic, Inc., www.medtronic.com/mri*	Safe	1.5, 3	84
Atrioventricular Valved Stent (AVS) *Navigate Cardiac Structures, Inc., Lake Forrest, CA*	Conditional 5	1.5, 3	
ATS Medical Open Pivot Aortic Valved Graft *Model # XX denotes size, 502AGxx* *ATS Medical, Minneapolis, MN*	Conditional 6	3	
ATS Medical Open Pivot Bileaflet Heart Valve *AP 360 Aortic, Model # XX denotes size, 505DAxx* *ATS Medical, Minneapolis, MN*	Conditional 6	3	
ATS Medical Open Pivot Bileaflet Heart Valve *AP 360 Mitral, Model # XX denotes size, 505DMxx* *ATS Medical, Minneapolis, MN*	Conditional 6	3	
ATS Medical Open Pivot, Bileaflet Heart Valve *AP Aortic, Model # XX denotes size, 501DAxx* *ATS Medical, Minneapolis, MN*	Conditional 6	3	
ATS Medical Open Pivot, Bileaflet Heart Valve *AP Mitral, Model # XX denotes size, 501DMxx* *ATS Medical, Minneapolis, MN*	Conditional 6	3	
ATS Medical Open Pivot, Bileaflet Heart Valve *Apex Aortic, Model # XX denotes size, 503DAxx* *ATS Medical, Minneapolis, MN*	Conditional 6	3	
ATS Medical Open Pivot, Bileaflet Heart Valve *Apex Mitral, Model # XX denotes size, 503DMxx* *ATS Medical, Minneapolis, MN*	Conditional 6	3	
ATS Medical Open Pivot, Bileaflet Heart Valve *Standard Aortic, Model # XX denotes size, 500FAxx* *ATS Medical, Minneapolis, MN*	Conditional 6	3	

Object	Status	Field Strength (T)	Reference
ATS Medical Open Pivot, Bileaflet Heart Valve *Standard Mitral* *Model # XX denotes size, 500DMxx* *ATS Medical, Minneapolis, MN*	Conditional 6	3	
ATS Medical Open Pivot, BiLeaflet Heart Valve *Mitral, Model 500DM29, Standard Valve* *ATS Medical, Minneapolis, MN*	Conditional 5	1.5	75
ATS Medical Open Pivot, BiLeaflet Heart Valve *Aortic, Model 501DA18* *ATS Medical, Minneapolis, MN*	Conditional 5	1.5	75
Attune Flexible Annuloplasty Ring *St. Jude Medical, www.sjm.com*	Conditional 5	3	
Autogenics Autologous *Model APHV, Eligoy, Heart Valve* *Autogenics Europe Ltd, Glasgow, Scotland*	Safe	1.5	75
Autogenics Autologous *Model ATCV, Eligoy, Heart Valve* *Autogenics Europe Ltd, Glasgow, Scotland*	Safe	1.5	75
Beall Heart Valve *Coratomic Inc., Indiana, PA*	Conditional 5	2.35	17
Beall Mitral Pyrolitic Carbon Heart Valve *Coratomic Inc., Indianapolis, IN*	Conditional 5	1.5	75
Bicarbon Fitline Mechanical Mitral Valve *Sorin Biomedica Cardio, www.sorin.com*	Conditional 6	3	
Bicarbon Heart Valve Prosthesis *Sorin Group, www.sorin.com*	Conditional 6	3	
Bicarbon Slimline Aortic Mechanical Heart Valve *Sorin Biomedica Cardio, www.sorin.com*	Conditional 6	3	
Bileaflet, Model A7760, 29-mm, Heart Valve *Medtronic, Inc., www.medtronic.com/mri*	Safe	1.5	
Biocor Valve, Aortic *Model H3636, Heart Valve* *St. Jude Medical, www.sjm.com*	Conditional 5	3	
Biocor Valve, Mitral *Model B10-35M, Heart Valve* *St. Jude Medical, www.sjm.com*	Conditional 5	3	
Bjork-Shiley (Convexo/Concave) Heart Valve *Shiley Inc., Irvine, CA*	Safe	1.5	3
Bjork-Shiley (Universal/Spherical) Heart Valve *Shiley Inc., Irvine, CA*	Conditional 5	1.5	3
Bjork-Shiley, Model 22 MBRC 11030, Heart Valve *Shiley Inc., Irvine, CA*	Conditional 5	1.5	18

Object	Status	Field Strength (T)	Reference
Bjork-Shiley, Model MBC Heart Valve *Shiley Inc., Irvine, CA*	Conditional 5	1.5	18
Bjork Shiley Monostrut, Aortic *Model ABMS, Heart Valve* *Pfizer, Inc., Cincinnati, OH*	Safe	1.5	75
Bjork Shiley Monostrut, Mitral *Model MBRMS, Heart Valve* *Pfizer, Inc., Cincinnati, OH*	Safe	1.5	75
Bjork Shiley Monostrut, Mitral *Model MBUM, Heart Valve* *Pfizer, Inc., Cincinnati, OH*	Conditional 5	1.5	75
Bjork Shiley Pyrolitic Carbon Conical Disc *Mitral, Model MBRP, Heart Valve* *Pfizer, Inc., Cincinnati, OH*	Conditional 5	1.5	75
Bjork Shiley Pyrolitic Carbon Conical Disc *Mitral, Model MBUP, Heart Valve* *Pfizer, Inc., Cincinnati, OH*	Safe	1.5	75
Bovine Pericardial Patch *Edwards Lifesciences, www.edwards.com*	Safe	1.5, 3	
Carbomedics Annuloflex Annuloplasty Ring *Sorin Group, www.sorin.com*	Safe	1.5	
Carbomedics Annuloflo AR-7XX Annuloplasty Ring *Sorin Group, www.sorin.com*	Conditional 6	3	
Carbomedics Carbo-Seal Conduit *with Mechanical Valve* *Sorin Biomedica Cardio, www.sorin.com*	Conditional 6	3	
Carbomedics Carbo-Seal Valsalva *Heart Valve Prosthesis* *Sorin Group, www.sorin.com*	Conditional 6	3	
Carbomedics Heart Valve Prosthesis *Annuloflo Annuloplasty Ring, Size 26* *Carbomedics and www.sorin.com*	Safe	1.5	
Carbomedics Heart Valve Prosthesis *Annuloflo Annuloplasty Ring, Size 36* *Carbomedics and www.sorin.com*	Safe	1.5	
CarboMedics Heart Valve Prosthesis *Aortic Reduced, Model R500, Size 19* *Carbomedics and www.sorin.com*	Safe	1.5	19
CarboMedics Heart Valve Prosthesis *Aortic Reduced, Model R500, Size 21* *Carbomedics and www.sorin.com*	Safe	1.5	19
CarboMedics Heart Valve Prosthesis *Aortic Reduced, Model R500, Size 23* *Carbomedics and www.sorin.com*	Safe	1.5	19

Object	Status	Field Strength (T)	Reference
CarboMedics Heart Valve Prosthesis *Aortic Reduced, Model R500, Size 25* *Carbomedics and www.sorin.com*	Safe	1.5	19
CarboMedics Heart Valve Prosthesis *Aortic Reduced, Model R500, Size 27* *Carbomedics and www.sorin.com*	Safe	1.5	19
CarboMedics Heart Valve Prosthesis *Aortic Reduced, Model R500, Size 29* *Carbomedics and www.sorin.com*	Safe	1.5	19
CarboMedics Heart Valve Prosthesis *Aortic Standard, Model 500, Size 31* *Carbomedics and www.sorin.com*	Safe	1.5	19
Carbomedics Heart Valve Prosthesis *Aortic Valve, Size 16* *Carbomedics and www.sorin.com*	Safe	1.5	
Carbomedics Heart Valve Prosthesis *Carbo-Seal, Size 31* *Carbomedics and www.sorin.com*	Safe	1.5	
CarboMedics Heart Valve Prosthesis *Mitral Standard, Model 700, Size 23* *Carbomedics and www.sorin.com*	Safe	1.5	19
CarboMedics Heart Valve Prosthesis *Mitral Standard, Model 700, Size 25* *Carbomedics and www.sorin.com*	Safe	1.5	19
CarboMedics Heart Valve Prosthesis *Mitral Standard, Model 700, Size 27* *Carbomedics and www.sorin.com*	Safe	1.5	19
CarboMedics Heart Valve Prosthesis *Mitral Standard, Model 700, Size 29* *Carbomedics and www.sorin.com*	Safe	1.5	19
CarboMedics Heart Valve Prosthesis *Mitral Standard, Model 700, Size 31* *Carbomedics and www.sorin.com*	Safe	1.5	19
CarboMedics Heart Valve Prosthesis *Mitral Standard, Model 700, Size 33* *Carbomedics and www.sorin.com*	Safe	1.5	19
Carbomedics Heart Valve Prosthesis *Mitral Valve, Size 33* *Carbomedics and www.sorin.com*	Safe	1.5	
Carbomedics Prosthetic Heart Valve (CPHV) *Sorin Group, www.sorin.com*	Conditional 6	3	
Carbo-Seal, Ascending Aortic Prosthesis *Size 33-mm, Model AP 33* *Carbomedics and www.sorin.com*	Safe	1.5, 3	

Object	Status	Field Strength (T)	Reference
Carbo-Seal, Ascending Aortic Valve Conduit *Size 33-mm, Model AP-033, Nitinol* *Carbomedics and www.sorin.com*	Safe	1.5, 3	83
Carbo-Seal, Ascending Aortic Valve Conduit *Size 33-mm, Model AP-033, Titanium* *Carbomedics and www.sorin.com*	Safe	1.5, 3	83
Carbomedics Synergy PC Aortic Pericardial *Heart Valve* *Sorin Biomedica Cardio, www.sorin.com*	Conditional 6	3	
CardiAQ TMV (Transcatheter Mitral Valve) *CardiAQ Valve Technologies, www.cardiaq.com*	Conditional 8	1.5, 3	
CardiAQ Transcatheter Mitral Valve *CardiAQ Valve Technologies, www.cardiaq.com*	Conditional 8	1.5, 3	
CardioValve Implant L, All Sizes *MitralTech Ltd.*	Conditional 8	1.5, 3	
Carpentier-Edwards Aortic and Mitral bioprostheses *Models 2625, 6625* *Edwards Lifesciences, www.edwards.com*	Conditional 5	1.5, 3	
Carpentier-Edwards BioPhysio Heart Valve Prosthesis *Model 3100, 29M* *Nitinol, Silicone* *Edwards Lifesciences, www.edwards.com*	Safe	1.5, 3	
Carpentier-Edwards Biophysio Valve *Models 3100TFX, Heart Valve Prosthesis* *Edwards Lifesciences, www.edwards.com*	Conditional 5	3	
Carpentier-Edwards Bioprosthetic Valved Conduit *Model 4300* *Edwards Lifesciences, www.edwards.com*	Conditional 5	1.5, 3	
Carpentier-Edwards Classic Annuloplasty Ring *Mitral Model 4400, Size 40-mm* *Edwards Lifesciences, www.edwards.com*	Safe	1.5, 3	77, 83
Carpentier-Edwards Classic Annuloplasty *Mitral and Tricuspid rings with Duraflo treatment, Models 4425, 4525* *Edwards Lifesciences, www.edwards.com*	Safe	1.5, 3	
Carpentier-Edwards Classic Annuloplasty *Mitral and Tricuspid rings, Models 4400, 4500* *Edwards Lifesciences, www.edwards.com*	Safe	1.5, 3	
Carpentier-Edwards (porcine) Heart Valve *American Edwards Laboratories* *Santa Ana, CA*	Conditional 5	1.5	18
Carpentier-Edwards, Annuloplasty Ring, Model 4400 *Baxter Healthcare Corporation, Santa Ana, CA*	Safe	1.5, 3	

Object	Status	Field Strength (T)	Reference
Carpentier-Edwards, Annuloplasty Ring, Model 4500 *Baxter Healthcare Corporation, Santa Ana, CA*	Safe	1.5, 3	
Carpentier-Edwards, Annuloplasty Ring, Model 4600 *Baxter Healthcare Corporation Santa Ana, CA*	Safe	1.5, 3	
Carpentier-Edwards, Bioprosthesis *Model 2625, Heart Valve* *Baxter Healthcare Corporation, Santa Ana, CA*	Safe	1.5, 3	
Carpentier-Edwards, Bioprosthesis *Model 6625, Heart Valve* *Baxter Healthcare Corporation, Santa Ana, CA*	Safe	1.5, 3	
Carpentier-Edwards Duraflex *low pressure porcine, mitral bioprosthesis* *with extended sewing ring* *6625-ESR-LP* *Edwards Lifesciences, www.edwards.com*	Conditional 5	1.5, 3	
Carpentier-Edwards Duraflex *low pressure, porcine mitral bioprosthesis, Model 6625LP* *Edwards Lifesciences, www.edwards.com*	Conditional 5	1.5, 3	
Carpentier-Edwards Low Pressure Bioprosthesis *Porcine, Mitral Model 6625-LP, Size 35-mm* *Edwards Lifesciences, www.edwards.com*	Safe	1.5, 3	77, 83
Carpentier-Edwards Magna II Pericardial *Aortic Heart Valve Prosthesis, Model 3300/3300TFX* *Edwards Lifesciences, www.edwards.com*	Conditional 6	3	
Carpentier-Edwards-McCarthy-Adams IMR ETlogic *Mitral Annuloplasty Ring Model 4100* *Edwards Lifesciences, www.edwards.com*	Conditional 5	1.5	
Carpentier-Edwards Pericardial Bioprosthesis *Model 2700, Heart Valve* *Baxter Healthcare Corporation, Santa Ana, CA*	Safe	1.5	
Carpentier-Edwards PERIMOUNT Pericardial *Bioprosthesis Mitral Model 6900, Size 33-mm, Heart Valve* *Edwards Lifesciences, www.edwards.com*	Conditional 5	1.5, 3	77, 83
Carpentier-Edwards PERIMOUNT Magna *Mitral Ease pericardial bioprosthesis, Model 7200TFX* *Edwards Lifesciences, www.edwards.com*	Conditional 6	3	
Carpentier-Edwards PERIMOUNT Magna *Mitral Ease pericardial bioprosthesis, Model 7300TFX* *Edwards Lifesciences, www.edwards.com*	Conditional 6	3	
Carpentier-Edwards PERIMOUNT Magna *Mitral pericardial bioprosthesis, Models 7000, 7000TFX* *Edwards Lifesciences, www.edwards.com*	Conditional 6	3	

Object	Status	Field Strength (T)	Reference
Carpentier-Edwards PERIMOUNT Magna *Pericardial aortic bioprostheses, Models 3000, 3000TFX* *Edwards Lifesciences, www.edwards.com*	Conditional 6	3	
Carpentier-Edwards PERIMOUNT Plus *Mitral pericardial bioprosthesis, Model 6900P* *Edwards Lifesciences, www.edwards.com*	Conditional 5	3	
Carpentier-Edwards PERIMOUNT Theon *Pericardial aortic bioprostheses, Models 2700TFX,* *2800TFX* *Edwards Lifesciences, www.edwards.com*	Conditional 5	3	
Carpentier-Edwards PERIMOUNT *Pericardial aortic bioprostheses, Models 2700, 2800* *Edwards Lifesciences, www.edwards.com*	Conditional 5	3	
Carpentier-Edwards Physio Annuloplasty Ring *Mitral Model 4450, Size 40-mm* *Edwards Lifesciences, www.edwards.com*	Conditional 5	1.5, 3	77, 83
Carpentier-Edwards Physio Annuloplasty Ring *Model 4450* *Baxter Healthcare Corporation, Santa Ana, CA*	Safe	1.5	77
Carpentier-Edwards *Physio Annuloplasty Ring* *Model 4450* *Elgiloy alloy* *Edwards Lifesciences, www.edwards.com*	Conditional 6	3	
Carpentier-Edwards Physio II Mitral *Annuloplasty Ring, Model 5200* *Edwards Lifesciences, www.edwards.com*	Conditional 6	3	
Carpentier-Edwards *Model 2650, Heart Valve* *American Edwards Laboratories, Santa Ana, CA*	Conditional 5	1.5	18
Carpentier-Edwards S.A.V. Aortic Bioprosthesis *Model 2650* *Edwards Lifesciences, www.edwards.com*	Conditional 5	1.5, 3	
CG Future Annuloplasty Ring *Colvin-Galloway Future Band 638B* *638B Band & 638R Ring* *Medtronic, Inc., www.medtronic.com/mri*	Conditional 5	3	
Colvin-Galloway Future Band 638B *Annuloplasty Device* *Medtronic, Inc., www.medtronic.com/mri*	Safe	1.5, 3	84
Contegra 200 Heart Valve *Medtronic, Inc., www.medtronic.com/mri*	Safe	1.5, 3	84
Contegra 200S, Heart Valve *Medtronic, Inc., www.medtronic.com/mri*	Safe	1.5, 3	84

Object	Status	Field Strength (T)	Reference
CoreValve Bioprosthesis *Medtronic, Inc., www.medtronic.com/mri*	Conditional 5	1.5, 3	
CoreValve Evolut R Transcatheter Aortic Valve *Medtronic, Inc., www.medtronic.com/MRI*	Conditional 6	3	
Cosgrove-Edwards Annuloplasty Ring *Model 4600* *Baxter Healthcare Corporation, Santa Ana, CA*	Safe	1.5	
Cosgrove-Edwards Annuloplasty *Mitral and Tricuspid band, Model 4600* *Edwards Lifesciences, www.edwards.com*	Safe	1.5, 3	
Cosgrove-Edwards Annuloplasty *Mitral and Tricuspid band with Duraflo treatment,* *Model 4625* *Edwards Lifesciences, www.edwards.com*	Safe	1.5, 3	
CPHV Annuloplasty Ring *Sulzer Medica and Sulzer Carbomedics*	Safe	1.5	
Cribier Aortic Bioprosthesis *Percutaneous Heart Valve, 316LVM SS* *Edwards Lifesciences, www.edwards.com*	Safe	3	
Cribier-Edwards Aortic Bioprosthesis *Model 9000 (PHV1A-26)* *combined with Carpentier-Edwards Porcine Bioprosthesis,* *Model 6650, 31-mm* *Heart Valve prostheses* *Edwards Lifesciences, www.edwards.com*	Conditional 6	3	
Cribier-Edwards Aortic Bioprosthesis (PHV) *Models 9000, 9000PHV* *Edwards Lifesciences, www.edwards.com*	Conditional 6	3	
Crown PRT Aortic Pericardial Heart Valve *LivaNova, www.livanova.sorin.com*	Conditional 8	1.5, 3	
dETlogix Mitral Annuloplasty Ring *Edwards Lifesciences, www.edwards.com*	Conditional 6	3	
Direct Flow Medical 18F Bioprosthesis *Direct Flow Medical, Inc., www.directflowmedical.com*	Conditional 5	3	
Durafic, Aortic, Model AD Heart Valve	Conditional 5	1.5	75
Durafic, Mitral, Model MD Heart Valve	Conditional 5	1.5	75
Duraflex Low Pressure Bioprosthesis *Model 6625E6R-LP, Heart Valve* *Baxter Healthcare Corporation, Santa Ana, CA*	Safe	1.5	
Duraflex Low Pressure Bioprosthesis *Model 6625LP Heart Valve* *Baxter Healthcare Corporation, Santa Ana, CA*	Safe	1.5	

Object	Status	Field Strength (T)	Reference
Duran AnCore, Models 620B, 620R *620RG & 620BG* *Medtronic, Inc., www.medtronic.com/mri*	Conditional 5	3	
Duran Ring, Model H601H Annuloplasty Device *Medtronic, Inc., www.medtronic.com/mri*	Safe	1.5, 3	84
Duran Ring, Model H608H Annuloplasty Device *Medtronic, Inc., www.medtronic.com/mri*	Safe	1.5, 3	84
Duran Ring, Model 610R Annuloplasty Device *Medtronic, Inc., www.medtronic.com/mri*	Safe	1.5, 3	84
Duran Annuloplasty Ring, Model H601H, 35-mm *Medtronic, Inc., www.medtronic.com/mri*	Safe	1.5	
Dynamic Remodeller Annuloplasty Ring *MiCardia Corporation, Irvine, CA*	Conditional 6	3	
Dynaplasty MiCardia Annuloplasty Device *Annuloplasty Ring* *MiCardia Corporation, Irvine, CA*	Conditional 6	3	
Edwards-Duromedics *Aortic and Mitral Bileaflet Prosthesis* *Models 3160, 9120* *Edwards Lifesciences, www.edwards.com*	Safe	1.5	
Edwards Intuity Aortic Valve, Heart Valve Prosthesis *Edwards Lifesciences, www.edwards.com*	Conditional 5	3	
Edwards MC3 Tricuspid Annuloplasty Ring, *Model 4900* *Edwards Lifesciences, www.edwards.com*	Safe	1.5, 3	
Edwards MIRA Aortic and Mitral Mechanical Valves *Models 3600, 3600f, 3600u, 9600* *Edwards Lifesciences, www.edwards.com*	Safe	1.5, 3	
Edwards MIRA Mechanical Valve, Mitral, Model 9600 *Edwards Lifesciences, www.edwards.com*	Safe	1.5	
Edwards Myxo ETlogix Annuloplasty Ring, *Model 5100* *Edwards Lifesciences, www.edwards.com*	Conditional 6	3	
Edwards Prima Aortic Stentless Bioprosthesis, *Model 2500* *Edwards Lifesciences, www.edwards.com*	Safe	1.5, 3	
Edwards Prima Plus Aortic Stentless Bioprosthesis, *Model 2500P* *Edwards Lifesciences, www.edwards.com*	Safe	1.5, 3	
Edwards SAPIEN 3 *Transcatheter Heart Valve* *Edwards Lifesciences, www.edwards.com*	Conditional 8	1.5, 3	
Edwards SAPIEN Transcatheter Heart Valve (THV) *Edwards Lifesciences, www.edwards.com*	Conditional 8	1.5, 3	

Object	Status	Field Strength (T)	Reference
Edwards SAPIEN XT Transcatheter Heart Valve *(THV)* *Edwards Lifesciences, www.edwards.com*	Conditional 8	1.5, 3	
Edwards TEKNA Bileaflet Valve Model 3200, *Heart Valve* *Baxter Healthcare Corporation, Santa Ana, CA*	Safe	1.5	
Edwards TEKNA Bileaflet Valve, Model 9200, *Heart Valve* *Baxter Healthcare Corporation, Santa Ana, CA*	Safe	1.5	
Edwards-Duromedics Bileaflet Valve *Model 3160, Heart Valve* *Baxter Healthcare Corporation, Santa Ana, CA*	Safe	1.5	
Edwards-Duromedics Bileaflet Valve *Model 9120, Heart Valve* *Baxter Healthcare Corporation, Santa Ana, CA*	Safe	1.5	
FlexForm Annuloplasty Ring *Genesee BioMedical, Inc.,* *www.geneseebiomedical.com*	Conditional 8	1.5, 3	
Freedom Solo Biological Valve, Heart Valve *Sorin Group, www.sorin.com*	Safe	1.5	
Freestyle Aortic Root *Model 995, Heart Valve* *Medtronic, Inc., www.medtronic.com/mri*	Safe	1.5, 3	84
Freestyle Model 995 *27-mm, Heart Valve* *Medtronic, Inc., www.medtronic.com/mri*	Safe	1.5	
GeoForm Mitral Annuloplasty Ring, Model 4200 *Edwards Lifesciences, www.edwards.com*	Conditional 5	1.5	
HAART Aortic Annuloplasty Ring *BioStable Science & Engineering, Inc.,* *www.biostable-s-e.com*	Conditional 6	3	
Hall-Kaster, Model A7700, Heart Valve *Medtronic, Inc., www.medtronic.com/mri*	Conditional 5	1.5	3
Hancock Apical Connector *Left Ventricular Connector, Model 174A* *Medtronic, Inc., www.medtronic.com/mri*	Conditional 5	3	
Hancock Low Porosity Conduit, Model 150 *Medtronic, Inc., www.medtronic.com/mri*	Conditional 5	3	
Hancock, Model 100, Pulmonic Conduit *Medtronic, Inc., www.medtronic.com/mri*	Safe	1.5, 3	84
Hancock, Model 105, Low Porosity Conduit *Medtronic, Inc., www.medtronic.com/mri*	Safe	1.5, 3	84
Hancock, Model 150, Pulmonic Conduit *Medtronic, Inc., www.medtronic.com/mri*	Safe	1.5, 3	84

Object	Status	Field Strength (T)	Reference
Hancock, Model 242, Aortic Valve *Medtronic, Inc., www.medtronic.com/mri*	Safe	1.5, 3	84
Hancock, Model 342, Mitral Valve *Medtronic, Inc., www.medtronic.com/mri*	Safe	1.5, 3	84
Hancock 342, 35-mm, Model 342 *Heart Valve* *Medtronic, Inc., www.medtronic.com/mri*	Safe	1.5	
Hancock Conduit *Model 100, 30-mm, Heart Valve* *Medtronic, Inc., www.medtronic.com/mri*	Safe	1.5	
Hancock Extracorporeal *Model 242R, Heart Valve* *Johnson & Johnson, Anaheim, CA*	Conditional 5	1.5	19
Hancock Extracorporeal *Model M 4365-33, Heart Valve* *Johnson & Johnson, Anaheim, CA*	Conditional 5	1.5	19
Hancock I (Porcine) Heart Valve *Johnson & Johnson, Anaheim, CA*	Conditional 5	1.5	3
Hancock II (Porcine) Heart Valve *Johnson & Johnson, Anaheim, CA*	Conditional 5	1.5	3
Hancock II, Model T505 *Aortic Valve, Heart Valve* *Medtronic, Inc., www.medtronic.com/mri*	Safe	1.5, 3	84
Hancock II, Model T510 *Mitral Valve, Heart Valve* *Medtronic, Inc., www.medtronic.com/mri*	Safe	1.5, 3	84
Hancock II, Model T510, 33-mm *Heart Valve* *Medtronic, Inc., www.medtronic.com/mri*	Safe	1.5	
Hancock MO II, Model 250 *Aortic Valve, Heart Valve* *Medtronic, Inc., www.medtronic.com/mri*	Safe	1.5, 3	84
Hancock MO II, Model 250B *Aortic Valve, Heart Valve* *Medtronic, Inc., www.medtronic.com/mri*	Safe	1.5, 3	84
Hancock MO II, Model 250C *Aortic Valve, Heart Valve* *Medtronic, Inc., www.medtronic.com/mri*	Safe	1.5, 3	84
Hancock MO II, Model 250D *Aortic Valve, Heart Valve* *Medtronic, Inc., www.medtronic.com/mri*	Safe	1.5, 3	84
Hancock MO II, Model 250E *Aortic Valve, Heart Valve* *Medtronic, Inc., www.medtronic.com/mri*	Safe	1.5, 3	84

Object	Status	Field Strength (T)	Reference
Hancock MO II, Model 250H *Aortic Valve, Heart Valve* *Medtronic, Inc., www.medtronic.com/mri*	Safe	1.5, 3	84
Hancock Pericardial Mitral *Model T410, Haynes alloy, Heart Valve* *Medtronic Inc.* *www.medtronic.com/mri*	Safe	1.5	75
Hancock Pericardial Patch *Models 710, 710L* *Medtronic, Inc., www.medtronic.com/mri*	Conditional 5	3	
Hancock Pulmonic Conduit, Model 105 *Medtronic, Inc., www.medtronic.com/mri*	Conditional 5	3	
Hancock Vascor, Model 505 *Heart Valve* *Johnson & Johnson, Anaheim, CA*	Safe	1.5	19
Highlife Medical Mitral Valve *Highlife Medical, Inc., Irvine, CA*	Conditional 5	1.5, 3	
HLT Transcatheter Aortic Heart Valve *Heart Leaflet Technologies, Inc (HLT),* *Maple Grove, MN*	Conditional 6	3	
Hydra Aortic Valve, Percutaneous Heart Valve *Prosthesis, TAVR* *Vascular Innovations Co. Ltd.*	Conditional 8	1.5, 3	127
IMR Annuloplasty Ring, Model 4100 *Edwards Lifesciences, www.edwards.com*	Conditional 6	3	
Inonescu-Shiley, Universal ISM *Heart Valve*	Conditional 5	1.5	19
Intact Aortic, Model A805 *Size 19-mm, Heart Valve* *Medtronic, Inc., www.medtronic.com/mri*	Safe	1.5	75
Intact Model 705, Mitral Valve, Heart Valve *Medtronic, Inc., www.medtronic.com/mri*	Safe	1.5, 3	84
Intact Model 750, Mitral Valve, Heart Valve *Medtronic, Inc., www.medtronic.com/mri*	Safe	1.5, 3	
Intact Model 805, Aortic Valve, Heart Valve *Medtronic, Inc., www.medtronic.com/mri*	Safe	1.5, 3	84
Intact Mitral, Model M705 *Size 25-mm, Heart Valve* *Medtronic Inc., www.medtronic.com/mri*	Safe	1.5	75
JenvaValve Pericardial THV *(Transcatheter Heart Valve)* *JenaValve Technology, www.jenavalve.com*	Conditional 5	1.5, 3	
JenaValve Transapical Prosthesis *JenaValve Technology, www.jenavalve.com*	Conditional 6	3	

Object	Status	Field Strength (T)	Reference
Jyros Aortic, Model J1A *carbon alloy, Heart Valve* *Axion Medical Ltd.*	Safe	1.5	75
Jyros Mitral, Model J1M *carbon alloy, Heart Valve* *Axion Medical Ltd.*	Safe	1.5	75
Labcor Porcine Stented Bioprosthesis Heart Valve, *TLPB - A Supra and TLPB - M (Size 31)* *Labcor Laboratorios Ltda., www.labcor.com*	Safe	1.5, 3	
Labcor Stented Bovine Pericardial Bioprosthesis, *Heart Valve, Dokimos Plus-A (Size 29)* *Labcor Laboratorios Ltda., www.labcor.com*	Safe	1.5, 3	
Lillehi-Kaster, Model 300S Heart Valve *Medical Inc., Inver Grove Heights, MN*	Conditional 5	2.35	17
Lillehi-Kaster, Model 5009 Heart Valve *Medical Inc., Inver Grove Heights, MN*	Conditional 5	1.5	19
Liotta *Aortic, Model MA783* *Delrin, Heart Valve* *St. Jude Medical, www.sjm.com*	Conditional 5	3	
Lotus Valve *Boston Scientific, www.bostonscientific.com*	Conditional 5	1.5, 3	
Magis Mitral Ring for Valve Annuloplasty *Labcor Laboratorios Ltda., www.labcor.com*	Safe	1.5, 3	
Magna Mitral, Model 7000 *Bioprosthetic tissue valve, Heart Valve* *Bovine pericardium, PTFE fabric, Elgiloy frame,* *polyester support* *Edwards Lifesciences, www.edwards.com*	Conditional 6	3	
Med Hall Conduit, Model R7700 *33-mm, Heart Valve* *Medtronic, Inc., www.medtronic.com/mri*	Safe	1.5	
Medtronic Advantage, Model A7760 *Aortic Valve, Heart Valve* *Medtronic, Inc., www.medtronic.com/mri*	Safe	1.5, 3	84
Medtronic Advantage, Model M7760 *Mitral Valve, Heart Valve* *Medtronic, Inc., www.medtronic.com/mri*	Safe	1.5, 3	84
Medtronic Hall, Heart Valve *Medtronic, Inc., www.medtronic.com/mri*	Conditional 5	1.5	18
Medtronic Hall, Model 7700 *33-mm, Heart Valve* *Medtronic, Inc., www.medtronic.com/mri*	Safe	1.5	

Object	Status	Field Strength (T)	Reference
Medtronic Hall, Model A7700 *Aortic Valve, Heart Valve* *Medtronic, Inc., www.medtronic.com/mri*	Safe	1.5, 3	84
Medtronic Hall, Model A7700-D-16 *Heart Valve* *Medtronic, Inc., www.medtronic.com/mri*	Conditional 5	1.5	18
Medtronic Hall, Model C7700 *Valved Conduit, Heart Valve* *Medtronic, Inc., www.medtronic.com/mri*	Safe	1.5, 3	84
Medtronic Hall, Model M7700 *Mitral Valve, Heart Valve* *Medtronic, Inc., www.medtronic.com/mri*	Safe	1.5, 3	84
Medtronic Hall, Model R7700 *Low Porosity Valved Conduit, Heart Valve* *Medtronic, Inc., www.medtronic.com/mri*	Safe	1.5, 3	84
Medtronic Hall, Model Z7700 *Low Porosity Valved Conduit, Heart Valve* *Medtronic, Inc., www.medtronic.com/mri*	Safe	1.5, 3	84
Melody Transcatheter Pulmonary Valve *Medtronic, Inc., www.medtronic.com/mri*	Conditional 5	3	
MEMO 3D ReChord Annuloplasty Ring *Sorin Group, www.sorin.com*	Conditional 6	3	
MEMO 3D Semirigid Annuloplasty Ring *CarboMedics, a Sorin Group Co., www.sorin.com*	Conditional 6	3	
MiCardia Annuloplasty Device *Annuloplasty Ring* *MiCardia Corporation, Irvine, CA*	Conditional 6	3	
Mitral Prosthetic Heart Valve *Model 2100* *TRI Technologies, Brazil*	Safe	1.5	70
Mitra-Spacer *Cardiosolutions, Inc., www.cardiosolutionsinc.com*	Conditional 8	1.5, 3	
MitraSpan TASRA (Trans Apical Segmented Reduction Annuloplasty) System *MitraSpan, Inc., www.mitraspan-inc.com*	Conditional 5	1.5, 3	
Mitral Valve, Size 33-mm, A307504F *Carbomedics and www.sorin.com*	Safe	1.5, 3	
Mitroflow, Aortic, Model 11A *Delrin, Heart Valve* *Mitroflow Sulzer CarboMedics, U.K.*	Safe	1.5	75
Mitroflow, Aortic, Model 14A *Delrin, Heart Valve* *Mitroflow Sulzer CarboMedics, U.K.*	Safe	1.5	75

Object	Status	Field Strength (T)	Reference
Mitroflow, Mitral, Model 11M *Delrin, Heart Valve* *Mitroflow Sulzer CarboMedics, U.K.*	Safe	1.5	75
Mitroflow Pericardial Heart Valve, Model 12 *Sulzer-Medica and Mitroflow International*	Safe	1.5	70
Mosaic, Model 305, Aortic Valve *Heart Valve* *Medtronic, Inc., www.medtronic.com/mri*	Conditional 5	1.5, 3	84
Mosaic, Model 310, Mitral Valve *Heart Valve* *Medtronic, Inc., www.medtronic.com/mri*	Conditional 5	1.5, 3	84
Mosaic, Model 310, 33-mm *Heart Valve* *Medtronic, Inc., www.medtronic.com/mri*	Conditional 5	1.5, 3	
Mosaic, All Models, Heart Valve *Medtronic, Inc., www.medtronic.com/mri*	Conditional 5	1.5, 3	
Mosaic Ultra, Heart Valve *Medtronic, www.medtronic.com/mri*	Conditional 5	3	
Omnicarbon, Model 35231029 *Heart Valve* *Medical Inc., Inver Grove Heights, MN*	Conditional 5	1.5	18
Omniscience, Model 6522 *Heart Valve* *Medical Inc., Inver Grove Heights, MN*	Conditional 5	1.5	18
On-X Valve, Model 6816 *Heart Valve* *Medical Carbon Research Institute, Austin, TX*	Safe	1.5	
On-X Prosthetic Heart Valve, Aortic *Aortic with Conform-X Sewing Ring* *Mitral, Mitral with Conform-X Sewing Cuff* *Sizes 25-33* *On-X Life Technologies, Inc., Austin, TX*	Conditional 6	3	
On-X Prosthetic Heart Valve *Conform-X Mitral Heart Valve Prosthesis* *Sizes 25-33* *On-X Life Technologies, Inc., Austin, TX*	Conditional 6	3	
Open Pivot Heart Valve, Mitral (Model 500) *ATS Medical, Inc., Lake Forest, CA*	Conditional 6	3	
Open Pivot Heart Valve, Aortic AP 360 (Model 505) *ATS Medical, Inc., Lake Forest, CA*	Conditional 6	3	
P-2010 Aortic and Mitral Bovine Pericardium *Heart Valve Prosthesis* *Labcor Laboratorios Ltda., www.labcor.com*	Safe	1.5, 3	

Object	Status	Field Strength (T)	Reference
Perceval S Sutureless Aortic Heart Valve *Sorin Biomedica Cardio, www.sorin.com*	Conditional 6	3	
Percutaneous Heart Valve, 316LMV SS *Percutaneous Valve Technologies, Ltd., Israel*	Safe	1.5, 3	
Percutaneous Mitral Annuloplasty Device (PMAD) *Cardiac Dimensions, Inc., Kirkland, WA*	Safe	3	
Pericarbon Freedom Stentless Biological Valve *Heart Valve Prosthesis* *Sorin Group, www.sorin.com*	Safe	1.5	
Pericarbon MORE Stented Heart Valve *Sorin Biomedica Cardio, www.sorin.com*	Conditional 6	3	
Pericardial Stented Bioprosthesis Heart Valve *Labcor Laboratorios Ltda., www.labcor.com.br*	Conditional 6	3	
Physio II Annuloplasty Ring *Edwards Lifesciences, www.edwards.com*	Conditional 6	3	
Porcine Synergy ST, Aortic, Size 19-mm *Carbomedics and www.sorin.com*	Safe	1.5, 3	
Porcine Synergy ST, Mitral, Size 33-mm *Carbomedics and www.sorin.com*	Safe	1.5, 3	
Portico Transcatheter Aortic Valve, Heart Valve *St. Jude Medical, www.sjm.com*	Conditional 5	1.5, 3	
Posterior Annuloplasty Band *Annuloplasty Device, Model H607* *Medtronic, Inc., www.medtronic.com/mri*	Safe	1.5, 3	84
Posterior Annuloplasty Band *Model 610B, Annuloplasty Device* *Medtronic, Inc., www.medtronic.com/mri*	Safe	1.5, 3	84
Profile 3D Annuloplasty Ring *Medtronic, Inc., www.medtronic.com/mri*	Conditional 5	3	
Pulmonic Bioprosthesis *9000TFXP Cribier-Edwards* *Pulmonic Bioprosthesis and Palmaz XL P3110* *Combined prostheses* *Edwards Lifesciences, www.edwards.com*	Conditional 6	3	
Reduced Aortic CPHV Carbomedics Prosthetic *Model R5-029, Size 29-mm, Heart Valve, Nitinol* *Carbomedics and www.sorin.com*	Safe	1.5, 3	83
Reduced Aortic CPHV Carbomedics Prosthetic *Model R5-029, Size 29-mm, Heart Valve, Titanium* *Carbomedics and www.sorin.com*	Safe	1.5, 3	83
Regent Mechanical Heart Valve *Model 27AG-701, 27-mm* *St. Jude Medical, www.sjm.com*	Conditional 5	3	

Object	Status	Field Strength (T)	Reference
Rigid Tilting Disc *Aortic/Mitral TTK, Chitra Heart Valve Substitute Models TC1, TC2, Heart Valve Prosthesis TTK Healthcare Limited, www.ttkhealthcare.com*	Conditional 6	3	
Sapiens XT Transcatheter Heart Valve *Edwards Lifesciences, www.edwards.com*	Conditional 8	1.5, 3	
Sculptor Ring, Model 605M *Annuloplasty Device Medtronic, Inc., www.medtronic.com/mri*	Safe	1.5, 3	84
Sculptor Ring, Model 605T *Annuloplasty Device Medtronic, Inc., www.medtronic.com/mri*	Safe	1.5, 3	84
Sculptor Annuloplasty Ring, Model 605M *Medtronic, Inc., www.medtronic.com/mri*	Safe	1.5	
Simulus Adjustable Annuloplasty Ring/Band *Medtronic, Inc., www.Medtronic.com/MRI*	Safe	1.5, 3	
Simulus Semi-Rigid Annuloplasty Ring *Medtronic, Inc., www.medtronic.com/mri*	Conditional 6	3	
Simplici-T Model 670 *Medtronic, Inc., www.medtronic.com/mri*	Conditional 5	3	
SJM Masters Series Valve, Mitral, Size 37-mm *St. Jude Medical, www.sjm.com*	Conditional 5	3	
SJM Regent Heart Valve, Aortic, Size 29-mm *St. Jude Medical, www.sjm.com*	Conditional 5	3	
SJM Regent Heart Valve, Rotatable, *Aortic Standard Cuff-Polyester St. Jude Medical, www.sjm.com*	Conditional 5	3	
SJM Rigid Saddle Ring, All Models *St. Jude Medical, www.sjm.com*	Conditional 8	1.5, 3	
SJM, St. Jude Medical Tissue Valves *Epic Stented Tissue Valves Epic Models include EL-xxA and EL-xxM for aortic and mitral valves ELS-xxA ELS-xxM for the silicon coated variety EPIC valve product numbers are listed at www.sjm.com/devices/modelNumbers.aspx Note: "-xx" denotes different sizes available St. Jude Medical, www.sjm.com*	Conditional 5	3	
SJM Tailor Annuloplasty Ring *Size 35-mm, Model TARP-35 St. Jude Medical, www.sjm.com*	Conditional 5	3	
Smelloff Cutter, Aortic Heart Valve *Sorin Biomedica, Italy*	Conditional 5	1.5	75

Object	Status	Field Strength (T)	Reference
Smeloff-Cutter, Heart Valve *Cutter Laboratories, Berkeley, CA*	Conditional 5	1.5	18
Split Ring, Posterior Band *Model H607* *Medtronic, Inc., www.medtronic.com/mri*	Conditional 5	3	
Solo Smart Heart Valve Prosthesis *Sorin Group, www.sorin.com*	Safe	1.5, 3	
Soprano Armonia Heart Valve Prosthesis *Sorin Group, www.sorin.com*	Conditional 6	3	
Sorin Allcarbon, AS *Model MTR-29AS, 29-mm, pyrolitic carbon, Heart Valve* *Sorin Biomedica Cardio S.p.A., Saluggia, Italy*	Conditional 5	1.5	75
Sorin, No. 23 *Heart Valve*	Conditional 5	1.5	20
Sorin Pericarbon (Stented) Mitral Heart Valve *Sorin Biomedica, Italy*	Conditional 5	1.5	75
Sovering Annuloplasty Ring *Sorin Group, www.sorin.com*	Safe	1.5	
Sovering Miniband Annuloplasty Ring *Sorin Group, www.sorin.com*	Safe	1.5	
St. Jude Medical *Mechanical Heart Valve* *SJM Masters Series Rotatable,* *Aortic Model 25AJ-501* *Heart Valve* *St. Jude Medical, www.sjm.com*	Conditional 5	3	
St. Jude Medical *Mechanical Heart Valve* *Model 33MECS-602* *33-mm* *St. Jude Medical, www.sjm.com*	Conditional 5	3	
St. Jude, Model A-100 *Heart Valve* *St. Jude Medical Inc., www.SJM.com*	Conditional 5	1.5	19
St. Jude, Model M-101 *Heart Valve* *St. Jude Medical Inc., www.SJM.com*	Conditional 5	3	
St. Jude Medical, Annuloplasty Rings *Models include* *AFR-xx, RSAR-xx* *SARP-xx, TARP-xx, TAB-xx* *Note: "xx" denotes different sizes available (e.g. 23A-101)* *St. Jude Medical, www.sjm.com*	Conditional 5	3	

Object	Status	Field Strength (T)	Reference
St. Jude Medical, Mechanical Heart Valves *Models include* *xxAGN-751, xxAGFN-756* *xxAHPJ-505 or xxMHPJ-505* *xxAEHPJ-505, xxAFHPJ-505* *xxAJ-501 or xxMJ-501* *xxAECJ-502 or xxMECJ-502* *xxATJ-503 or xxMTJ-503* *xxMETJ-504, xxA-101 or xxM-101* *xxVAVGJ-515, xxCAVGJ-514* **Note: "xx" denotes different sizes available (e.g. 23A-101)* *St. Jude Medical, www.sjm.com*	Conditional 5	3	
St. Jude Medical, Tissue Valves *Models include* *E100-xxA-00 or E100-xxM-00* *ESP100-xx-00* *B100-xxA-00 or B100-xxM-00* *BSP100-xx* *B10-xxA-00 or B10-xxM-00, B10SP-xx, TF-xxA** *Note: "xx" denotes different sizes available (e.g. 23A-101)* *St. Jude Medical, www.sjm.com*	Conditional 5	3	
Standard Mitral CPHV Carbomedics Prosthetic *Model R5-029* *Size 29-mm, Heart Valve, Nitinol* *Carbomedics and www.sorin.com*	Safe	1.5, 3	83
Standard Mitral CPHV Carbomedics Prosthetic *Model M7-033* *Size 33-mm, Heart Valve, Titanium* *Carbomedics and www.sorin.com*	Safe	1.5, 3	83
Starr-Edwards Aortic and Mitral Prostheses *Models 1000, 1200, 2300, 2310, 2400,* *6000, 6120, 6300, 6310, 6320, 6400* *Edwards Lifesciences, www.edwards.com*	Safe	1.5	
Starr-Edwards, Model 1000, Heart Valve *Baxter Healthcare Corporation, Santa Ana, CA*	Conditional 5	1.5	
Starr-Edwards, Model 1200, Heart Valve *Baxter Healthcare Corporation, Santa Ana, CA*	Conditional 5	1.5	
Starr-Edwards, Model 1260, Heart Valve *Baxter Healthcare Corporation, Santa Ana, CA*	Conditional 5	2.35	17
Starr-Edwards, Model 2300, Heart Valve *Baxter Healthcare Corporation, Santa Ana, CA*	Conditional 5	1.5	
Starr-Edwards, Model 2310, Heart Valve *Baxter Healthcare Corporation, Santa Ana, CA*	Conditional 5	1.5	
Starr-Edwards, Model 2320, Heart Valve *American Edwards Laboratories* *Baxter Healthcare Corporation, Santa Ana, CA*	Conditional 5	2.35	17

Object	Status	Field Strength (T)	Reference
Starr-Edwards, Model 2400, Heart Valve *American Edwards Laboratories* *Baxter Healthcare Corporation, Santa Ana, CA*	Safe	1.5	3
Starr-Edwards, Model 6000, Heart Valve *Baxter Healthcare Corporation, Santa Ana, CA*	Conditional 5	1.5	
Starr-Edwards, Model 6120, Heart Valve *Baxter Healthcare Corporation, Santa Ana, CA*	Conditional 5	1.5	
Starr-Edwards, Model 6300, Heart Valve *Baxter Healthcare Corporation, Santa Ana, CA*	Conditional 5	1.5	
Starr-Edwards, Model 6310, Heart Valve *Baxter Healthcare Corporation, Santa Ana, CA*	Conditional 5	1.5	
Starr-Edwards, Model 6320, Heart Valve *Baxter Healthcare Corporation, Santa Ana, CA*	Conditional 5	1.5	
Starr-Edwards, Model 6400, Heart Valve *Baxter Healthcare Corporation, Santa Ana, CA*	Conditional 5	1.5	
Starr-Edwards, Model 6520, Heart Valve *Baxter Healthcare Corporation, Santa Ana, CA*	Conditional 5	1.5	
Starr-Edwards, Model Pre 6000, Heart Valve *American Edwards Laboratories* *Baxter Healthcare Corporation, Santa Ana, CA*	Conditional 5	1.5	
Star Valvular Annuloplasty Ring *Tricuspid Model* *Labcor Laboratorios Ltda., www.labcor.com.br*	Conditional 5	3	
Sulzer/Carbomedics Synergy PC *Pericardial Heart Valve* *Sulzer-Medica and Mitroflow International* *Richmond, B.C., Canada*	Safe	1.5	70
Supra G Porcine Aortic Valve Conduit *Labcor Laboratorios Ltda., www.labcor.com*	Safe	1.5, 3	
Tascon Aortic, Elgiloy, Heart Valve *Medtronic, Inc., www.medtronic.com/mri*	Safe	1.5	75
TAVR Valve, All Sizes *Valve Medical Ltd., www.valcaremedical.com*	Conditional 8	1.5, 3	
THV2, Model 9300TFX-29 *Aortic Heart Valve Prosthesis* *Edwards Lifesciences, www.edwards.com*	Conditional 6	3	
Tiara Mitral Heart Valve *Neovasc, Inc., www.neovasc.com*	Conditional 5	1.5, 3	
Tiara Transcatheter Mitral Heart Valve, 35-mm *Neovasc, Inc., www.neovasc.com*	Conditional 6	3	
TIV Pericardial Aortic Valve Conduit *Labcor Laboratorios Ltda., www.labcor.com*	Safe	1.5, 3	

Object	Status	Field Strength (T)	Reference
TLPB Porcine Valve, Aortic and Mitral Valves *Labcor Laboratorios Ltda., www.labcor.com*	Safe	1.5, 3	
Toronto SPV Valve *Stentless Porcine, Aortic Model SPA-101-25,* *Heart Valve* *St. Jude Medical, www.sjm.com*	Conditional 5	3	
Tri-AdT, Tricuspid Annuloplasty Ring *Models 900SFC-XX* *Medtronic, Inc., www.medtronic.com/mri*	Conditional 6	3	
Trifecta Valve, Heart Valve Prosthesis, All Models *St. Jude Medical, www.sjm.com*	Conditional 8	1.5, 3	
TS 3f Enable Aortic Bioprosthesis, Model 6000 *ATS Medical, Inc., Lake Forest, CA*	Conditional 6	3	
Valtech Cardinal Annuloplasty Ring, Mitral *Valtech Cardio LTD*	Conditional 6	3	
Valve Medical Transcatheter Aortic Valve *Replacement (TAVR) Device* *Valve Medical Ltd, Israel*	Conditional 5	1.5, 3	
Wessex Aortic, Model WAV10, Heart Valve *Sorin Biomedica, Italy*	Safe	1.5	75
Wessex Mitral, Model WMV20, Heart Valve *Sorin Biomedica, Italy*	Safe	1.5	75
Xenofic Aortic, Model AP80, Size 23 *Heart Valve*	Safe	1.5	75

Hemostatic Clips, Other Clips, Fasteners, and Staples

Object	Status	Field Strength (T)	Reference
Absolok Plus, Large Hemostatic Clip *Ethicon, www.ethicon.com*	Safe	1.5	71
Absolok Plus, Medium Hemostatic Clip *Ethicon, www.ethicon.com*	Safe	1.5	71
Absolok Plus, Small Hemostatic Clip *Ethicon, www.ethicon.com*	Safe	1.5	71
AC2 System Clip, Anastomotic Clip System *Rox Medical, San Clemente, CA*	Conditional 6	3	
AcuClip Hemostatic Clip *Origin Medsystems, Menlo Park, CA*	Safe	1.5	71
C-Port Clip *Cardica, Inc. and Dextera Surgical, Inc.,* *www.dexterasurgical.com*	Conditional 6	3	
CONTOUR Curved Cutter Staplers *Staple, CR40B, CR40G, CS40B,* *CS40G, STR5G, OUS only* *Ethicon, www.ethicon.com*	Conditional 5	3	

Object	Status	Field Strength (T)	Reference
Cosgrove-Gillinov Vascular Occlusion Clip *AtriCure, Inc., www.atricure.com*	Conditional 6	3	
DuraClip *Conmed Corporation, www.conmed.com*	Conditional 8	1.5, 3	
ECHELON (45 and 60) ENDOPATH *Linear Cutter Staplers, Staple* *ECR60G, ECR60W, ECR60B, ECR60D, ECR45W,* *ECR45B, ECR45D, ECR45G, ECR45M* *Ethicon, www.ethicon.com*	Conditional 5	3	
Echelon Flex 60 Linear Cutter Staplers *Ethicon, www.ethicon.com*	Conditional 5	3	
ECR60T Clip, Hemostatic Clip/Staple *Ethicon, www.ethicon.com*	Conditional 6	3	
Endo GIA Reloads Extra Thick, Staple *Covidien, www.covidien.com*	Conditional 6	3	
ENDOPATH EMS Endoscopic Multifeed Stapler *EMS* *Ethicon, www.ethicon.com*	Conditional 5	3	
ENDOPATH Endoscopic Curved Intraluminal *Circular Staplers, Staple* *ECS21, ECS25, ECS29, ECS33* *Ethicon, www.ethicon.com*	Conditional 5	3	
ENDOPATH Endoscopic Linear Cutters *and Staplers, Staple* *ATB45, TSB45, SCB45, ZR45B, ATG45,* *TR45B, TR45G, TSG45, SCG45, ZR45G,* *NK45B, NAB45, NSB45, NSG45, NK45G* *Ethicon, www.ethicon.com*	Conditional 5	3	
ENDOPATH Endoscopic Linear Cutters *and Staplers, Staple* *TR60W, TR60B,TR60G, 6R45M, 6R45B,* *6SB45, 6CB45, 6TB45, ATW35, TSW35,* *TSB35, TR35W, TR35B, ET45B, EZ45B* *Ethicon, www.ethicon.com*	Conditional 5	3	
ENDOPATH Endoscopic Linear Cutters *and Staplers, Staple* *ZR45B, ZR45G, ATW45, TSW45,* *SCW45, TR45W* *Ethicon, www.ethicon.com*	Conditional 5	3	
Endostaple, Surgical Fastener, MP35N *MedSource Technologies, Newton, MA*	Safe	1.5, 3	83
Endostaple, Surgical Fastener, Nitinol *MedSource Technologies, Newton, MA*	Safe	1.5, 3	83

Object	Status	Field Strength (T)	Reference
ES-830 Microcutter Green Staple *Cardica, Inc., and Dextera Surgical, Inc.,* *www.dexterasurgical.com*	Conditional 6	3	
EVALVE Clip *Cardiovascular Valve Repair System* *Elgiloy* *EVALVE, Redwood City, CA*	Safe	3	
EVS Vascular Closure Staple *AngioLINK Corporation, Tauton, MA*	Safe	3	
EZ Clip, E Z Clip *Olympus, www.olympus-europa.com/endoscopy*	Unsafe 1	1.5	
Fascia Staple, 316L SS *United States Surgical, North Haven, CT*	Safe	1.5, 3	83
Filshie Clip *Avalon Medical Corporation, Williston, VT*	Safe	1.5	
Filshie Clip (Filshie Tubal Ligation System) *CooperSurgical, www.coopersurgical.com*	Conditional 6	3	
Gastrointestinal Anastomosis Clip *Auto Suture SGIA, SS* *United States Surgical Corp., Norwalk, CT*	Safe	1.5	3
Gemini Ligation Clip *Microline Surgical, www.microlinesurgical.com*	Conditional 5	1.5, 3	
GIA 4.8 Staple, Titanium *United States Surgical, North Haven, CT*	Safe	1.5, 3	83
GIA 4.8 Formed Titanium Staple *Multifire Endo GIA* *Covidien, www.covidien.com*	Conditional 6	3	
Gillinov-Cosgrove LAA Clip *AtriCure Incorporated, www.atricure.com*	Conditional 6	3	
Hemoclip, #10, 316L SS, Hemostatic Clip *Edward Weck, Triangle Park, NJ*	Safe	1.5	3
Hemoclip, Hemostatic Clip *Teleflex Medical, www.teleflex.com*	Conditional 6	3	
Hemoclip, Tantalum, Hemostatic Clip *Edward Weck, Triangle Park, NJ*	Safe	1.5	3
Hem-o-lok Polymer Clip, Nonmetallic *Teleflex Medical, www.teleflexmedical.com*	Safe	1.5, 3	
Hem-o-lok Polymer Ligation Clip *All Sizes, All Versions* *Teleflex Medical Inc., www.teleflex.com*	Safe	1.5, 3	
Hemostasis Clip, DHC-7-230, Hemostatic Clip *Cook Medical, www.cookmedical.com*	Conditional 6	3	

Object	Status	Field Strength (T)	Reference
Hulka Clip *Richard Wolf Medical Instruments, Vernon Hills, IL*	Conditional 6	3	
Implantable Ligation Clip *Applied Medical, www.appliedmedical.com*	Conditional 8	1.5, 3	
Instinct Endoscopic Hemoclip *Hemostatic Clip* *Cook Medical, Inc., www.cookmedical.com*	Conditional 5	1.5, 3	
IVC Venous Clip, Teflon *Pilling Weck Co.*	Safe	1.5	
LIGACLIP, Extra Ligating Clips *LT100, LT200, LT300, LT400* *Ethicon, www.ethicon.com*	Conditional 5	3	
LIGACLIP ERCA, ER320, ER420 *Ethicon, www.ethicon.com*	Conditional 5	3	
LIGACLIP Extra Ligating Clips *LS400, LS100, LS200, LS300* *Ethicon, www.ethicon.com*	Conditional 5	3	
LIGACLIP Extra LT 100, C.P. Titanium, *Hemostatic Clip* *Ethicon, www.ethicon.com*	Safe	1.5	71
LIGACLIP Extra LT 200, C.P. Titanium, *Hemostatic Clip* *Ethicon, www.ethicon.com*	Safe	1.5	71
LIGACLIP Extra LT 300, C.P. Titanium, *Hemostatic Clip* *Ethicon, www.ethicon.com*	Safe	1.5	71
LIGACLIP Extra LT 400, C.P. Titanium, *Hemostatic Clip* *Ethicon, www.ethicon.com*	Safe	1.5	71
LIGACLIP Extra, Ligating Clip, Hemostatic Clip *Ethicon, www.ethicon.com*	Conditional 6	3	
LIGACLIP, MCA Multiple Clip Applier *MCS20, MCM20, MCL20* *Ethicon, www.ethicon.com*	Conditional 5	3	
LIGACLIP, Tantalum, Hemostatic Clip *Ethicon, www.ethicon.com*	Safe	1.5	3
LIGACLIP, #6, 316L SS Hemostatic Clip *Ethicon, www.ethicon.com*	Safe	1.5	3
LIGAMAX, Endoscopic Multiple Clip Applier *Ethicon, www.ethicon.com*	Conditional 5	3	
Ligating Clip, Small, C.P. Titanium *Horizon Surgical, Evergreen, CO*	Safe	1.5	71

Object	Status	Field Strength (T)	Reference
Ligating Clip, Medium, C.P. Titanium *Horizon Surgical, Evergreen, CO*	Safe	1.5	71
Long Clip HX-600-090L *Olympus Medical Systems Corporation, Japan*	Unsafe 1	1.5	
MCS 20, C.P. Titanium, Hemostatic Clip *Ethicon, www.ethicon.com*	Safe	1.5	71
MCM 20, C.P. Titanium, Hemostatic Clip *Ethicon, www.ethicon.com*	Safe	1.5	71
Micro SurgiClips, Titanium *U.S. Surgical Corporation, North Haven, CT*	Safe	1.5	
ML-10 Ligation Clip *Microline Surgical, www.microlinesurgical.com*	Conditional 5	1.5, 3	
MultApplier Clip, Titanium *United States Surgical, North Haven, CT*	Safe	1.5, 3	83
MultApplier Clip *500-28 Endoclip Multapplier* *Covidien, www.covidien.com*	Conditional 6	3	
Ogden Suture Anchor, Titanium *United States Surgical, North Haven, CT*	Safe	1.5, 3	83
Olympus Single-use Rotating Clip *Olympus Medical Systems Corporation,* *www.medical.olympusamerica.com*	Unsafe 1	1.5	
OTSC Clip, Over The Scope Clip *Ovesco Endoscopy GmbH, Germany*	Conditional 6	3	
Premium SurgiClip, L-13, C.P. Titanium *United States Surgical, North Haven, CT*	Safe	1.5	71
Premium SurgiClip, M-11, C.P. Titanium *United States Surgical, North Haven, CT*	Safe	1.5	71
Premium SurgiClip, S-9, C.P. Titanium *United States Surgical, North Haven, CT*	Safe	1.5	71
PROXIMATE Curved and Straight *Intraluminal Staplers, Staple* *CDH21, SDH21, CDH25, SDH25, CDH29,* *SDH29, CDH33, SDH33* *Ethicon, www.ethicon.com*	Conditional 5	3	
PROXIMATE HCS Hemorrhoidal *Circular Stapler, PPH01, STR10* *Ethicon, www.ethicon.com*	Conditional 5	3	
PROXIMATE Linear Cutters, Clip, Staple *TLC10, TRT10,* *TLC55, TRT55, TCT55, TRC55, TVC55,* *TRV55, TCT75, TRT75, TCD75,* *TRD75, TLC75, TCR75, TCT10, TCR10* *Ethicon, www.ethicon.com*	Conditional 5	3	

Object	Status	Field Strength (T)	Reference
PROXIMATE Linear Stapler *Staple, AX55B, AX55G, TLV30, TRV30,* *TL30, TR30, TL60, TR60, TL90,* *TR90, TLH30, TRH30, TLH60, TRH60,* *TLH90, TRH90, TX30V, XR30V,* *TX30B, XR30B, TX30G, XR30G,* *TX60B, XR60B, TX60G, XR60G* *Ethicon, www.ethicon.com*	Conditional 5	3	
PROXIMATE PPH Hemorrhoidal Circular Stapler, *Staple, PPH03* *Ethicon, www.ethicon.com*	Conditional 5	3	
PROXIMATE Skin Staplers, Staple, *PXW35, PRR35, PRW35,* *PMR35, PMW35, PMW55, PXR35* *Ethicon, www.ethicon.com*	Conditional 5	3	
QuickClip2 Long, HX-201LR-135L *Olympus Medical Systems Corporation,* *www.medical.olympusamerica.com*	Unsafe 1	1.5	
QuickClip2 Long, HX-201UR-135L *Olympus Medical Systems Corporation,* *www.medical.olympusamerica.com*	Unsafe 1	1.5	
QuickClip Pro Clip *Olympus Medical Systems Corporation,* *www.medical.olympusamerica.com*	Conditional 5	3	
Resolution Clip *Boston Scientific, www.bostonscientific.com*	Conditional 5	1.5, 3	
Royal Staple *United States Surgical, North Haven, CT*	Safe	1.5, 3	83
SECQURE Reach Titanium Staple *SECQURE Surgical Corporation*	Conditional 8	1.5, 3	
Spider Fastener *I.B.I Israel Biomedical, www.ibimedical.com*	Conditional 6	3	
Staple, 3M Precise Vista Lite W Type *Mani, Inc., www.mani.co.jp/en/*	Conditional 6	3	
Staple Commercial, Hemostatic Clip *Teleflex Medical, www.teleflex.com*	Conditional 6	3	
StarClose Clip *Abbott Vascular, www.abbottvascular.com*	Conditional 5	3	
Starclose Surgical Clip *Nitinol* *Abbott Vascular, Santa Clara, CA*	Conditional 6	3	
Sterile Repositionable Hemostasis Clipping Device *SureClip* *Micro-Tech Co., Ltd., www.micro-tech.com.cn/en*	Conditional 8	1.5, 3	

Object	Status	Field Strength (T)	Reference
Sternal Closure Device *Vitalitec International, www.vitalitecusa.com*	Conditional 8	1.5, 3	
SurgiClip *Medtronic, www.medtronic.com*	Conditional 8	1.5, 3	
Surgiclip, M-9.5, C.P. Titanium *United States Surgical, North Haven, CT*	Safe	1.5	71
Surgiclip, M-11, C.P. Titanium *United States Surgical, North Haven, CT*	Safe	1.5	71
Surgiclip, Auto Suture M-9.5 *United States Surgical, North Haven, CT*	Safe	1.5	3
Suture Anchor with Titanium Nitride Coating *Herculon Soft Tissue Anchor* *Covidien, www.covidien.com*	Conditional 6	3	
T-Bar Assembly, T-Fastener *Kimberly-Clark Health Care, Roswell, GA*	Conditional 6	3	
TA 90-4.8 Directional Staples, Titanium *United States Surgical, North Haven, CT*	Safe	1.5, 3	83
Tacker Helical Fastener, Titanium *United States Surgical, North Haven, CT*	Safe	1.5, 3	83
Tacker Titanium Helical Clip *Tacker 5-mm Mesh Fixation Device* *Covidien, www.covidien.com*	Conditional 6	3	
Tack-It Endovascular Staple, Hemostatic Clip *Intact Vascular, www.intactvascular.com*	Conditional 6	3	
Titanium Hemostatic Clip, Vessel Occlusion *Vitalitec International, www.vitalitecusa.com*	Conditional 6	3	
Titanium Ligation Clip *Vesocclude Medical, Inc., www.vesoccludemedical.com*	Conditional 6	3	
TriClip Endoscopic Clipping Device *Cook Medical, www.cookmedical.com*	Unsafe 1	1.5	118
U-CLIP, (B180) *Represents largest version of following U-CLIP products:* *S15, S18, S20, S25, S35,* *S50, S60, V45, V50, V60,* *V100D, S70, S90, S105,* *S120, B140, B160, B180* *Medtronic, www.medtronic.com*	Conditional 6	3	
Ultraclip, 316 SS *INRAD, Inc., Grand Rapids, MI*	Safe	1.5	
Ultraclip, Titanium alloy *INRAD, Inc., Grand Rapids, MI*	Safe	1.5	
Vesocclude Ligating Clip *Vesocclude Medical, LLC, Mebane, NC*	Conditional 6	3	

Object	Status	Field Strength (T)	Reference
Visistat Skin Stapler (Staple) *Hemostatic Clip* *Teleflex Medical, www.teleflex.com*	Conditional 6	3	
Visu-loc Ligation clip, hemostatic clip *Microline Surgical, www.microlinesurgical.com*	Conditional 6	3	
Weck Horizon, Titanium Clip, Large *Teleflex Medical, www.teleflex.com*	Conditional 6	3	
Weck Horizon, Titanium Clip, Medium *Teleflex Medical, www.teleflex.com*	Conditional 6	3	

Miscellaneous

Object	Status	Field Strength (T)	Reference
"J" Hook Bracket *816* *Amerex Corporation, Trussville, AL*	Conditional 7	3	
3/4" Socket Wrench, 3/4" x 41-mm *Newmatic Medical, www.newmaticmedical.com*	Conditional 7	3	
357 Magnum Revolver, Model 66-3 *Smith and Wesson, Springfield, MA*	Unsafe 1	1.5	46
3D Interstitial Ring Applicator with Plastic Needles *Varian Medical Systems, www.varian.com*	Conditional 5	1.5, 3	
3D Interstitial Ring Applicator 90° *with Plastic Needles* *Varian Medical Systems, www.varian.com*	Conditional 5	1.5, 3	
3M Kind Removal Silicone Tape *3M, www.3m.com*	Safe	1.5, 3	
3M PICC/CVC Securement Device + Tegaderm I.V. *Advanced Securement Dressing* *3M, www.3m.com*	Safe	1.5, 3	
3M Tegaderm CHG Chlorhexidine Gluconate I.V. *Securement Dressing* *3M, www.3m.com*	Safe	1.5, 3	
3M Tegaderm Silicone Foam Border Dressing *3M, www.3m.com*	Safe	1.5, 3	
4D Dome Semi-resorbable Parietal Reinforcement *Implant* *Cousin Biotech, www.cousin-biotech.com*	Safe	1.5, 3	
4D Mesh Semi-resorbable Parietal Reinforcement *Implant* *Cousin Biotech, www.cousin-biotech.com*	Safe	1.5, 3	
4D Ventral Semi-resorbable Parietal Reinforcement *Implant* *Cousin Biotech, www.cousin-biotech.com*	Safe	1.5, 3	
4-Leg Base IV Stand, Stainless Steel *Pryor Products, Oceanside, CA*	Conditional 7	3	

Object	Status	Field Strength (T)	Reference
5-Leg Base IV Stand, Aluminum *Pryor Products, Oceanside, CA*	Conditional 7	3	
11" Microfiber Flexi Frame, FGQ85500BK00 *Rubbermaid, www.rubbermaidhealthcare.com*	Safe	1.5, 3	
18" Quick Connect Wet/Dry Frame, FGQ56000YL00 *Rubbermaid, www.rubbermaidhealthcare.com*	Conditional 7	3	
50 PSI PRESET OXY REG 15LPM CGA 870 BLU *Ohio Medical Corporation, www.ohiomedical.com*	Conditional 7	3	
880 MRI Compatible Anaesthesia Machine *Mechanical Ventilation Pneupac* *Not available in the US or Canada* *Smiths Medical, www.smiths-medical.com*	Conditional 5	1.5, 3	
AB5000 Ventricle *with In-Flow Cannula and Out-Flow Cannula* *Cardiac assist device* *Abiomed, Inc., Danvers MA*	Conditional 6	3	113
Abbvie J Gastrostomy Tube *AbbVie, Inc., www.abbvie.com*	Conditional 8	1.5, 3	
Abiliti System, Neurostimulation System *Intrapace, www.abiliti.com*	Unsafe 1	1.5	
Accucinch Implant *Guided Delivery Systems, www.gdsmed.com*	Conditional 5	1.5, 3	
AccuDrain External CSF Drainage System *Integra NeuroSciences, www.integralife.com*	Safe	1.5, 3	
Accusite pH *Enteral Feeding System pH Site Locator* *Zinetics Medical, Salt Lake City, UT*	Unsafe 2	1.5	
ACTICOAT 7 Antimicrobial Barrier Dressing *Smith and Nephew, www.global.smith-nephew.com*	Unsafe 1	1.5	
ActiGait Implantable Drop Foot Stimulator *Neurostimulation system* *Ottobock, www.ottobock.com*	Conditional 5	1.5, 3	
ActiFlo Indwelling Bowel Catheter System *also known as Zassi Bowel Management System* *Hollister Incorporated, Libertyville, IL*	Conditional 5	3	
ActiPatch Drug Delivery Patch *BioElectronics Corporation, Frederick, MD*	Unsafe 1	1.5	
AcuMed Advanced Magnetic Patches *Acumed, www.acumedpatches.com*	Unsafe 1	1.5	
Acuvance Jelco (FEP Radiopaque) Intravenous *(I.V.) Catheter* *Smiths Medical, www.smiths-medical.com*	Safe	1.5, 3	

Object	Status	Field Strength (T)	Reference
Acuvance Plus (PUR Radiopaque) Intravenous (I.V.) Catheter *Smiths Medical, www.smiths-medical.com*	Safe	1.5, 3	
Acuvance Plus W (PUR Radiopaque) Intravenous (I.V.) Catheter *Smiths Medical, www.smiths-medical.com*	Safe	1.5, 3	
ACX Tissue Expander, Integrated Magnetic Injection Port *(various models)* *Sientra, www.sientra.com*	Unsafe 1	1.5	
Adapter used for ICP *Aesculap, Inc., www.aesculapusa.com*	Safe	1.5, 3	
Adhesix Bioring, Adjustable Gastric Band with Self-Adhesive Port *Cousin Biotech, www.cousin-biotech.com*	Safe	1.5, 3	
Adiana Radiopaque Implant *Adiana Permanent Contraception System* *Hologic, Inc., www.hologic.com*	Conditional 6	3	
Adiana Silicone Implant *permanent female contraception device* *Adiana, Inc., Redwood City, CA*	Safe	3	
Adjustable Combination Pliers, 152-mm *Newmatic Medical, www.newmaticmedical.com*	Conditional 7	3	
Adjustable Combination Pliers, P-30 *Ampco Safety Tools, www.amcosafetytools.com*	Conditional 7	3	
Adjustable-End Wrench, 3/4" *NGK Metals Corporation, Sweetwater, TN*	Conditional 7	3	
Adjustable-End Wrench, 1 1/8" *NGK Metals Corporation, Sweetwater, TN*	Conditional 7	3	
Adjustable Esophageal Reconstruction Tube *Hood Laboratories, www.hoodlabs.com*	Safe	1.5, 3	
Adjustable Pipe Wrench, W-212AL *Ampco Safety Tools, www.amcosafetytools.com*	Conditional 7	3	
Adjustable Pipe Wrench 10" *NGK Metals Corporation, Sweetwater, TN*	Conditional 7	3	
Adjustable Wrench, 24 x 200-mm *Newmatic Medical, www.newmaticmedical.com*	Conditional 7	3	
Adjustable Wrench, W-70 *Ampco Safety Tools, www.amcosafetytools.com*	Conditional 7	3	
Adson Tissue Forcep, Ti6Al4V *Johnson & Johnson, www.depuysynthes.com*	Safe	1.5	62
Adult Walker, FAHWA *Newmatic Medical, www.newmaticmedical.com*	Conditional 7	3	

Object	Status	Field Strength (T)	Reference
Advance Implant System, Model 10403 *Aspire Medical, Sunnyvale, CA*	Conditional 6	3	
AdVance Male Sling System *AMS, American Medical Systems,* *www.americanmedicalsystems.com*	Safe	1.5, 3	
AdVance XP Male Incontinence Sling System *American Medical Systems,* *www.americanmedicalsystems.com*	Safe	1.5, 3	
Advanta VXT Vascular Graft *Maquet, www.maquet.com*	Safe	1.5, 3	
Advantiv (PUR Radiopaque) Intravenous *(I.V.) Catheter* *Smiths Medical, www.smiths-medical.com*	Safe	1.5, 3	
Agile Patency System, Capsule Device *Given Imaging, www.givenimaging.com*	Unsafe 1	1.5	
AgX100, I-125 Brachytherapy Seed *Theragenics Corporation, www.theragenics.com*	Conditional 8	1.5, 3	
AirLife Bypass HME *Cardinal Health, www.cardinalhealth.com*	Conditional 6	3	
AirLife Positive End Expiratory Pressure *(PEEP) Valve* *CareFusion, www.carefusion.com*	Conditional 7	3	
Air-Lon Laryngectomy Tube *Premier Medical Products, www.premusa.com*	Safe	1.5	
Air-Lon Tracheal Tube *Premier Medical Products, www.premusa.com*	Safe	1.5	
Air-Q Disposable Masked Laryngeal Airway *Mercury Medical, www.mercurymed.com*	Conditional 5	3	
Algovita Spinal Cord Stimulation (SCS) System *Neuromodulation System* *Nuvectra, www.nuvectra.com*	Unsafe 1	1.5	
Allen Wrench, WH-1/4 *Ampco Safety Tools, www.amcosafetytools.com*	Conditional 7	3	
Aleve Direct Therapy *Bayer, www.aleve.com/aleve-direct-therapy/*	Unsafe 1	1.5	
AlloMax Surgical Graft *Bard Plastic Surgery, www.bardps.com*	Safe	1.5, 3	
AltaSeal Tubal Occlusion Implant (TOI) *Alta Science, www.altascience.ie*	Conditional 6	3	
American Macintosh Size 4 Laryngoscope Blade *(Greenline F/O Amer Mac Size 4)* *Newmatic Medical, www.newmaticmedical.com*	Conditional 7	3	

Object	Status	Field Strength (T)	Reference
Ambu Disposable PEEP Valve *Ambu, www.ambu.com*	Conditional 7	3	
Ambu Mark IV Baby Resuscitator *Ambu, www.ambu.com*	Conditional 7	3	
Ambu King Mask *Ambu, www.ambu.com*	Safe	1.5	
Ambu SPUR II Infant Resuscitator *Ambu, ww.ambu.com*	Conditional 7	3	
AMS 800 Urinary Control System *American Medical Systems Inc.,* *www.americanmedicalsystems.com*	Conditional 6	3	
AMS Acticon Neosphincter Prosthesis *AMS, American Medical Systems,* *www.americanmedicalsystems.com*	Safe	1.5, 3	
AMS Artificial Urinary Sphincter 791 *AMS, American Medical Systems,* *www.americanmedicalsystems.com*	Safe	1.5, 3	
AMS Mainstay Urologic Soft-Tissue Anchor *AMS, American Medical Systems,* *www.americanmedicalsystems.com*	Safe	1.5, 3	
AMS Sphincter 800 Urinary Control System *AMS, American Medical Systems,* *www.americanmedicalsystems.com*	Safe	1.5, 3	3
Anatomical Chin Implant *Implantech Associates, Inc., www.implantech.com*	Safe	1.5, 3	
Anatomical Nasal Implant *Implantech Associates, Inc., www.implantech.com*	Safe	1.5, 3	
Anesthesia Machine MR Magellan-2200 *Model 1 Pneumatically Powered* *Anesthesia Machine* *Oceanic Medical Products, Inc., Atchison, KS*	Conditional 7	3	
Anesthesia Machine MR Magellan-2200 *Model-3 Pneumatically Powered* *Anesthesia Machine* *Oceanic Medical Products, Inc., Atchison, KS*	Conditional 7	3	
Annular Occlusion Device, AOD *AtriCure, Inc., www.atricure.com*	Safe	3	
Annular Occlusion Device, AOD1, 50-mm *AtriCure, Inc., www.atricure.com*	Conditional 8	1.5, 3	
Annular Occlusion Device, AOD2 *AtriCure, Inc., www.atricure.com*	Conditional 5	1.5, 3	
Apogee Vaginal Vault Prolapse Repair System *AMS, American Medical Systems,* *www.americanmedicalsystems.com*	Safe	1.5, 3	

Object	Status	Field Strength (T)	Reference
Appendage Occlusion System Implant *Coherex Medical, www.coherex.com*	Conditional 5	1.5, 3	
Applicator Set GammaMedplus *Varian Medical Systems, www.varian.com*	Safe	1.5, 3	
AQUACEL Ag+, All Sizes *ConvaTec, www.convatec.com*	Safe	1.5, 3	
Aquacel Ag Foam Dressing *ConvaTec, www.convatec.com*	Safe	1.5, 3	
Aquacel Ag Foam Dressing, Non Adhesive *ConvaTec, www.convatec.com*	Safe	1.5, 3	
Aquacel Ag Dressing *Aquacel AG Hydrofiber Wound Dressing with Ionic Silver ConvaTec, www.convatec.com*	Safe	1.5, 3	115
Aquacel Ag Surgical Dressing *ConvaTec, www.convatec.com*	Safe	1.5, 3	
Arctic Sun Temperature Management System *No metallic components, controller not allowed in MRI environment Bard Medical, www.bardmedical.com*	Safe	3	
ARGOS 11-mm Restrictor *Pulmonx, Palo Alto, CA*	Conditional 6	3	
Aria MRI Drill System *Stryker, www.stryker.com*	Conditional 5	3	
Aris Trans-Obturator Tape *Coloplast, www.coloplast.com*	Safe	3	
Armboard, Dale, #650 Large *Dale Medical Products, Inc., www.dalemed.com*	Conditional 6	3	
Arnett LeFort Implant *Implantech Associates, Inc., www.implantech.com*	Safe	1.5, 3	
ARO Anchor, ARO Ti Anchor, ForceFiber Suture *ARO Medical, Denmark*	Conditional 8	1.5, 3	
Arto Implant *MVRx, Inc., www.mvrxinc.com*	Conditional 8	1.5, 3	
Asept Drainage Catheter System *PFM Medical, Inc.*	Safe	3	
Aspire Medical Advance Implant System *Aspire Medical, Sunnyvale, CA*	Conditional 6	3	
Assembly, Bolt *Depuy Synthes, www.depuysynthes.com*	Conditional 8	1.5, 3	
Atrial Flow Regulator, AFR *Occlutech, www.occlutech.com*	Conditional 8	1.5, 3	

Object	Status	Field Strength (T)	Reference
Atrostim Phrenic Nerve Stimulator *Neurostimulation System* *ATROTECH OY, Tampere, Finland*	Unsafe 1	1.5	
AuraGen Cortical Surface Electrodes, *Cortical Grid Electrodes, Cortical Strip Electrodes,* *Platinum Depth Electrodes, Integra NeuroSciences,* *www.integralife.com*	Conditional 5	1.5	
Autoflush Device *Vygon, www.vygon.com*	Safe	1.5	
Azure, AZ500, Positioning/Comfort Pad *Trulife, www.Trulife.com*	Safe	1.5, 3	
B. Braun PERIFIX FX *Epidural Springwound Catheter* *B. Braun Medical Inc., www.bbraunusa.com*	Unsafe 1	1.5	
babyPac 100 Ventilator *Smiths Medical PM Inc., Waukesha, WI*	Conditional 5	3	
BACTISEAL Antimicrobial Catheter System *Codman, www.depuysynthes.com*	Safe	3	
Badger MRI Model B5V MR	Conditional 7	3	
Ball Peen Hammer, H-00FG *Ampco Safety Tools, www.amcosafetytools.com*	Conditional 7	3	
BandIt Clip *AtriCure Inc., West Chester, OH*	Conditional 6	3	
Bard Edwards Outflow Tract Fabric *Bard Peripheral Vascular, www.bardpv.com*	Safe	1.5	
Bard Kugal Patch, polypropylene *Davol, A Bard Company, www.davol.com*	Safe	1.5	
Bard Mesh *Davol, A Bard Company, www.davol.com*	Safe	1.5	
Bard Sauvage Filamentous Fabric *Bard Peripheral Vascular, www.bardpv.com*	Safe	1.5	
Bard Soft Mesh *Davol, A Bard Company, www.davol.com*	Safe	1.5	
Bard Urinary Drainage Bag *C.R. Bard, www.crbard.com*	Conditional 7	3	
Bariatric Walker, FAHWB *Newmatic Medical, www.newmaticmedical.com*	Conditional 7	3	
BAROnova GEN III Transpyloric Shuttle (TPS) *BAROnova, Inc., www.baronova.com*	Conditional 6	3	
Barricaid ARD, Annular Reconstruction Device *Intrinsic Therapeutics, Inc., Woburn, MA*	Conditional 6	3	
Barton-Mayo Tracheostoma Button *Atos Medical, www.atosmedical.com*	Safe	1.5	

Object	Status	Field Strength (T)	Reference
Battery for Laryngoscope Handle *Stubby Size* *Scope Medical Devices, www.scopemedical.in*	Conditional 7	3	
Battery, Lithium, 3.9 Volt, 304 SS and 316L SS, *Nickel* *Greatbatch Scientific, Clarence, NY*	Conditional 7	1.5	
Battery, Low Magnetic Signature *"C" Sized, Spiral Wound Lithium- Bromine Chloride Cell* *Wilson Greatbatch Technologies, Inc., Clarence NY*	Conditional 7	3	
Battery, Model CR26500 *Anaesthetics India Pvt Ltd., ww.anaesthaids.com*	Unsafe 1	1.5	
B-D PosiFlow *needleless IV access connector* *Becton Dickinson, Sandy, Utah*	Safe	1.5	
Beacon Transponder *Calypso Medical Technologies, Inc.,* *www.calypsomedical.com*	Conditional 5	1.5, 3	
Binder Submalar I Implant *Implantech Associates, Inc., www.implantech.com*	Safe	1.5, 3	
Binder Submalar II Implant *Implantech Associates, Inc., www.implantech.com*	Safe	1.5, 3	
BioArc SP Sling System *AMS, American Medical Systems,* *www.americanmedicalsystems.com*	Safe	1.5, 3	
BioArc TO Subfascial Hammock *AMS, American Medical Systems,* *www.americanmedicalsystems.com*	Safe	1.5, 3	
BioClip, Beurosurgery Fixation *Codman, www.depuysynthes.com*	Safe	1.5, 3	
Bioclip, Neurosurgical Implant, Titanium alloy *Bioplate, Inc., Los Angeles, CA*	Conditional 6	3	
BioMesh, Neurosurgery Fixation, C.P. Titanium *Codman, www.depuysynthes.com*	Safe	1.5, 3	
BioMesh, Neurosurgical Implant, Titanium *Bioplate, Inc., Los Angeles, CA*	Conditional 6	3	
Biomesh Soft Prolaps Cystocele Implant *Cousin Biotech, www.cousin-biotech.com*	Safe	1.5, 3	
Biomesh Soft Prolap Rectocele Implant *Cousin Biotech, www.cousin-biotech.com*	Safe	1.5, 3	
Biomesh Synthetic Dura-Matter Substitute *Cousin Biotech, www.cousin-biotech.com*	Safe	1.5, 3	
Bionector Device *Vygon, www.vygon.com*	Safe	1.5, 3	

Object	Status	Field Strength (T)	Reference
Bionector, Needleless Connector *Vygon SA, www.vygon.com*	Conditional 6	3	
Biosearch Endo-Feeding Tube	Safe	1.5	
Biomet EBI Bone Healing System *Neurostimulation System* *Biomet, www.biomet.com*	Unsafe 1	1.5	
BIORING Adjustable Gastric Banding *Cousin Biotech, www.cousin-biotech.com*	Safe	1.5, 3	
BioValsalva Porcine Aortic Valved Conduit *Vascutech and Terumo Medical Corporation,* *www.terumomedical.com*	Safe	1.5, 3	
Bipolar Coagulation Forceps, *For use in intraoperative MRI systems* *Aesculap AG & CO.KG, Tuttlingen, Germany*	Safe	1.5, 3	83
Blip Implanted Fiducial Marker, Platinum/Iridium *Navotek Medical Ltd., Yokneam, Israel*	Conditional 6	3	
Blom-Singer Adjustable Bi-Flanged Fistula Prosthesis *InHealth Technologies, www.inhealth.com*	Safe	1.5, 3	
Blom-Singer Advantage Indwelling Voice Prosthesis *Hard Valve Assembly* *InHealth Technologies, www.inhealth.com*	Conditional 8	1.5, 3	
Blom-Singer Advantage Indwelling Voice Prosthesis *Soft Valve Assembly* *InHealth Technologies, www.inhealth.com*	Conditional 8	1.5, 3	
Blom-Singer ClassicFlow HME for Tracheostomy *InHealth Technologies, www.inhealth.com*	Safe	1.5, 3	
Blom-Singer Classic Indwelling Voice Prosthesis *InHealth Technologies, www.inhealth.com*	Safe	1.5, 3	
Blom-Singer Dual Valve Indwelling Voice Prosthesis *InHealth Technologies, www.inhealth.com*	Conditional 8	1.5, 3	
Blom-Singer Duckbill Voice Prosthesis *InHealth Technologies, www.inhealth.com*	Safe	1.5, 3	
Blom-Singer EasyFlow HME for Tracheostomy *InHealth Technologies, www.inhealth.com*	Safe	1.5, 3	
Blom-Singer HumidiFilter System for Tracheostomy *InHealth Technologies, www.inhealth.com*	Safe	1.5, 3	
Blom-Singer Low Pressure Voice Prosthesis *InHealth Technologies, www.inhealth.com*	Safe	1.5, 3	
Blom-Singer Special Order Classic Indwelling *Voice Prosthesis* *InHealth Technologies, www.inhealth.com*	Safe	1.5, 3	

Object	Status	Field Strength (T)	Reference
Blom-Singer Special Order Low Pressure *Voice Prosthesis* *InHealth Technologies, www.inhealth.com*	Safe	1.5, 3	
Blood Collection Set, SS *United States Surgical, North Haven, CT*	Safe	1.5, 3	83
Bone Anchored Port (BAP) *Cendres+Metaux, www.cmsa.ch*	Conditional 6	3	
Boston Keratoprosthesis, Lucia Type I *Massachusetts Eye and Ear, www.masseyeandear.org*	Conditional 8	1.5, 3	
Bovine Pericardial Patch, Model 4700 *Edwards Lifesciences, www.edwards.com*	Safe	1.5, 3	
BrachySource, Radioactive Seed *Bard Brachytherapy, Inc., Carol Stream, IL*	Conditional 6	3	
Bracket, Model 801 NM 17737 *Amerex Corporation, Trussville, AL*	Conditional 7	3	
Bracket, Model 810 NM 06572 *Amerex Corporation, Trussville, AL*	Conditional 7	3	
Bracket, Model 816 NM 14315 *Amerex Corporation, Trussville, AL*	Conditional 7	3	
Bravo pH Monitoring System *Given Imaging, www.givenimaging.com*	Unsafe 1	1.5	
Bung Wrench, W-56 *Ampco Safety Tools, www.amcosafetytools.com*	Conditional 7	3	
Burr Hole Cover, Neurosurgery Fixation *C.P. Titanium* *Codman, www.depuysynthes.com*	Safe	1.5	
Burr Hole Cover, Neurosurgical Implant *Titanium* *Bioplate, Inc., Los Angeles, CA*	Conditional 6	3	
B.Y. Fix Anastomotic Device, Phynox *HDH Medical Ltd, Israel*	Conditional 6	3	
B.Y. Fix Anastomotic Device, Stainless Steel *HDH Medical Ltd, Israel*	Conditional 6	3	
CA.B.S. Air Composite Parieral Prosthesis *Cousin Biotech, www.cousin-biotech.com*	Safe	1.5, 3	
CA.B.S. Air Light Non-resorbable Parietal Implant *Cousin Biotech, www.cousin-biotech.com*	Safe	1.5, 3	
CA.B.S. Air Semi-resorbable Semi-resorbable *Parietal Reinforcement Implant* *Cousin Biotech, www.cousin-biotech.com*	Safe	1.5, 3	
Calf Implant, Silicone *Groupe SEBBIN SAS, www.sebbin.com/en/*	Safe	1.5, 3	

Object	Status	Field Strength (T)	Reference
Camino Flex Ventricular Catheter *Integra NeuroSciences, www.integralife.com*	Conditional 5	1.5, 3	
Cannon Catheter II, Chronic Hemodialysis Catheter *Arrow International, www.arrowintl.com*	Safe	1.5, 3	
CAPSURE Permanent Fixation System *Bard (Davol, Inc.), www.davol.com*	Conditional 5	3	
CardioBand *Valtech Cardio Ltd., www.valtechcardio.com*	Conditional 6	1.5, 3	
Cardioband Mitral Reconstruction System Implant *Valtech Cardio Ltd., www.valtechcardio.com*	Conditional 8	1.5, 3	
CardioBand Trans-Femoral, for Mitral Valve Repair *Valtech Cardio Ltd., www.valtechcardio.com*	Conditional 6	3	
CardioClose Ventricular Closure System *Entourage Medical, Menlo Park, CA*	Conditional 6	3	
CardioKinetix Parachute *CardioKinetix, Inc., www.cardiokinetix.com*	Conditional 8	1.5, 3	
Cardioroot Vascular Graft *Maquet, www.maquet.com*	Safe	1.5, 3	
Caresite Luer Access Device *B. Braun Medical Inc., www.bbraunusa.com*	Conditional 6	3	
CAREvent MRI Ventilator *O-Two Medical Technologies, Inc., www.otwo.com*	Conditional 5	3	
Carillon Implant, Mitral Contour System *Cardiac Dimensions Inc., Kirkland, WA*	Conditional 6	3	
Cart, 6 Drawer Breakaway Locking MR Cart *with Emergency Cart Package* *Model: MR6B-EMG* *The Harloff Company, Colorado Springs, CO*	Conditional 7	3	
Cart, 7 Drawer Keylocking MR Cart *with Anesthesia Accessory Package* *Model: MR7K-MAN* *The Harloff Company, Colorado Springs, CO*	Conditional 7	3	
Cart, 7 Drawer Narrow Body Keylocking MR Cart *with Emergency Cart* *Model: MRN7K-EMG* *The Harloff Company, Colorado Springs, CO*	Conditional 7	3	
Celsius Control Accutrol Catheter, 10.7 Fr. *INNERCOOL Therapies, San Diego, CA*	Conditional 5	1.5	
Celsius Control Accutrol Catheter, 14 Fr. *INNERCOOL Therapies, San Diego, CA*	Conditional 5	1.5	
Celsius Control Standard Catheter, 10.7 Fr. *INNERCOOL Therapies, San Diego, CA*	Conditional 5	1.5	

Object	Status	Field Strength (T)	Reference
Celsius Control Standard Catheter, 14 Fr. *INNERCOOL Therapies, San Diego, CA*	Conditional 5	1.5	
CenterPointLock, Drainable Irrigator Sleeve *Hollister Incorporated, www.hollister.com*	Unsafe 1	1.5	
CGA 870 Regulator *The Respiratory Group, www.respiratorygroup.com*	Conditional 7	3	
Champion HF Pressure Sensor, *CardioMEMS HF System* *CardioMEMS, www.sjm.com/cardiomems*	Conditional 8	1.5, 3	
CHEMETRON ADAPTER US AIR *DC CHECK INLET* *Ohio Medical Corporation, www.ohiomedical.com*	Conditional 7	3	
CHEMETRON COUPLER DISS H.T. VAC USA *Ohio Medical Corporation, www.ohiomedical.com*	Conditional 7	3	
Chin Implant, Silicone *Groupe SEBBIN SAS, www.sebbin.com/en/*	Safe	1.5, 3	
Chin Implant, Styles 1 to 11 *Implantech Associates, Inc., www.implantech.com*	Safe	1.5, 3	
Cianna Passive Tag *Cianna Medical, Inc., www.ciannamedical.com*	Conditional 6	3	
Cingular Bovine Pericardial Bioprosthesis *Shanghai Cingular Biotech Corporation,* *www.cingularbio.com*	Conditional 8	1.5, 3	
Claw Hammer, 1 lb head, 13" handle *NGK Metals Corporation, Sweetwater, TN*	Conditional 7	3	
Claw Hammer with Handle, 680-g *Newmatic Medical, www.newmaticmedical.com*	Conditional 7	3	
Claw Hammer, H-19FG *Ampco Safety Tools, www.amcosafetytools.com*	Conditional 7	3	
CleanScene MRI Fixture, 4 x 4 LED, CSMRI44 *Kenall Lighting, Gurnee, IL*	Conditional 7	3	
ClearCount RFID Tag *ClearCount Medical Solutions, www.clearcount.com*	Conditional 5	3	
Clip Board *Newmatic Medical, www.newmaticmedical.com*	Conditional 7	3	
Codman EDS 3, CSF External Drainage System *Codman, www.depuysynthes.com*	Conditional 6	3	
Codman Microsensor ICP Transducer *Note: MRI labeling is different for the United States* *versus Outside of the United States* *Codman, www.depuysynthes.com*	Conditional 5	1.5	
Codman Microsensor Skull Bolt, Skull Bolt *Codman, www.depuysynthes.com*	Safe	3	

Object	Status	Field Strength (T)	Reference
Coherex WaveCrest Left Atrial Appendage Occluder *Coherex Medical, www.coherex.com*	Conditional 6	3	
Combination Pliers, slip joint *NGK Metals Corporation, Sweetwater, TN*	Conditional 7	3	
Combination Wrench, 1304 *Ampco Safety Tools, www.amcosafetytools.com*	Conditional 7	3	
Combined Submalar Shell Implant *Implantech Associates, Inc., www.implantech.com*	Safe	1.5, 3	
Common Knife, K-1 *Ampco Safety Tools, www.amcosafetytools.com*	Conditional 7	3	
COMPASS Headframe (Complete) *using fixation, carbon fiber pin, Delrin Sleeve, Carbon Fiber Pin, Delrin Collet w/Nut COMPASS International, Inc., Rochester, MN*	Conditional 8	1.5, 3	
COMPASS Headframe (Complete) *using fixation, sharp pin, Delrin Sleeve w/ Titanium Tip Insert and Delrin Collet w/Nut COMPASS International, Inc., Rochester, MN*	Conditional 8	1.5, 3	
Compat 12 Fr. Nasogastric Tube *Nestle HealthCare Nutrition, Inc., www.nestle-nutrition.com*	Conditional 6	3	
Compat MRI S Feeding Tube *Nestle HealthCare Nutrition, www.nestle-nutrition.com*	Conditional 8	1.5, 3	
Compatible StarBurst XL Device *MRI Compatible StarBurst, Electrosurgical Device Angiodynamics, www.angiodynamics.com/products/starburst-mri*	Conditional 5	1.5	
Complete Care Urine Collection Bag *C.R. Bard, www.crbard.com*	Conditional 5	3	
Composite Anatomical Chin *Implantech Associates, Inc., www.implantech.com*	Safe	1.5, 3	
Composite Curvilinear Chin *Implantech Associates, Inc., www.implantech.com*	Safe	1.5, 3	
Composite Extended Anatomical Chin *Implantech Associates, Inc., www.implantech.com*	Safe	1.5, 3	
Composite Flowers Dorsal Nasal *Implantech Associates, Inc., www.implantech.com*	Safe	1.5, 3	
Composite Sinus Stent *S.T. Stent Ltd, www.ststent.com*	Conditional 8	1.5, 3	
Composite Voloshin Columella *Implantech Associates, Inc., www.implantech.com*	Safe	1.5, 3	
Concealed Sprinkler, Model VK462 *The Viking Corporation, Hastings, MI*	Conditional 7	3	

Object	Status	Field Strength (T)	Reference
Conform Binder Submalar Implant *Implantech Associates, Inc., www.implantech.com*	Safe	1.5, 3	
Conform Extended Anatomical Chin Implant *Implantech Associates, Inc., www.implantech.com*	Safe	1.5, 3	
Conform Midfacial Implant *Implantech Associates, Inc., www.implantech.com*	Safe	1.5, 3	
Conform Terino Malar Shell Implant *Implantech Associates, Inc., www.implantech.com*	Safe	1.5, 3	
Contoured Carving Block *Implantech Associates, Inc., www.implantech.com*	Safe	1.5, 3	
Contraceptive Diaphragm, All Flex *Ortho Pharmaceutical, Raritan, NJ*	Conditional 5	1.5	3
Contraceptive Diaphragm, Flat Spring *Ortho Pharmaceutical, Raritan, NJ*	Conditional 5	1.5	3
Contraceptive Diaphragm, Gyne T	Safe	1.5	47
Contraceptive Diaphragm, Koroflex *Young Drug Products, Piscataway, NJ*	Conditional 5	1.5	3
Contraceptive IUD/IUS, MIRENA, *intrauterine system (IUS)* *Berlex Laboratories, Montville, NJ*	Safe	1.5, 3	
Contraceptive IUD, Multiload Cu375 *Copper, Silver*	Safe	1.5	47
Contraceptive IUD, Nova T *Copper, Silver*	Safe	1.5	47
COOK-SWARTZ Doppler Flow Probe *Cook Medical, www.cookmedical.com*	Unsafe 1	1.5	
Cool Line Catheter *Alsius Heat Exchange Catheter* *Zoll, www.zoll.com*	Conditional 5	1.5	
CoolGuard 3000 Thermoregulation System *Alsius Heat Exchange Catheter* *Zoll, www.zoll.com*	Unsafe 1	1.5	
Core Temperature Ingestible Capsule *Temperature Device* *VitalSense Integrated Physiological Monitoring System* *Mini Mitter Company, Inc., Bend, OR*	Unsafe 1	1.5	
CORFLO Ultra, Non-weighted *Feeding Tube, Stylet Removed* *Viasys Healthcard Systems, Wheeling, IL*	Conditional 6	3	
CORFLO, ULTRA 7, Enteral Feeding Tube *Viasys MedSystems, Wheeling, IL*	Conditional 6	3	
Corolla TAA Device *CorAssist Cardiovascular Ltd., www.corassist.com*	Conditional 8	1.5, 3	

Object	Status	Field Strength (T)	Reference
Coronary Vein Marker *Med-Edge, Inc., www.med-edge.info*	Conditional 6	3	
CO-Set Room Temperature Injectate Kit *Edwards Lifesciences, www.edwards.com*	Conditional 7	3	
corVCD (implant for vessel coupling) *corLife GBR, www.corlife.eu*	Conditional 5	1.5, 3	124
CPR Infant Patient Valve, Infant/Child *Patient Valve w/Pop-Off & PEEP Adapter* *Mercury Medical, www.mercurymed.com*	Conditional 5	3	
Craftsman's Knife, 4 1/4" blade *NGK Metals Corporation, Sweetwater, TN*	Conditional 7	3	
Cranial Ceramic Drill bit *ceramic* *MicroSurgical Techniques Inc., Fort Collins, CO*	Safe	1.5	48
Cranial Screw, Neurosurgery Fixation *Codman, www.depuysynthes.com*	Safe	1.5	
Cranial Screw, Neurosurgery Fixation *Codman, www.depuysynthes.com*	Safe	1.5	
CranioFix, Bone Flap Fixation System, Titanium alloy *Aesculap, Inc., www.aesculapusa.com*	Safe	1.5	50
CranioFix, Burr Hole Clamp, FF0997, 20-mm *Titanium* *Aesculap, Inc., www.aesculapusa.com*	Safe	1.5, 3	83
CranioFix, Burr Hole Clamp, FF100T, 11-mm *Titanium* *Aesculap, Inc., www.aesculapusa.com*	Safe	1.5, 3	83
CranioFix, Burr Hole Clamp, FF101T, 16-mm *Titanium* *Aesculap, Inc., www.aesculapusa.com*	Safe	1.5, 3	83
CranioFix Titanium Clamps *Models including FF099T, FF100T,* *FF101T, FF490T, FF491T, FF492T* *Aesculap, Inc., www.aesculapusa.com*	Safe	3	
CranioFix 2 *Aesculap, Inc., www.aesculapusa.com*	Conditional 8	1.5, 3	
CranioFix 2 Titanium Clamps *Models including FF099T, FF100T,* *FF101T, FF490T, FF491T, FF492T* *Aesculap, Inc., www.aesculapusa.com*	Safe	3	
CranioFix Absorbable *Aesculap, Inc., www.aesculapusa.com*	Safe	1.5, 3	
CranioFix PEEK Radiolucent Clamp System *B. Braun, www.bbraun.com*	Safe	1.5, 3	

Object	Status	Field Strength (T)	Reference
CranioPlate, 6" x 5" *Aesculap, Inc., www.aesculapusa.com*	Conditional 8	1.5, 3	
Crate Opener, 70 x 230-mm *Newmatic Medical, www.newmaticmedical.com*	Conditional 7	3	
Crate Opener, CJ-1-ST *Ampco Safety Tools, www.amcosafetytools.com*	Conditional 7	3	
Curvilinear Silicone Chin Implant *Implantech Associates, Inc., www.implantech.com*	Safe	1.5, 3	
CV-1 CapsoCam, Pill Camera *Capso Vision, Inc., Saratoga, CA*	Unsafe 1	1.5	
Cytocan Needle *B. Braun, www.bbraunusa.com*	Conditional 5	1.5, 3	
CYTOGUARD Closed Male Luer Connector *B. Braun, www.bbraunusa.com*	Safe	1.5, 3	
Deck Scraper, 45 x 300-mm *Newmatic Medical, www.newmaticmedical.com*	Conditional 7	3	
Deck Scraper, S-11G *Ampco Safety Tools, www.amcosafetytools.com*	Conditional 7	3	
Denver Ascites Shunt, Double Valve *with 15.5 Fr. Venous Catheter* *CareFusion, www.carefusion.com*	Safe	1.5, 3	
Deponit, Nitroglycerin *transdermal delivery system, aluminized plastic* *Schwarz Pharma, Milwaukee, WI*	Unsafe 1	1.5	
Diagonal Cutting Pliers, 200-mm *Newmatic Medical, www.newmaticmedical.com*	Conditional 7	3	
DIGNISHIELD Stool Management System (SMS) *C.R. Bard, www.crbard.com*	Conditional 7	3	
Dilatator Brusis *Kurz Medical, www.kurzmed.com/en/products/mri-safety/*	Conditional 5	1.5, 3	
Disetronic Pump *Disetronic Medical Systems, Inc., St. Paul, MN*	Unsafe 1	1.5	
Disposable Laryngoscope, Blade Mac 3 *Scope Medical Devices, www.scopemedical.in*	Conditional 7	3	
Disposable Laryngoscope Handle with Super LED *Scope Medical Devices, www.scopemedical.in*	Conditional 7	3	
Disposable Laryngoscope Handle with Super LED *Combined with Laryngoscope Handle Battery Pack,* *Plastic Container Scope Medical Devices,* *www.scopemedical.in*	Conditional 7	3	
Disposable Sterile, Non-magnetic scalpel #11, *MRDS1* *Newmatic Medical, www.newmaticmedical.com*	Conditional 7	3	

Object	Status	Field Strength (T)	Reference
Disposable Sterile, Non-magnetic scalpel #21, MRDS21 *Newmatic Medical, www.newmaticmedical.com*	Conditional 7	3	
DISS H.T 1-1/2" STEM 1/8" MNPT O2 US MRI *Ohio Medical Corporation, www.ohiomedical.com*	Conditional 7	3	
Distflo Mini-Cuff Bypass Graft *Bard Peripheral Vascular, www.bardpv.com*	Safe	1.5	
Dobbhoff Gastro-Jejunal System *Covidien, www.covidien.com*	Conditional 6	3	
Dobbhoff Jejunal Feeding *Naso-Jejunal/Gastric Decompression System* *Covidien, www.covidien.com*	Conditional 6	3	
Dobbhoff Nasogastric Feeding Tube *Covidien, www.covidien.com*	Conditional 6	3	
Dobbhoff Naso-Jejunal/Gastric *Decompression System* *Covidien, www.covidien.com*	Conditional 6	3	
Dorsal Columella Implant Firm *Implantech Associates, Inc., www.implantech.com*	Safe	1.5, 3	
Dorsal Nasal Implant *Implantech Associates, Inc., www.implantech.com*	Safe	1.5, 3	
Double Box End Wrench, W-3130 *Ampco Safety Tools, www.amcosafetytools.com*	Conditional 7	3	
Double Box Ended Wrench, 14 X 15-mm *Newmatic Medical, www.newmaticmedical.com*	Conditional 7	3	
Double Open End Wrench *Titanium* *EMAREI Ltd. & Co, www.emarei.info/english*	Conditional 7	3	
Double Open End Wrench *Beryllium Copper* *EMAREI Ltd. & Co, www.emarei.info/english*	Conditional 7	3	
Double Open Ended Wrench, 18 x 19-mm *Newmatic Medical, www.newmaticmedical.com*	Conditional 7	3	
Double Open Ended Wrench, 5.5 x 7-mm *Newmatic Medical, www.newmaticmedical.com*	Conditional 7	3	
Double Open-end Wrench, WO-17X19 *Ampco Safety Tools, www.amcosafetytools.com*	Conditional 7	3	
Double Step Stool *Newmatic Medical, www.newmaticmedical.com*	Conditional 7	3	
Doyle Airwayless Nasal Splint *Hood Laboratories, www.hoodlabs.com*	Safe	1.5, 3	
Doyle Shark Nasal Splint *Hood Laboratories, www.hoodlabs.com*	Safe	1.5, 3	

Object	Status	Field Strength (T)	Reference
Dressing, PriMatrix Ag Antimicrobial *Dressing, 25-cm x 13-cm* *TEI Biosciences Inc., Boston, MA*	Safe	1.5, 3	
Dry Pad 9 x 9 with Silver Antimicrobial Agent *Newmatic Medical, www.newmaticmedical.com*	Conditional 7	3	
DURAFORM Dural Graft Implant *Depuy Synthes, www.depuysynthes.com*	Safe	1.5, 3	
Duet External Drainage System, Model 46914 *Medtronic, Inc., www.medtronic.com/mri*	Conditional 7	3	
Dura-Guard Dural Repair Patch *Synovis Surgical Innovations, www.synovissurgical.com*	Safe	1.5, 3	
DVS, Dose Verification System *Implantable Radiation Dosimeter* *Sicel Technologies, Inc., Morrisville, NC*	Conditional 5	1.5, 3	
E Cylinder Aluminum Construction *Newmatic Medical, www.newmaticmedical.com*	Conditional 7	3	
EchoSpark Tray Kit *Halyard Health, www.halyardhealth.com*	Safe	1.5, 3	
E/D Cylinder Rack 6 *Newmatic Medical, www.newmaticmedical.com*	Conditional 7	3	
E/D Dual Cylinder Hand Cart *Newmatic Medical, www.newmaticmedical.com*	Conditional 7	3	
EEG Electrodes, Adult E-6-GH *Grass Co., Quincy, MA*	Safe	0.3	51
EEG Electrodes, Pediatric E-5-GH *Grass Co., Quincy, MA*	Safe	0.3	51
Elana Ring, Platinum *ELANA BV, Utrecht, The Netherlands*	Safe	3	
Electronic Pressure Gauge Walk-O2-Bout system *(EPG WOB)* *Essex Industries, www.essexindustries.com*	Conditional 7	3	
Elevate Female Prolapse Systems *AMS, American Medical Systems,* *www.americanmedicalsystems.com*	Safe	1.5, 3	
Eliachar Nasal Splint *Hood Laboratories, www.hoodlabs.com*	Safe	1.5, 3	
Emergency Medical Cot, Model 30-NM *Ferno-Washington, Inc., Wilmington, OH*	Conditional 7	3	
Emergency Medical Cot, Model 33-NM *Ferno-Washington, Inc., Wilmington, OH*	Conditional 7	3	
Emergency Medical Cot, Model 35-ANM *Ferno-Washington Inc., Wilmington, OH*	Conditional 7	3	

Object	Status	Field Strength (T)	Reference
EmpowerMR Contrast Injector System *Product Number: 102901* *Bracco Diagnostics, Inc., Princeton, NJ*	Conditional 7	7	
EndoBarrier, EndoBarrier Gastrointestinal Liner *GI Dynamics, Lexington, MA*	Conditional 6	3	
Endo Capsule, Capsule Endoscope System *Olympus Medical Systems Corporation, Japan*	Unsafe 1	1.5	
Endobronchial Valve, EBV-6.5 *Emphasys Medical Inc., Redwood City, CA*	Safe	3	
EndoVive 3S Low Profile Balloon *Xeridiem, www.xeridiem.com*	Conditional 5	3	
Endoluminal Occlusion System (EOS) *ArtVentive Medical Group, Inc.,* *www.artventivemedical.com*	Conditional 8	1.5, 3	
Endoscope, 30000-10 Endoscope *Shakani Malleable Endoscopic Stylet,* *Clarus Medical, Golden Valley, MN*	Conditional 7	3	
Endoscope, 30000-GLS Scope *Levitan Endoscope* *Clarus Medical, Golden Valley, MN*	Conditional 7	3	
Endoscope, 30001-10 Endoscope *Malleable Pediatric Endoscopic Stylet* *Clarus Medical, Golden Valley, MN*	Conditional 7	3	
Endoscope, rigid, 2.7-mm (Sinuscope) *Greatbatch Scientific, Clarence, NY*	Safe	1.5	59
Endoscope, rigid, 8.0-mm (Laryngoscope) *Greatbatch Scientific, Clarence, NY*	Safe	1.5	59
EndoSure s2 Wireless AAA *Abdominal Aortic Aneurysm Pressure Sensor* *CardioMEMS, www.sjm.com/cardiomems*	Conditional 5	1.5, 3	
EndoSure Wireless AAA *(Abdominal Aortic Aneurysm) Pressure Sensor* *CardioMEMS, www.sjm.com/cardiomems*	Conditional 5	1.5, 3	
Endotracheal (ET) Tube *polyurethane coating with silver* *Bard Medical, www.bardmedical.com*	Safe	1.5	
Endotracheal Tube with Metal Ring Marker *Trachmate*	Safe	1.5	
Endotracheal Tube, Agento IC *Silver Coated Endotracheal Tube* *Bard Medical, www.bardmedical.com*	Conditional 8	1.5, 3	
ENDO-TUBE, Naso-Jejunal Feeding Tube *Covidien, www.covidien.com*	Conditional 6	3	

Object	Status	Field Strength (T)	Reference
Engineer Hammer, H-14FG *Ampco Safety Tools, www.amcosafetytools.com*	Conditional 7	3	
ENTRI-FLEX Nasogastric (NG) Feeding Tube *Covidien, www.covidien.com*	Conditional 6	3	
Equine Pericardial Patch, Model XAG *Edwards Lifesciences, www.edwards.com*	Safe	1.5, 3	
EquipLite blade *Truphatek International LTD., www.truphatek.com*	Conditional 7	3	
ESTRING, Estradiol Vaginal Ring *Pfizer, www.pfizer.com*	Safe	1.5	
ENTRISTAR *Jejunum Feeding Tube/Gastric Depression Tube* *Covidien, www.covidien.com*	Conditional 6	3	
Esophageal Reconstruction Tube *Hood Laboratories, www.hoodlabs.com*	Safe	1.5, 3	
ESSURE Device, 316L SS, *Platinum, Iridium, Nickel, Titanium* *Conceptus, www.conceptus.com*	Safe	1.5, 3	76, 83
ESSURE Device, Nickel-Titanium *outer and inner coils* *Conceptus, Inc., www.conceptus.com*	Conditional 6	3	
ESSURE Device, Nickel-Titanium outer coil *with a SS inner coil* *Conceptus, Inc., www.conceptus.com*	Conditional 6	3	
Essure ESS505 Micro-Insert With Hydrogel *Conceptus Inc., www.conceptus.com*	Conditional 6	3	
Essure Micro-insert, Permanent *contraception device* *Conceptus, Inc., Mountain View, CA*	Conditional 6	3	
Esteem, Hearing Implant *Envoy Medical, www.envoymedical.com*	Unsafe 1	1.5	
eSVS Mesh *Kips Bay Medical, www.kipsbaymedical.com*	Conditional 5	1.5, 3	
ETHILON Black Monofilament Nylon *with Surgical Bolster 1 3/4" Long 3/16" Diameter* *1/32" Wall and Lead Shot* *Ethicon, Inc., www.ethicon.com*	Conditional 6	3	
EVAHEART, Left Ventricular Assist Device (LVAD) *www.evaheart-usa.com*	Unsafe 1	1.5	
EVERPOINT Cardiovascular Needle *Ethicon, www.ethicon.com*	Conditional 6	3	

Object	Status	Field Strength (T)	Reference
Express Chest Drain, Models 001140-302SS	Conditional 7	3	
001317-302SS, 342135-302SS			
Atrium Medical, www.atriummed.com			
EXOSEAL Vascular Closure Device	Safe	1.5	
Cordis, www.cordis.com			
Extended Anatomical Chin Implant	Safe	1.5, 3	
Implantech Associates, Inc., www.implantech.com			
Extended Tear Trough Implant	Safe	1.5, 3	
Implantech Associates, Inc., www.implantech.com			
Extension Set with Caresite Luer Access Device	Conditional 6	3	
and Spin-Lock Connector			
B. Braun Medical Inc., www.bbraunusa.com			
Extension Set with ULTRASITE Injection Site	Conditional 6	3	
and Spin-Lock Connector			
B. Braun Medical Inc., www.bbraunusa.com			
Extinguisher, Model B270NM 6-Liter	Conditional 7	7	
Water Mist Extinguisher			
Amerex Corporation, Trussville, AL			
Extinguisher, Model B272NM 2.5-Gallon	Conditional 7	7	
Water Mist Extinguisher			
Amerex Corporation, Trussville, AL			
Extinguisher, Model 322NM 5.0-LB CO_2	Conditional 7	7	
Extinguisher			
Amerex Corporation, Trussville, AL			
Eyelid Weight, gold	Safe	1.5	52
EZ Huber Safety Infusion Set	Conditional 6	3	
PFM Medical, Inc., Oceanside, CA			
Fanous Premaxillary Implant	Safe	1.5, 3	
Implantech Associates, Inc., www.implantech.com			
Fastrac Device, Long-term Enteral Feeding	Conditional 6	3	
Management Device			
Bard Access Systems, www.bardaccess.com			
Fastrac Gastric Access Port, Silicone, 316LVM SS	Safe	1.5	
Bard Endoscopic Technologies, Billerica, MA			
Feeding Tube	Safe	3	
C-FMT-8.0-120, Frederick Miller Feeding Tube			
Cook Medical, Inc., www.cookmedical.com			
Feeding Tube	Safe	3	
C-FMT-8.0-70, Frederick Miller Feeding Tube			
Cook Medical, Inc., www.cookmedical.com			
Feeding Tube	Safe	3	
Gastrostomy Feeding Tube, Jejunal			
Kimberly-Clark, Draper, UT			

Object	Status	Field Strength (T)	Reference
Feeding Tube *McClean-Ring Feeding Tube* *Cook Medical, Inc., www.cookmedical.com*	Unsafe 1	1.5	
FenoTEX-2060, Textile UHF RFID Tag *Fenotag, www.fenotag.com*	Unsafe 1	1.5	
FenoTEX-2060A, Textile UHF RFID Tag *Fenotag, www.fenotag.com*	Conditional 8	1.5, 3	
Fiber-Optic Cardiac Pacing Lead *Photonic Device* *Biophan Technologies, Inc., Rochester, NY*	Safe	1.5, 3	81
Fiber-optic Intubating Laryngoscope Blade *Greatbatch Scientific, Clarence, NY*	Safe	1.5	
Fiber-optic Intubating Laryngoscope Handle *Greatbatch Scientific, Clarence, NY*	Safe	1.5	
Fiber-Optic Laryngoscope Blade, Stainless Steel *PriMedCo, St. Petersburg, FL*	Conditional 7	3	
Fiber-Optic Laryngoscope Handle, Stainless Steel *with Battery from Electrohem* *PriMedCo, St. Petersburg, FL*	Conditional 7	3	
Fire Extinquisher, Ansul Cleanguard Fire *Extinguisher, FE13NM* *Ansul, www.ansul.com*	Conditional 7	3	
Fire Extinguisher *Dry Chemical Fire Extinguisher, OVAL-10JABC* *Oval Brand Fire Products, www.ovalfireproducts.com*	Conditional 7	3	
Fire Extinguisher, Model 322, 5.0 lb. CO_2 *Amerex Corporation, Trussville, AL*	Conditional 7	3	
Fire Extinguisher, Model B270NM, *1 3/4 gallon Water Mist* *Amerex Corporation, Trussville, AL Note: Tested prior to* *new terminology in 2005. The correct labeling is MR* *Conditional for this product.*	Safe	3	
Fire Extinguisher, Model B272NM, *2 1/2 gallon Water Mist* *Amerex Corporation, Trussville, AL Note: Tested prior to* *new terminology in 2005. The correct labeling is MR* *Conditional for this product.*	Safe	3	
Fire Extinguisher, Model XL 5 MR, *Multipurpose Dry Chemical* *Portable Fire Extinguisher* *Kidde Fire Safety, www.kidde.com*	Conditional 7	7	
Firestar 9-mm Semiautomatic *Star Bonifacio Echeverria, Eibar, Spain*	Unsafe 1	1.5	46

Object	Status	Field Strength (T)	Reference
Flat Plate Concealed Sprinkler *Tyco Fire Protection Products, www.tyco-fire.com*	Conditional 7	3	
Fletcher CT/MR Shielded Applicator, (Set #110.950) *Nucletron, An Elekta Company, www.nucletron.com*	Conditional 5	1.5, 3	
FlexBlock Continuous Peripheral Nerve Block *Catheter* *Teleflex Medical, www.teleflex.com*	Conditional 5	3	
FlexTip Plus Epidural Catheter, 304V SS *Arrow International Inc., Reading, PA*	Unsafe 2	1.5	
FlexTip Plus Epidural Catheter, 19-gauge x 90-cm, *Nonmagnetic SS Version* *Teleflex Medical, Inc., www.teleflex.com*	Conditional 8	1.5, 3	
Flixene Vascular Graft *Maquet, www.maquet.com*	Safe	1.5, 3	
Flow Re-direction Endoluminal Device, FRED *MicroVention, Inc., www.microvention.com*	Conditional 8	1.5, 3	
FloTrac Sensor *Edwards Lifesciences, www.edwards.com*	Conditional 5	3	
FLOWMETER 15LPM BM PROBE OXY USA MRI *Ohio Medical Corporation, www.ohiomedical.com*	Conditional 7	3	
FLOWMETER, 15LPM DIAL FLOWMETER *GM OXY USA* *Ohio Medical Corporation, www.ohiomedical.com*	Conditional 7	3	
Flowmeter, Quick Click, CFMXXX-XX *Western Scott Fetzer, Inc., Westlake, OH*	Conditional 7	3	
Flowmeter, Slim-Line Flowmeter, FMAX0X *Western Scott Fetzer, Inc., Westlake, OH*	Conditional 7	3	
Flowmeter, Slim-Line Flowmeter, FMEX0X *Western Scott Fetzer, Inc., Westlake, OH*	Conditional 7	3	
Flowmeter, Slim-Line Flowmeter, FMR100 *Western Scott Fetzer, Inc., Westlake, OH*	Conditional 7	3	
Flow-Safe CPAP System with Large *Adult Deluxe Contoured Mask* *Mercury Medical, www.mercurymed.com*	Conditional 5	3	
Forceps, Ceramic *MicroSurgical Techniques Inc., Fort Collins, CO*	Safe	1.5	48
Forceps, Titanium	Safe	1.5	
Fortius Catheter Alsius Heat Exchange Catheter *Zoll, www.zoll.com*	Conditional 5	1.5	
FREEHAND System Implantable Functional *Neurostimulator (FNS)* *NeuroControl Corporation, Cleveland, OH*	Conditional 5	1.5	

Object	Status	Field Strength (T)	Reference
FREKA Intestinal Tube *Long Term Intestinal Feeding* *Animech Technologies AB, Uppsala, Sweden*	Conditional 6	3	
Fusion Positioning/Comfort Pad *Trulife, www.Trulife.com*	Safe	1.5, 3	
Fusion Vascular Graft *Maquet, www.maquet.com*	Safe	1.5, 3	
G-JET Feeding Tube Device Device *Applied Medical Technology, Inc.,* *www.appliedmedical.net*	Conditional 5	1.5, 3	
Gabriel Feeding Tube Magnetically-Guided *Feeding Tube, 12-Fr, GFT112 Neo-dymium magnets* *imbedded in distal tip of the Tube* *Syncro Medical Innovations, Inc., Canton, OH*	Unsafe 1	1.5	
GaleMed PEEP Valve *CareFusion, www.carefusion.com*	Conditional 7	3	
GammaTile *IsoRay Medical, Inc., www.IsoRay.com*	Conditional 8	1.5, 3	
GAS REG 50PSI PRST OXY CGA 870 INLET MRI *Ohio Medical Corporation, www.ohiomedical.com*	Conditional 7	3	
Gel Pad, Various shapes *AADCO Medical, Inc., Randolph, VT*	Conditional 7	3	
Gelseal Polyester Vascular Prosthesis *Vascutek, www.vascutek.com*	Safe	1.5, 3	
Gelsoft Polyester Vascular Prosthesis *Vascutek, www.vascutek.com*	Safe	1.5, 3	
Gelsoft ERS Polyester Vascular Prosthesis *Vascutek, www.vascutek.com*	Safe	1.5, 3	
Gelsoft Plus Polyester Vascular Prosthesis *Vascutek, www.vascutek.com*	Safe	1.5, 3	
Gelsoft Plus ERS Polyester Vascular Prosthesis *Vascutek, www.vascutek.com*	Safe	1.5, 3	
Gelweave Polyester Vascular Prosthesis *Vascutek, www.vascutek.com*	Safe	1.5, 3	
Gelweave Valsalva Polyesther Vascular Prosthesis *Vascutek, www.vascutek.com*	Safe	1.5, 3	
Gen 6.0 HeRO, The Adapter *Hemosphere, Inc., Eden Prairie, MN*	Conditional 8	3	
Genesys Cross-FT Suture Anchor with Four Sutures *ConMed Linvatec Biomaterials, Inc., www.conmed.com*	Safe	1.5, 3	
Glasgold Wafer for the Extended Anatomical Chin *Implantech Associates, Inc., www.implantech.com*	Safe	1.5, 3	

Object	Status	Field Strength (T)	Reference
GlucoClear System including GlucoClear *Peripheral IV Sensor, GlucoClear Flush Line,* *GlucoClear Cassette* *Edwards Laboratories, www.edwards*	Conditional 5	1.5, 3	
Gluteal Implant Silione *Groupe SEBBIN SAS, www.sebbin.com/en/*	Safe	1.5, 3	
GOLDBAL2 Tracheal Occlusion Balloon *Balt Extrusion, www.balt.fr*	Conditional 6	3	
GORE ACUSEAL Cardiovascular Patch *W.L. Gore & Associates, www.goremedical.com*	Safe	1.5, 3	
GORE BIO-A Fistula Plug *W.L. Gore & Associates, www.goremedical.com*	Safe	1.5, 3	
GORE BIO-A Hernia Plug *W.L. Gore & Associates, www.goremedical.com*	Safe	1.5, 3	
GORE BIO-A Tissue Reinforcement *W.L. Gore & Associates, www.goremedical.com*	Safe	1.5, 3	
GORE DUALMESH Biomaterial *W.L. Gore & Associates, www.goremedical.com*	Safe	1.5, 3	
GORE DUALMESH PLUS Biomaterial *DUALMESH PLUS Biomaterial with Holes* *W.L. Gore & Associates, www.goremedical.com*	Safe	1.5, 3	
GORE INFINIT Mesh *W.L. Gore & Associates, www.goremedical.com*	Safe	1.5, 3	
GORE PRECLUDE Peritoneal Membrane *W.L. Gore & Associates, www.goremedical.com*	Safe	1.5, 3	
GORE Pulmonary Valved Conduit (PVC) *W. L. Gore and Associates, Inc., www.wlgore.com*	Conditional 8	1.5, 3	
GORE RESOLUT ADAPT Regenerative Membrane *W.L. Gore & Associates, www.goremedical.com*	Safe	1.5, 3	
GORE RESOLUT ADAPT LT Regenerative Membrane *W.L. Gore & Associates, www.goremedical.com*	Safe	1.5, 3	
GORE RESOLUT XT Regenerative Membrane *W.L. Gore & Associates, www.goremedical.com*	Safe	1.5, 3	
GORE SEAMGUARD Staple Line Reinforcement *W.L. Gore & Associates, www.goremedical.com*	Safe	1.5, 3	
GORE-TEX Cardiovascular Patch *GORE-TEX Expanded Polytetrafluoroethylene* *Cardiovascular Patch* *W.L. Gore and Associates, www.goremedical.com*	Safe	1.5, 3	
GORE-TEX Regenerative Membrane *W.L. Gore & Associates, www.goremedical.com*	Safe	1.5, 3	

Object	Status	Field Strength (T)	Reference
Grab 'n Go Heliox Portable Medical Heliox System *Aluminum Cylinder* *CAUTION: DO NOT USE STEEL CYLINDERS* *Praxair, www.praxair.com*	Conditional 7	3	
Grab 'n Go Vantage Portable Oxygen System *Aluminum D Cylinder* *CAUTION: DO NOT USE STEEL CYLINDERS* *Praxair, www.praxair.com*	Conditional 7	3	
Grab 'n Go Vantage Portable Oxygen System *Aluminum E Cylinder* *CAUTION: DO NOT USE STEEL CYLINDERS* *Praxair, www.praxair.com*	Conditional 7	3	
Grab 'n Go Vantage Regulator/Pressure Gauge *CAUTION: DO NOT USE STEEL CYLINDERS* *Praxair, www.praxair.com*	Conditional 7	3	
Grab 'n Go Vantage D Cylinder, Oxygen Tank *CAUTION: DO NOT USE STEEL CYLINDERS* *Praxair, www.praxair.com*	Conditional 7	3	
Grab 'n Go Vantage E Cylinder, Oxygen Tank *CAUTION: DO NOT USE STEEL CYLINDERS* *Praxair, www.praxair.com*	Conditional 7	3	
Green System Fiber-optic Laryngoscope Blade *Anaesthetics India Pvt Ltd., ww.anaesthaids.coms*	Conditional 7	3	
Green System Fiber-optic LED Laryngoscope *Handle* *Anaesthetics India Pvt Ltd., ww.anaesthaids.com*	Conditional 7	3	
Groove Joint Pliers, 2 1/2" *NGK Metals Corporation, Sweetwater, TN*	Conditional 7	3	
Groove Joint Pliers, 10" *Newmatic Medical, www.newmaticmedical.com*	Conditional 7	3	
Groove Joint Pliers, 300-mm *Newmatic Medical, www.newmaticmedical.com*	Conditional 7	3	
Groove Joint Pliers, P-39 *Ampco Safety Tools, www.amcosafetytools.com*	Conditional 7	3	
Guardian Cranial Burr Hole Cover System *St. Jude Medical and Abbott, www.abbott.com*	Unsafe 1	1.5	
Gurney *Newmatic Medical, www.newmaticmedical.com*	Conditional 7	3	
Gurney with IV Pole *Newmatic Medical, www.newmaticmedical.com*	Conditional 7	3	
Hamper, HAMPF *Newmatic Medical, www.newmaticmedical.com*	Conditional 7	3	

Object	Status	Field Strength (T)	Reference
Hand Tool Kit, Six piece, NF-240 *Standard screw driver, Philips Screw Driver* *Wrench, Pliers, Adjustable pliers, Crate opener* *AADCO Medical, Inc., Randolph, VT*	Conditional 7	3	
HDH SureConnect Patient Connector *Baxa Corp., www.baxa.com*	Conditional 6	3	
HeartMate 3 Left Ventricular Assist Device (LVAD) *St. Jude Medical, www.SJM.com*	Unsafe 1	1.5	
Heine Gamma Sphygmomanometer *Newmatic Medical, www.newmaticmedical.com*	Conditional 7	3	
Hemacarotid Heparin Knitted Ultrathin Patch *Maquet, www.maquet.com*	Safe	1.5, 3	
Hemacarotid Knitted Patch *Maquet, www.maquet.com*	Safe	1.5, 3	
Hemacarotid Knitted Ultrathin Patch *Maquet, www.maquet.com*	Safe	1.5, 3	
Hemacarotid Vascular Patch *Maquet, www.maquet.com*	Safe	1.5, 3	
Hemagard Knitted Vascular Patch *Maquet, www.maquet.com*	Safe	1.5, 3	
Hemagard Vascular Patch *Maquet, www.maquet.com*	Safe	1.5, 3	
Hemapatch Knitted Vascular Patch *Maquet, www.maquet.com*	Safe	1.5, 3	
Hemapatch Silver Knitted Ultrathin Vascular Patch *Maquet, www.maquet.com*	Safe	1.5, 3	
Hemapatch Woven Vascular Patch *Maquet, www.maquet.com*	Safe	1.5, 3	
Hemapatch Vascular Patch *Maquet, www.maquet.com*	Safe	1.5, 3	
Hemashield Finesse Ultra-Thin, Knitted *Cardiovascular Patch, Vascular Graft, Polyester* *Boston Scientific, www.bostonscientific.com*	Safe	1.5, 3	
Hemashield Gold Microvel *Knitted Double Velour, Vascular Graft, Polyester* *Boston Scientific, www.bostonscientific.com*	Safe	1.5, 3	
Hemashield Gold Vascular Graft *Maquet, www.maquet.com*	Safe	1.5, 3	
Hemashield Gold Vascular Patch *Maquet, www.maquet.com*	Safe	1.5, 3	
Hemashield Gold Woven 3 Branch Vascular Graft *Maquet, www.maquet.com*	Safe	1.5, 3	

Object	Status	Field Strength (T)	Reference
Hemashield Platinum Finesse Knitted *Cardiovascular Patch* *Maquet, www.maquet.com*	Safe	1.5, 3	
Hemashield Platinum Finesse Vascular Patch *Maquet, www.maquet.com*	Safe	1.5, 3	
Hemashield Platinum Woven Double Velour *Vascular Graft* *Maquet, www.maquet.com*	Safe	1.5, 3	
Hemashield Platinum Vascular Graft *Maquet, www.maquet.com*	Safe	1.5, 3	
Hemashield Platinum Vascular Patch *Maquet, www.maquet.com*	Safe	1.5, 3	
Hermetic Plus External CSF Drainage System *Integra NeuroSciences, www.integralife.com*	Safe	1.5, 3	
HemoDraw Plus LogiCal Triple Line *Smiths Medical, www.smiths-medical.com*	Conditional 6	3	
HemoDraw Plus TranStar Triple Line *Smiths Medical, www.smiths-medical.com*	Conditional 6	3	
HeRO Graft System *Merit Medical Systems, Inc., www.merit.com*	Conditional 8	1.5, 3	
Hex Key Wrench, 1.5-mm *Newmatic Medical, www.newmaticmedical.com*	Conditional 7	3	
Hex Key Wrench, 1-1/16" *Newmatic Medical, www.newmaticmedical.com*	Conditional 7	3	
Horizontal-Vertical (H-V) Lumbar Valve System *Integra LifeSciences Corporation, www.Integralife.com*	Conditional 5	1.5, 3	
HoverMatt, HM34DC - 34"x 78" *HoverTech International, Bethlehem, PA*	Conditional 6	3	
HoverMatt, HM34HS - 34"x 78" *HoverTech International, Bethlehem, PA*	Conditional 6	3	
Huang Inner Ear Shunt *Hood Laboratories, www.hoodlabs.com*	Safe	1.5, 3	
Hummingbird Parenchyma, ICP Monitoring *InnerSpace, www.innerspacemedical.com*	Conditional 5	1.5, 3	
Hyperinflation System, Hyperinflation *Valve Assembly with Pop-Off Valve and Manometer* *Mercury Medical, www.mercurymed.com*	Conditional 5	3	
IBV Valve, Nitinol *Spiration Inc., Redmond, WA*	Conditional 6	3	
Icy Catheter, Alsius Heat Exchange Catheter *Zoll, www.zoll.com*	Conditional 5	1.5	
Icy Hot Smart Relief Tens Therapy *Chattem, Inc., www.icyhot.com/smartrelief-back/*	Unsafe 1	1.5	

Object	Status	Field Strength (T)	Reference
IMPEDE Embolization Plug Device *Shape Memory Medical Inc., www.shapemem.com*	Conditional 8	1.5, 3	
Impella Ventricular Support System, All Versions *Abiomed, www.abiomed.com*	Unsafe 1	1.5	
IMPLANON Contraceptive Implant *Organon USA Inc., Roseland, NJ*	Safe	1.5	109
Implantable Spinal Fusion Stimulator *Bone Fusion Stimulator, Model SpF-100* *Electro-Biology, Inc. (EBI) and Biomet, www.biomet.com*	Conditional 5	1.5	63
Implantable Spinal Fusion Stimulator *Bone Fusion Stimulators* *Models SpF-XL IIb and SpF PLUS-Mini* *Electro-Biology, Inc. (EBI) and Biomet, www.biomet.com*	Conditional 5	1.5	
Indwelling Fecal Diverter *Consure Medical, consuremedical.com*	Conditional 5	1.5, 3	
In-Fast Bone Screw, Titanium alloy *AMS, American Medical Systems,* *www.americanmedicalsystems.com*	Safe	3	
In-Fast Loop Screw, Titanium alloy *AMS, American Medical Systems,* *www.americanmedicalsystems.com*	Safe	3	
In-Fast Sling System *AMS, American Medical Systems,* *www.americanmedicalsystems.com*	Safe	1.5, 3	
In-Fast Swivel Screw *Titanium alloy* *AMS, American Medical Systems,* *www.americanmedicalsystems.com*	Safe	3	
In-Fast Ultra Sling System *AMS, American Medical Systems,* *www.americanmedicalsystems.com*	Safe	1.5, 3	
InfuseIT Pressure Infuser, 1,000-ml *Zefon International, Inc., www.zefon.com*	Conditional 7	3	
Infusion Set, MMT-11X *Medtronic, Inc., www.medtronicdiabetes.com*	Safe	1.5	
Infusion Set, MMT-31X *Medtronic, Inc., www.medtronicdiabetes.com*	Safe	1.5	
Infusion Set, MMT-32X *Medtronic, Inc., www.medtronicdiabetes.com*	Safe	1.5	
Infusion Set, MMT-37X *Medtronic, Inc., www.medtronicdiabetes.com*	Safe	1.5	
Infusion Set, MMT-39X *Medtronic, Inc., www.medtronicdiabetes.com*	Safe	1.5	

Object	Status	Field Strength (T)	Reference
Infusion Set, Polyfin, MMT-106 *Medtronic, Inc., www.medtronicdiabetes.com*	Unsafe 1	1.5	
Infusion Set, Polyfin, MMT-107 *Medtronic, Inc., www.medtronicdiabetes.com*	Unsafe 1	1.5	
Infusion Set, Polyfin, MMT-16X *Medtronic, Inc., www.medtronicdiabetes.com*	Unsafe 1	1.5	
Infusion Set, Polyfin, MMT-30X *Medtronic, Inc., www.medtronicdiabetes.com*	Unsafe 1	1.5	
Infusion Set, Polyfin, MMT-36X *Medtronic, Inc., www.medtronicdiabetes.com*	Unsafe 1	1.5	
Initial Placement Feeding Tube, 24-Fr. *Cook Medical, www.cookmedical.com*	Conditional 8	1.5, 3	
Inner Ear Valved Shunt *Hood Laboratories, www.hoodlabs.com*	Safe	1.5, 3	
Instar Stentless Endoluminal Aortic Prosthesis *Labcor Laboratorios Ltda., www.labcor.com*	Safe	1.5, 3	
Insert Earphones for fMRI Model S14 *Sensimetrics Corporation, www.sens.com*	Conditional 5	1.5, 3	
Insulin Pump, Animas 2020 Insulin Pump *Animas Corporation, www.animas.com*	Unsafe 1	1.5	
Insulin Pump, La Fenice Insulin Pump *Microport, www.microport.com.cn/*	Unsafe 1	1.5	
Insulin Pump, IR 1000 Insulin Pump *Animas Corporation, www.animas.com*	Unsafe 1	1.5	
Insulin Pump, IR 1100 Insulin Pump *Animas Corporation, www.animas.com*	Unsafe 1	1.5	
Insulin Pump, IR 1200 Insulin Pump *Animas Corporation, www.animas.com*	Unsafe 1	1.5	
Insulin Pump, IR Animas 1200 *Animas Corporation, www.animas.com*	Unsafe 1	1.5	
InterAtrial Shunt Device (IASD) *Corvia Medical, www.corviamedical.com*	Conditional 5	1.5, 3	
Intergard Heparin Vascular Graft *Maquet, www.maquet.com*	Safe	1.5, 3	
Intergard Heparin Vascular Patch *Maquet, www.maquet.com*	Safe	1.5, 3	
Intergard Knitted Ultrathin Vascular Graft *Maquet, www.maquet.com*	Safe	1.5, 3	
Intergard Knitted Vascular Graft *Maquet, www.maquet.com*	Safe	1.5, 3	

Object	Status	Field Strength (T)	Reference
Intergard Silver Ultrathin Vascular Graft *Maquet, www.maquet.com*	Safe	1.5, 3	
Intergard Silver Vascular Graft *Maquet, www.maquet.com*	Safe	1.5, 3	
Intergard Synergy Vascular Graft *Maquet, www.maquet.com*	Safe	1.5, 3	
Intergard Synergy Ultrathin Vascular Graft *Maquet, www.maquet.com*	Safe	1.5, 3	
Intergard Woven Vascular Graft *Maquet, www.maquet.com*	Safe	1.5, 3	
Intervascular InterGard Woven Polyester Graft *W.L. Gore and Associates, www.goremedical.com*	Safe	1.5, 3	
Intima-II I.V. Catheter System *BD Medical Systems* *Becton Dickinson, Sandy, Utah*	Safe	1.5, 3	
Intracranial Depth Electrodes (EEG) *Superior Tube Company, Norristown, NY*	Safe	1.5	53
Intracranial Pressure Monitor (ICP) *Pressio ICP Monitoring Device* *Sophysa, www.sophysa.com*	Unsafe 1	1.5	
Intracranial Pressure Monitoring Catheter *with Licox IMC Bolt Fitting* *Integra NeuroSciences, www.integralife.com*	Unsafe 1	1.5	
Intracranial Pressure Monitoring Catheter *with Licox IMC Bolt Fitting with Cranial Access Kit* *Integra NeuroSciences, www.integralife.com*	Unsafe 1	1.5	
Intracranial Pressure Monitoring Kit *with Cranial Access* *Integra NeuroSciences, www.integralife.com*	Unsafe 1	1.5	
Intracranial Pressure-Temperature Monitoring Kit *Integra NeuroSciences, www.integralife.com*	Unsafe 1	1.5	
Intraflex Feeding Tube	Safe	1.5, 3	
Intramesh T1 Non resorbable Double Sided *Parietal Reinforcement Implant* *Cousin Biotech, www.cousin-biotech.com*	Safe	1.5, 3	
Intrauterine Contraceptive Device (IUD), Copper T *Searle Pharmaceuticals, Chicago, IL*	Safe	1.5	54
Intrauterine Contraceptive Device, Copper T 380A *ParaGard* *FEI, North Tanawanda, NY*	Conditional 5	3	111
Intrauterine Contraceptive Device (IUD), *Flexi-T 300, Flex-T +300, Flexi-T-380 IUD* *Trimedica, www.trimedic.com*	Conditional 5	3	

Object	Status	Field Strength (T)	Reference
Intrauterine Contraceptive Device (IUD), *Intrauterine System (IUS), Kyleena* *Bayer, www.bayer.com*	Conditional 5	1.5, 3	
Intrauterine Contraceptive Device (IUD) *Lippey Loop*	Safe	1.5, 3	
Intrauterine Contraceptive Device (IUD), Jaydess *Bayer, www.bayer.com*	Conditional 5	1.5, 3	
Intrauterine Contraceptive Device (IUD), LCS, *Ultra Low Dose Levonorgestrel Contraceptive System* *Bayer, www.bayer.com*	Conditional 6	3	
Intrauterine System, LCS12 IUS, *Contraceptive Device* *Bayer, www.bayer.com*	Conditional 6	3	
Intrauterine Contraceptive Device (IUD) *Liletta Intrauterine System* *Allergan, www.liletta.com*	Safe	1.5, 3	
InVance Male Sling System *AMS, American Medical Systems,* *www.americanmedicalsystems.com*	Safe	1.5, 3	
iPro2 Continuous Glucose Monitoring (CGM) *Medtronic, Inc., www.medtronic.com*	Unsafe 1	1.5	
IsoMed Implantable Drug Infusion System *Medtronic, Inc., www.medtronic.com/mri*	Conditional 5	1.5	
Integra Camino Complete Intracranial Pressure Kit, *1104BC* *Integra, www.integralife.com*	Unsafe 1	1.5	
Integra Camino Complete Micro Ventricular Bolt Kit, *110-4HMC* *Integra, www.integralife.com*	Unsafe 1	1.5	
Integra Camino Flex Ventricular Intracranial *Pressure Monitoring Kit* *Integra, www.integralife.com*	Conditional 8	1.5, 3	
Integra Camino Intracranial Pressure Monitoring Kit, *110-4L* *Integra, www.integralife.com*	Unsafe 1	1.5	
Integra Camino Intracranial Pressure Monitoring Kit, *110-4LC* *Integra, www.integralife.com*	Unsafe 1	1.5	
Integra Camino Micro Ventricular Bolt Intracranial *Pressure Monitoring Kit, 110-4HM* *Integra, www.integralife.com*	Unsafe 1	1.5	
Integra Camino Micro Ventricular Bolt Intracranial *Pressure Temperature Monitoring Kit, 110-4HMT* *Integra, www.integralife.com*	Unsafe 1	1.5	

Object	Status	Field Strength (T)	Reference
Integra Camino Parenchymal Intracranial *Pressure Monitoring Kit, 110-4B* *Integra, www.integralife.com*	Unsafe 1	1.5	
Integra Camino Parenchymal Intracranial *Pressure Temperature Kit, 110-4BT* *Integra, www.integralife.com*	Unsafe 1	1.5	
Integra Camino Post Craniotomy Subdural *Intracranial Pressure Kit, 110-4G* *Integra, www.integralife.com*	Unsafe 1	1.5	
Intubation Device, Avant with Regular Blade, *Guided Intubation Device* *Airtraq, airtraq.com*	Conditional 7	3	
Intubation Device, Double Lumen, *Guided Intubation Device* *Airtraq, airtraq.com*	Conditional 7	3	
Intubation Device, Infant Nasal, *Guided Intubation Device* *Airtraq, airtraq.com*	Conditional 7	3	
IsoRay Model CS-1 Brachytherapy Seed *IsoRay Medical, Inc., www.isoray.com*	Conditional 5	1.5, 3	
iStent Inject Trabecular Micro-Bypass System *G2-W* *Glaukos Corporation, www.glaukos.com*	Conditional 6	3	
IV Pole, HD NM, Model 513-10 *Ferno Washington Inc., Wilmington, Ohio*	Conditional 7	3	
IV Pole, Large Base *Newmatic Medical, www.newmaticmedical.com*	Conditional 7	3	
IV Pole, PN R&D#0556 *Pryor Products, Oceanside, CA*	Conditional 7	3	
IV Pole, Small Base *Newmatic Medical, www.newmaticmedical.com*	Conditional 7	3	
IV Stand 4 Hook with Casters, Aluminum *Newmatic Medical, www.newmaticmedical.com*	Conditional 7	3	
IV Stand 4 Hook with Casters *Newmatic Medical, www.newmaticmedical.com*	Conditional 7	3	
IV Stand, IVS-7004-MRI *MAC Medical, Inc., www.macmedical.com*	Conditional 7	3	
Jacobs Frontal Sinus Cannula *Hood Laboratories, www.hoodlabs.com*	Safe	1.5, 3	
Janitorial Cleaning Cart *Continental Commercial Products, Bridgeton, MO*	Conditional 7	3	
Jelco (FEP Radiopaque) Intravenous (I.V.) Catheter *Smiths Medical, www.smiths-medical.com*	Safe	3	

Object	Status	Field Strength (T)	Reference
Jelco (FEP) Intravenous (I.V.) Catheter *Smiths Medical, www.smiths-medical.com*	Safe	3	
Jelco 2 (FEP) Intravenous (I.V.) Catheter *Smiths Medical, www.smiths-medical.com*	Safe	3	
Jelco IntuitIV Safety IV Catheter, *(FEP Radiopaque)* *Safety IV Catheter with Straight Hub* *Smiths Medical International Ltd., www.smiths-medical.com*	Conditional 6	3	
Jelco IntuitIV Safety IV Catheter, (FEP Radiopaque) *Safety IV Catheter with Side Injection Port Hub* *Smiths Medical International Ltd., www.smiths-medical.com*	Conditional 6	3	
Jelco IntuitIV Safety IV Catheter, (PUR Radiopaque) *Safety IV Catheter with Straight Hub* *Smiths Medical International Ltd., www.smiths-medical.com*	Conditional 6	3	
Jelco IntuitIV Safety IV Catheter, (PUR Radiopaque) *Safety IV Catheter with Side Injection Port Hub* *Smiths Medical International Ltd., www.smiths-medical.com*	Conditional 6	3	
Jelco W (FEP) Intravenous (I.V.) Catheter *Smiths Medical, www.smiths-medical.com*	Safe	3	
Jejunal Feeding Tube, 12-Fr. *Cook Medical, www.cookmedical.com*	Conditional 8	1.5, 3	
Kangaroo Feeding Tube with IRIS Technology *Covidien, www.covidien.com*	Conditional 5	1.5, 3	
KerraContact Dressing *Crawford Healthcare Ltd, www.crawfordhealthcare.com*	Safe	1.5, 3	
Kick Bucket, KB-1000-MRI *MAC Medical, Inc., www.macmedical.com*	Conditional 7	3	
KimVent Multi Access Port Closed Suction Catheter *Kimberly Clark, Roswell, GA*	Conditional 6	3	
KimVent Percutaneous Dilatational *Tracheostomy Tube* *Kimberly Clark, Roswell, GA*	Conditional 6	3	
K.D. Chin Implant *Implantech Associates, Inc., www.implantech.com*	Safe	1.5, 3	
L-Chord *Corpus Medical, Inc., www.corpusmed.com*	Conditional 8	1.5, 3	
Ladder, 8-ft *Newmatic Medical, www.newmaticmedical.com*	Conditional 7	3	
Ladder, Aluminum, L-2431-08MR *Cuprum S.A. de C.V., www.cuprum.com*	Conditional 7	3	

Object	Status	Field Strength (T)	Reference
Ladder, Aluminum, TIA 6-ft, Twin Front *Cuprum S.A. de C.V., www.cuprum.com*	Conditional 7	3	
Ladder, Fiberglass Ladder, L-3431-08MR *Cuprum S.A. de C.V., www.cuprum.com*	Conditional 7	3	
Ladder, Fiberglass, TIA 6-ft, Twin Front *Cuprum S.A. de C.V., www.cuprum.com*	Conditional 7	3	
Laminate External Support *Laminate Medical Technologies Ltd., Israel*	Conditional 8	1.5, 3	
Langenbeck Periosteal Elevator, 304 SS *Johnson & Johnson Professional, Inc.,* *www.depuysynthes.com*	Safe	1.5	62
Laparoscopic Graspers *Greatbatch Scientific, Clarence, NY*	Safe	1.5	
LAP-BAND (Lapband), Adjustable Gastric Band *INAMED, Goleta, CA*	Safe	3	
LAP-BAND (Lapband) AP System *Adjustable Gastric Banding System* *with OMNIFORM Design* *Allergan, Inc., www.allergan.com*	Conditional 5	3	
LAP-BAND (Lapband) AP Adjustable Gastric *Banding System with OMNIFORM Design* *Allergan, www.allergan.com*	Conditional 5	3	
Large Flexible Burr Hole Cover, *Neurosurgery Fixation* *Codman, www.depuysynthes.com*	Safe	1.5	
Large Rigid Burr Hole Cover, Neurosurgery Fixation *Codman, www.depuysynthes.com*	Safe	1.5	
LaryButton *Atos Medical, www.atosmedical.com*	Safe	1.5	
Laryngeal White Umbrella Keel *Hood Laboratories, www.hoodlabs.com*	Safe	1.5, 3	
Laryngoscope Blade, Fiber-Optic *Sun-Flex, MAC 4, 304 SS* *PriMedCo*	Conditional 7	3	
Laryngoscope Blade, Fiber-Optic *Straight, 304 SS* *PriMedCo*	Conditional 7	3	
Laryngoscope Blade Miller 00, LRYM00 *Newmatic Medical, www.newmaticmedical.com*	Conditional 7	3	
Laryngoscope Blade Miller 04, LRYM4 *Newmatic Medical, www.newmaticmedical.com*	Conditional 7	3	

Object	Status	Field Strength (T)	Reference
Laryngoscope Chrome Plated Brass Handle *(Greenline F/O C/P Handle)* *Newmatic Medical, www.newmaticmedical.com*	Conditional 7	3	
Laryngoscope Fiber Optic Blade, Size Mac 2 *Scope Medical Devices, www.scopemedical*	Conditional 7	3	
Laryngoscope Fiber Optic Blade, Size Mac 3 *Scope Medical Devices, www.scopemedical*	Conditional 7	3	
Laryngoscope Fiber Optic Blade, Size Mac 4 *Scope Medical Devices, www.scopemedical*	Conditional 7	3	
Laryngoscope Fiber Optic Blade, Size Mill 1 *Scope Medical Devices, www.scopemedical*	Conditional 7	3	
Laryngoscope Fiber Optic Blade, Size Mill 2 *Scope Medical Devices, www.scopemedical*	Conditional 7	3	
Laryngoscope Fiber Optic Blade, Size Mill 3 *Scope Medical Devices, www.scopemedical*	Conditional 7	3	
Laryngoscope Fiber Optic, Handle Medium Size *Scope Medical Devices, www.scopemedical*	Conditional 7	3	
Laryngoscope Handle Battery Pack, *Plastic Container* *Scope Medical Devices, www.scopemedical.in*	Conditional 7	3	
Laryngoscope Handle, Model 15-MRI-HMED- *Blade - Mac 3, Model 15-MRI-MAC3* *Lithium Battery, Model 15-MRI-L1* *NovaMed, LLC, Rye, New York*	Conditional 7	3	
Laryngoscope Handle, Size Stubby *Scope Medical Devices, www.scopemedical.in*	Conditional 7	3	
Laryngoscope Handle *Size Stubby and Battery, Combined* *Scope Medical Devices, www.scopemedical*	Conditional 7	3	
Laryngoscope Handle, Standard, LRYH *Newmatic Medical, www.newmaticmedical.com*	Conditional 7	3	
LaryTube *Atos Medical, www.atosmedical.com*	Safe	1.5, 3	
Left Atrial Appendage Occlusion System Implant *Coherex Medical, www.coherex.com*	Conditional 5	1.5, 3	
LED Downlight Fixture, MRIDL6VL *Kenall Lighting, Gurnee, Illinois*	Conditional 7	3	
Licox CC1.P1 Oxygen and Temperature Probe *Brain Tissue Oxygen Monitoring System* *Integra NeuroSciences, www.integralife.com*	Conditional 5	1.5	
LifeGuard Safety Infusion Set *ANGIODYNAMICS Inc., Manchester, GA*	Conditional 6	3	

Object	Status	Field Strength (T)	Reference
Lift Treatment of Urinary Stress Incontinence *Cousin Biotech, www.cousin-biotech.com*	Safe	1.5, 3	
Light Source *for Malleable Pediatric Endoscopic Stylet,* *Malleable Pediatric Endoscopic Stylet,* *and Levitan Endoscope* *5197-201 Turbo LED Light Source* *nonmagnetic power source is needed* *Clarus Medical, Golden Valley, MN*	Conditional 7	3	
Lightweight Aluminum Gurney *Newmatic Medical, www.newmaticmedical.com*	Conditional 7	3	
Lineman's Pliers, 200-mm *Newmatic Medical, www.newmaticmedical.com*	Conditional 7	3	
Lineman's Pliers, P-35 *Ampco Safety Tools, www.amcosafetytools.com*	Conditional 7	3	
Linen Hamper 18-inch D-Casters *Newmatic Medical, www.newmaticmedical.com*	Conditional 7	3	
Linen Tag, RFID *Fujitsu WT-A52x UHD RFID Linen Tag* *Fujitsu Frontech North America, www.fujitsu.com*	Conditional 5	1.5, 3	
Linen Tag, RFID *Fujitsu WT-A53x UHD RFID Linen Tag* *Fujitsu Frontech North America, www.fujitsu.com*	Conditional 5	1.5, 3	
LINTRAK C, RFID Tag *Invengo Technologies, www.invengo.com*	Conditional 5	1.5, 3	
LINX Reflux Management System Implant *LINX System* *Note: Two different devices exist, 0.7- and 1.5-T MR* *Conditional Labeling* *Torax Medical, www.toraxmedical.com*	Conditional 5	0.7, 1.5	
Lite Blade *Truphatek International LTD., www.truphatek.com*	Conditional 7	3	
LMA Endoscopy *Teleflex Medical Asia Pte. Ltd., www.teleflex.com*	Safe	1.5, 3	
LMA Fastrach, ETT Size 8 *The Laryngeal Mask Company, Singapore*	Conditional 5	3	
LMA Fastrach Endotracheal Tube *Size 8-mm, endotracheal Tube* *LMA North America, Inc., San Diego, CA*	Conditional 5	1.5	
LMA Classic, Size 5, large adult *, laryngeal mask airway* *LMA North America, Inc., San Diego, CA*	Conditional 5	1.5	
LMA Flexible, Size 6 *The Laryngeal Mask Company, Singapore*	Conditional 5	3	

Object	Status	Field Strength (T)	Reference
LMA Flexible, Size 2, larygeal mask airway *LMA North America, Inc., San Diego, CA*	Conditional 5	1.5	
LMA Flexible (Silicone) *Teleflex, Inc., www.teleflex.com*	Conditional 5	3	
LMA Gastro Cuff Pilot *Teleflex, Inc., www.teleflex.com*	Safe	1.5, 3	
LMA Guardian *Teleflex, Inc., www.teleflex.com*	Safe	1.5, 3	
LMA ProSeal *LMA North America, Inc., San Diego*	Conditional 5	3	
LMA ProSeal, Size 5 *The Laryngeal Mask Company, Singapore*	Conditional 5	1.5	
LMA Protector *Teleflex Medical Asia Pte. Ltd., www.teleflex.com*	Safe	1.5, 3	
LMA Protector Cuff Pilot *Teleflex, Inc., www.teleflex.com*	Safe	1.5, 3	
LMA SureSeal PreCurved with Metallic Spring *Teleflex Medica, www.teleflex.com*	Conditional 6	3	
LMA SureSeal PreCurved *Teleflex Medical, www.teleflex.com*	Safe	1.5, 3	
LMA SureSeal PreCurved with CPV *Teleflex, Inc., www.teleflex.coms*	Safe	1.5, 3	
LMA Supreme, Size 5 *The Laryngeal Mask Company, Singapore*	Conditional 5	3	
LMA Unique (Silicone) with CPV *Teleflex, Inc., www.teleflex.com*	Safe	1.5, 3	
LMA Unique (Silicone Cuff) with CPV *Teleflex, Inc., www.teleflex.com*	Safe	1.5, 3	
LMA WydeGlyde with CPV *Teleflex, Inc., www.teleflex.com*	Safe	1.5, 3	
Lock Rings and Balloon Construct *MicroAire Surgical Instruments LLC, www.microaire.com*	Conditional 5	1.5, 3	
Long Nose Side Cut Pliers, P-326 *Ampco Safety Tools, www.amcosafetytools.com*	Conditional 7	3	
Low Magnetic Signature, Lithium Battery (C Size) *Greatbatch Scientific, Clarence, NY*	Safe	1.5	
Low Magnetic Signature Lithium Battery, *Part # BTRY* *Newmatic Medical, www.newmaticmedical.com*	Conditional 7	3	
LUNA PVO *NFOCUS Neuromedical, Palo Alto, CA*	Conditional 6	3	

Object	Status	Field Strength (T)	Reference
LVIS Device, Low Profile Visualized Intraluminal *Support Device* *Microvention, www.microvention.com*	Conditional 5	3	
Lyoplant Biological Dura Substitute *B. Braun, www.bbraun.com*	Safe	1.5, 3	
Mac 4, 15-MRI-FOD-Mac 4, Plastic, *Laryngoscope Part NovaMed, LLC, Rye, New York*	Conditional 7	3	
Mac 5, 15-MRI-Mac 5, Laryngoscope Part *NovaMed, LLC, Rye, New York*	Conditional 7	3	
Maestro Aria Intraoperative MRI Drill System *Stryker, www.stryker.com*	Conditional 7	3	
Maestro Neuroregulator, Model 1002 *Neurostimulator, Obesity Treatment* *EnteroMedics Inc., www.enteromedics.com*	Unsafe 1	1.5	
Maestro, vBloc Maestro System, vBloc Therapy *Neuromodulation System* *Obesity Treatment* *EnteroMedics Inc., www.enteromedics.com*	Unsafe 1	1.5	
Magill Forceps, Non-magnetic Titanium *EMAREI Ltd. & Co. KG, www.emarei.info/english/*	Conditional 7	3	
Malar Implant, Silicone *Groupe SEBBIN SAS, www.sebbin.com/en/*	Safe	1.5, 3	
Malar Implant, Styles 3, 5, 6 *Implantech Associates, Inc., www.implantech.com*	Safe	1.5, 3	
Mallinckrodt Laser Oral Tracheal Tube, Cuffless *Covidien, www.covidien.com*	Safe	1.5	
Mallinckrodt Laser Oral Tracheal Tub, Dual Cuffed *Covidien, www.covidien.com*	Safe	1.5	
Mallinckrodt Oral/Nasal Tracheal Tube, Cuffless *Covidien, www.covidien.com*	Safe	1.5	
Mallinckrodt Reinforced Endotracheal Tube, Cuffless *Covidien, www.covidien.com*	Safe	1.5	
Mandibular Glove *Implantech Associates, Inc., www.implantech.com*	Safe	1.5, 3	
Manometer, Disposable Manometer Assembly *Mercury Medical, www.mercurymed.com*	Conditional 5	3	
Manometer, NF-121, for mounting on IV pole *AADCO Medical, Inc., Randolph, VT*	Conditional 7	3	
Manual Jet Ventilator (P/N 00-325-MRI) *Anesthesia Associates, Inc., San Marcos, CA*	Conditional 7	3	
Marked Polyamide Epidural Catheter, *19-Gauge, Closed Tip* *B. Braun Medical, Inc., www.bbraunusa.com*	Conditional 8	1.5, 3	

Object	Status	Field Strength (T)	Reference
May Hegar Needle, Holder, Ti6Al-4V *Johnson & Johnson Professional, Inc.,* *www.depuysynthes.com*	Safe	1.5, 3	62
Mayo Stand, MYO-4001-MRI *MAC Medical, Inc., www.macmedical.com*	Conditional 7	3	
Mayo Stand 16-inch x 21-inch *Newmatic Medical, www.newmaticmedical.com*	Conditional 7	3	
Mechanical Ventilator, MR Magellan *Pneumatically Powered, Mechanical Ventilator* *Oceanic Medical Products, Inc., Atchison, KS*	Conditional 7	3	
Medex 3000 Series MRI Syringe Infusion Pump *Medex, Dublin, OH*	Conditional 5	1.5	
Medfusion 3500 Syringe Infusion Pump *Smiths Medical, www.smiths-medical.com*	Conditional 5	1.5	
Medical M Cylinder Hand Cart *Newmatic Medical, www.newmaticmedical.com*	Conditional 7	3	
Medium Handle, 15-MRI-HMED-2 *Laryngoscope part* *NovaMed, LLC, Rye, New York*	Conditional 7	3	
Medium Handle, 15-MRI-HMED-3 *Laryngoscope part* *NovaMed, LLC, Rye, New York*	Conditional 7	3	
Medivance Nasogastric Sump Tube *with YSI Series 400 Temperature Sensor* *Medivance, Inc., Louisville, CO*	Conditional 5	3	
MEDRAD Continuum MR Infusion System *MEDRAD, Inc., Indianola, PA*	Conditional 5	1.5, 3	
Melo-Labial Fold Implant, Small *Implantech Associates, Inc., www.implantech.com*	Safe	1.5, 3	
Mepilex Ag Antimicrobial Dressing *Molnlycke Health Care AB, www.molnlycke.com*	Safe	1.5, 3	
Mepitel Ag with Safetec Technology *Antimicrobial Dressing* *Molnlycke Health Care AB, www.molnlycke.com/us/*	Safe	1.5, 3	
Mepilex Transfer Ag Antimicrobial Dressing *Molnlycke Health Care AB, www.molnlycke.com*	Safe	1.5, 3	
Mepitel Film AM *Molnlycke Health Care AB, www.molnlycke.com*	Safe	1.5, 3	
Merit Peritoneal Dialysis Catheter *Merit Medical Systems, www.merit.com*	Conditional 8	1.5, 3	
Mercury DuoTube-Feeding, Feeding Tube	Safe	1.5	
Mic-Key SF Low Profile Gastronomy Tube *Kimberly Clark Corp., www.kimberly-clark.com*	Conditional 6	3	

Object	Status	Field Strength (T)	Reference
MIC Gastro-Enteric (GE) Enteral Feeding Tube *Halyard Health, www.halyardhealth.com*	Conditional 5	1.5, 3	
MIC Gastric-Jejunal (GJ) Enteral Feeding Tube *Halyard Health, www.halyardhealth.com*	Conditional 5	1.5, 3	
Micro Needle Holder *Greatbatch Scientific, Clarence, NY*	Safe	1.5	
Micro Plug *KA Medical, LLC, Roseville, MN*	Conditional 5	1.5, 3	
Micro Round Handled Scissors *Greatbatch Scientific, Clarence, NY*	Safe	1.5	
Micro Tissue Forceps *Greatbatch Scientific, Clarence, NY*	Safe	1.5	
Micro Tying Forceps *Greatbatch Scientific, Clarence, NY*	Safe	1.5	
Micro Vascular Plug (MVP), Model - MVP5 *Reverse Medical Corporation, www.reversemed.com*	Conditional 5	3	
Mil 4, 15-MRI-FOMD-Mil 4, Laryngoscope Part *NovaMed, LLC, Rye, New York*	Conditional 7	3	
Miller Size 4 Laryngoscope Blade *(Greenline F/O Miller Size 4)* *Newmatic Medical, www.newmaticmedical.com*	Conditional 7	3	
MiniArc Precise Single-Incision Sling System *AMS, American Medical Systems,* *www.americanmedicalsystems.com*	Safe	1.5	
MiniMed 2007, Implantable Insulin Pump *Medtronic, Inc., www.medtronicdiabetes.com*	Unsafe 1	1.5	
MiniMed 407C, Infusion Pump *Medtronic, Inc., www.medtronicdiabetes.com*	Unsafe 1	1.5	
MiniMed 530G System, Insulin Pump *Medtronic, Inc., www.medtronicdiabetes.com*	Unsafe 1	1.5	
MiniMed 508, Insulin Pump *Medtronic, Inc., www.medtronicdiabetes.com*	Unsafe 1	1.5	
MiniMed 640G, Insulin Pump System *Medtronic, Inc., www.medtronicdiabetes.com*	Unsafe 1	1.5	
Mini ONE Balloon Button *Applied Medical Technology, Inc.,* *www.appliedmedical.net*	Conditional 8	1.5, 3	
Mitek anchor *Mitek Products, www.depuysynthes.com*	Safe	1.5	
MitraClip Device *Abbott Vascular Devices, www.abbottvascular.com*	Conditional 5	3	
Mitroflow Valsalva Conduit *Sorin Group, www.sorin.com*	Conditional 6	3	

Object	Status	Field Strength (T)	Reference
Mittelman Pre-Jowl Chin Implant *Implantech Associates, Inc., www.implantech.com*	Safe	1.5, 3	
Mittelman Pre-Jowl Implant *Implantech Associates, Inc., www.implantech.com*	Safe	1.5, 3	
Mobile Lead Acrylic Barrier, NS-602 NF *for use in MRI and Image Guided Therapy* *AADCO Medical, Inc., Randolph, VT*	Conditional 7	3	
Molnlycke Tortoise Turning & Positioning System *Molnlycke Health Care AB, www.molnlycke.com*	Safe	1.5, 3	
Molnlycke Z-Flo Fluidized Positioner *Molnlycke Health Care AB, www.molnlycke.com*	Safe	1.5, 3	
Monarc Subfascial Hammock *AMS, American Medical Systems,* *www.americanmedicalsystems.com*	Safe	1.5	
MONARC System *Edwards Lifesciences* *www.edwards.com*	Conditional 5	3	
Monkey Wrench, 58 x 305-mm *Newmatic Medical, www.newmaticmedical.com*	Conditional 7	3	
MR Bone Punch, Dismantalable *Aesculap, Inc., www.aesculapusa.com*	Safe	1.5	74
MR Compatible Laryngoscope Handle, Short *MINRAD INC., Buffalo, NY*	Conditional 7	3	
MR Compatible Laryngoscope Handle, Standard *MINRAD INC., Buffalo, NY*	Conditional 7	3	
MR Compatible WISCONSIN 4 Laryngoscope Blade *MINRAD INC., Buffalo, NY*	Conditional 7	3	
MR Conditional Disposable EEG *(Electroencephalography) Cup Electrodes* *Rhythmlink, https://rhythmlink.com*	Conditional 5	1.5, 3	
MR Conditional Disposable EEG *(Electroencephalography) Webbed Electrodes* *Rhythmlink, https://rhythmlink.com*	Conditional 5	1.5, 3	
MR Conditional PressOn Electrode, for EEG *Rhythmlink, https://rhythmlink.com*	Conditional 5	1.5, 3	
MR Currette, Curved, 90 degree Blunt Ring *Aesculap, Inc., www.aesculapusa.com*	Safe	1.5	74
MR Brain Spatula with Silicone, Model FF408K *Aesculap AG & CO., Tuttlingen, Germany*	Safe	1.5	83
MRI Conditional Flashlight, FLSH *Newmatic Medical, www.newmaticmedical.com*	Conditional 7	3	
MRI Conditional Pen, Part # MRPEN2 *Newmatic Medical, www.newmaticmedical.com*	Conditional 7	3	

Object	Status	Field Strength (T)	Reference
MRI Conditional Roller Ball Pen, Part # MRPEN1 *Newmatic Medical, www.newmaticmedical.com*	Conditional 7	3	
MRI Disposable Scalpel, Titanium *QSUM Biopsy Disposables LLC, Boulder, CO*	Conditional 7	3	
MRidium 3850 MRI IV Pump *MRidium Corporation, www.iradimed.com*	Conditional 5	3	
MRidium 3860 MRI IV Pump *MRidium Corporation, www.iradimed.com*	Conditional 5	3	
MRI FastSystem Retractor System *Omni-Tract Surgical, Minneapolis, MN*	Safe	1.5	83
MRI Integrated Regulator/Post Valve *on Aluminum Medical D Cylinder* *WOB-p/n 2526-25* *Essex Industries, www.essexindustries.com*	Conditional 7	3	
MRI Integrated Regulator/Post Valve *with Swivel Fitting on Aluminum Medical D Cylinder* *WOB-p/n 2526-25* *Essex Industries, www.essexindustries.com*	Conditional 7	3	
MRI IV Pole, adjustable, NF-110 *AADCO Medical, Inc., Randolph, VT*	Conditional 7	3	
MRI Laryngoscope LED Handle *Newmatic Medical, www.newmaticmedical.com*	Conditional 7	3	
MRI Needle, Inconel *QSUM Biopsy Disposables LLC, Boulder, CO*	Conditional 7	3	
MRI Non-Magnetic 1.5v Dry Cell Battery *Newmatic Medical, www.newmaticmedical.com*	Conditional 7	3	
MRI Walk - O2 - Bout Regulator *The Respiratory Group, www.respiratorygroup.com*	Conditional 7	3	
MRI Wheelchair 18 " wide, NF-500 *AADCO Medical, Inc., Randolph, VT*	Conditional 7	3	
MR-Kocher-Langenbeck Retractor, 70 X 14-mm *Aesculap, Inc., www.aesculapusa.com*	Safe	1.5	74
MR-Mallet with Alloy Handle, 50 grams *Aesculap, Inc., www.aesculapusa.com*	Safe	1.5	74
MR IV Pole *MRidium Corporation, www.iradimed.com*	Conditional 5	3	
MR-Septum Speculum *Aesculap, Inc., www.aesculapusa.com*	Safe	1.5	74
MR Suction Cannula, with Suction Stop *Aesculap, Inc., www.aesculapusa.com*	Safe	1.5	74
MR-Weil-Blakesley Ethmoid Forceps *Aesculap, Inc., www.aesculapusa.com*	Safe	1.5	74

Object	Status	Field Strength (T)	Reference
MR Wheelchair, 26 x 20 DP *Gendron, www.gendroninc.com*	Conditional 7	1.5, 3	
MVP Micro Vascular Plug Mechanical Detachment *Reverse Medical Corporation, www.reversemed.com*	Conditional 6	3	
Nasal Implant, Styles 1 to 12 *Implantech Associates, Inc., www.implantech.com*	Safe	1.5, 3	
Nasal Jejunal Feeding Tube, 10-Fr. *Cook Medical, www.cookmedical.com*	Conditional 8	1.5, 3	
Nasal Septal Button *Hood Laboratories, www.hoodlabs.com*	Safe	3	
Nasal Splint *Hood Laboratories, www.hoodlabs.com*	Safe	3	
Neo-Fit Neonatal Endotracheal Tube Grip/Holder *Cooper Surgical, www.coopersurgical.com*	Conditional 6	3	
Neo-Tee Infant T-Piece Resuscitator *Mercury Medical, www.mercurymed.com*	Conditional 5	3	
NephroMax High Pressure *Nephrostomy Balloon Catheter* *Boston Scientific, www.bostonscientific.com*	Safe	1.5	
Neucrylate, Liquid Embolic System *Valor Medical, www.valormedical.com*	Conditional 8	1.5, 3	122
NeuGuide Anchor *POP Medical Solutions, Tel Aviv, Israel*	Conditional 6	3	
Neulasta OnPro *Amgen, www.amgen.com*	Unsafe 1	1.5	
Neuro Arch *Pulsar Vascular, www.pulsarvascular.com*	Conditional 6	3	
Neuro-Patch Synthetic Dura Substitute *B. Braun, www.bbraun.com*	Safe	1.5	
Neurostimulation System *Activa PC Deep Brain Neurostimulator (Model 37601)* *DBS System* *Medtronic, Inc., www.medtronic.com/mri*	Conditional 5	1.5	
Neurostimulation System *Activa RC Deep Brain Neurostimulator (Model 37612)* *DBS System* *Medtronic, Inc., www.medtronic.com/mri*	Conditional 5	1.5	
Neurostimulation System *Activa SC Deep Brain Neurostimulator (Model 37602)* *DBS System* *Medtronic, Inc., www.medtronic.com/mri*	Conditional 5	1.5	

Object	Status	Field Strength (T)	Reference
Neurostimulation System *Activa SC Deep Brain Neurostimulator (Model 37603)* *DBS System* *Medtronic, Inc., www.medtronic.com/mri*	Conditional 5	1.5	
Neurostimulation System *Axonics Sacral Neuromodulation System* *Axonics Neurostimulator, Model 1101,* *Tined Lead, Model 1201* *Axonics Neuromodulation, www.axonicsmodulation.com*	Conditional 5	1.5, 3	
Neurostimulation System *Deep Brain Stimulation, Activa System* *includes Model 7426 Soletra and Model 7424* *neurostimulators* *Model 3387 and Model 3389 DBS leads* *Medtronic, Inc., www.medtronic.com/mri*	Conditional 5	1.5	79, 80, 100
Neurostimulation System *Deep Brain Stimulation Itrel II* *Medtronic, Inc., www.medtronic.com/mri*	Conditional 5	1.5	99, 101
Neurostimulation System *Deep Brain Stimulation Libra, Libra XP, Brio* *St. Jude Medical, www.sjm.com/MRI*	Unsafe 2	1.5	
Neurostimulation System *Deep Brain Stimulation, Kinetra* *Medtronic, Inc., www.medtronic.com/mri*	Conditional 5	1.5	99, 100
Neurostimulation System *Deep Brain Stimulation, Soletra* *Medtronic, Inc., www.medtronic.com/mri*	Conditional 5	1.5	92, 99
Neurostimulation System *EndoStim Lower Esophagus Stimulation* *(LES) Stimulation System* *EndoStim BV, www.endostim.com*	Conditional 5	1.5	
Neurostimulation System *Enterra Therapy, Gastric Electrical Stimulation* *(GES) System* *Models: Enterra Model 3116, Enterra II Model 37800* *Medtronic, Inc., www.medtronic.com/mri*	Unsafe 2	1.5	
Neurostimulation System *Eon (IPG), Spinal Cord Stimulation System* *St. Jude Medical, www.sjm.com*	Unsafe 1	1.5	
Neurostimulation System *Eon C, Spinal Cord Stimulation System* *St. Jude Medical, www.sjm.com*	Unsafe 1	1.5	
Neurostimulation System *Eon Mini, Spinal Cord Stimulation* *St. Jude Medical, www.sjm.com*	Unsafe 1	1.5	

Object	Status	Field Strength (T)	Reference
Neurostimulation System, External *L3000 Foot Drop System, Must be removed before MRI* *Bioness, www.bioness.com*	Unsafe 1	1.5	
Neurostimulation System, External *L3000 Plus Foot Drop System,* *Must be removed before MRI* *Bioness, www.bioness.com*	Unsafe 1	1.5	
Neurostimulation System, External *H200 Wireless Hand Rehabilitation System* *Must be removed before MRI* *Bioness. www.bioness.com*	Unsafe 1	1.5	
Neurostimulation System *Genesis, Spinal Cord Stimulation* *St. Jude Medical, www.sjm.com*	Unsafe 1	1.5	
Neurostimulation System *GenesisRC, Spinal Cord Stimulation System* *St. Jude Medical, www.sjm.com*	Unsafe 1	1.5	
Neurostimulation System *GenesisXP, Spinal Cord Stimulation System* *St. Jude Medical, www.sjm.com*	Unsafe 1	1.5	
Neurostimulation System *Inspire Upper Airway Stimulation (UAS)* *Inspire Therapy, IPG Model, 3024* *Inspire Medical Systems, Inc.,* *http://manuals.inspiresleep.com/*	Unsafe 1	1.5	
Neurostimulation System *Inspire Upper Airway Stimulation (UAS)* *Inspire Therapy, IPG Model, 3028* *Inspire Medical Systems, Inc.,* *http://manuals.inspiresleep.com/*	Conditional 5	1.5	
Neurostimulation System *InterStim Therapy Sacral Nerve Stimulation* *for Urinary Control* *InterStim Models 3058 and 3023* *Medtronic, Inc., www.medtronic.com/mri*	Conditional 5	1.5	99
Neurostimulation System *InterStim II* *InterStim Models 3058 and 3023* *Medtronic, Inc., www.medtronic.com/mri*	Conditional 5	1.5	
Neurostimulation System *Itrel 4, Models 37703 and 37704* *Spinal Cord Stimulation System* *Medtronic, Inc. www.medtronic.com/mri*	Conditional 5	1.5	

Object	Status	Field Strength (T)	Reference
Neurostimulation System *Neurostep* *Neurostream Technologies,* *www.neurostream-technologies.com*	Unsafe 1	1.5	
Neurostimulation System *NeuRx Diaphragm Pacing System DPS* *Synapse Biomedical, www.synapsebiomedical.com*	Unsafe 1	1.5	
Neurostimulation System *Nevro Senza Spinal Cord Stimulation System* *Nevro Corporation, www.nevrocorp.com*	Conditional 5	1.5, 3	
Neurostimulation System *PrimeAdvanced Spinal Cord Neurostimulator* *PrimeAdvanced, Model 37702* *Medtronic, Inc., www.medtronic.com/mri*	Conditional 5	1.5	
Neurostimulation System *PrimeAdvanced SureScan MRI, Model 97702* *Spinal Cord Stimulation System* *Important Note: This device is a "full-body eligible system"* *if all specific MRI conditions and device requirements are* *carefully followed. Please refer to the labeling documents* *available at www.medtronic.com/mri* *Medtronic, Inc., www.medtronic.com/mri*	Conditional 5	1.5	
Neurostimulation System *Protégé MRI Spinal Cord Stimulation System* *St. Jude Medical, www.sjm.com*	Conditional 5	1.5	
Neurostimulation System *Pulsante SPG (Sphenopalatine Ganglion) Microstimulator* *Autonomic Technologies, Inc., www.ati-spg.com*	Conditional 5	3	
Neurostimulation System *Reclaim Deep Brain Neurostimulator,* *Model 3760 DBS System* *Medtronic, Inc., www.medtronic.com/mri*	Conditional 5	1.5	
Neurostimulation System *Remede' (remede) System* *Respicardia Inc., www.respicardia.com*	Unsafe 1	1.5	
Neurostimulation System *Renew, Spinal Cord Stimulation* *St. Jude Medical, www.sjm.com*	Unsafe 1	1.5	
Neurostimulation System *Renova Cortical Stimulation System* *Northstar Neuroscience, Seattle, WA*	Unsafe 1	1.5	
Neurostimulation System *Responsive Neurostimulation Device, RNS System* *Ncuropace, Inc., www.neuropace.com*	Unsafe 1	1.5	

Object	Status	Field Strength (T)	Reference
Neurostimulation System *RestoreAdvanced Spinal Cord Neurostimulator* *RestoreAdvanced, Model 37713* *Medtronic, Inc., www.medtronic.com/mri*	Conditional 5	1.5	
Neurostimulation System *RestoreAdvanced SureScan MRI, Model 97713* *Spinal Cord Stimulation System* *Important Note: This device is a "full-body eligible system"* *if all specific MRI conditions and device requirements are* *carefully followed. Please refer to the labeling documents* *available at www.medtronic.com/mri* *Medtronic, Inc., www.medtronic.com/mri*	Conditional 5	1.5	
Neurostimulation System *RestoreSensor Spinal Cord Neurostimulator, Model 37714* *Medtronic, Inc., www.medtronic.com/mri*	Conditional 5	1.5	
Neurostimulation System *RestoreSensor SureScan MRI, Model 97714* *Spinal Cord Stimulation System* *Important Note: This device is a "full-body eligible system"* *if all specific MRI conditions and device requirements are* *carefully followed. Please refer to the labeling documents* *available at www.medtronic.com/mri* *Medtronic, Inc., www.medtronic.com/mri*	Conditional 5	1.5	
Neurostimulation System *RestoreUltra Spinal Cord Neurostimulator* *RestoreUltra, Model 37712* *Medtronic, Inc., www.medtronic.com/mri*	Conditional 5	1.5	
Neurostimulation System *RestoreUltra SureScan MRI, Model 97712* *Spinal Cord Stimulation System* *Important Note: This device is a "full-body eligible system"* *if all specific MRI conditions and device requirements are* *carefully followed. Please refer to the labeling documents* *available at www.medtronic.com/mri* *Medtronic, Inc., www.medtronic.com/mri*	Conditional 5	1.5	
Neurostimulation System *Spinal Cord Stimulation, Freedom Spinal Cord Stimulator* *(SCS) System* *Models: FRT4-A001, FRE4-A001* *Stimwave Technologies, Inc., www.stimwave.com*	Conditional 5	1.5, 3	126
Neurostimulation System *Spinal Cord Stimulation* *Freedom-4A Stimulator* *Stimwave Technologies, Inc., www.stimwave.com*	Conditional 5	1.5, 3	

Object	Status	Field Strength (T)	Reference
Neurostimulation System *Spinal Cord Stimulation* *Freedom-8A Stimulator* *Stimwave Technologies, Inc., www.stimwave.com*	Conditional 5	1.5, 3	
Neurostimulation System *Spinal Cord Stimulation, Itrel 3* *Medtronic, Inc., www.medtronic.com/mri*	Conditional 5	1.5	99
Neurostimulation System *Spinal Cord Stimulation, Mattrix* *Medtronic, Inc., www.medtronic.com/mri*	Unsafe 1	1.5	99
Neurostimulation System *Spinal Cord Stimulation, Restore* *Medtronic, Inc., www.medtronic.com/mri*	Conditional 5	1.5	99
Neurostimulation System *Spinal Cord Stimulation (SCS) StimQ* *Peripheral Nerve Stimulator (PNS) System* *Freedom-4A (StimQ) Spare Lead with RF Stylet* *Stimwave Technologies, Inc., www.stimwave.com*	Conditional 5	1.5, 3	
Neurostimulation System *Spinal Cord Stimulation (SCS)* *StimQ Peripheral Nerve Stimulator (PNS) System* *Freedom-4A (StimQ) Stimulator with Receiver* *Stimwave Technologies, Inc., www.stimwave.com*	Conditional 5	1.5, 3	
Neurostimulation System *Spinal Cord Stimulation, Synergy* *Medtronic, Inc., www.medtronic.com/mri*	Conditional 5	1.5	99
Neurostimulation System *Spinal Cord Stimulation, SynergyCompact* *Medtronic, Inc., www.medtronic.com/mri*	Conditional 5	1.5	99
Neurostimulation System *Spinal Cord Stimulation, SynergyPlus* *Medtronic, Inc., www.medtronic.com/mri*	Conditional 5	1.5	99
Neurostimulation System *Spinal Cord Stimulation, Versitrel* *Medtronic, Inc., www.medtronic.com/mri*	Conditional 5	1.5	99
Neurostimulation System *StimRouter Neuromodulation System* *Bioness, www.bioness.com*	Conditional 5	1.5, 3	
Neurotimulation System *Targeted Hypoglossal Neurostimulation* *(THN) Sleep Therapy, aura6000 system* *ImThera Medical Inc. www.imtheramedical.com*	Unsafe 1	1.5	

Object	Status	Field Strength (T)	Reference
Neurostimulation System *Vagus Nerve Stimulation, Vagal Nerve Stimulator* *VNS Therapy, NeuroCybernetic Prosthesis (NCP) System* *Cyberonics, Inc., www.cyberonics..com*	Conditional 5	1.5, 3	
Neurostimulation System *Vercise Deep Brain Stimulation System, DBS System* *Boston Scientific, www.bostonscientific.com*	Unsafe 2	1.5	
NeuroVentriClear, Ventricular Drainage Catheter Set *Cook Medical, Inc., www.cookmedical.com*	Safe	3	
Nexplanon Etonogestrel Implant *Contraceptive Implant* *Merck, www.nexplanon.com*	Safe	1.5, 3	
Nextus/Raz Soft Tissue Anchor, Straight, *Titanium alloy* *AMS, American Medical Systems,* *www.americanmedicalsystems.com*	Safe	3	
Nextus/Raz Soft Tissue Anchor, Curved, *Titanium alloy* *AMS, American Medical Systems,* *www.americanmedicalsystems.com*	Safe	3	
Nit-Occlud ASD-R *PFM S.R.L., www.pfmsrl.com*	Conditional 6	3	
Nitinol Anchor *Hairstetics Ltd, www.hairstetics.com*	Conditional 8	1.5, 3	
Non-Magnetic Adjustable Chair *Newmatic Medical, www.newmaticmedical.com*	Conditional 7	3	
Non-Magnetic Cylinder Cart *Newmatic Medical, www.newmaticmedical.com*	Conditional 7	3	
Non-Magnetic Floor Sweeper, SWPR *Newmatic Medical, www.newmaticmedical.com*	Conditional 7	3	
Non-Magnetic Prism Glasses *Newmatic Medical, www.newmaticmedical.com*	Conditional 7	3	
Non-Magnetic Sprague Rappaport Stethoscope *Newmatic Medical, www.newmaticmedical.com*	Conditional 7	3	
NORPLANT System, Levonorgestrel Implant *Silicone, Birth Control Implant* *Population Council*	Safe	1.5, 3	
NovaSilk, Synthetic Mesh *Coloplast, www.coloplast.com*	Safe	1.5, 3	
Nutriseal Nasogastric Aspiration Tube *Swing Medical Management Ltd., Israel*	Conditional 5	3	
NuvaRing, Contraceptive device *Schering Corporation, Kenilworth, NJ*	Safe	1.5, 3	

Object	Status	Field Strength (T)	Reference
OARtrac System *Prostate Immobilization Device* *Radiadyne, www.radiadyne.com*	Unsafe 1	1.5	
Oasis Chest Drain *Models 001317-302SS, 342135-302SS* *Atrium Medical, www.atriummed.com*	Conditional 7	3	
Oasis Elite, EL218, Positioning/Comfort Pad *Trulife, www.Trulife.com*	Safe	1.5, 3	
Oasis, OA053, Positioning/Comfort Pad *Trulife, www.Trulife.com*	Safe	1.5, 3	
Obalon Gastric Balloon System *Obalon, www.obalon.com*	Conditional 5	3	
Ocean Chest Drain *Models 342135-302SS* *Atrium Medical, www.atriummed.com*	Conditional 7	3	
Occlutech Muscular VSD (mVSD) Occluder *Occlutech Ltd., www.occlutech.com*	Conditional 5	1.5, 3	
Occlutech PLD Paravalvular Leak Device *Occlutech Ltd., www.occlutech.com*	Conditional 5	1.5, 3	
Ohmeda Adapter Diss Male Check Oxy *Ohio Medical Corporation, www.ohiomedical.com*	Conditional 7	3	
Ohmeda Coupler Diss Male Air *Ohio Medical Corporation, www.ohiomedical.com*	Conditional 7	3	
OLM Intracranial Pressure Monitoring Kit *Integra NeuroSciences, www.integralife.com*	Unsafe 1	1.5	
Omega Cuff *CT Resources, Inc.www.ctresources.com*	Conditional 8	1.5, 3	
OmniPod Insulin Management System *Insulin Pump, Controlling device must be removed* *Insulet Corporation, www.myomnipod.com*	Unsafe 1	1.5	
OncoSeed *GE Healthcare, www.gehealthcare.com*	Conditional 6	3	
ON-Q EchoSpark, Echogenic Non-Stimulating Catheter *Halyard Health, www.halyardhealth.com*	Conditional 8	1.5, 3	
ON-Q SilverDressing *I-Flow Corporation, www.iflo.com*	Conditional 6	3	
ON-Q T-Bloc Catheter, Epimed Catheter *Halyard Health and Epimed International,* *www.halyardhealth.com*	Unsafe 1	1.5	
Onyx HD-500 Liquid Embolic System *Covidien and ev3 Inc., www.ev3.net*	Conditional 8	1.5, 3	

Object	Status	Field Strength (T)	Reference
Onyx Liquid Embolic System *Covidien and ev3 Inc., www.ev3.net*	Conditional 8	1.5, 3	
Opti-Flo Tube Attachment Device (T.A.D.) *ConvaTec, www.convatec.com*	Conditional 6	3	
OptiStar Elite MR Contrast Delivery System *Mallinckrodt Pharmaceuticals, www.mallinckrodt.com*	Conditional 5	7	
Optiva (PUR Radiopaque) Intravenous *(I.V.) Catheter* *Smiths Medical, www.smiths-medical.com*	Conditional 6	3	
Optiva 2 (PUR Radiopaque) Intravenous *(I.V.) Catheter* *Smiths Medical, www.smiths-medical.com*	Conditional 6	3	
Optiva W (PUR Radiopaque) Intravenous *(I.V.) Catheter* *Smiths Medical, www.smiths-medical.com*	Conditional 6	3	
OsteoGen Implantable Bone Growth Stimulator *EBI, A Biomet Company, www.biomet.com*	Unsafe 1	1.5	
Oxygen Cylinder Cart, MRI Small Cylinder Cart *MADA Medical Products, Inc., www.madamedical.com*	Conditional 7	3	
OxyTOTE NG, All In One System, *Western MNS-603* *Western Enterprises, Westlake, OH*	Conditional 7	3	
p64 Flow Modulation Device *Phenox, www.phenox.net*	Conditional 5	1.5, 3	
P140 System Implant, HeartNet *Paracor Medical, Inc., Sunnyvale, CA*	Conditional 6	3	
P150 System Implant, HeartNet *Paracor Medical, Inc., Sunnyvale, CA*	Conditional 6	3	
Palatal System Implant Assembly *Pavad Medical, Inc., Fremont, CA*	Conditional 5	1.5	
Palindrome Chronic Catheter *Covidien, www.covidien.com*	Safe	1.5, 3	
Palindrome H Chronic Catheter *Covidien, www.covidien.com*	Safe	1.5, 3	
Palindrome HSI Chronic Catheter *Covidien, www.covidien.com*	Safe	1.5, 3	
Palindrome Precision Chronic Catheter *Covidien, www.covidien.com*	Safe	1.5, 3	
Palindrome Precision H Chronic Catheter *Covidien, www.covidien.com*	Safe	1.5, 3	
Palindrome Precision SI Chronic Catheter *Covidien, www.covidien.com*	Safe	1.5, 3	

Object	Status	Field Strength (T)	Reference
Palindrome SI Chronic Catheter *Covidien, www.covidien.com*	Safe	1.5, 3	
Panje Voice Button *Hood Laboratories, www.hoodlabs.com*	Safe	1.5, 3	
PAS-Port Proximal, Anastomosis System Implant *Cardica and Dextera Surgical, Inc.,* *www.dexterasurgical.com*	Conditional 6	3	
PAS-Port Shaped Implant *Dextera Surgical, www.dexterasurgical.com*	Conditional 5	3	
Patient Scoop, Model 65 EXL *Ferno-Washington, Inc., Wilmington, OH*	Conditional 7	3	
pCANVAS Bifurcation Aneurysm Implant *Phenox, www.phenox.net*	Conditional 5	1.5, 3	
pCONUS Bifurcation Aneurysm Implant *Phenox, www.phenox.net*	Conditional 5	1.5, 3	
Pediatric Tracheostomy Tube *Smiths Medical, www.smiths-medical.com*	Conditional 5	3	
PEDI-TUBE *Pediatric Nasogastric (NG) Feeding Tube* *Covidien, www.covidien.com*	Conditional 6	3	
Peep Valve *Mercury Medical, www.mercurymed.com*	Conditional 5	3	
Peep Valve with Filter *Mercury Medical, www.mercurymed.com*	Conditional 5	3	
Penfield Dissector, 304 SS *Johnson & Johnson Professional, Inc.,* *www.depuysynthes.com*	Safe	1.5	62
Percutaneous Intraspinal Catheter, Model 8516 *Medtronic, Inc., www.medtronic.com/mri*	Unsafe 2	1.5	
Pericardial Patch, Hancock, Model 710 *Medtronic, Inc., www.medtronic.com/mri*	Safe	1.5, 3	84
Pericardial Patch, Hancock, Model 710L *Medtronic, Inc., www.medtronic.com/mri*	Safe	1.5, 3	84
PERIFIX FX Springwound Epidural Catheter *B. Braun Medical, www.bbraunusa.com*	Unsafe 1	1.5	
PERIFIX ONE Marked Polyamide/Polyurethane *Epidural Catheter* *B. Braun Medical, Inc., www.bbraunusa.com*	Conditional 8	1.5, 3	
PERIFIX Polyamide Epidural Catheter *B. Braun Medical, Inc., www.bbraunusa.com*	Conditional 8	1.5, 3	

Object	Status	Field Strength (T)	Reference
Perigee Transobturator Anterior Prolapse *Repair System* *AMS, American Medical Systems,* *www.americanmedicalsystems.com*	Safe	1.5, 3	
Peri-Guard Repair Patch *Synovis Surgical Innovations, www.synovissurgical.com*	Safe	1.5, 3	
Peripheral Nerve Stimulator, MR-STIM, Model GN-013 *Greatbatch Scientific, Clarence, NY*	Safe	1.5	
Peri-Strips Dry with Veritas Collagen Matrix *Synovis Surgical Innovations, www.synovissurgical.com*	Safe	1.5, 3	
Peri-Pyriform Facial Implant *Implantech Associates, Inc., www.implantech.com*	Safe	1.5, 3	
Phillips Screwdriver, 200-mm *Newmatic Medical, www.newmaticmedical.com*	Conditional 7	3	
Piramal Critical Care-Minrad Mac 1 Blade *Truphatek International LTD., www.truphatek.com*	Unsafe 1	1.5	
Piramal Critical Care-Minrad. Medium Handle *Truphatek International LTD., www.truphatek.com*	Conditional 7	3	
PillCam, All models *Given Imaging, www.givenimaging.com*	Unsafe 1	1.5	
PillCam Colon2 Capsule Endoscopy *Given Imaging, www.givenimaging.com*	Unsafe 1	1.5	
PillCam M2A Capsule Endoscopy Device *Ingestible Capsule* *Given Imaging, www.givenimaging.com*	Unsafe 1	1.5	
PillCam ESO Capsule Endoscopy Device *Ingestible Capsule* *Given Imaging, www.givenimaging.com*	Unsafe 1	1.5	
PillCam ESO2 Capsule Endoscopy Device *Ingestible Capsule* *Given Imaging, www.givenimaging.com*	Unsafe 1	1.5	
PillCam Patency Capsule *Given Imaging, www.givenimaging.com*	Unsafe 1	1.5	
PillCam SB Capsule Endoscopy Device *Ingestible Capsule* *Given Imaging, www.givenimaging.com*	Unsafe 1	1.5	
PillCam SB2 Capsule Endoscopy Device *Ingestible Capsule* *Given Imaging, www.givenimaging.com*	Unsafe 1	1.5	
PillCam Patency Capsule Endoscopy Device *Given Imaging, www.givenimaging.com*	Unsafe 1	1.5	
Pinnacle Pelvic Floor Repair (PFR) Kit *Boston Scientific, www.bostonscientific.com*	Safe	1.5	

Object	Status	Field Strength (T)	Reference
Pipe Wrench, 50-mm *Newmatic Medical, www.newmaticmedical.com*	Conditional 7	3	
Plastic Interstitial Needles *Varian Medical Systems, www.varian.com*	Conditional 8	1.5, 3	
PliCath HF Cardiac Implant *BioVentrix, www.bioventrix.com*	Conditional 5	1.5, 3	
PneumRx Lung Volume Reduction Coil (LVRC) *PneumRx, Inc., www.pneumrx.com*	Conditional 6	3	
Pneupac babyPAC, Mechanical Ventilation *Smiths Medical, www.smiths-medical.com*	Conditional 5	1.5, 3	
Pneupac paraPAC, Mechanical Ventilation *Smiths Medical, www.smiths-medical.com*	Conditional 5	1.5, 3	
Pneupac ventiPAC, Mechanical Ventilation *Smiths Medical, www.smiths-medical.com*	Conditional 5	1.5, 3	
Pneupac VR1, Mechanical Ventilation *Smiths Medical, www.smiths-medical.com*	Conditional 5	1.5, 3	
pNeuton Mini Infant Ventilator *Airon Corporation, aironusa.com*	Conditional 7	3	
Polyform Mesh, Polypropylene *Boston Scientific, www.bostonscientific.com*	Safe	1.5	
Polyform Synthetic Mesh *Boston Scientific, www.bostonscientific.com*	Safe	1.5	
Polyurethane Flange *Biodesign Enterocutaneous Fistula Plug* *Cook Medical, Inc., www.cookmedical.com*	Conditional 6	3	
Ponto Wide Implant, Used With *Bone Conduction Hearing System* *Oticon Medical, www.oticonmedical.com*	Conditional 6	3	
PorousTi Family of Implants *OBL Paris, Materialise Medical, www.materialise.com*	Conditional 8	1.5, 3	
Port Delivery System (PDS) Implant *Forsight Vision, Menlo Park, CA*	Conditional 6	3	
Portex Bivona Flextend Tracheostomy Tube *All similar products* *Tracheostomy* *Smiths Medical International, England*	Conditional 6	3	
Portex Bivona Laryngectomy Tube, *All similar products* *Smiths Medical International, England*	Safe	3	

Object	Status	Field Strength (T)	Reference
Portex Bivona Non-Wire *Reinforced Cuffed Tracheostomy Tube* *All similar products* *Tracheostomy* *Smiths Medical International, England*	Conditional 6	3	
Portex Bivona Neonatal Tracheostomy Tube *Smiths Medical, www.smiths-medical.com*	Conditional 5	3	
Portex Bivona Sleep Apoea (Apnea) Tube *All similar products, Sleep Apoea (Apnea) Tube* *Smiths Medical International, England*	Safe	3	
Portex Bivona Uncuffed *Non-Reinforced Endotracheal Tube* *All similar products* *Smiths Medical International, England*	Safe	3	
Portex Bivona Uncuffed *Non-Wire Reinforced Tracheostomy Tube* *All similar products, Tracheostomy* *Smiths Medical International, England*	Safe	3	
Portex Bivona Wire, Reinforced Endotracheal Tube *All similar products, Endotracheal* *Smiths Medical International, England*	Conditional 6	3	
Portex Bivona Wire, Reinforced *Tracheostomy Tube, All similar products* *Smiths Medical International, England*	Conditional 6	3	
Portex Cricothyroidotomy Tube *Cricothyroidotomy* *Smiths Medical International, England*	Conditional 6	3	
Portex Cuffed Endotracheal Tube *All similar products* *Smiths Medical International, England*	Conditional 6	3	
Portex Guedel Airway *Airway, All similar products* *Smiths Medical International, England*	Safe	3	
Portex Heat and Moisture Exchanger *All similar products* *Smiths Medical International, England*	Safe	3	
Portex Mini-Trach, Tracheostomy *Smiths Medical International, England*	Safe	3	
Portex Nasal Oxygen Set *All similar products, Nasal Oxygen Set* *Smiths Medical International, England*	Safe	3	

Object	Status	Field Strength (T)	Reference
Portex Non-Wire Reinforced Cuffed	Conditional 6	3	
Tracheostomy Tube			
All similar products			
Tracheostomy			
Smiths Medical International, England			
Portex Orator Speaking Valve	Safe	3	
All similar products, Speaking Valve			
Smiths Medical International, England			
Portex Tracheal Tube Holder	Safe	3	
All similar products, Endotracheal Tube Holder			
Smiths Medical International, England			
Portex Uncuffed Non-Wire Reinforced Endotracheal Tube	Safe	3	
All similar products, Endotracheal			
Smiths Medical International, England			
Portex Uncuffed Non-reinforced Tracheostomy Tube	Safe	3	
All similar products			
Tracheostomy			
Smiths Medical International, England			
Portex, UniPerc Tracheostomy Tube	Conditional 5	3	
Tracheostomy			
Smiths Medical			
www.smiths-medical.com			
Portex Wire Reinforced Endotracheal Tube	Conditional 6	3	
All similar products			
Smiths Medical International, England			
PortIO, Intraosseous Infusion Device	Conditional 8	1.5, 3	
PAVmed, Inc., www.pavm.com			
Posterior Mandibular Angle Implant	Safe	1.5, 3	
Implantech Associates, Inc., www.implantech.com			
Post Craniotomy Subdural Pressure Monitoring Kit	Unsafe 1	1.5	
Integra NeuroSciences, www.integralife.com			
Post Valve and Aluminum E Cylinder	Conditional 7	3	
PX-8703-1CW			
Western Scott Fetzer, Inc., Westlake, OH			
Post Valve, MPV-5870	Conditional 7	3	
Western Scott Fetzer, Inc., Westlake, OH			
Pouchkins, Newborn Ostomy Pouch	Conditional 8	1.5, 3	
Hollister Incorporated, www.hollister.com/en			
PPS Quick Safety Huber Needle	Conditional 6	3	
Perouse Medical.com, www.perousemedical.com			
Precision Montage MRI Spinal Cord Stimulation	Conditional 5	1.5	
(SCS) System			
Boston Scientific, www.bostonscientific.com			

Object	Status	Field Strength (T)	Reference
Precision Plus Spinal Cord Stimulation *(SCS) System, Neurostimulation System* *Boston Scientific, www.bostonscientific.com*	Unsafe 1	1.5	
Precision Spectra Spinal Cord Stimulator *(SCS) System, Neurostimulation System* *Boston Scientific, www.bostonscientific.com*	Conditional 5	1.5	
Premier Closed Pouch with Filter *Hollister Incorporated, www.hollister.com/en*	Safe	1.5, 3	
Premium Lightweight Polypropylene Implant *Cousin Biotech, www.cousin-biotech.com*	Safe	1.5, 3	
PREVAIL Paragastric Implant System *Vibrynt Inc., www.vibrynt.com*	Conditional 6	3	
ProAct, Male Adjustable Continence Therapy *Uromedica Inc., www.uromedica-inc.com*	Conditional 6	3	
Procellera Antimicrobial Wound Dressing *Bioelectric, antimicrobial device* *Vomaris, Inc., www.vomaris.com*	Unsafe 1	1.5	
Pro Pierce Safety Huber Needle Infusion Set *Medcomp, www.medcompnet.com*	Conditional 6	3	
Protectiv (FEP Radiopaque) Intravenous *(I.V.) Catheter* *Smiths Medical, www.smiths-medical.com*	Safe	3	
Protectiv Acuvance 2 (PUR Radiopaque) *Intravenous (I.V.) Catheter* *Smiths Medical, www.smiths-medical.com*	Safe	3	
Protectiv Jelco (FEP Radiopaque) Intravenous *(I.V.) Catheter* *Smiths Medical, www.smiths-medical.com*	Safe	3	
Protectiv Plus (PUR Radiopaque) Intravenous *(I.V.) Catheter* *Smiths Medical, www.smiths-medical.com*	Safe	3	
Protectiv Plus W (PUR Radiopaque) Intravenous *(I.V.) Catheter* *Smiths Medical, www.smiths-medical.com*	Safe	3	
Protectiv W (FEP Radiopaque) Intravenous *(I.V.) Catheter* *Smiths Medical, www.smiths-medical.com*	Safe	3	
Provox 1 Voice Prosthesis *Atos Medical, www.atosmedical.com*	Safe	1.5	
Provox 2 Voice Prosthesis *Atos Medical, www.atosmedical.com*	Safe	1.5	
Provox ActiValve *Atos Medical, www.atosmedical.com*	Unsafe 1	1.5	

Object	Status	Field Strength (T)	Reference
Provox Adhesive, *Flexiderm, Optiderm, Regular, XtraBase* *Atos Medical, www.atosmedical.com*	Safe	1.5	
Provox BasePlate Adaptor *Atos Medical, www.atosmedical.com*	Safe	1.5	
Provox HME Cassettes *Atos Medical, www.atosmedical.com*	Safe	1.5	
Provox HME Compact *Atos Medical, www.atosmedical.com*	Safe	1.5	
Provox HME *Atos Medical, www.atosmedical.com*	Safe	1.5	
Provox Indwelling Voice Prostheses *Atos Medical, www.atosmedical.com*	Safe	1.5	
Provox LaryClip *Atos Medical, www.atosmedical.com*	Safe	1.5	
Provox Micron HME *Atos Medical, www.atosmedical.com*	Safe	1.5	
Provox NID, Non-indwelling Voice Prosthesis *Atos Medical, www.atosmedical.com*	Safe	1.5	
Provox Stom Vent *Atos Medical, www.atosmedical.com*	Safe	1.5	
Provox Trach-HME *Atos Medical, www.atosmedical.com*	Safe	1.5	
Provox Vega Voice Prosthesis *Atos Medical, www.atosmedical.com*	Safe	1.5	
Provox Voice Prosthesis *Atos Medical, www.atosmedical.com*	Safe	1.5	
Provox XtraFlow HME *Atos Medical, www.atosmedical.com*	Safe	1.5	
Provox XtraHME *Atos Medical, www.atosmedical.com*	Safe	1.5	
Provox XtraMoist HME *Atos Medical, www.atosmedical.com*	Safe	1.5	
PulseRider Implant *Pulsar Vascular and Codman, www.pulsarvascular.com*	Conditional 5	1.5, 3	
Putty Knife, 40 x 200-mm *Newmatic Medical, www.newmaticmedical.com*	Conditional 7	3	
Putty Knife, K-20 *Ampco Safety Tools, www.amcosafetytools.com*	Conditional 7	3	
Putty Knife, Wooden Handle *NGK Metals Corporation, Sweetwater, TN*	Conditional 7	3	

Object	Status	Field Strength (T)	Reference
PVC Sling Bariatric Gurney *Newmatic Medical, www.newmaticmedical.com*	Conditional 7	3	
Quick Connect Ergo Adjustable Handle, *FGQ760000000* *Rubbermaid, www.rubbermaidhealthcare.com*	Conditional 7	3	
Quick Connect Flexible Dusting Wand *with Microfiber Sleeve, FGQ85000BK00* *Rubbermaid, www.rubbermaidhealthcare.com*	Conditional 7	3	
Qora AIM Stool Management System *Consure Medical, www.consuremedical.com*	Conditional 8	1.5, 3	
Radiopaque T-Tubes *Hood Laboratories, www.hoodlabs.com*	Safe	1.5, 3	
RapidFlap LS, Resorbable Cranial Flap Fixation *Biomet Microfixation, www. www.lorenzsurgical.com*	Safe	1.5, 3	
Ratchet Wrench, 3/4" x 320-mm *Newmatic Medical, www.newmaticmedical.com*	Conditional 7	3	
Realize Adjustable Gastric Band *also known as Swedish Adjustable Gastric Band* *Ethicon, www.ethicon.com*	Conditional 5	3	
REALIZE Adjustable Gastric Band-C *Ethicon, www.ethicon.com*	Conditional 5	3	
Rebound HRD, Hernia Repair Device, Nitinol *Minnesota Medical, Plymouth, MN*	Conditional 6	3	
Reducing Diameter T-Tube *Hood Laboratories, www.hoodlabs.com*	Safe	1.5, 3	
Regulator and Aluminum Cylinder System *AirTOTE, MTS-303* *Western Scott Fetzer, Inc., Westlake, OH*	Conditional 7	3	
Regulator and Aluminum Cylinder System *OxyTOTE, MTS-603* *Western Scott Fetzer, Inc., Westlake, OH*	Conditional 7	3	
Regulator and Aluminum Cylinder System *OxyTOTE, MTS-803* *Western Scott Fetzer, Inc., Westlake, OH*	Conditional 7	3	
Regulator and Aluminum Cylinder System *PediaTOTE, MTS-103* *Western Scott Fetzer, Inc., Westlake, OH*	Conditional 7	3	
Regulator, NMR-540-15FM *Western Scott Fetzer, Inc., Westlake, OH*	Conditional 7	3	
Regulator, NMR-870-15FM *Western Scott Fetzer, Inc., Westlake, OH*	Conditional 7	3	
Regulator, NMR-870-P *Western Scott Fetzer, Inc., Westlake, OH*	Conditional 7	3	

Object	Status	Field Strength (T)	Reference
Regulator, Western NMR-870-15FM *MR Conditional Regulator on* *Aluminum M6A cylinder* *Western Enterprises, Westlake, OH*	Conditional 7	3	
Regulator, Western NMR-870-15FM *MR Conditional Regulator with non-conforming* *G-2-4000N inlet gauge on Aluminum M6A cylinder* *Western Enterprises, Westlake, OH*	Conditional 7	3	
Regulator, Western NMR-540-15FM *MR Conditional Regulator with non-conforming* *G-2-4000N inlet gauge on Aluminum M6A cylinder* *Western Enterprises, Westlake, OH*	Conditional 7	3	
Relieva Stratus Microflow Spacer *Acclarent, Inc., Menlo Park, CA*	Conditional 6	3	
RePneu Coil, Lung Volume Reduction Coil *PneumRx, Inc., www.pneumrx.com*	Conditional 8	1.5, 3	
Repliform Tissue Regeneration Matrix *Boston Scientific, www.bostonscientific.com*	Safe	1.5, 3	
ReSolve Biliary Drainage Catheter *Merit Medical, www.merit.com*	Conditional 6	3	
RespiCardia System *neurostimulation system* *phrenic nerve stimulator* *Cardiac Concepts, Inc., www.cardiacconcepts.com*	Unsafe 1	1.5	
Revision Vascular Reconstruction Device (RVRD), *Model - RVRD-4580* *Reverse Medical Corporation, www.reversemed.com*	Conditional 5	3	
RF BION Microstimulator *Neurostimulation System* *Alfred E. Mann Foundation for Scientific Research,* *Valencia, CA*	Conditional 5	1.5	89
RFID Tag, WT-A533 UHF RFID Tag for Linens *MRI information applies to Fujitsu WT-A53x UHD RFID* *Linen Tag and Fujitsu WT-A52x UHD RFID Linen Tag* *Fujitsu Frontech North America, www.fujitsu.com*	Conditional 5	1.5, 3	
Rheos Baroreflex System *Rheos Hypertension (HT) Therapy* *CVRx Inc., www.cvrx.com*	Unsafe 1	1.5	
Rizzo Dorsal Nasal Implant *Implantech Associates, Inc., www.implantech.com*	Safe	1.5, 3	
Robotic Radiosurgery Tumor Marking Seed *Tumor marking device* *RADONTEK LTD., Ankara, Turkey*	Conditional 6	3	

Object	Status	Field Strength (T)	Reference
Rosch-Uchida Transjugular Liver Access Set *Cook Medical, www.cookmedical.com*	Unsafe 2	1.5	
Round Wire Brush, B-399 *Ampco Safety Tools, www.amcosafetytools.com*	Conditional 7	3	
Rusch Larygoscope Handle *Teleflex Medical, Durham, NC*	Conditional 7	3	
Rusch Macintosh Size 4 *Fiber-optic Laryngoscope Blade* *Teleflex Medical, Durham, NC*	Conditional 7	3	
S-3 Implant *Javelin Medical LTD., www.javelin-mrp.com/medical*	Conditional 8	1.5, 3	
S-ICD System, Subcutaneous Implantable *Cardioverter Defibrillator* *Boston Scientific, www.bostonscientific.com*	Unsafe 1	1.5	
Sacromesh Mesh for Sacrocolpopexy *Cousin Biotech, www.cousin-biotech.com*	Safe	1.5, 3	
Salivary Bypass Tube *Hood Laboratories, www.hoodlabs.com*	Safe	1.5, 3	
SAM Sling *SAM Medical Products, www.sammedical.com*	Conditional 6	3	
SAM Splint, Large *SAM Medical Products, www.sammedical.com*	Conditional 5	1.5, 3	
Sancuso, Granisetron Transdermal System *Transdermal Patch* *ProStrakan*	Safe	1.5	
Sand bag *12 pound, Vinyl Silica Sand Bag* *Newmatic Medical Systems, Inc.*	Conditional 7	3	
Scalpel, Microsharp Ceramic Scalpels, *Sizes #10, #11, #11c, #15* *MicroSurgical Techniques, Inc., Fort Collins, CO*	Safe	1.5	48
Scalpel, SS	Unsafe 1	1.5	
Schaitkin Salivary Duct Cannula *Hood Laboratories, www.hoodlabs.com*	Safe	1.5, 3	
Scissors, Ceramic *Microsurgical Techniques, Inc., Fort Collins, CO*	Safe	1.5	48
Scissors, 225-mm *Newmatic Medical, www.newmaticmedical.com*	Conditional 7	3	
SCRAM Continuous Alcohol Monitoring (CAM) *SCRAM Systems, www.scramsystems.com*	Unsafe 1	1.5	
Scraper, S-10G *Ampco Safety Tools, www.amcosafetytools.com*	Conditional 7	3	

Object	Status	Field Strength (T)	Reference
Screw Driver, Phillips, S-1099A *Ampco Safety Tools, www.amcosafetytools.com*	Conditional 7	3	
Screw Driver, Slot, Flat Head *NGK Metals Corporation, Sweetwater, TN*	Conditional 7	3	
Screw Driver, Standard, S-49 *Ampco Safety Tools, www.amcosafetytools.com*	Conditional 7	3	
Screw, Titanium alloy *Bioplate, Inc., Los Angeles, CA*	Conditional 6	3	
SecurAcath Universal Version *Interrad Medical, Inc., St. Paul, MN*	Conditional 6	3	
SecurAcath Universal Version 1.1 *Interrad Medical, Inc., St. Paul, MN*	Conditional 6	3	
SENSIMED Triggerfish, *Intraocular Pressure Monitor* *Sensimed, www.sensimed.ch*	Unsafe 1	1.5	
SERVO-i Ventilator, MRI Version *Maquet, Inc., www.maquet.com*	Conditional 5	1.5, 3	
Seven System Continuous Glucose *Monitoring System* *DexCom, Inc., San Diego, CA*	Unsafe 1	1.5	
ShapeLoc Soft Tissue Fastener *MedShape Solutions, Inc., Atlanta, GA*	Conditional 6	3	
Shelhigh Injectable Pulmonic Valve *Shelhigh Inc., Union, NJ*	Conditional 6	3	
Sherwood Post-Valve *Praxair, Inc., www.praxair.com*	Conditional 7	3	
Shirakabe Nasal Implant *Implantech Associates, Inc., www.implantech.com*	Safe	1.5, 3	
Shoe Handle Wire-brush, 4 x 17 rows *NGK Metals Corporation, Sweetwater, TN*	Conditional 7	3	
Side Cutting Pliers, P-36 *Ampco Safety Tools, www.amcosafetytools.com*	Conditional 7	3	
Silicone Block *Implantech Associates, Inc., www.implantech.com*	Safe	1.5, 3	
Silver Graft Helix Vascular Prosthesis *B. Braun, www.bbraunusa.com*	Conditional 5	1.5, 3	
Silver Graft Vascular Graft *B. Braun, www.bbraun.com*	Conditional 5	1.5, 3	
Silver Nitrate Coated Pleural Catheter *CareFusion, www.carefusion.com*	Safe	1.5, 3	
SilverSite Access Site Dressing, 4-mm opening *Tri-State Hospital Supply Corporation, Howell, MI*	Conditional 6	3	

Object	Status	Field Strength (T)	Reference
Silver Stump Shrinker *Juzo Silver* *Juzo, www.juzo.com*	Unsafe 1	1.5	
Single PVC Hamper Cart *Newmatic Medical, www.newmaticmedical.com*	Conditional 7	3	
Skyla Intrauterine Device, IUD *Bayer, www.bayer.com*	Conditional 5	3	
Slimband Adjustable Gastric Banding *Cousin Biotech, www.cousin-biotech.com*	Safe	1.5, 3	
Slim Lite *Truphatek International LTD., www.truphatek.com*	Conditional 7	3	
Slot Screwdriver, 11 x 300-mm *Newmatic Medical, www.newmaticmedical.com*	Conditional 7	3	
Slot Screwdriver, 3 x 50-mm *Newmatic Medical, www.newmaticmedical.com*	Conditional 7	3	
Smartpatch MicroLead Percutaneous Lead, *Fragmented* *NDI Medical, www.ndimedical.com*	Conditional 5	1.5, 3	
Snowshoe Suture Anchor Pair *USGI Medical, Inc., www.usgimedical.com*	Conditional 8	1.5, 3	
Soft Lift Treatment of Urinary Stress Incontinence *Cousin Biotech, www.cousin-biotech.com*	Safe	1.5, 3	
Solyx SIS, Single Incision Sling System *Boston Scientific, www.bostonscientific.com*	Safe	1.5, 3	
SONIC Micro-Catheter *Balt, www.balt.fr/en*	Unsafe 1	1.5	
Space Station MRI *B. Braun, www.bbraun.com*	Conditional 5	1.5, 3	
SPARC Sling System *AMS, American Medical Systems,* *www.americanmedicalsystems.com*	Safe	1.5, 3	
Spectris MR Injection System *Medrad, Inc., Indianola, PA*	Conditional 5	1.5, 3	
Spetzler Lumbar-Peritoneal Shunt System, *Spetzler Lumbar-Peritoneal (LP) Kit* *Integra LifeSciences Corporation, www.Integralife.com*	Conditional 5	1.5, 3	
Spiegelberg System Bolt, SS *Aesculap, Inc., www.aesculapusa.com*	Safe	1.5, 3	83
Spine Fusion Stimulator, SpF PLUS-Mini *Biomet, www.biomet.com*	Conditional 5	1.5	
Spine Fusion Stimulator, SpF-XL IIb *Biomet, www.biomet.com*	Conditional 5	1.5	

Object	Status	Field Strength (T)	Reference
Spirol Continuous Peripheral Nerve Block Catheter *Halyard Health and Epimed International,* *www.halyardhealth.com*	Unsafe 1	1.5	
Sponge Forcep, Ti6Al-4V *Johnson & Johnson Professional, Inc.,* *www.depuysynthes.com*	Safe	1.5	62
Sprinkler, Model F4FR-NF *Non-Ferrous Quick Response Concealed Automatic* *Sprinkler for MRI Type Applications* *The Reliable Automatic Sprinkler Co., Inc., Elmsford, NY*	Conditional 7	3	
Spirol Continuous Peripheral Nerve Block Catheter *Halyard Health and Epimed International,* *www.halyardhealth.com*	Unsafe 1	1.5	
Stainless Steel Laryngectomy Tube *Premier Medical Products, www.premusa.com*	Unsafe 1	1.5	
Stainless Steel Tracheal Tube *Premier Medical Products, www.premusa.com*	Unsafe 1	1.5	
Standard G-Tube with PG-Lock Connectors *Xeridiem, www.xeridiem.com*	Conditional 6	3	
StarClose SE Vascular Closure System *Abbott Vascular, www.abbottvascular.com*	Conditional 5	3	
StarClose Vascular Closure System *Abbott Vascular, www.abbottvascular.com*	Conditional 5	3	
Step Stool, STS-241616-2SMRI *MAC Medical, Inc., www.macmedical.com*	Conditional 7	3	
Sternum Band *Johnson & Johnson, www.depuysynthes.com*	Conditional 8	1.5, 3	
Stereotactic Headframe with Removable Mouthpiece *Compass International, Inc., Rochester, MN*	Safe	1.5	
Stool, Foot Stool, 7445MR-C *Blickman, Inc., www.blickman.com*	Conditional 7	3	
Stool, Foot Stool, 7757MR *Blickman, Inc., www.blickman.com*	Conditional 7	3	
Stool, Foot Stool, No Frame, 7757MR *Blickman, Inc., www.blickman.com*	Conditional 7	3	
Stool Management, Bard DigniShield *Stool Management System* *Bard Medical, www.bardmedical.com*	Conditional 7	3	
Stool, Step Stool with Handrail *Newmatic Medical, www.newmaticmedical.com*	Conditional 7	3	
Storage Cart *Starsys Single Wide Non-Locking Cart for MRI* *InterMetro Industries Corp., Wilkes-Barre, PA*	Conditional 7	3	

Object	Status	Field Strength (T)	Reference
Straight-In Sacral Colpopexy System *AMS, American Medical Systems,* *www.americanmedicalsystems.com*	Safe	1.5, 3	
Stretcher, 35-XNM Cot/Gurney *Ferno Washington, Inc., www.ferno.com*	Conditional 7	3	
Stretcher, 1000 MR *Gendron, Inc., Archbold, OH*	Conditional 7	3	
Stryker PainPump 2 Infusion Pump *Stryker Instruments, www.stryker.com*	Unsafe 1	1.5	
Stryker PainPump Infusion Pump *Stryker Instruments, www.stryker.com*	Unsafe 1	1.5	
Subcutaneous Evacuating Port System, SEPS *Medtronic, Inc., www.medtronic.com/mri*	Unsafe 1	1.5	
Suction/Irrigation Handle for Sinuscope *Greatbatch Scientific, Clarence, NY*	Safe	1.5, 3	
Suction Regulator, Model Number 881VR *Genstar Technologies Co., Inc., Chino, CA*	Conditional 7	3	
Super ArrowFlex PSI *10 Fr. x 65-cm* *304V SS* *Arrow International Inc., Reading, PA*	Unsafe 2	1.5	
Super ArrowFlex PSI *9 Fr. x 11-cm* *304 V SS* *Arrow International Inc., Reading, PA*	Unsafe 2	1.5	
Supple Peri-Guard Repair Patch *Synovis Surgical Innovations, www.synovissurgical.com*	Safe	1.5, 3	
SUPPRELIN Long Acting (LA) Implant *Endo Pharmaceuticals, www.supprelinla.com*	Safe	1.5, 3	
Supris, Suprapubic Mesh Sling *Coloplast, www.coloplast.com*	Safe	3	
Surecan Needle *B. Braun, www.bbraunusa.com*	Conditional 5	1.5, 3	
Surecan Safety II, Safety Needle *B. Braun, www.bbraunusa.com*	Conditional 6	3	
SureConnect Patient Connector *Baxa Corporation, Englewood, CO*	Conditional 5	3	
Swedish Adjustable Gastric Band (SAGB) *Ethicon, Inc., www.ethicon.com*	Safe	1.5, 3	
Symphony, Counter Pulsation *Device for Heart Failure Patient* *Abiomed, Inc., Danvers, MA*	Conditional 5	3	

Object	Status	Field Strength (T)	Reference
Symphony Glucose Monitoring System *Echo Therapeutics, www.echotx.com*	Unsafe 1	1.5	
SynchroMed Implantable Drug Infusion System *Medtronic, Inc., www.medtronic.com/mri*	Conditional 5	1.5, 3	
SynchroMed EL Implantable Drug Infusion System *Medtronic, Inc., www.medtronic.com/mri*	Conditional 5	1.5, 3	
SynchroMed II Implantable Drug Infusion System *Medtronic, Inc., www.medtronic.com/mri*	Conditional 5	1.5, 3	
T07 Stentless Valved Pulmonary Conduit *Labcor Laboratorios Ltda., www.labcor.com*	Safe	1.5, 3	
T12 Tack, Tack Endovascular System *Intact Vascular, Inc., www.intactvascular.com*	Conditional 8	1.5, 3	
Table Model Mercury Blood Pressure Manometer *Table model* *NF-120* *AADCO Medical, Inc., Randolph, VT*	Conditional 7	3	
Tantalum powder	Safe	1.5	
Tape Mechanical Occlusive Device (TMOD) *Implantable Artificial Urinary Sphincter* *GT Urological, Minneapolis, MN*	Conditional 7	3	
Taylor Lateral Mandibular Angle Implant *Implantech Associates, Inc., www.implantech.com*	Safe	1.5, 3	
Tears Naturale Port Punctal Occluder *Alcon, www.alcon.com*	Safe	1.5	
Telemetric ICP (Intracranial Pressure) Sensor Probe *Neckarate GmbH & Co KG, www.neckarate.com*	Unsafe 1	1.5	
Tellez Nasal Splint *Hood Laboratories, www.hoodlabs.com*	Safe	1.5, 3	
Temporal Shell Implant *Implantech Associates, Inc., www.implantech.com*	Safe	1.5, 3	
Terino Extended Anatomical Chin Implant *Implantech Associates, Inc., www.implantech.com*	Safe	1.5, 3	
Terino Shell Implant *Implantech Associates, Inc., www.implantech.com*	Safe	1.5, 3	
Terino Square Chin, Style I *Implantech Associates, Inc., www.implantech.com*	Safe	1.5, 3	
Terino Square Chin, Style II *Implantech Associates, Inc., www.implantech.com*	Safe	1.5, 3	
Terino Vertical Chin Implant *Implantech Associates, Inc., www.implantech.com*	Safe	1.5, 3	
Testicular Prosthesis, Implant, Gel-filled *Coloplast, www.coloplast.com*	Safe	3	

Object	Status	Field Strength (T)	Reference
Testicular Prosthesis, Implant, Saline-filled *Coloplast, www.coloplast.com MR*	Safe	3	
Testicular Prosthesis, Implant, Torosa *Coloplast, www.coloplast.com*	Safe	3	
TESTOPEL, Testosterone Pellet *Endo Pharmaceuticals, www.testopel.com*	Safe	1.5, 3	
TheraCath, 304 V SS *Arrow International Inc., Reading, PA*	Unsafe 2	1.5	
TheraSeed, Model 200 Pd-103, Brachytherapy Seed *Theragenics Corporation, www.theragenics.com*	Conditional 8	1.5, 3	
TheraSeed Radioactive Seed Implant *Theragenics Corporation, www.theragenics.com*	Safe	1.5, 3	
ThinSeed *GE Healthcare, www.gehealthcare.com*	Conditional 6	3	
TigerPaw System *LAAx, Inc., Livermore, CA*	Conditional 8	1.5, 3	
Tin Snips *S-1144, W-212AL* *Ampco Safety Tools, www.amcosafetytools.com*	Conditional 7	3	
Titan Wireless Implantable Hemodynamic Monitoring (WIHM) System *Integrated Sensing Systems, Inc., www.mems-issys.com*	Conditional 8	1.5, 3	
Titanium Adjustable Wrench *Newmatic Medical, www.newmaticmedical.com*	Conditional 7	3	
Titanium Bengolea Haemostatic Forceps *Curved* *Newmatic Medical, www.newmaticmedical.com*	Conditional 7	3	
Titanium Gerald Dissecting Forceps *Newmatic Medical, www.newmaticmedical.com*	Conditional 7	3	
Titanium Knot *LSI Solutions Inc., Victor, NY*	Conditional 6	3	
Titanium Potts Micro Scissors *Newmatic Medical Systems, www.newmaticmedical.com*	Conditional 7	3	
Tornado, Pulmonary Vein Isolation Device (PVID) *Medical Device Innovations, www.mdi-md.com*	Conditional 8	1.5, 3	
Trachea Support Ring *Kurz Medical, www.kurzmed.com/en/products/mri-safety/*	Conditional 5	1.5, 3	
Tracheal T-Tube *Hood Laboratories, www.hoodlabs.com*	Safe	1.5, 3	
Transport Chair 20-inch *Newmatic Medical, www.newmaticmedical.com*	Conditional 7	3	
TransWarmer Infant Transport Mattress *Cooper Surgical, www.coopersurgical.com*	Conditional 6	3	

Object	Status	Field Strength (T)	Reference
Trapezoidal Malar *Implantech Associates, Inc., www.implantech.com*	Safe	1.5, 3	
TriCinch 2 Coil, All Sizes *4TECH Cardio Ireland Ltd, www.4techtricuspid.com*	Conditional 8	1.5, 3	
TruMRI Blade *Truphatek International LTD., www.truphatek.com*	Unsafe 1	1.5	
TruMRI Handle (Brass Head) *Truphatek International LTD., www.truphatek.com*	Conditional 7	3	
TruMRI Handle (SAE 303 Head) *Truphatek International LTD., www.truphatek.com*	Conditional 7	3	
TruScan Surface Electrode, EEG Electrode *PMT Corporation, www.pmtcorp.com*	Conditional 5	1.5	
TruScan Surface Electrode, Model 2305 series, *EEG Electrode* *PMT Corporation, www.pmtcorp.com*	Conditional 5	1.5	
TruWave Disposable Pressure Transducer *Edwards Lifesciences, www.edwards.com*	Conditional 5	3	
t:slim Insulin Pump *Tandem Diabetes Care, Inc., www.tandemdiabetes.com*	Unsafe 1	1.5	
TS System Arterial Closure Device *Arterial Closure Device (ACD)* *Vasorum Ltd, Ireland*	Conditional 6	3	
TVFMI, Titanium Vocal Fold Medializing Implant *Kurz Medical, www.kurzmed.com/en/products/mri-safety/*	Conditional 5	1.5, 3	
Tweezers, Ceramic, prototype, ceramic *MicroSurgical Techniques, Inc., Fort Collins, CO*	Safe	1.5	48
Tweezers, 8340 *Ampco Safety Tools, www.ampcosafetytools.com*	Conditional 7	3	
ULT - Drainage Catheter *Cook Medical, www.cookmedical.com*	Conditional 6	3	
UltraSeal Disposable Anesthesia Face Mask *With and Without Check Valve* *Ambu Ltd., www.ambuusa.com*	Safe	1.5, 3	
ULTRASITE Valve *B. Braun Medical Inc., www.bbraunusa.com*	Conditional 6	3	
UroLift Anchor, 316L SS *NeoTract, Inc., www.neotract.com*	Conditional 5	3	
Uni-Graft K DV Patch *B. Braun, www.bbraun.com*	Safe	1.5	
Uni-Graft K DV, Vascular Graft *B. Braun, www.bbraun.com*	Safe	1.5	
Uni-Graft W Aortic Arch, Vascular Graft *B. Braun, www.bbraun.com*	Safe	1.5	

Object	Status	Field Strength (T)	Reference
Uni-Graft W Sinus, Vascular Graft *B. Braun, www.bbraun.com*	Safe	1.5	
Uni-Graft W, Vascular Graft *B. Braun, www.bbraun.com*	Safe	1.5	
Universal Cylinder Family Sets *Universal Cylinder Applicator with Cervix Probe* *Varian Medical Systems, www.varian.com*	Conditional 8	1.5, 3	
Upper Eyelid Implant, Gold *Kurz Medical, www.kurzmed.com/en/products/mri-safety/*	Conditional 5	1.5, 3	
Upper Eyelid Implant, Platinum/Iridium *Kurz Medical, www.kurzmed.com/en/products/mri-safety/*	Conditional 5	1.5, 3	
UroLift Implant *NeoTract, Inc., www.neotract.com*	Conditional 6	3	
Urolume Endoprosthesis *AMS, American Medical Systems,* *www.americanmedicalsystems.com*	Safe	1.5, 3	
V-Chordal Surgical *Valtech Cardio Ltd., Israel*	Conditional 6	3	
V-Go Disposable Insulin Delivery Device *Valeritas, www.valeritas.com*	Unsafe 1	1.5	
VK462 *UNS-S43000 Pins* *The Viking Corporation, www.vikinggroupinc.com*	Conditional 7	3	
V-Wave Implant *V Wave Ltd., www.iati.co.il/company*	Conditional 6	3	
V.A.C. GranuFoam Silver *V.A.C. Dressing* *KCI USA, Inc., San Antonio, TX*	Conditional 6	3	
VANTAS Implant, Histrelin Implant *Endo Pharmaceuticals, www.vantasimplant.com*	Safe	1.5	
VASCADE Vascular Closure System (VCS) *Cardiva Medical, Inc., www.cardivamedical.com*	Safe	1.5, 3	
VascuGraft PTFE, Vascular Graft *B. Braun, www.bbraun.com*	Safe	1.5	
VascuGraft Soft, Vascular Graft *B. Braun, www.bbraun.com*	Safe	1.5	
Vascu-Guard Vascular Patch *Peripheral Vascular Patch* *Synovis Surgical Innovations, www.synovissurgical.com*	Safe	1.5, 3	
Vascular Marker, O-Ring washer *PIC Design, Middlebury, CT*	Conditional 5	1.5	
Vascular Occlusion Device *MicroVention, Inc., www.microvention.com*	Conditional 5	1.5, 3	

Object	Status	Field Strength (T)	Reference
Vascular Patch *B. Braun, www.bbraun.com*	Safe	1.5	
Vasti Cardiovascular Valved Vein Graft *Labcor Laboratorios Ltda., www.labcor.com*	Safe	1.5, 3	
Vectra Vascular Access Graft (VAG) *Bard Peripheral Vascular, www.bardpv.com*	Safe	1.5	
Velox CD Vascular Closure Device *Transluminal Technologies, www.transluminal.net*	Conditional 6	3	
Vehicle Bracket, 810NM *Amerex Corporation, Trussville, AL*	Conditional 7	3	
Velum Pulmonary Valved Conduit with L-Hydro *Labcor Laboratorios Ltda., www.labcor.com*	Safe	3	
Venaflo II Vascular Graft *Bard Peripheral Vascular, www.bardpv.com*	Safe	1.5	
VenoPatch *B. Braun, www.bbraun.com*	Safe	1.5	
Ventricular Bolt Pressure Monitoring Kit *Integra NeuroSciences, www.integralife.com*	Unsafe 1	1.5	
Ventricular Bolt Pressure Monitoring Kit *with Cranial Access Kit* *Integra NeuroSciences, www.integralife.com*	Unsafe 1	1.5	
Ventricular Partitioning Implant, VPD *CardioKinetix Inc., Redwood City, CA*	Conditional 6	3	
VeriChip Microtransponder, RFID *VeriChip Corporation*	Conditional 5	7	
Veritas Collagen Matrix *Synovis Surgical Innovations, www.synovissurgical.com*	Safe	1.5, 3	
Viadur *Bayer HealthCare Pharmaceuticals, West Haven, CT*	Safe	1.5	
Vitallium Implant	Safe	1.5	
Vivendi Bovine Pericardium Patch with L-Hydro *Labcor Laboratorios Ltda., www.labcor.com*	Safe	3	
V-Link Luer Activated Device *with VitalShield Protective Coating,* *Non-DEHP Y-Type Catheter Extension Set,* *Non-DEHP Y-Type Catheter Extension Set* *Baxter Healthcare, Round Lake, IL*	Conditional 6	3	
VOCARE Bladder System *Implantable Functional Neuromuscular Stimulator (FNS)* *NeuroControl Corporation and* *www.finetech-medical.co.uk/*	Conditional 5	1.5	
Voloshin Dorsal Columella Implant *Implantech Associates, Inc., www.implantech.com*	Safe	1.5, 3	

Object	Status	Field Strength (T)	Reference
VPASS Implant *Percardia Inc., Merrimack, NH*	Safe	3	
Vygon AutoFlush *Vygon Coporation, Norristown, PA*	Conditional 6	3	
Vygon Bionector, Needle Access Device *Vygon Corporation, Norristown, PA*	Conditional 6	3	
Walk-O2-Bout 2.0 System (WOB 2.0) *Essex Industries, www.essexindustries.com*	Conditional 7	3	
Wall Bracket, 17737 (801) *Amerex Corporation, Trussville, AL*	Conditional 7	3	
Watchman Gen 4 Implant *Atritech Inc. and Boston Scientific, www.bostonscientific.com*	Conditional 6	3	
WATCHMAN Left Atrial Appendage Closure Device *Atritech Inc. and Boston Scientific, www.bostonscientific.com*	Conditional 6	3	
WayPoint Anchor *FHC, Inc., Bowdoin, ME*	Conditional 6	3	
WedgeLoc Suture Anchor *MedShape Solutions, Inc., Atlanta, GA*	Conditional 6	3	
Western EZ-OX Plus System *ALQ-2342 on an Aluminum D cylinder Western Enterprises, Westlake, OH*	Conditional 7	3	
Western EZ-OX Plus System *ALQ-2342 on an Aluminum D cylinder Western Enterprises, Westlake, OH*	Conditional 7	3	
Wheelchair, 18-inch Detachable Foot Rest *Newmatic Medical, www.newmaticmedical.com*	Conditional 7	3	
Wheelchair, 20-inch *SS Heavy Duty Folding Aquatic Wheelchair Aqua Creek Products, LLC, Missoula, MT*	Conditional 7	3	
Wheelchair, 22-inch Detachable Foot Rest *Newmatic Medical, www.newmaticmedical.com*	Conditional 7	3	
Wheelchair, 26-inch Detachable Foot Rest *Newmatic Medical, www.newmaticmedical.com*	Conditional 7	3	
Wheelchair, 4850 MR Wheelchair *Gendron, Inc., www.gendroninc.com*	Conditional 7	3	
Wheelchair, IV/Oxygen Tank Holder *Newmatic Medical, www.newmaticmedical.com*	Conditional 7	3	
Wheelchair, Merlexi Craft Liberty *MRI Synthetic Resin Manual Wheelchair Turbo Wheelchair Co., Beaufort, SC*	Conditional 7	3	

Object	Status	Field Strength (T)	Reference
Wheelchair, MR 18, 4000 MR *SPORTLITE* *Gendron, Inc., Archbold, OH*	Conditional 7	3	
Winged Infusion Set, MRI Compatible *E-Z-EM, Inc., Westbury, NY*	Safe	1.5	58
Wisefix Implant *Novogate Medical Ltd., Israel*	Conditional 8	1.5, 3	
Woodson Elevator, 304 SS *Johnson & Johnson Professional, Inc.,* *www.depuysynthes.com*	Safe	1.5	62
Wristband, Soft Infant Wristband *Zebra Technologies, Vernon Hills, IL*	Safe	1.5, 3	
Wristband, Z-Band 4000 *Zebra Technologies, Vernon Hills, IL*	Safe	1.5, 3	
Wristband, Z-Band Comfort *Zebra Technologies, Vernon Hills, IL*	Safe	1.5, 3	
Wristband, Z-Band Direct (no color) *Zebra Technologies, Vernon Hills, IL*	Safe	1.5, 3	
Wristband, Z-Band Direct with Color (Red) *Zebra Technologies, Vernon Hills, IL*	Safe	1.5, 3	
Wristband, Z Band Quick Clip & Red Clip *Zebra Technologies, Vernon Hills, IL*	Safe	1.5, 3	
Xenform Soft Tissue Repair Matrix *Boston Scientific, www.bostonscientific.com*	Safe	1.5, 3	
XenMatrix Surgical Graft *Bard Plastic Surgery, www.bardps.com*	Safe	1.5, 3	
XL 5 MR- Multipurpose Dry Chemical Portable *Fire Extinguisher* *Kidde Fire Safety, www.kidde.com*	Conditional 7	3	
Xseal *Essential Medical, Wayne, PA*	Conditional 6	3	
YD Post-Valve *Praxair, Inc., www.praxair.com*	Conditional 7	3	
Z-Band Wristband, HC100 *All models* *Zebra Technologies, www.zebra.com*	Safe	1.5, 3	
Zephyr Endobronchial Valve (EBV) *Pulmonx, Inc., www.pulmonx.com*	Conditional 6	3	
Zephyr Transcopic Endobronchial Valve *Emphasys Medical Inc., Redwood City, CA*	Conditional 6	3	
Zip Implant Device, Titanium alloy *Bioplate, Inc., Los Angeles, CA*	Conditional 6	3	

Object	Status	Field Strength (T)	Reference

Ocular Implants, Lens Implants, and Devices

Object	Status	Field Strength (T)	Reference
Afinity Collamer Aspheric IOL (Intraocular Lens) *STAAR Surgical Company, Staar www.staar.com*	Safe	1.5	
Ahmed Glaucoma Valve *Glaucoma Drainage Implant, Nonmetallic* *New World Medical, Rancho Cucamonga, CA*	Safe	3	105
ARGOS-IO, Eye Implant, Ocular Implant *Implandata Ophthalmic Products GmbH,* *www.implandata.com*	Conditional 6	3	
AquaFlow Collagen Drainage Device *Glaucoma Drainage* *STAAR Surgical Company, Staar www.staar.com*	Safe	1.5	
ATTRACTOR Screw, 17-4 SS *Porex Surgical, Newnan, GA*	Unsafe 1	1.5	
Baerveldt Glaucoma Drainage Implant *Glaucoma Drainage Implant, nonmetallic* *Pharmacia Co., Kalamazoo, MI*	Safe	3	
Boston Keratoprosthesis *Massachusetts Eye and Ear Infirmary,* *www.masseyeandear.org*	Conditional 6	3	
Clip 250, Double Tantalum Clip *Mira Inc.*	Safe	1.5	29
Clip 50, Double Tantalum Clip *Mira Inc.*	Safe	1.5	29
Clip 51, Single Tantalum Clip *Mira Inc.*	Safe	1.5	29
Clip 52, Single Tantalum Clip *Mira Inc.*	Safe	1.5	29
Collamer ICL (Implantable Contact Lens) *STAAR Surgical Company, Staar www.staar.com*	Safe	1.5	
Double Tantalum Clip *Storz Instrument Co.*	Safe	1.5	29
Double Tantalum Clip Style 250 *Storz Instrument Co.*	Safe	1.5	29
DuraPlug, Temporary Canalicular Insert *EagleVision, Memphis, TN*	Safe	3	
EaglePlug Punctum Plug *EagleVision, Memphis, TN*	Safe	3	
Eagle FlexPlug Punctum Plug *EagleVision, Memphis, TN*	Safe	3	
Elastimide Silicone Aspheric IOL (Intraocular Lens) *STAAR Surgical Company, Staar www.staar.com*	Safe	1.5, 3	

Object	Status	Field Strength (T)	Reference
EX-PRESS Glaucoma Filtration Device *Alcon, www.alcon.com*	Conditional 5	3	
EX-PRESS Mini Glaucoma Shunt *Alcon, www.alcon.com*	Conditional 5	3	117
Fatio Eyelid Spring/Wire, Ocular	Unsafe 1	1.5	30
Forsight Vision4 Port Delivery System Implant *Forsight Vision4, Menlo Park, CA*	Conditional 6	3	
Gelansert *Temporary Canalicular Insert* *EagleVision, Memphis, TN*	Safe	1.5, 3	
Gold Eyelid Spring, Ocular	Safe	1.5, 3	
Gold Eyelid Implant *MedDev Corporation, www.meddev-corp.com*	Conditional 6	3	
Hydrus Aqueous Implant, Ocular Implant *Ivantis, Inc. www.ivantisinc.com*	Conditional 6	3	
Hydrus Microstent *Ivantis, Inc., www.ivantisinc.com*	Conditional 6	3	
Implantable Miniature Telescope *VisionCare Ophthalmic Technologies, Inc., www.visioncareinc.net*	Conditional 8	1.5, 3	
Intraocular Lens, Binkhorst, Iridocapsular Lens *Platinum-Iridium Loop*	Safe	1.5, 3	
Intraocular Lens, Binkhorst, Iiridocapsular Lens *Titanium Loop*	Safe	1.5, 3	31
Intraocular Lens, Hoya AF-1 (UV) *Hoya Surgical Optics, www.hoyasurgicaloptics.com*	Safe	1.5, 3	
Intraocular Lens, Hoya AF-1 (UY) *Hoya Surgical Optics, www.hoyasurgicaloptics.com*	Safe	1.5, 3	
Intraocular Lens, Hoya PS (UV) *Hoya Surgical Optics, www.hoyasurgicaloptics.com*	Safe	1.5, 3	
Intraocular Lens, Hoya PS (UY) *Hoya Surgical Optics, www.hoyasurgicaloptics.com*	Safe	1.5, 3	
Intraocular Lens, Models 12A, 12P, 12S, 24P, 31P, 42P, 61P, 71, 71B, 71M, 71P, 71PC, 71R, 75M, 75P, EXP D *Bausch & Lomb, www.bausch.com*	Unsafe 1	1.5	
Intraocular Lens, Worst, Platinum Clip Lens	Safe	1.5, 3	31
Intraocular Lens, ISert Geometric Preloaded *IOL System, Model 751* *Hoya Surgical Optics, www.hoyasurgicaloptics.com*	Safe	1.5, 3	
Intraocular Lens, ISert Preloaded IOL System, *Model 230* *Hoya Surgical Optics, www.hoyasurgicaloptics.com*	Safe	1.5, 3	

Object	Status	Field Strength (T)	Reference
Intraocular Lens, ISert Preloaded IOL System, Model 231 *Hoya Surgical Optics, www.hoyasurgicaloptics.com*	Safe	1.5, 3	
Intraocular Lens, ISert Preloaded IOL System, Model 250 *Hoya Surgical Optics, www.hoyasurgicaloptics.com*	Safe	1.5, 3	
Intraocular Lens, ISert Preloaded IOL System, Model 251 *Hoya Surgical Optics, www.hoyasurgicaloptics.com*	Safe	1.5, 3	
Intraocular Lens, ISert Preloaded IOL System, Model PC-60AD *Hoya Surgical Optics, www.hoyasurgicaloptics.com*	Safe	1.5, 3	
Intraocular Lens, ISert Preloaded IOL System, Model PY-60AD *Hoya Surgical Optics, www.hoyasurgicaloptics.com*	Safe	1.5, 3	
Intraocular Lens, ISert Preloaded IOL System, Model PY-60R *Hoya Surgical Optics, www.hoyasurgicaloptics.com*	Safe	1.5, 3	
Intraocular Lens, ISpherical IOL, Model YA-60BB *Hoya Surgical Optics, www.hoyasurgicaloptics.com*	Safe	1.5, 3	
Intraocular Lens, ISpherical IOL, Model YA-60BR *Hoya Surgical Optics, www.hoyasurgicaloptics.com*	Safe	1.5, 3	
Intraocular Lens, ISymm IOL, Model FC-60AD *Hoya Surgical Optics, www.hoyasurgicaloptics.com*	Safe	1.5, 3	
Intraocular Lens, ISymm IOL, Model FY-60AD *Hoya Surgical Optics, www.hoyasurgicaloptics.com*	Safe	1.5, 3	
Intraocular Lens, Optimized Aspheric IOL *Hoya Surgical Optics, www.hoyasurgicaloptics.com*	Safe	1.5, 3	
iStent Trabecular Micro-Bypass Stent *Models GTS100R and GTS100L* *Glaukos, www.glaukos.com*	Conditional 5	3	
Joseph Valve, Glaucoma Drainage Implant *Valve Implants Limited, Hertford, England*	Safe	1.5, 3	31
Krupin-Denver Eye Valve to Disc Implant *Glaucoma Drainage Implant* *E. Benson Hood Laboratories, Pembroke, MA*	Safe	1.5, 3	
Lacriflow Lacrimal Duct Tube *Kaneka Corporation, www.kaneka-eye.com*	Conditional 8	1.5, 3	
Lens Implant, CR5BUO *Alcon, www.alcon.com*	Safe	1.5, 3	
Lens Implant, CZ60BD *Alcon, www.alcon.com*	Safe	1.5, 3	

Object	Status	Field Strength (T)	Reference
Lens Implant, CZ70BD *Alcon, www.alcon.com*	Safe	1.5, 3	
Lens Implant, LC80BD *Alcon, www.alcon.com*	Safe	1.5, 3	
Lens Implant, LX10BD *Alcon, www.alcon.com*	Safe	1.5, 3	
Lens Implant, LX90BD *Alcon, www.alcon.com*	Safe	1.5, 3	
Lens Implant, MA30AC *Alcon, www.alcon.com*	Safe	1.5, 3	
Lens Implant, MA60AC *Alcon, www.alcon.com*	Safe	1.5, 3	
Lens Implant, MA30BA *Alcon, www.alcon.com*	Safe	1.5, 3	
Lens Implant, MA50BM *Alcon, www.alcon.com*	Safe	1.5, 3	
Lens Implant, MA60BM *Alcon, www.alcon.com*	Safe	1.5, 3	
Lens Implant, MA60MA *Alcon, www.alcon.com*	Safe	1.5, 3	
Lens Implant, MC30BA *Alcon, www.alcon.com*	Safe	1.5, 3	
Lens Implant, MA40BD *Alcon, www.alcon.com*	Safe	1.5, 3	
Lens Implant, MC50BD *Alcon, www.alcon.com*	Safe	1.5, 3	
Lens Implant, MC60BD *Alcon, www.alcon.com*	Safe	1.5, 3	
Lens Implant, MC50BM *Alcon, www.alcon.com*	Safe	1.5, 3	
Lens Implant, MC51BM *Alcon, www.alcon.com*	Safe	1.5, 3	
Lens Implant, MC60BM *Alcon, www.alcon.com*	Safe	1.5, 3	
Lens Implant, MC61BM *Alcon, www.alcon.com*	Safe	1.5, 3	
Lens Implant, MC60CM *Alcon, www.alcon.com*	Safe	1.5, 3	
Lens Implant, MC61CM *Alcon, www.alcon.com*	Safe	1.5, 3	
Lens Implant, MC70CM *Alcon, www.alcon.com*	Safe	1.5, 3	

Object	Status	Field Strength (T)	Reference
Lens Implant, MC71CM *Alcon, www.alcon.com*	Safe	1.5, 3	
Lens Implant, MN20BD *Alcon, www.alcon.com*	Safe	1.5, 3	
Lens Implant, MN30BD *Alcon, www.alcon.com*	Safe	1.5, 3	
Lens Implant, MN40BD *Alcon, www.alcon.com*	Safe	1.5, 3	
Lens Implant, MN60BD *Alcon, www.alcon.com*	Safe	1.5, 3	
Lens Implant, MN60D3 *Alcon, www.alcon.com*	Safe	1.5, 3	
Lens Implant, MTA2UO *Alcon, www.alcon.com*	Safe	1.5, 3	
Lens Implant, MTA3UO *Alcon, www.alcon.com*	Safe	1.5, 3	
Lens Implant, MTA4UO *Alcon, www.alcon.com*	Safe	1.5, 3	
Lens Implant, MTA5UO *Alcon, www.alcon.com*	Safe	1.5, 3	
Lens Implant, MTA6UO *Alcon, www.alcon.com*	Safe	1.5, 3	
Lens Implant, MZ20BD *Alcon, www.alcon.com*	Safe	1.5, 3	
Lens Implant, MZ30BD *Alcon, www.alcon.com*	Safe	1.5, 3	
Lens Implant, MZ40BD *Alcon, www.alcon.com*	Safe	1.5, 3	
Lens Implant, MZ60BD *Alcon, www.alcon.com*	Safe	1.5, 3	
Lens Implant, MZ70BD *Alcon, www.alcon.com*	Safe	1.5, 3	
Lens Implant, MZ20CD *Alcon, www.alcon.com*	Safe	1.5, 3	
Lens Implant, MZ60CD *Alcon, www.alcon.com*	Safe	1.5, 3	
Lens Implant, MZ60MD *Alcon, www.alcon.com*	Safe	1.5, 3	
Lens Implant, MZ60PD *Alcon, www.alcon.com*	Safe	1.5, 3	
Lens Implant, SA30AL *Alcon, www.alcon.com*	Safe	1.5, 3	

Object	Status	Field Strength (T)	Reference
Lens Implant, SA30AT *Alcon, www.alcon.com*	Safe	1.5, 3	
Lens Implant, SA60AT *Alcon, www.alcon.com*	Safe	1.5, 3	
Lens Implant, SN60AT *Alcon, www.alcon.com*	Safe	1.5, 3	
Lens Implant, SA60D3 *Alcon, www.alcon.com*	Safe	1.5, 3	
Lens Implant, SN60D3 *Alcon, www.alcon.com*	Safe	1.5, 3	
Lens Implant, SN60T3 *Alcon, www.alcon.com*	Safe	1.5, 3	
Lens Implant, SN60T4 *Alcon, www.alcon.com*	Safe	1.5, 3	
Lens Implant, SN60T5 *Alcon, www.alcon.com*	Safe	1.5, 3	
Lens Implant, SN60WF *Alcon, www.alcon.com*	Safe	1.5, 3	
Lens Implant, SN6AD3 *Alcon, www.alcon.com*	Safe	1.5, 3	
Lens Implant, SN60WS *Alcon, www.alcon.com*	Safe	1.5, 3	
Malhotra Platinum Segment *Altomed Limited, www.altomed.com*	Conditional 8	1.5, 3	
MEDPOR Oculoplastic Implant *Stryker, www.stryker.com*	Safe	1.5, 3	
Molteno Drainage Device, *Glaucoma Drainage Implant* *Molteno Ophthalmic Ltd., Dunedin, New Zealand*	Safe	1.5, 3	
MORCHER Capsular Tension Ring *Ocular Implant* *Morcher GmbH, www.morcher.com*	Safe	1.5, 3	
nanoFLEX Collamer Aspheric Single-Piece IOL *(Intraocular Lens)* *STAAR Surgical Company, Staar www.staar.com*	Safe	1.5	
OZURDEX Implant, dexamethasone *intravitreal implant* *Allergan, Inc., www.allergan.com*	Safe	1.5, 3	
Platinum Eyelid Implant *MedDev Corporation, www.meddev-corp.com*	Conditional 6	3	
Retisert Implant, Ocular Implant *Bausch and Lomb, www.bausch.com*	Safe	1.5, 3	

Object	Status	Field Strength (T)	Reference
Retinal Tack, 303 SS, Ocular *Bascom Palmer Eye Institute*	Safe	1.5	32
Retinal Tack, 303 SS, Ocular *Duke*	Safe	1.5	32
Retinal Tack, Aluminum Textraoxide, Ocular, Ruby	Safe	1.5	32
Retinal Tack, Cobalt, Nickel, Ocular *Greishaber, Fallsington, PA*	Safe	1.5	32
Retinal Tack, Martensitic SS, Ocular *Western European*	Unsafe 1	1.5	32
Retinal Tack, Titanium alloy, Ocular *Coopervision, Irvine, CA*	Safe	1.5	32
Retinal Tack, Norton Staple *Platinum, Rhodium, Ocular* *Norton*	Safe	1.5	32
Single Tantalum Clip, Ocular	Safe	1.5	29
SOLX Gold Shunt *SOLX, Inc, www.solx.com*	Conditional 8	1.5, 3	
STAAR Elastic Lens (Intraocular Lens) *STAAR Surgical Company, Staar www.staar.com*	Safe	1.5, 3	
STAAR Elastimide Lens, 3-piece silicone IOL *(Intraocular Lens)* *STAAR Surgical Company, Staar www.staar.com*	Safe	1.5, 3	
STAAR Surgical AquaFlow Collagen Glaucoma *Drainage Device* *STAAR Surgical Company, Staar www.staar.com*	Safe	1.5, 3	
STAAR Surgical Collamer Ultraviolet Absorbing *Posterior Chamber 1-Piece Intraocular Lens* *STAAR Surgical Company, Staar www.staar.com*	Safe	1.5, 3	
STAAR Surgical Collamer Ultraviolet Absorbing *Posterior Chamber 3-Piece Intraocular Lens* *STAAR Surgical Company, Staar www.staar.com*	Safe	1.5, 3	
STAAR Surgical Elastic Ultraviolet Absorbing Posterior *Chamber Intraocular Lens with Toric Optic* *STAAR Surgical Company, Staar www.staar.com*	Safe	1.5, 3	
STAAR Surgical Elastic Ultraviolet Absorbing *Posterior Chamber Intraocular Lens* *STAAR Surgical Company, Staar www.staar.com*	Safe	1.5, 3	
STAAR Surgical Elastimide Posterior Chamber *Intraocular Lens* *STAAR Surgical Company, Staar www.staar.com*	Safe	1.5, 3	
STAAR Surgical Elastimide Posterior Chamber *Intraocular Lens* *STAAR Surgical Company, Staar www.staar.com*	Safe	1.5, 3	

Object	Status	Field Strength (T)	Reference
STAAR Surgical Elastimide Ultraviolet Absorbing *Posterior Chamber Aspheric Intraocular Lens* *STAAR Surgical Company, Staar www.staar.com*	Safe	1.5, 3	
STAAR Surgical Elastimide Ultraviolet Absorbing *Posterior Chamber Intraocular Lens* *STAAR Surgical Company, Staar www.staar.com*	Safe	1.5, 3	
STAAR Toric IOL (Intraocular Lens) *STAAR Surgical Company, Staar www.staar.com*	Safe	1.5, 3	
STAAR Visian Implantable Collamer Lens for Myopia *STAAR Surgical Company, Staar www.staar.com*	Safe	1.5, 3	
SuperEagle Punctum Plug *EagleVision, Memphis, TN*	Safe	3	
SuperFlex Punctum Plug *EagleVision, Memphis, TN*	Safe	3	
Tapered Shaft Flow Controller *EagleVision, Memphis, TN*	Safe	3	
Troutman Magnetic Ocular Implant	Unsafe 1	1.5	
Unitech Round Wire Eye Spring, Ocular	Unsafe 1	1.5	
Visian ICL (Implantable Contact Lens) *STAAR Surgical Company, Staar www.staar.com*	Safe	1.5, 3	
Visian TICL (Toric version, Implantable Contact Lens) *STAAR Surgical Company, Staar www.staar.com*	Safe	1.5, 3	
Wide Angle Implantable Miniature Telescope *Lens Implant, VisionCare Ophthalmic Technologies, Inc., Saratoga, CA*	Conditional 6	3	

Orthopedic Implants, Materials, and Devices

3D ProFuse Bioscaffold Safe *Alphatec Spine Inc., www.alphatecspine.com*	Safe	1.5, 3	
Absolute Absorbable Interference Screw	Safe	1.5, 3	
Ace-Fischer External Fixation System *Depuy Synthes, www.depuysynthes.com*	Unsafe 1	1.5	
active L Lumbar Disc Implant *B. Braun, www.bbraun.com*	Conditional 5	1.5, 3	
Adjustable External Fixation Device *External Fixation Device* *Biomet, www.Biomet.com*	Conditional 5	3	
ADVANCE, Total Knee Assembly *MicroPort Orthopedics Inc., www.ortho.microport.com*	Conditional 5	1.5, 3	
Advent Cervical Disc *Blackstone Medical, Inc., Wayne, NJ*	Conditional 8	1.5, 3	

Object	Status	Field Strength (T)	Reference
Aequalis Humeral Plate *and component parts, 120-mm plate 4.0-mm x 60-mm length self tapping cancellous locking screw, 3.5-mm x 50-mm length self tapping cortical compression screw 3.5-mm x 40-mm length self tapping cortical locking screw, 19-gauge cerclage wire Tornier, Inc., Stafford, TX*	Conditional 6	3	
Agility Total Ankle *Titanium alloy tibial, CoCrMo alloy talus Depuy Synthes, www.depuysynthes.com*	Conditional 6	3	
AlphaGRAFT Demineralized Bone Matrix *Alphatec Spine Inc., www.alphatecspine.com*	Safe	1.5, 3	
AML Hip Stem, CoCrMo Alloy with CoCrMo *Alloy Head Depuy Synthes, www.depuysynthes.com*	Conditional 6	3	
AML Femoral Component Bipolar Hip Prosthesis *Zimmer, www.zimmer.com*	Safe	1.5	3
AmnioShield Amniotic Tissue Barrier *Alphatec Spine Inc., www.alphatecspine.com*	Safe	1.5, 3	
Anchor FS Facet Screw *Medtronic, Inc., www.medtronic.com/mri*	Conditional 6	3	
Anterior Cervical Body Interbody Spacer (ACIS) *All versions Depuy Synthes, www.depuysynthes.com*	Conditional 8	1.5, 3	
APERIUS PercLID System *Medtronic, www.medtronic.com/mri*	Conditional 5	3	
Arcos Femoral Revision System *with BoneMaster Coating Biomet, www.biomet.com*	Conditional 5	1.5, 3	
Arsenal Degenerative Spinal Fixation System *Alphatec Spine Inc., www.alphatecspine.com*	Conditional 8	1.5, 3	
ARTISAN Space Maintenance System *Medtronic, Inc., www.medtronic.com/mri*	Conditional 5	1.5, 3	
Aspida Anterior Lumbar Plating System *Alphatec Spine Inc., www.alphatecspine.com*	Conditional 8	1.5, 3	
ASR-Surface Replacement Hip *CoCrMo alloy acetabulum and head Depuy Synthes, www.depuysynthes.com*	Conditional 6	3	
ATLAS Knee System *Moximed Inc., www.moximed.com*	Conditional 8	1.5, 3	

Object	Status	Field Strength (T)	Reference
Atrix-C Cervical Allograft Interbody Spacer *Xtant Medical, www.xtantmedical.com*	Safe	1.5, 3	
Avalon Occipital Fixation System *Alphatec Spine Inc., www.alphatecspine.com*	Conditional 8	1.5, 3	
AVN Cage *Depuy Synthes, www.depuysynthes.com*	Conditional 6	3	
BacFast, BacFast HD Facet Stabilization Dowel *Xtant Medical, www.xtantmedical.com*	Safe	1.5, 3	
Battalion PC Universal Spacer System *Alphatec Spine Inc., www.alphatecspine.com*	Conditional 6	3	
Battalion PS Universal Spacer System *Alphatec Spine Inc., www.alphatecspine.com*	Conditional 6	3	
Biocomposite Interference Screw, Cannulated, *Delta Tapered* *Arthrex, www.arthrex.com*	Safe	1.5, 3	
Biocryl Interference Screw, Nonmetallic *Depuy Synthes, www.depuysynthes.com*	Safe	1.5, 3	
Bio-Intrafix Tapered Screw, Nonmetallic *Depuy Synthes, www.depuysynthes.com*	Safe	1.5, 3	
Bio-Intrafix Tibial Sheath, Nonmetallic *Depuy Synthes, www.depuysynthes.com*	Safe	1.5, 3	
BioKnotless Anchor w/Ethibond *Nonmetallic* *Depuy Synthes, www.depuysynthes.com*	Safe	1.5, 3	
BioKnotless Anchor w/Panacryl *Nonmetallic* *Depuy Synthes, www.depuysynthes.com*	Safe	1.5, 3	
BioKnotless BR Anchor w/Orthocord *Nonmetallic* *Depuy Synthes, www.depuysynthes.com*	Safe	1.5, 3	
BioKnotless BR Anchor w/Panacryl *Nonmetallic* *Depuy Synthes, www.depuysynthes.com*	Safe	1.5, 3	
BioKnotless Plus Anchor w/Ethibond *Nonmetallic* *Depuy Synthes, www.depuysynthes.com*	Safe	1.5, 3	
BioKnotless Plus Anchor w/Orthocord *Nonmetallic* *Depuy Synthes, www.depuysynthes.com*	Safe	1.5, 3	
BioKnotless Plus Anchor w/Panacryl *Nonmetallic* *Depuy Synthes, www.depuysynthes.com*	Safe	1.5, 3	

Object	Status	Field Strength (T)	Reference
BioKnotless RC Anchor w/Ethibond *Nonmetallic* *Depuy Synthes, www.depuysynthes.com*	Safe	1.5, 3	
BioKnotless RC Anchor w/Panacryl *Nonmetallic* *Depuy Synthes, www.depuysynthes.com*	Safe	1.5, 3	
Biomet Bio-Modular Reverse Shoulder Products *Biomet, www.Biomet.com*	Conditional 5	1.5, 3	
Biomet Metal on Metal Hip Device *Biomet, www.Biomet.com*	Conditional 5	1.5, 3	
Biomet MRI SAFE SLM Rapid Rod-to-Rod Clamp *Biomet, www.biomet.com*	Safe	1.5, 3	
Biomet MRI SAFE SLM Rapid Rod-to-Screw Clamp *Biomet, www.biomet.com*	Safe	1.5, 3	
Biomet Oxford Partial Knee Implants *Biomet, www.Biomet.com*	Conditional 5	1.5, 3	
Biomet Sports Medicine JuggerKnot Mini Soft Anchor *Biomet, www.Biomet.com*	Safe	1.5, 3	
Biomet Sports Medicine Sternal Fixation Device *Biomet, www.Biomet.com*	Conditional 5	1.5, 3	
Biomet Upper Extremity Fixation Devices *Biomet, www.Biomet.com*	Conditional 5	1.5, 3	
Biomet Plating Systems *Biomet, www.Biomet.com*	Conditional 5	1.5, 3	
Biomet Vanguard Knee Joint Replacement *Prostheses* *Biomet, www.Biomet.com*	Conditional 5	1.5, 3	
Bio-Modular Shoulder System Reverse *Conversion Option* *Biomet, www.Biomet.com*	Conditional 5	1.5, 3	
BioPro Great Toe M-P Joint, Cobalt Chrome *BioPro, Inc., Port Huron, MI*	Safe	1.5	
BioROC EZ, Nonmetallic *Depuy Synthes, www.depuysynthes.com*	Safe	1.5, 3	
Biosymetric P.P. (Finger) Fixator *External Fixation Device* *Biomet, www.Biomet.com*	Conditional 6	3	
Biomet Ziploop *Biomet, www.Biomet.com*	Conditional 5	1.5, 3	
BIRMINGHAM Hip Resurfacing (BHR) *System Implant* *Smith & Nephew, www.smith-nephew.com*	Conditional 5	1.5, 3	

Object	Status	Field Strength (T)	Reference
Bone Tendon Bio-TransFix *Arthrex, www.arthrex.com*	Safe	1.5, 3	
BOOMERANG II PEEK Body Spacer *Medtronic, Inc., www.medtronic.com/mri*	Conditional 6	3	
BridgePoint Spinous Process Fixation System *Alphatec Spine Inc., www.alphatecspine.com*	Conditional 8	1.5, 3	
Bryan Cervical Disc System *Medtronic, Inc., www.medtronic.com/mri*	Conditional 8	1.5, 3	
BTB Cross Pins, 2.7-mm x 42-mm BIOCRYL *(TCP/PLA), Nonmetallic* *Depuy Synthes, www.depuysynthes.com*	Safe	1.5, 3	
BRYAN Cervical Disc System *Medtronic, Inc., www.medtronic.com/mri*	Conditional 6	3	
C-Leg Microprocessor Knee, Compact Version *Otto Bock HealthCare, www.ottobockus.com*	Unsafe 1	1.5	
C-Leg Microprocessor Knee *Otto Bock HealthCare, www.ottobockus.com*	Unsafe 1	1.5	
C Stem, Small and Large Assembly *Depuy Synthes, www.depuysynthes.com*	Conditional 8	1.5, 3	
C-Stem with CoCrMo Head, CoCrMo, *High Strength SS* *Depuy Synthes, www.depuysynthes.com*	Conditional 6	3	
CADISC-C, Artificial Disc *Ranier Technology Limited, www.ranier.co.uk*	Conditional 6	3	
CAISKIT, Nonmetallic *Depuy Synthes, www.depuysynthes.com*	Safe	1.5, 3	
CAIS Scaffold *DePuy Mitek, www.depuysynthes.com*	Safe	1.5, 3	
CAIS Staple *DePuy Mitek, www.depuysynthes.com*	Safe	1.5, 3	
Calix-C Cervical Interbody Spacer *Xtant Medical, www.xtantmedical.com*	Safe	1.5, 3	
CALYPSO-JAZZ Spine Construct *Implanet, www.implanet.com*	Conditional 8	1.5, 3	
Cannulated Cancellous Screw, 6.5 x 50-mm *Titanium alloy* *Depuy Synthes, www.depuysynthes.com*	Safe	1.5	
Captured Screw Assembly, 100-mm *Titanium alloy* *Depuy Synthes, www.depuysynthes.com*	Safe	1.5	
Cerclage Wires *Depuy Synthes, www.depuysynthes.com*	Conditional 5	1.5, 3	

Object	Status	Field Strength (T)	Reference
Cervical Wire, 18 gauge, 316L SS	Safe	0.3	33
CerviCore Intervertebral Disc *Stryker Spine, www.stryker.com*	Conditional 6	3	
Charite Artificial Disc *Depuy Synthes, www.depuysynthes.com*	Safe	3	
Charnley-Muller Hip Prosthesis, Protasyl-10 alloy	Safe	0.3	
Clearfix Meniscal PLA Absorbable Screw, Nonmetallic *Depuy Synthes, www.depuysynthes.com*	Safe	1.5, 3	
Clearfix Meniscal Screw Driver, Nonmetallic *Depuy Synthes, www.depuysynthes.com*	Safe	1.5, 3	
CLYDESDALE PEEK (polyetheretherketone) *Vertebral Body Spacer* *Medtronic, www.medtronic.com/mri*	Conditional 5	1.5, 3	
Cobalt Chrome Staple, Cobalt Chrome, ASTM F75 *Smith & Nephew, www.smith-nephew.com*	Safe	1.5, 3	83
Comprehensive Segmental Revision System *Biomet, www.biomet.com*	Conditional 5	1.5, 3	
Compression Hip Screw Plate *and Lag Screw (tested as assembly)* *Smith & Nephew, www.smith-nephew.com*	Safe	1.5, 3	83
CoNextions TR *CoNextions Medical, Inc., www.conextionsmed.com*	Conditional 8	1.5, 3	
Conserve BFH Total Hip System *Wright Medical Technology, www.wmt.com*	Conditional 8	1.5, 3	
Contiguous Fusion and Dynamic Spinal Fixation *from S1-TH10, Spine Construct* *SpineLab AG, www.spinelab.com*	Conditional 8	1.5, 3	
Converge Nitinol Bone Plate System *Biomedical Enterprises, www.bme.com*	Conditional 8	1.5, 3	
Coflex Interlaminar Technology *Paradigm Spine, www.paradigmspine.com*	Conditional 5	1.5, 3	
CORNERSTONE PSR Implant *Medtronic, Inc., www.medtronic.com/mri*	Conditional 5	1.5, 3	
Cortical Bone Screw, 4.5 x 36-mm *Titanium alloy* *Depuy Synthes, www.depuysynthes.com*	Safe	1.5	
Cortical Bone Screw, Large, Titanium alloy *Zimmer, www.zimmer.com*	Safe	1.5	34
Cortical Bone Screw, Small, Titanium alloy *Zimmer, www.zimmer.com*	Safe	1.5	34

Object	Status	Field Strength (T)	Reference
Cotrel Rod, SS-ASTM, Grade 2	Safe	1.5	
Cotrel Rods, with Hooks, 316L SS	Safe	0.3	33
Cougar Lateral Cage System *Depuy Synthes, www.depuysynthes.com*	Conditional 5	3	
Cuff Link Bone Tunnel Device, Nonmetallic *Depuy Synthes, www.depuysynthes.com*	Safe	1.5, 3	
CyclaPlex Implant *Cycla Orthopedics, www.cycla-or.com*	Conditional 8	1.5, 3	
Dall-Miles Cable System *Stryker, www.stryker.com*	Conditional 8	1.5, 3	
Delta Tapered PEEK Interference Screw *Arthrex, www.arthrex.com*	Safe	1.5, 3	
Delta Total Shoulder, SS *Depuy Synthes, www.depuysynthes.com*	Conditional 6	3	
DePuy Mitek Metal Anchors *DePuy Mitek, www.depuysynthes.com*	Conditional 5	3	
Disposable Titanium Skull Pin *Integra LifeSciences, www.integralife.com*	Conditional 6	3	
Distal Radius Fixator *External Fixation System* *Depuy Synthes, www.depuysynthes.com*	Conditional 5	1.5, 3	
Distraction Osteogenesis Ring System *Femur Frame, External Fixation System* *Depuy Synthes, www.depuysynthes.com*	Conditional 5	1.5, 3	
Divide Absorbable Adhesion Barrier, Nonmetallic *Depuy Synthes, www.depuysynthes.com*	Safe	1.5, 3	
Drummond Wire, 316L SS	Safe	0.3	33
DTT, Device for Transverse Traction	Safe	0.3	33
E1 Implant *Biomet Inc., www.biomet.com*	Safe	1.5, 3	
Elbow Hinge Fixator *External Fixation System* *Depuy Synthes, www.depuysynthes*	Conditional 5	1.5, 3	
Elite Nitinol Fixation System *BioMedical Enterprises, www.bme-tx.com*	Conditional 5	1.5, 3	
Emergency Bone Screw *Titanium alloy* *Biomet, www.Biomet.com*	Conditional 6	3	
Endoscopic Noncannulated *Interference Screw, Titanium* *Acufex Microsurgical, Norwood, MA*	Safe	1.5	34

Object	Status	Field Strength (T)	Reference
EOI Spinal System EPPS *(Expanding Polyaxial Pedicle Screw)* *Expanding Orthopedics Inc., Israel*	Conditional 8	1.5, 3	
Epicage *Alphatec Spine Inc., www.alphatecspine.com*	Conditional 6	3	
Episealer Knee Condyle *Episurf Medical AB, www.episurf.com*	Conditional 6	3	
ExoToe Plate, All Sizes *ExoToe, LLC, Grimes, IA*	Conditional 8	1.5, 3	
Expedium Implant System *Depuy Synthes, www.depuysynthes.com*	Conditional 5	1.5, 3	
Expert TN Tibial Nail *Depuy Synthes, www.depuysynthes.com*	Conditional 5	3	
External Fixation Device, Hoffmann II MRI *External Fixation System* *Stryker Trauma AG, www.stryker.com*	Conditional 5	1.5, 3	
External Fixation Device, Hoffmann II (Standard) *External Fixation System* *Stryker Trauma AG, www.stryker.com*	Unsafe 1	1.5	
External Fixation Device, *JET-X BAR External Fixation System* *Smith & Nephew, www.smith-nephew.com*	Conditional 5	1.5, 3	
Facet-Link, Bilateral Device *Facet-Link, Inc., Rockaway, NJ*	Conditional 6	3	
Facet-Link, Facet Screw *Facet-Link, Inc., Rockaway, NJ*	Conditional 6	3	
Facet-Link, Standard Device *Facet-Link, Inc., Rockaway, NJ*	Conditional 8	1.5, 3	
Facet Screw *Medtronic, www.medtronic.com/mri*	Conditional 5	3	
Facet Screw and Polyaxial Washer *and Polyaxial Washer* *Facet-Link, Inc., Rockaway, NJ*	Conditional 8	1.5, 3	
FD Tibial Intramedullary Nail, 316 SS *Biomet, www.Biomet.com*	Conditional 6	3	
Femoral Intrafix, Hard, Nonmetallic *Depuy Synthes, www.depuysynthes.com*	Safe	1.5, 3	
Femoral Intrafix, Standard, Nonmetallic *Depuy Synthes, www.depuysynthes.com*	Safe	1.5, 3	
Femoral Head Implant, Cobalt Chromium *Biomet, www.Biomet.com*	Conditional 6	3	
FibuLink Ankle Syndesmosis Fixation Device *Akros Medical, www.akrosmedical.com*	Conditional 8	1.5, 3	

Object	Status	Field Strength (T)	Reference
Fixation Staple, Orthopedic Implant *Richards Medical Co., Memphis, TN*	Safe	1.5	34
FlexiCore Intervertebral Disc *Stryker Spine-Summit, www.stryker.com*	Conditional 6	3	
Focal Femoral Condyle Resurfacing System, *HemiCAP* *Arthrosurface, Inc., www.arthrosurface.com*	Conditional 5	3	
Fracture Fixation System *Conventus Orthopaedics, Inc.,* *www.conventusortho.com*	Conditional 8	1.5, 3	
Furlong H-AC THR System *Joint Replacement Instrumentation Limited (JRI Ltd),* *Sheffield, U.K.*	Conditional 6	3	
Furlong Modular Revision System Hemiarthroplasty *Joint Replacement Instrumentation Limited (JRI Ltd),* *Sheffield, U.K.*	Conditional 6	3	
Galaxy System Fixator Components, *External Fixation System* *Orthofix, www.orthofix.com*	Conditional 5	1.5, 3	
Galaxy UNYCO Diaphyseal Tibia Kit *Orthofix, www.orthofix.com*	Conditional 5	1.5, 3	
Genium Bionic Prosthetic System *Otto Bock HealthCare, www.ottobockus.com*	Unsafe 1	1.5	
GII Titanium Anchor, Titanium *Mitek Products, www.depuysynthes.com*	Safe	1.5	
Global Total Shoulder, CoCrMo head and *stem/poly bearing component* *Depuy Synthes, www.depuysynthes.com*	Conditional 6	3	
Gryphon P BR Anchor w/Orthocord, Nonmetallic *Depuy Synthes, www.depuysynthes.com*	Safe	1.5, 3	
Gryphon P BR DS Anchor w/Orthocord, Nonmetallic *Depuy Synthes, www.depuysynthes.com*	Safe	1.5, 3	
Gryphon T BR Anchor w/Orthocord, Nonmetallic *Depuy Synthes, www.depuysynthes.com*	Safe	1.5, 3	
Gryphon T BR DS Anchor w/ Orthocord, Nonmetallic *Depuy Synthes, www.depuysynthes.com*	Safe	1.5, 3	
Halifax Clamps *American Medical Electronics, Richardson, TX*	Safe	1.5	
Hallmark Anterior Cervical Plate System *Blackstone Medical, Inc., Wayne, NJ*	Conditional 8	1.5, 3	
HammerLock 2, All Sizes *Depuy Synthes, www.depuysynthes.com*	Conditional 8	1.5, 3	

Object	Status	Field Strength (T)	Reference
Harrington Compression Rod *with Hooks and Nuts*	Safe	0.3	33
Harrington Distraction Rod with Hooks	Safe	0.3	33
Harris Hip Prosthesis *Zimmer, www.zimmer.com*	Safe	1.5	3
Healix BR 3-Suture Anchor w/Orthocord, Nonmetallic *Depuy, www.Depuy.com*	Safe	1.5, 3	
Healix BR Anchor w/Ethibond, Nonmetallic *Depuy Synthes, www.depuysynthes.com*	Safe	1.5, 3	
Healix BR Anchor w/Orthocord, Nonmetallic *Depuy Synthes, www.depuysynthes.com*	Safe	1.5, 3	
Healix BR Anchor w/Orthocord and Needles, *Nonmetallic* *Depuy Synthes, www.depuysynthes.com*	Safe	1.5, 3	
Healix BR Anchor w/Panacryl, Nonmetallic *Depuy Synthes, www.depuysynthes.com*	Safe	1.5, 3	
Healix PEEK 3-Suture Anchor w/Orthocord, *Nonmetallic* *Depuy Synthes, www.depuysynthes.com*	Safe	1.5, 3	
Healix PEEK Anchor w/Orthocord, Nonmetallic *Depuy Synthes, www.depuysynthes.com*	Safe	1.5, 3	
Healix PEEK Anchor w/Panacryl, Nonmetallic *Depuy Synthes, www.depuysynthes.com*	Safe	1.5, 3	
HeliFix Interspinous Spacer System *Alphatec Spine Inc., www.alphatecspine.com*	Conditional 6	3	
Helix3D Hip Joint System *Otto Bock HealthCare, www.ottobockus.com*	Unsafe 1	1.5	
HEMI 8-mm Large Buttress, *Left and Two Facet Screws (5-mm x 55-mm)* *Facet-Link, Inc., Rockaway, NJ*	Conditional 8	1.5, 3	
Hip Implant, Austenitic SS *DePuy, www.Depuy.com*	Safe	1.5, 3	83
Hybrid Ring Fixator *External Fixation System* *Depuy Synthes, www.depuysynthes.com*	Unsafe 1	1.5	
iBalance Femoral Knee Implant *Arthrex, www.arthrex.com*	Conditional 8	1.5, 3	
iForma, Orthopedic Implant *CONFORMIS, Inc., Lexington, MA*	Conditional 6	3	
IFuse Implant, L Implant *SI Bone, www.si-bone.com*	Conditional 8	1.5, 3	
Ilizarov-Taylor Spatial Frame, metal version *Smith and Nephew*	Unsafe 1	1.5	

Object	Status	Field Strength (T)	Reference
Illico Facet Fixation System *Alphatec Spine Inc., www.alphatecspine.com*	Conditional 8	1.5, 3	
IMF Wire, 316 SS *Biomet, www.Biomet.com*	Conditional 6	3	
Inbone Total Ankle System *Wright Medical Technology, www.wmt.com*	Conditional 8	1.5, 3	
Interbody Cage System, Including Anatomic Cage, Lordotic Cage *Titanium Coated Anatomic Cage,* *Titanium Coated Lordotic Cage* *LDR Spine, www.ldrspine.com*	Conditional 5	1.5, 3	
Intrafix Tapered Screw, Nonmetallic *Depuy Synthes, www.depuysynthes.com*	Safe	1.5, 3	
Intrafix Tibial Sheath, Nonmetallic *Depuy Synthes, www.depuysynthes.com*	Safe	1.5, 3	
Intramedullary Nail *Titanium Nail and Polymer Composite* *Smith and Nephew*	Conditional 8	1.5, 3	
Ionic Spine Spacer System, Titanium alloy *EBI, L.P., Parsippany, NJ*	Safe	1.5	
Iridium *Alphatec Spine Inc., www.alphatecspine.com*	Conditional 6	3	
Isobar Top Loading Degenerative Module *Alphatec Spine Inc., www.alphatecspine.com*	Conditional 8	1.5, 3	
iTotal CR (Cruciate Retaining) *KRS (Knee Replacement System)* *ConforMIS, Inc., www.conformis.com*	Conditional 8	1.5, 3	
Jewett Nail *Zimmer, www.zimmer.com*	Safe	1.5	3
JuggerKnot Soft Anchor *Biomet, www.Biomet.com*	Safe	1.5, 3	
Kirschner Intermedullary Rod *Kirschner Medical, Timonium, MD*	Safe	1.5	3
Kirschner Wires *Depuy Synthes, www.depuysynthes.com*	Conditional 5	1.5, 3	
KneeSpring Knee Implant System *Moximed, Inc., www.moximed.com*	Conditional 8	1.5, 3	
Large External Fixation System *Depuy Synthes, www.depuysynthes.com*	Conditional 5	1.5, 3	
Large External Fixator *Basic Modular Frame, External Fixation Device* *Depuy Synthes, www.depuysynthes.com*	Conditional 5	1.5, 3	

Object	Status	Field Strength (T)	Reference
Large External Fixator *Delta Frame Ankle Bridge, External Fixation Device* *Depuy Synthes, www.depuysynthes.com*	Conditional 5	1.5, 3	
Large External Fixator *Knee Arthrodesis Frame, External Fixation System* *Depuy Synthes, www.depuysynthes.com*	Conditional 5	1.5, 3	
Large External Fixator *Modular Knee Bridge, External Fixation System* *Depuy Synthes, www.depuysynthes.com*	Conditional 5	1.5, 3	
Large External Fixator *Modular Rod System, External Fixation Device* *Depuy Synthes, www.depuysynthes.com*	Conditional 5	1.5, 3	
Large External Fixator *Pelvic Frame, External Fixation System* *Depuy Synthes, www.depuysynthes.com*	Conditional 5	1.5, 3	
Latella Knee Implant System *Cotera, Inc., Menlo Park, CA*	Conditional 5	1.5, 3	
LCS Complete Assembly, Small and Large *Depuy Synthes, www.depuysynthes.com*	Conditional 8	1.5, 3	
LCP Anterolateral Distal Tibial Plate *Depuy Synthes, www.depuysynthes.com*	Conditional 5	3	
LCP Metalphyseal Plates *Depuy Synthes, www.depuysynthes.com*	Conditional 5	3	
Leucadia Autolok Pedicle Screw System *Alphatec Spine Inc., www.alphatecspine.com*	Conditional 8	1.5, 3	
LimiFlex Spinal Stabilization System *Simpirica Spine, Inc., www.simpirica.com*	Conditional 8	1.5, 3	
Linx HT Ligament Fastener, Nonmetallic *Depuy Synthes, www.depuysynthes.com*	Safe	1.5, 3	
L Plate, 6-hole, Titanium alloy *Depuy Synthes, www.depuysynthes.com*	Safe	1.5	
L Rod, Cobalt-Nickel alloy *Richards Medical Co., Memphis, TN*	Safe	1.5	
Locking Compression Plate (LCP) *Clavicle Hook Plate* *Depuy Synthes, www.depuysynthes.com*	Conditional 5	3	
Locking Compression Plate (LCP) *Extra-articular Distal Humerus Plate* *DePuy Synthes, www.depuysynthes.com*	Conditional 5	3	
Locking Compression Plate (LCP) *Olecranon Plate* *DePuy Synthes, www.depuysynthes.com*	Conditional 5	3	

Object	Status	Field Strength (T)	Reference
Low Profile MTP Plate *Arthrex, www.arthrex.com*	Conditional 8	1.5, 3	
Low Profile Screw, Cannulated, SS *Arthrex, www.arthrex.com*	Conditional 8	1.5, 3	
Low Profile Screw, Cannulated, Titanium *Arthrex, www.arthrex.com*	Conditional 8	1.5, 3	
Luna 360 Spinal Implant *Benvenue Medical, www.benvenuemedical.com*	Conditional 8	1.5, 3	
Lupine Loop Anchor, Nonmetallic *Depuy Synthes, www.depuysynthes.com*	Safe	1.5, 3	
Lupine Loop BR Anchor w/DS Orthocord, Nonmetallic *Depuy Synthes, www.depuysynthes.com*	Safe	1.5, 3	
Lupine Loop Dual Suture (DS) Anchor, Nonmetallic *Depuy Synthes, www.depuysynthes.com*	Safe	1.5, 3	
Lupine Loop Plus Anchor w/Ethibond, Nonmetallic *Depuy Synthes, www.depuysynthes.com*	Safe	1.5, 3	
Lupine Loop Plus Anchor w/Orthocord, Nonmetallic *Depuy Synthes, www.depuysynthes.com*	Safe	1.5, 3	
Lupine Loop Plus Anchor w/Panacryl, Nonmetallic *Depuy Synthes, www.depuysynthes.com*	Safe	1.5, 3	
Lupine Loop Plus Dual Suture (DS) *Anchor w/Orthocord, Nonmetallic* *Depuy Synthes, www.depuysynthes.com*	Safe	1.5, 3	
Luque Wire	Safe	0.3	33
M. KUROSAKA ADVANTAGE Cannulated *Fixation Screw* *Depuy Synthes, www.depuysynthes.com*	Conditional 6	3	
M. KUROSAKA ADVANTAGE Cannulated *Fixation Screw* *MRI information applies to many other similar implants* *Depuy Synthes, www.depuysynthes.com*	Conditional 6	3	
M6-C Artificial Cervical Disc *All Sizes* *Spinal Kinetics, www.spinalkinetics.com*	Conditional 8	1.5, 3	
M6-L Artificial Lumbar Disc *All Sizes* *Spinal Kinetics, www.spinalkinetics.com*	Conditional 8	1.5, 3	
MAGEC System *Ellipse Technologies and Nuvasive, www.nuvasive.com*	Conditional 5	1.5	
Mandibular Locking Bone Plate, 316 SS *Biomet, www.Biomet.com*	Conditional 6	3	

Object	Status	Field Strength (T)	Reference
MatrixMIDFACE (Matrix MIDFACE) Plate *and Screw System* *Depuy Synthes, www.depuysynthes.com*	Conditional 5	1.5, 3	
MaxFire with ZipLoop Meniscal Repair Device *MaxFire, MarXmen with ZipLoop Meniscal Repair Device* *Biomet, www.biomet.com*	Conditional 5	1.5, 3	
MAXFRAME Multi-Axial Correction System *External Fixation System* *Depuy Synthes, www.depuysynthes.com*	Conditional 5	1.5, 3	
Medial Pivot Knee System *MicroPort Medial, www.microportmedial.com*	Conditional 5	1.5, 3	
Medium External Fixator *Humeral Shaft Frame, External Fixation System* *Depuy Synthes, www.depuysynthes.com*	Conditional 5	1.5, 3	
Medium External Fixator *Modular Rod System, External Fixation System* *Depuy Synthes, www.depuysynthes.com*	Conditional 5	1.5, 3	
Medium External Fixator *Pediatric Femoral Shaft Frame* *External Fixation System* *Depuy Synthes, www.depuysynthes.com*	Conditional 8	1.5, 3	
MENISCAL FASTENER, Nonmetallic *Depuy Synthes, www.depuysynthes.com*	Safe	1.5, 3	
Meta-Lock Suture Anchor System *Tarsus Medical, Inc., www.tarsusmedical.com*	Conditional 6	3	
MICROFIX QUICKANCHOR Plus, Nonmetallic *Depuy Synthes, www.depuysynthes.com*	Safe	1.5, 3	
MILAGRO Interference Screw, Nonmetallic *Depuy Synthes, www.depuysynthes.com*	Safe	1.5, 3	
MiniLok QUICKANCHOR Plus, Nonmetallic *Depuy Synthes, www.depuysynthes.com*	Safe	1.5, 3	
MR Safe Clamps *for use with Large External Fixation System* *Synthes, www.synthes.com*	Conditional 5	1.5, 3	
MOBIS Spinal Implant, PEEK, Tantalum Pins *SIGNUS Medizintechnik GmbH, www.signus-med.de*	Conditional 6	3	
MOBIS Spinal Implant, PEEK, Titanium Pins *SIGNUS Medizintechnik GmbH, www. www.signus-med.de*	Conditional 6	3	
MOBIS II ST Spinal Implant *SIGNUS Medizintechnik GmbH, www.signus-med.de*	Conditional 8	1.5, 3	
Moe spinal instrumentation *Zimmer, www.zimmer.com*	Safe	1.5	

Object	Status	Field Strength (T)	Reference
Monoblock Neolif Intersomatic Cage *Biomet, www.Biomet.com*	Conditional 6	3	
Neo Cage System *All Sizes* *Neo Medical SA, www.neo-medical.com*	Conditional 8	1.5, 3	
Neocore Osteoconductive Matrix *Alphatec Spine Inc., www.alphatecspine.com*	Safe	1.5, 3	
Neo Pedicle Screw System, All Sizes *Neo Medical SA, www.neo-medical.com*	Conditional 8	1.5, 3	
NGage Surgical Mesh System *Blackstone Medical, Inc., Wayne, NJ*	Conditional 8	1.5, 3	
NOVAL Spinal Implant *SIGNUS Medizintechnik GmbH, www.signus-med.de*	Conditional 6	3	
Novel Anterior Lumbar Spacer (ALS) *Spinal Spacer System* *Alphatec Spine Inc., www.alphatecspine.com*	Conditional 6	3	
Novel Cervical Interbody System (CIS) *Alphatec Spine Inc., www.alphatecspine.com*	Conditional 6	3	
Novel Corpectomy (CP) Vertebral Body *Replacement System* *Alphatec Spine Inc., www.alphatecspine.com*	Conditional 6	3	
Novel DL Spinal Spacer System *Alphatec Spine Inc., www.alphatecspine.com*	Conditional 6	3	
Novel SD Spinal Spacer System *Alphatec Spine Inc., www.alphatecspine.com*	Conditional 6	3	
Novel Tapered DL Spinal Spacer System *Alphatec Spine Inc., www.alphatecspine.com*	Conditional 6	3	
Novel XS Spinal Spacer System *Alphatec Spine Inc., www.alphatecspine.com*	Conditional 6	3	
NUBIC Spinal Implant, PEEK, Titanium Pins *SIGNUS Medizintechnik GmbH, www.signus-med.de*	Conditional 6	3	
NUBIC XL Spinal Implant, PEEK, Titanium Pins *SIGNUS Medizintechnik GmbH, www.signus-med.de*	Conditional 6	3	
OrthoFuzIon Cannulated Screw System *Silver Bullet Therapeutics Inc., San Jose, CA*	Conditional 8	1.5, 3	
OsseoScrew Spinal Fixation System *Alphatec Spine Inc., www.alphatecspine.com*	Conditional 8	1.5, 3	
OsteoSelect Allograft *Xtant Medical, www.xtantmedical.com*	Safe	1.5, 3	
OsteoSponge Allograft *Xtant Medical, www.xtantmedical.com*	Safe	1.5, 3	
OsteoVive Allograft *Xtant Medical, www.xtantmedical.com*	Safe	1.5, 3	

Object	Status	Field Strength (T)	Reference
OsteoWrap, Human Cortical Bone *Xtant Medical, www.xtantmedical.com*	Safe	1.5, 3	
Panalok Anchor *Mitek Products, www.depuysynthes.com*	Safe	1.5, 3	
Patellofemoral joint (PFJ) Reconstruction System *IBalance PFJ, Entire Family, All Sizes* *Arthrex, Inc., www.arthrex.com*	Conditional 8	1.5, 3	
PCB Evolution *Alphatec Spine Inc., www.alphatecspine.com*	Conditional 6	3	
Pectus Bar Implant, Part# 01-3707 *Biomet, www.Biomet.com*	Conditional 8	1.5, 3	
Pectus Bar Implant, Part# 01-3717 *Biomet, www.Biomet.com*	Conditional 8	1.5, 3	
Pedicle Screw and Locking Clip *for use in the Elaspine Implant System* *SpineLab AG, Switzerland*	Conditional 6	3	
Pedimax II Construct *GMReis, www.gmreis.com*	Conditional 8	1.5, 3	
PEEKPower, Distal Radius Plate (DRP), *3-hole, right* *Arthrex, www.arthrex.com*	Conditional 5	1.5, 3	
PEEKPower, HTO Plate *Arthrex, www.arthrex.com*	Conditional 5	1.5, 3	
PEEK PREVAIL Cervical Interbody Device *Medtronic, www.medtronic.com/mri*	Conditional 5	1.5, 3	
Piccolo Composite Femoral *and Tibial Nailing System* *N.M.B. Medical Applications Ltd., Israel*	Conditional 8	1.5, 3	
Piccolo Composite Plate System *N.M.B. Medical Applications Ltd., Israel*	Conditional 8	1.5, 3	
POWER KNEE *Ossur, www.ossur.com*	Unsafe 1	1.5	
PRECICE Intramedullary Limb Lengthening System *Ellipse Technologies and Nuvasive, www.nuvasive.com*	Unsafe 1	1.5	
PRESTIGE LP Cervical Disc *Medtronic, Inc., www.Medtronic.com*	Conditional 5	3	
ProDisc-C Total Disc Replacement *DePuy Synthes, www.depuysynthes.com*	Conditional 5	1.5, 3	
ProDisc-L Total Disc Replacement *DePuy Synthes, www.depuysynthes.com*	Conditional 5	1.5, 3	
Pro-Flex Prosthetic Foot *Ossur, www.ossur.com*	Unsafe 1	1.5	

Object	Status	Field Strength (T)	Reference
Propio Foot *Ossur, www.ossur.com*	Unsafe 1	1.5	
Pro-Toe C2 Compression Implant *Compression Implant* *Wright Medical, www.wright.com*	Conditional 5	1.5, 3	
Opus Magnum Implant *ArthroCare, ArthroCare.com*	Conditional 5	1.5, 3	
OPUS SpeedFix *ArthroCare, ArthroCare.com*	Safe	1.5, 3	
OPUS SpeedLock Knotless Fixation Device *ArthroCare, ArthroCare.com*	Safe	1.5, 3	
OPUS SpeedScrew Device *ArthroCare, ArthroCare.com*	Safe	1.5, 3	
Orthocord, Nonmetallic *DePuy Synthes, www.depuysynthes.com*	Safe	1.5, 3	
Orthocord Suture, Size #2 *DePuy Mitek, www.depuysynthes.com*	Safe	1.5, 3	
OSS Distal Femoral Replacement Prosthesis *Biomet, www.Biomet.com*	Conditional 6	3	
OsseoFix, Titanium *Alphatec Spine Inc., www.alphatecspine.com*	Conditional 6	3	
Osseotite Dental Post Implant, Titanium alloy *Biomet, www.Biomet.com*	Conditional 6	3	
OsteoGen Implantable Bone Growth Stimulator *No MRI Info* *Biomet, www.Biomet.com*	Unsafe 1	1.5	
Otto Bock Microprocessor Knee *Otto Bock HealthCare, Minneapolis, MN*	Unsafe 1	1.5	
Oxidized Zirconium Knee, Femoral Component *Smith & Nephew, www.smith-nephew.com*	Safe	1.5, 3	83
PANALOK #2 ETHIBOND, Nonmetallic *Depuy Synthes, www.depuysynthes.com*	Safe	1.5, 3	
Panalok Absorbable Anchor, Nonmetallic *Depuy Synthes, www.depuysynthes.com*	Safe	1.5, 3	
Panalok Loop Anchor, Nonmetallic *Depuy Synthes, www.depuysynthes.com*	Safe	1.5, 3	
Panalok RC Loop Anchor, Nonmetallic *Depuy Synthes, www.depuysynthes.com*	Safe	1.5, 3	
Panalok RC QA+DS Suture Orthocord, Nonmetallic *Depuy Synthes, www.depuysynthes.com*	Safe	1.5, 3	
Panalok RC QuickAnchor Plus, Nonmetallic *Depuy Synthes, www.depuysynthes.com*	Safe	1.5, 3	

Object	Status	Field Strength (T)	Reference
Perfix Interence Screw, 17-4 SS *Instrument Makar, Okemos, MI*	Conditional 5	1.5	34
PERIMETER C Spinal System *Medtronic, Inc., www.medtronic.com/mri*	Conditional 5	3	
PERIMETER PEEK Vertebral Body Spacer *Medtronic, Inc., www.medtronic.com/mri*	Conditional 5	3	
Piccolo Composite Femoral Nailing System *N.M.B. Medical Applications Ltd., www.carbo-fix.com*	Conditional 8	1.5, 3	
Piccolo Composite Tibial Nailing System *N.M.B. Medical Applications Ltd., www.carbo-fix.com*	Conditional 8	1.5, 3	
Pinnacle MOM Acetabular Cup System *Titanium alloy shell, CoCrMo insert* *DePuy Synthes, www.depuysynthes.com*	Conditional 6	3	
Profile Plate System *Depuy Synthes, www.depuysynthes.com*	Conditional 8	1.5, 3	
Propeller Head Small Cannulated Screw *Biomet, www.Biomet.com*	Conditional 6	3	
PRESTIGE LP Cervical Disc *Medtronic, Inc., www.Medtronic.com*	Conditional 5	3	
Pyrocarbon Implant Replacement (PIR) System *Moirai Orthopaedics, Inc., Metairie, LA*	Conditional 6	3	
PyroTitan Humeral Resurfacing *Arthroplasty Implant* *Ascension Humeral Resurfacing Arthroplasty* *(HRA) System* *Ascension Orthopedics, Inc., Austin, TX*	Conditional 6	3	
RHEO KNEE 3 *Ossur, www.ossur.com*	Unsafe 1	1.5	
Quantum Composite Nailing System *N.M.B. Medical Applications Ltd., Israel*	Conditional 8	1.5, 3	
RABEA Cervical Cage, Titanium *SIGNUS Medizintechnik GmbH, www.signus-med.de*	Conditional 6	3	
RABEA Cervical Cage, PEEK, Titanium Pins *SIGNUS Medizintechnik GmbH, www.signus-med.de*	Conditional 6	3	
Radiopaque Implant *IlluminOss, www.illuminoss.com*	Conditional 5	1.5, 3	
RapidFlap *Biomet, www.Biomet.com*	Safe	1.5, 3	
RapidLoc Meniscal Repair-PLA Tophat, Nonmetallic *Depuy Synthes, www.depuysynthes.com*	Safe	1.5, 3	
RapidLoc PDS Meniscal Repair System, Nonmetallic *Depuy Synthes, www.depuysynthes.com*	Safe	1.5, 3	

Object	Status	Field Strength (T)	Reference
Ratcheting Compression Plate, Compression Staple *Acumed, www.acumed.net*	Conditional 8	1.5, 3	
Reef Stem/Octopus Acetabular Assembly *Depuy Synthes, www.depuysynthes.com*	Conditional 8	1.5, 3	
Restoration Modular Hip System *Stryker Orthopaedics, www.stryker.com*	Conditional 8	1.5, 3	
Reusable Titanium Skull Pin *Integra LifeSciences, www.integralife.com*	Conditional 6	3	
RigidFix Biocryl Tibial ST Cross Pin Kit, Nonmetallic *Depuy Synthes, www.depuysynthes.com*	Safe	1.5, 3	
RigidFix Biocryl Femoral ST Cross Pin Kit, Nonmetallic *Depuy Synthes, www.depuysynthes.com*	Safe	1.5, 3	
RigidFix BTB Cross Pin Kit, Nonmetallic *Depuy Synthes, www.depuysynthes.com*	Safe	1.5, 3	
RigidFix FEM/TIB BTB Cross Pin Kit, Nonmetallic *Depuy Synthes, www.depuysynthes.com*	Safe	1.5, 3	
RigidFix Femoral ST Cross Pin Kit, Nonmetallic *Depuy Synthes, www.depuysynthes.com*	Safe	1.5, 3	
RigidFix Kit, Nonmetallic *Depuy Synthes, www.depuysynthes.com*	Safe	1.5, 3	
RigidFix Tibial ST Cross Pin Kit, Nonmetallic *Depuy Synthes, www.depuysynthes.com*	Safe	1.5, 3	
RigidLoop Adjustable Cortical Fixation Implant *Depuy Synthes, www.depuysynthes.com*	Conditional 8	1.5, 3	
ROC XS, Nonmetallic *Depuy Synthes, www.depuysynthes.com*	Safe	1.5, 3	
Rod-To-Rod Clamp *Biomet, www.Biomet.com*	Safe	1.5	
ROI-A ALIF Cage, Spinal Implant *Zimmer Biomet, www.zimmerbiomet.com*	Conditional 5	1.5, 3	
ROI-C Cervical Cage *LDR Spine, www.ldrspine.com*	Conditional 5	1.5, 3	
Rusch Rod	Safe	1.5	
Samarys RF Cage *Alphatec Spine Inc., www.alphatecspine.com*	Conditional 6	3	
SECURE-C Cervical Artificial Disc *Globus Medical, Inc., www.globusmedical.com*	Conditional 8	1.5, 3	
SEMIAL Spinal Implant *PEEK, Titanium* *SIGNUS Medizintechnik GmbH, www.signus-med.de*	Conditional 6	3	
Side plate, 6-hole, Titanium alloy *Depuy Synthes, www.depuysynthes.com*	Safe	1.5	

Object	Status	Field Strength (T)	Reference
Sigma RP Total Knee *CoCrMo alloy and polyethylene* *Depuy Synthes, www.depuysynthes.com*	Conditional 6	3	
Silent Stem Assembly *Depuy Synthes, www.depuysynthes.com*	Conditional 8	1.5, 3	
Sleeve with ZipLoop Fixation Device *Biomet, www.biomet.com*	Safe	1.5, 3	
SLM Pin-To-Rod Clamp *Biomet, www.Biomet.com*	Safe	1.5	
Small External Fixator *External Fixation Device* *Biomet, www.biomet.com*	Conditional 5	1.5, 3	
Small External Fixator *External Fixation System* *Depuy Synthes, www.depuysynthes.com*	Conditional 5	1.5, 3	
Solanas Posterior Cervico-Thoracic Fixation System *Alphatec Spine Inc., www.alphatecspine.com*	Conditional 8	1.5, 3	
Solus Anterior Lumbar Interbody Fusion (ALIF) *Alphatec Spine Inc., www.alphatecspine.com*	Conditional 6	3	
Solus Lumbar Spacer *MRI information pertains to the following:* *Helifix, Novel CIS, Samarys, Novel X, Novel CP,* *Novel SD, Novel Tapered TL, Novel TL, Epicage,* *CC Cages, CO Cages, Iridium, and Novel ALS* *Alphatec Spine, Inc., www.alphatecspine.com*	Conditional 6	3	
Soteira Kyphoplasty System, Cement Director *Soteira, Inc., Natick, MA*	Conditional 6	3	
SOVEREIGN Spinal Interbody System *Medtronic, Inc., www.medtronic.com/mri*	Conditional 5	1.5, 3	
SOVEREIGN Spinal System *Medtronic, www.medtronic.com/mri*	Conditional 5	1.5, 3	
SpineAlign, Nitinol *SpineWorks, Santa Clara, CA*	Conditional 6	3	
Spinal L-Rod *Depuy Synthes, www.depuysynthes.com*	Safe	1.5, 3	
SpineJack *VEXIM SA, www.vexim.fr*	Conditional 8	1.5, 3	
Spiralok w/o Needles - Ethibond, Nonmetallic *Depuy Synthes, www.depuysynthes.com*	Safe	1.5, 3	
Spiralok w/o Needles - Panacryl, Nonmetallic *Depuy Synthes, www.depuysynthes.com*	Safe	1.5, 3	
Spiralok w/Orthocord, Nonmetallic *Depuy Synthes, www.depuysynthes.com*	Safe	1.5, 3	

Object	Status	Field Strength (T)	Reference
Spiralok with Needles - Ethibond, Nonmetallic *Depuy Synthes, www.depuysynthes.com*	Safe	1.5	
Spiralok with Needles - Panacryl, Nonmetallic *Depuy Synthes, www.depuysynthes.com*	Safe	1.5, 3	
Sports Medicine Allograft *Xtant Medical, www.xtantmedical.com*	Safe	1.5, 3	
Stainless Steel Mesh *Zimmer, www.zimmer.com*	Safe	1.5	3
Stainless Steel Plate *Zimmer, www.zimmer.com*	Safe	1.5	3
Stainless Steel Screw *Zimmer, www.zimmer.com*	Safe	1.5	3
Stainless Steel Wire *Zimmer, www.zimmer.com*	Safe	1.5	3
Stalif Midline Spinal Implant *Centinel Spine, www.centinelspine.com*	Conditional 6	3	
Staple Plate, Large, Zimaloy *Zimmer, www.zimmer.com*	Safe	1.5	3
Stryker Hoffmann III *Modular External Fixation Device* *Stryker, www.stryker.com*	Conditional 5	1.5, 3	
Summit Basic *Depuy Synthes, www.depuysynthes.com*	Conditional 6	3	
Summit Hip Stem, Titanium alloy *with CoCrMo alloy head* *Depuy Synthes, www.depuysynthes.com*	Conditional 6	3	
SuperAnchor *MRI information applies to other similar implants* *Depuy Synthes, www.depuysynthes.com*	Conditional 6	3	
SYMBIONIC LEG 3 *Ossur, www.ossur.com*	Unsafe 1	1.5	
Synde-Lock Fixation Device *Tarsus Medical, Inc., www.tarsusmedical.com*	Conditional 6	3	
Synthes AO DCP 2, 3, 4, 5 Hole Plate *Synthes, www.synthes.com*	Safe	1.5	
T2 ALTITUDE Expandable Corpectomy System *with 25-mm expandable centerpiece with 15 degree endcaps* *Medtronic, www.medtronic.com/mri*	Conditional 5	1.5, 3	
T2 XVBR Spinal System, *Expandable Centerpiece Device with T2 Spinal System 25-mm Extended Endcaps, 8 Degree* *Medtronic, Inc., www.medtronic.com/mri*	Conditional 6	3	

Object	Status	Field Strength (T)	Reference
T2 XVBR Spinal System *generation 1.5, with 25-mm expandable centerpiece with 15 degree endcaps Medtronic, www.medtronic.com/mri*	Conditional 5	1.5, 3	
Tapered Hip Stem *Arthrex, www.arthrex.com*	Conditional 8	1.5, 3	
Taylor Spatial Frame, Metal Version *Smith and Nephew, Memphis, TN*	Unsafe 1	1	
TeCorp VBR System *Telescopic Corpectomy System Alphatec Spine Inc., www.alphatecspine.com*	Conditional 8	1.5, 3	
Teno Fix Tendon Repair System *Ortheon Medical, LLC, Winter Park, FL*	Safe	1.5	
TETRIS Round Shape, Spinal Implant, PEEK, *Tantalum Pins SIGNUS Medizintechnik GmbH, www.signus-med.de*	Conditional 6	3	
TETRIS Spinal Implant, PEEK *SIGNUS Medizintechnik GmbH, www.signus-med.de*	Conditional 6	3	
TETRIS Spinal Implant, Titanium *SIGNUS Medizintechnik GmbH, www.signus-med.de*	Conditional 6	3	
TETRIS II Spinal Implant, PEEK, Tantalum Pins *SIGNUS Medizintechnik GmbH, www.signus-med.de*	Conditional 6	3	
TETRIS II Spinal Implant, Titanium *SIGNUS Medizintechnik GmbH, www.signus-med.de*	Conditional 6	3	
TiMesh Cranial Plating System *Medtronic, Inc., www.medtronic.com/mri*	Safe	1.5	
Tibial Intramedullary Nail *with Transfixation Screws, Titanium alloy Depuy Synthes, www.depuysynthes.com*	Conditional 6	3	
Tibial Nail, 9-mm, Titanium alloy *Depuy Synthes, www.depuysynthes.com*	Safe	1.5	
Titanium Femoral Reconstruction Nail, *Titanium alloy Biomet, www.Biomet.com*	Conditional 6	3	
Titanium Intramedullary Nail, Titanium alloy *Smith & Nephew, www.smith-nephew.com*	Safe	1.5, 3	83
Toe Joint, All Models *Biopro, Inc., www.bioproimplants.com*	Conditional 6	3	
TOPS (Total Posterior Arthroplasty System) *and VersaLink System Impliant Ltd.*	Conditional 6	3	
Total Hip System *MicroPort Orthopedics Inc., www.ortho.microport.com*	Conditional 5	1.5, 3	

Object	Status	Field Strength (T)	Reference
Total Knee Arthroplasty (TKA) *IBalance TKA, Entire Family, All Sizes* *Arthrex, Inc., www.arthrex.com*	Conditional 8	1.5, 3	
Transcarpal Hand with DMC Plus *Otto Bock HealthCare, www.ottobockus.com*	Unsafe 1	1.5	
Trestle Anterior Cervical Plating System *Alphatec Spine Inc., www.alphatecspine.com*	Conditional 8	1.5, 3	
Trestle Luxe Anterior Cervical Plating System *Alphatec Spine Inc., www.alphatecspine.com*	Conditional 8	1.5, 3	
Tri-Lobe Total Cervical Disc, cTDR *Dimicron, Inc., www.dimicron.com*	Conditional 8	1.5, 3	
TunneLoc Tibial Fixation Device Implant, PEEK *Biomet, www.Biomet.com*	Safe	1.5, 3	
Ultima Tri-Flange Acetabulum Cage, Titanium alloy *Depuy Synthes, www.depuysynthes.com*	Conditional 6	3	
UltraFix RC Suture Anchor *Linvatec Corporation*	Safe	1.5	
Unicondylar Knee Arthroplasty (UKA) *IBalance UKA, Entire Family, All Sizes* *Arthrex, Inc., www.arthrex.com*	Conditional 8	1.5, 3	
Univers II Humeral Stem *Arthrex, www.arthrex.com*	Conditional 8	1.5, 3	
Universal Reconstruction Ribbon *Depuy Synthes, www.depuysynthes.com*	Safe	1.5	
Variable Angle Compression Hip Screw *Biomet, www.Biomet.com*	Conditional 6	3	
VERTEX Reconstruction System *Medtronic, www.medtronic.com*	Conditional 5	1.5, 3	
Vertical Expandable Prosthetic Titanium Rib (VEPTR) *DePuy Synthes, www.depuysynthes.com*	Conditional 5	3	
Vertical Expandable Prosthetic Titanium Rib II (VEPTR II) *DePuy Synthes, www.depuysynthes.com*	Conditional 5	3	
Vertiflex Superion IDS, InterSpinous Spacer, *Spinal Implant* *Vertiflex, www.vertiflexspine.com*	Conditional 5	1.5, 3	
VSP Implant System *Depuy Synthes, www.depuysynthes.com*	Conditional 5	1.5, 3	
Wallis Posterior Dynamic Stabilization System *Zimmer, www.zimmer.com*	Safe	1.5, 3	
WedgeLoc Suture Anchor with Opti-Fiber Sutures *MedShape Solutions, Atlanta, GA*	Conditional 6	3	

Object	Status	Field Strength (T)	Reference
WOMBAT ST Spinal Implant *SIGNUS Medizintechnik GmbH, www.signus-med.de*	Conditional 8	1.5, 3	
Wristore Distal Radius Fracture Fixator *External Fixation Device* *Zimmer, Inc., Warsaw, IN*	Conditional 5	3	
Xenon Pedicle Screw System *Alphatec Spine Inc., www.alphatecspine.com*	Conditional 8	1.5, 3	
X-Mesh Expandable Cage System *Depuy Synthes, www.depuysynthes.com*	Conditional 8	1.5, 3	
X STOP Interspinous Process Decompression *(IPD) Implant* *Medtronic, Inc., www.medtronic.com/mri*	Conditional 6	3	
XtraFix External Fixation System *Extra Ortho, www.extraortho.com*	Conditional 5	1.5, 3	
Zielke Rod with Screw, Washer and Nut, 316L SS	Safe	0.3	33
Zodiac Deformity System *Alphatec Spine Inc., www.alphatecspine.com*	Conditional 8	1.5, 3	
Zodiac Direct Vertebral Rotation (DVR) System *Alphatec Spine Inc., www.alphatecspine.com*	Conditional 8	1.5, 3	
Zodiac Spinal Fixation System *Alphatec Spine Inc., www.alphatecspine.com*	Conditional 8	1.5, 3	
Zodiac Stainless Steel Construct *MRI information pertains to the following:* *Avalon, Solanas, Trestle, Trestle Luxe, Arsenal,* *Zodiac Degenerative System, Zodiac Deformity, Illico,* *Xenon, Osseoscrew, Leucadia Autolok, Isobar TTL-IN,* *Aspida, Bridgepoint, Illico FS, TeCorp,* *Novel Titanium Systems* *Alphatec Spine, Inc., www.alphatecspine.com*	Conditional 8	1.5, 3	

Otologic Implants, Cochlear Implants, and Others

Object	Status	Field Strength (T)	Reference
Applebaum Incus Replacement *Gyrus ACMI (Olympus Medical),* *www.medical.olympusamerica.com*	Safe	1.5	
Adjustable Length Titanium Ossicular *(ALTO) Partial Prostheses* *Grace Medical, www.gracemedical.com*	Conditional 5	1.5	
Adjustable Micron PORP, Otologic Implant, Titanium *Gyrus ACMI (Olympus Medical),* *www.medical.olympusamerica.com*	Conditional 5	3	
Adjustable Micron TORP, Otologic Implant, Titanium *Gyrus ACMI (Olympus Medical),* *www.medical.olympusamerica.com*	Conditional 5	3	

Object	Status	Field Strength (T)	Reference
Aerial Total Dusseldorf Titanium, Otologic Implant *Kurz Medical, www.kurzmed.com/en/products/mri-safety/*	Safe	1.5	
Aerial Total Tuebingen Titanium, Otologic Implant *Kurz Medical, www.kurzmed.com/en/products/mri-safety/*	Safe	1.5	
Aerial Total Vincent *Kurz Medical, www.kurzmed.com/en/products/mri-safety/*	Conditional 5	1.5, 3	
Alpha (M) Magnetic Implant, *Bone Conduction Hearing System* *Sophono, Inc. and Medtronic, www.sophono.com*	Conditional 5	1.5, 3	
ALTO Partial and Total Prostheses *Device Family, ALTO Partial and Total Prostheses;* *Family Product Number(s), 6XX, 612-001L, 612-002R;* *Device Material(s), Titanium, HA (hydroxyapatite), Silicone* *Grace Medical, www.gracemedical.com*	Conditional 6	3	
Angular Clip Prosthesis *Kurz Medical, www.kurzmed.com/en/products/mri-safety/*	Conditional 5	1.5, 3	
Angular Prosthesis *Kurz Medical, www.kurzmed.com/en/products/mri-safety/*	Conditional 5	1.5, 3	
Austin Mod TORP *Gyrus ACMI (Olympus Medical),* *www.medical.olympusamerica.com*	Safe	1.5	
Austin Tytan Piston *Titanium, Otologic Implant* *Treace Medical, Nashville, TN*	Safe	1.5	35
Baha, Bone Conduction Implant *Cochlear Corporation, www.cochlear.com*	Conditional 5	1.5, 3	
Bell Partial Dusseldorf Titanium, Otologic Implant *Kurz Medical, www.kurzmed.com/en/products/mri-safety/*	Safe	1.5	
Bell Partial Tuebingen Titanium, Otologic Implant *Kurz Medical, www.kurzmed.com/en/products/mri-safety/*	Safe	1.5	
Bell Partial Vincent *Kurz Medical, www.kurzmed.com/en/products/mri-safety/*	Conditional 5	1.5, 3	
Berger V Bobbin, Ventilation Tube *Richards Medical Co., Memphis, TN*	Safe	1.5	35
Berger V Bobbin VT, Ventilation Tube *Gyrus ACMI (Olympus Medical),* *www.medical.olympusamerica.com*	Conditional 5	3	
Black Oval *Gyrus ACMI (Olympus Medical),* *www.medical.olympusamerica.com*	Safe	3	
Blue Bobbin VT, Ventilation Tube *Gyrus ACMI (Olympus Medical),* *www.medical.olympusamerica.com*	Conditional 5	3	

Object	Status	Field Strength (T)	Reference
Bobbin VT, Ventilation Tube *Gyrus ACMI (Olympus Medical),* *www.medical.olympusamerica.com*	Conditional 5	3	
BONEBRIDGE BCI 601 *Bone Conduction Implant* *MED-EL, www.medel.com*	Conditional 5	1.5	
Bucket Handle, Stapes Prosthesis *Gyrus ACMI (Olympus Medical),* *www.medical.olympusamerica.com*	Conditional 5	3	
Bucket Type Stapes Prosthesis *Kurz Medical, www.kurzmed.com/en/products/mri-safety/*	Conditional 5	1.5, 3	
Causse Flex H/A, Partial Ossicular Prosthesis *Microtek Medical, Inc., Memphis, TN*	Safe	1.5	36
Causse Flex H/A, Total Ossicular Prosthesis *Microtek Medical Inc., Memphis, TN*	Safe	1.5	36
Chicago Bucket Handle Stapes Prosthesis *Gyrus ACMI (Olympus Medical),* *www.medical.olympusamerica.com*	Conditional 5	3	
Classic SS, Otologic Implant *Gyrus ACMI (Olympus Medical),* *www.medical.olympusamerica.com*	Conditional 5	3	
Classic Stapes Prosthesis, Otologic Implant *Gyrus ACMI (Olympus Medical),* *www.medical.olympusamerica.com*	Conditional 5	3	
Classic Stapes Prostheses, Otologic Implant *Gyrus ACMI (Olympus Medical),* *www.medical.olympusamerica.com*	Conditional 5	3	
Clip Partial Prosthesis *Kurz Medical, www.kurzmed.com/en/products/mri-safety/*	Conditional 5	1.5, 3	
Clip Partial Prosthesis Titanium *(Dresden type), Otologic Implant* *Kurz Medical, www.kurzmed.com/en/products/mri-safety/*	Conditional 5	1.5, 3	
Clip Piston aWengen Titanium, Otologic Implant *Kurz Medical, www.kurzmed.com/en/products/mri-safety/*	Conditional 5	1.5, 3	
Cochlear Implant, HiRes 90K Cochlear Implant *Advanced Bionics Corporation, Sylmar, CA*	Conditional 5	0.3, 1.5	
Cochlear Implant, HiRes 90K ADVANTAGE *Cochlear Implant* *Advanced Bionics Corporation, Sylmar, CA*	Conditional 5	1.5	
Cochlear Implant, Nucleus 24 ABI Cochlear *Implant System* *Cochlear Corporation, www.cochlear.com*	Conditional 5	1.5	
Cochlear Implant, Nucleus Mini 20-channel *Cochlear Corporation, www.cochlear.com*	Unsafe 1	1.5	38

Object	Status	Field Strength (T)	Reference
Cochlear Implant, Nucleus, Various Models *Cochlear Corporation, www.cochlear.com*	Conditional 5	1.5	
Cochlear Implant *3M/House*	Unsafe 1	0.6	37
Cochlear Implant *3M/Vienna*	Unsafe 1	0.6	37
Cody Tack, Otologic Implant	Safe	0.6	37
Collar Bobbin VT, Ventilation Tube *Gyrus ACMI (Olympus Medical),* *www.medical.olympusamerica.com*	Conditional 5	3	
CONCERT and CONCERT PIN Cochlear Implant *Med-El, www.medel.com*	Conditional 5	0.2, 1.5	
Custom Classic Stapes, Otologic Implant, 316L SS *Gyrus ACMI (Olympus Medical),* *www.medical.olympusamerica.com*	Conditional 5	3	
De La Cruz, Fluoroplastic, Platinum, Piston *Medtronic Xomed, www.medtronic.com*	Conditional 5	3	
Duesseldorf Type Aerial *Kurz Medical, www.kurzmed.com/en/products/mri-safety/*	Conditional 5	1.5, 3	
Duesseldorf Type Bell *Kurz Medical, www.kurzmed.com/en/products/mri-safety/*	Conditional 5	1.5, 3	
Dornhoffer Footplate Shoe, Otologic Implant, *Titanium* *Gyrus ACMI (Olympus Medical),* *www.medical.olympusamerica.com*	Conditional 5	3	
Dornhoffer Malleable PORP, Otologic Implant, *316L SS* *Gyrus ACMI (Olympus Medical),* *www.medical.olympusamerica.com*	Conditional 5	3	
Dornhoffer Titanium, Otologic Implant, Titanium *Gyrus ACMI (Olympus Medical),* *www.medical.olympusamerica.com*	Conditional 5	3	
Ehmke Hook Stapes Prosthesis, Platinum, *Otologic Implant* *Richards Medical Co., Memphis, TN*	Safe	1.5	35
Fisch Piston, Teflon, SS, Otologic Implant *Richards Medical Co., Memphis, TN*	Safe	1.5	38
Fisch Piston, Otologic Implant, 316L SS *Gyrus ACMI (Olympus Medical),* *www.medical.olympusamerica.com*	Conditional 5	3	
Fisch Teflon Piston, Otologic Implant, 316L SS *Gyrus ACMI (Olympus Medical),* *www.medical.olympusamerica.com*	Conditional 5	3	

Object	Status	Field Strength (T)	Reference
Flex H/A Notched, Offset Total Ossicular Prosthesis *Microtek Medical, Inc., Memphis, TN*	Safe	1.5	36
Flex H/A Offset Partial Ossicular Prosthesis *Microtek Medical, Inc., Memphis, TN*	Safe	1.5	36
FLPL Malleable Piston Otologic Implant *Gyrus ACMI (Olympus Medical),* *www.medical.olympusamerica.com*	Conditional 5	3	
FLPL/Titanium VT, Ventilation Tube *Gyrus ACMI (Olympus Medical),* *www.medical.olympusamerica.com*	Conditional 5	3	
Foot Shoes *Family Product Number(s), 636-XXX; Material, Titanium* *Grace Medical, www.gracemedical.com*	Conditional 6	3	
Goldenberg Mal Porp Otologic Implant *Gyrus ACMI (Olympus Medical),* *www.medical.olympusamerica.com*	Conditional 5	3	
Grote Canal *Gyrus ACMI (Olympus Medical),* *www.medical.olympusamerica.com*	Safe	1.5, 3	
Gyrus All Titanium Centered PORP *Partial Ossicular Replacement Prosthesis* *Gyrus ACMI (Olympus Medical),* *www.medical.olympusamerica.com*	Safe	3	106
Gyrus All Titanium Monolithic Centered TORP *Total Ossicular Replacement Prosthesis* *Gyrus ACMI (Olympus Medical),* *www.medical.olympusamerica.com*	Safe	3	106
Gyrus, PORP, Partial Ossicular Replacement Prosthesis *Gyrus ACMI (Olympus Medical),* *www.medical.olympusamerica.com*	Safe	3	106
Gyrus, TORP, Total Ossicular Replacement Prosthesis *Gyrus ACMI (Olympus Medical),* *www.medical.olympusamerica.com*	Safe	3	106
Gyrus SMart Stapes Piston, Titanium *Gyrus ACMI (Olympus Medical),* *www.medical.olympusamerica.com*	Safe	3	106
House Double Loop, ASTM-318- 76 Grade 2 SS, *Otologic Implant* *Storz, St. Louis, MO*	Safe	1.5	35
House Double Loop, Tantalum, Otologic Implant *Storz, St. Louis, MO*	Safe	1.5	35
House Single Loop, ASTM-318- 76, Grade 2 SS, *Otologic Implant* *Storz, St. Louis, MO*	Safe	1.5	31

Object	Status	Field Strength (T)	Reference
House Single Loop, Tantalum, Otologic Implant *Storz, St. Louis, MO*	Safe	1.5	35
House Wire Loop, Otologic Implant, 316LVM SS *Gyrus ACMI (Olympus Medical),* *www.medical.olympusamerica.com*	Conditional 5	3	
House wire, SS, Otologic Implant *Otomed*	Safe	0.5	39
House wire, Tantalum, Otologic Implant *Otomed*	Safe	0.5	39
House-type Incus Prosthesis *Otologic Implant*	Safe	0.6	
House-type SS, Piston and wire *ASTM-318-76 Grade 2 SS, Otologic Implant* *Xomed-Treace Inc., A Bristol-Myers Squibb Co.*	Safe	1.5	35
House-type wire loop, Stapes prosthesis, 316L SS, *Otologic Implant* *Richards Medical Co., Memphis, TN*	Safe	1.5	35
Incus Bridge Prosthesis *Kurz Medical, www.kurzmed.com/en/products/mri-safety/*	Conditional 5	1.5, 3	
InSound XT Series *InSound Medical, Newark, CA*	Unsafe 1	1.5	
Jahn Tube *Gyrus ACMI (Olympus Medical),* *www.medical.olympusamerica.com*	Safe	1.5, 3	
K-Helix Prosthesis *Device Family, K-Helix Prosthesis; Family Product* *Number(s),* *756-XXX, 757-XXX; Device Material(s), Titanium* *Grace Medical, www.gracemedical.com*	Conditional 6	3	
K Piston Titanium, Otologic Implant *Kurz Medical, www.kurzmed.com/en/products/mri-safety/*	Safe	3	
Kartush Incus Strut Prostheses *Gyrus ACMI (Olympus Medical),* *www.medical.olympusamerica.com*	Conditional 6	3	
Kurz Aerial, Titanium *Kurz Medical, www.kurzmed.com/en/products/mri-safety/*	Safe	3	106
Kurz Aerial-Total-Dusseldorf-Titanium *TORP, Total Ossicular Replacement Prosthesis* *Kurz Medical, www.kurzmed.com/en/products/mri-safety/*	Safe	3	106
Kurz Bell *Titanium* *Kurz Medical, www.kurzmed.com/en/products/mri-safety/*	Safe	3	106

Object	Status	Field Strength (T)	Reference
Kurz Bell-Partial-Dusseldorf-Titanium *PORP, Partial Ossicular Replacement Prosthesis* *Kurz Medical, www.kurzmed.com/en/products/mri-safety/*	Safe	3	106
Kurz Piston, Titanium *Kurz Medical, www.kurzmed.com/en/products/mri-safety/*	Safe	3	106
Kurz Piston-Titanium, Stapes *Kurz Medical, www.kurzmed.com/en/products/mri-safety/*	Safe	3	106
Lenticle Cup Prosthesis *Kurz Medical, www.kurzmed.com/en/products/mri-safety/*	Conditional 5	1.5, 3	
Lippy Modified Bucket Handle, Stapes Prosthesis *Gyrus ACMI (Olympus Medical),* *www.medical.olympusamerica.com*	Conditional 5	3	
Lippy Modified Stapes Prostheses *Gyrus ACMI (Olympus Medical),* *www.medical.olympusamerica.com*	Conditional 5	3	
Lyric Hearing Device *InSound Medical, Newark, CA*	Unsafe 1	1.5	
Malleus Notch Prosthesis *Kurz Medical, www.kurzmed.com/en/products/mri-safety/*	Conditional 5	1.5, 3	
MAXUM System, MAXUM Hearing Implant *Ototronix, www.ototronix.com*	Unsafe 1	1.5	
Matrix Stapes Prosthesis *Kurz Medical, www.kurzmed.com/en/products/mri-safety/*	Conditional 5	1.5, 3	
McGee Piston, Otologic Implant *Gyrus ACMI (Olympus Medical),* *www.medical.olympusamerica.com*	Conditional 5	3	
McGee Piston Stapes Prosthesis *Otologic Implant* *Richards Medical Co., Memphis, TN*	Safe	1.5	35
McGee Piston Stapes Prosthesis *Platinum, Otologic Implant* *Richards Medical Co., Memphis, TN*	Safe	1.5	35
McGee Piston Stapes Prosthesis *Platinum, Chromium-Nickel alloy, SS, Otologic Implant* *Richards Medical Co., Memphis, TN*	Unsafe 1	1.5	38
McGee Shepard's Crook Piston, *Otologic Implant, SS* *Gyrus ACMI (Olympus Medical),* *www.medical.olympusamerica.com*	Conditional 5	3	
McGee Sheperd's Crook Stapes prosthesis *316L SS, Otologic Implant* *Richards Medical Co., Memphis, TN*	Safe	1.5	35
MED-EL COMBI 40+, MED-EL Cochlear Implant *Med-El, www.medel.com*	Conditional 5	0.2, 1.5	

Object	Status	Field Strength (T)	Reference
MED-EL SONATA Cochlear Implant *Med-El, www.medel.com*	Conditional 5	0.2, 1.5	
Medtronic-Xomed PORP *Partial Ossicular Replacement Prosthesis, Titanium* *Medtronic Xomed, www.medtronic.com*	Safe	3	106
Medtronic-Xomed TORP *Total Ossicular Replacement Prosthesis, Titanium* *Medtronic Xomed, www.medtronic.com*	Safe	3	106
MEY Modified Lippy, Otologic Implant *Gyrus ACMI (Olympus Medical),* *www.medical.olympusamerica.com*	Conditional 5	3	
Micron Bobbin Blue VT, Ventilation Tube *Gyrus ACMI (Olympus Medical),* *www.medical.olympusamerica.com*	Conditional 5	3	
Micron Bobbin VT, Ventilation Tube *Gyrus ACMI (Olympus Medical),* *www.medical.olympusamerica.com*	Conditional 5	3	
Micron II Modular, PORP Otologic Implant *Gyrus ACMI (Olympus Medical),* *www.medical.olympusamerica.com*	Conditional 5	3	
Micron II Modular, TORP Otologic Implant *Gyrus ACMI (Olympus Medical),* *www.medical.olympusamerica.com*	Conditional 5	3	
Micron II Monolithic, PORP Otologic Implant *Gyrus ACMI (Olympus Medical),* *www.medical.olympusamerica.com*	Conditional 5	3	
Micron II Monolithic, TORP Otologic Implant *Gyrus ACMI (Olympus Medical),* *www.medical.olympusamerica.com*	Conditional 5	3	
Micron Plus VT, Ventilation Tube *Gyrus ACMI (Olympus Medical),* *www.medical.olympusamerica.com*	Conditional 5	3	
Micron Spoon Bobbin VT, Ventilation Tube *Gyrus ACMI (Olympus Medical),* *www.medical.olympusamerica.com*	Conditional 5	3	
Minimal Type Ventilation Tube *Kurz Medical, www.kurzmed.com/en/products/mri-safety/*	Unsafe 1	1.5	
Modified Lippy, Otologic Implant, 316L SS *Gyrus ACMI (Olympus Medical),* *www.medical.olympusamerica.com*	Conditional 5	3	
Moretz Type VT, Ventilation Tube *Gyrus ACMI (Olympus Medical),* *www.medical.olympusamerica.com*	Conditional 5	3	

Object	Status	Field Strength (T)	Reference
Munchen Aerial Total Prosthesis *Kurz Medical, www.kurzmed.com/en/products/mri-safety/*	Conditional 5	1.5, 3	
Munchen Bell Partial Prosthesis *Kurz Medical, www.kurzmed.com/en/products/mri-safety/*	Conditional 5	1.5, 3	
NitiBOND Stapes Prosthesis *Kurz Medical, www.kurzmed.com/en/products/mri-safety/*	Conditional 5	1.5, 3	
NitiFLEX Stapes Prosthesis *Kurz Medical, www.kurzmed.com/en/products/mri-safety/*	Conditional 5	1.5, 3	
Nucleus 22, Cochlear Implant *Without removable magnet* *Cochlear LTD, www.cochlear.com*	Unsafe 1	1.5	
Nucleus 22, Cochlear Implant *With removable magnet* *Cochlear LTD, www.cochlear.com*	Conditional 5	1.5	
Nucleus 24 Series, Cochlear Implant *Cochlear LTD, www.cochlear.com*	Conditional 5	1.5	
Nucleus Freedom, Cochlear Implant *Cochlear LTD, www.cochlear.com*	Conditional 5	1.5	
Offset ALTO Total Prosthesis *MRI information applies to Pistons,* *SS/Teflon, P/N 410-600;* *Titanium/Teflon, P/N 409-XXX, 417-XXX;* *Platinum/Titanium, P/N 418-XXX, 419-XXX;* *Grace Medical, www.gracemedical.com*	Conditional 6	3	
Offset ALTO Total Prosthesis *MRI information applies to Pistons,* *SS/Teflon, P/N 410-600;* *Titanium/Teflon, P/N 409-XXX, 417-XXX;* *Platinum/Titanium, P/N 418-XXX, 419-XXX;* *Grace Medical, www.gracemedical.com*	Conditional 6	3	
Offset ALTO Total Prosthesis *MRI information applies to* *Platinum/Teflon, P/N 411-XXX, 412-XXX,* *415-XXX, 452-XXX, 453-XXX;* *Nitinol/Teflon, P/N 465-XXX, 466-XXX,* *467-XXX, 468-XXX, 469-XXX;* *Grace Medical, www.gracemedical.com*	Conditional 6	3	
Offset ALTO Total Prosthesis *MRI information applies to Buckets* *Titanium, CP2 & CP4* *P/N 420-XXX through 430-XXX* *OCR's, Middle Ear Implants, Titanium CP2,* *other materials HA and Silicone* *ALTO 600 Series, Titanium CP2, Fixed Length 700 Series* *Grace Medical, www.gracemedical.com*	Conditional 6	3	

Object	Status	Field Strength (T)	Reference
Pacific Vent Tube *Gyrus ACMI (Olympus Medical),* *www.medical.olympusamerica.com*	Conditional 6	3	
Partial and Total Prostheses *Device Family, Partial and Total Prosthesis;* *Family Product Number(s), 1XX, 190-XXX, 749-XXX;* *Device Material(s), HA, hydroxyapatite* *Grace Medical, www.gracemedical.com*	Safe	3	
Partial and Total Prostheses *Device Family, Partial and Total Prosthesis;* *Family Product Number(s), 2XX, 193;* *Device Material(s), HA (hydroxyapatite), Silicone* *Grace Medical, www.gracemedical.com*	Safe	3	
Pediatric VT Ventilation Tube *Gyrus ACMI (Olympus Medical),* *www.medical.olympusamerica.com*	Conditional 5	3	
Piston Teflon Wire Otologic Implant, 316L SS *Gyrus ACMI (Olympus Medical),* *www.medical.olympusamerica.com*	Conditional 5	3	
Plasti-pore Piston, 316L SS, Plasti-pore material *Richards Medical Co., Memphis, TN*	Safe	1.5	35
Platinum Ribbon Loop Stapes Prosthesis *Richards Medical Co., Memphis, TN*	Safe	1.5	35
Ponto Implant Assembly *Oticon Medical, www.oticonmedical.com*	Conditional 8	1.5, 3	
Precise and other Ossicular Prostheses *Device Family, Precise Prosthesis;* *Family Product Number(s),* *602-XXX, 652-XXX, 700-XXX, 705-XXX, 706-XXX, 707-* *XXX, 720-XXX, 750-XXX, 751-XXX, 765-XXX, 770-XXX;* *Device Material(s), Titanium, HA (hydroxyapatite)* *Grace Medical, www.gracemedical.com*	Conditional 6	3	
Pulsar Cochlear Implant, PULSARCI100 *Med-El, www.medel.com*	Conditional 5	0.2, 1.5	98
Regensberg Type Prosthesis *Kurz Medical, www.kurzmed.com/en/products/mri-safety/*	Conditional 5	1.5, 3	
Reuter Bobbin, Ventilation Tube *Richards Medical Co., Memphis, TN*	Safe	1.5	35
Reuter Bobbin VT, Ventilation Tube *Gyrus ACMI (Olympus Medical),* *www.medical.olympusamerica.com*	Conditional 5	3	
Reuter Bobbin Vent Tube *Gyrus ACMI (Olympus Medical),* *www.medical.olympusamerica.com*	Conditional 5	3	

Object	Status	Field Strength (T)	Reference
Reuter Drain Tube, Otologic Implant	Safe	1.5	35
Richards Bucket Handle Stapes Prosthesis *Richards Medical Co., Memphis, TN*	Safe	1.5	35
Richard's Bucket Handle, Otologic Implant, *Tantalum* *Gyrus ACMI (Olympus Medical),* *www.medical.olympusamerica.com*	Conditional 5	3	
Richards Piston Stapes Prosthesis, *Platinum, Fluoroplastic, Otologic Implant* *Richards Medical Co., Memphis, TN*	Safe	1.5	35
Richards Plasti-pore with Armstrong-style *Platinum, Otologic Implant* *Richards Medical Co., Memphis, TN*	Safe	1.5	35
Richards Platinum Teflon Piston *0.6-mm, Teflon, Platinum, Otologic Implant* *Richards Medical Co., Memphis, TN*	Safe	1.5	38
Richards Platinum Teflon Piston *0.8-mm, Teflon, Platinum, Otologic Implant* *Richards Medical Co., Memphis, TN*	Safe	1.5	38
Richards Shepherd's crook *Platinum, Otologic Implant* *Richards Medical Co., Memphis, TN*	Safe	0.5	39
Richards Teflon Piston *Teflon, Otologic Implant* *Richards Medical Co., Memphis, TN*	Safe	1.5	38
Roberson Stapes Prosthesis, Titanium *Medtronic Xomed, www.medtronic.com*	Safe	3	
Roberts Universal Prosthesis, PORP *Otologic Implant, Titanium* *Gyrus ACMI (Olympus Medical),* *www.medical.olympusamerica.com*	Conditional 5	3	
Roberts Universal Prosthesis, TORP *Otologic Implant, Titanium* *Gyrus ACMI (Olympus Medical),* *www.medical.olympusamerica.com*	Conditional 5	3	
Robinson incus replacement Prosthesis *ASTM-318-76 Grade 2 SS, Otologic Implant* *Storz, St. Louis, MO*	Safe	1.5	35
Robinson Stapes Prosthesis *ASTM-318-76 Grade 2 SS, Otologic Implant* *Storz, St. Louis, MO*	Safe	1.5	35
Robinson-Moon offset Stapes Prosthesis *ASTM-318-76 Grade 2 SS, Otologic Implant* *Storz, St. Louis, MO*	Safe	1.5	35

Object	Status	Field Strength (T)	Reference
Robinson-Moon-Lippy offset Stapes Prosthesis *ASTM- 318-76 Grade 2 SS, Otologic Implant Storz, St. Louis, MO*	Safe	1.5	35
Ronis Piston Stapes Prosthesis *Richards Medical Co., Memphis, TN*	Safe	1.5	35
Ronis Piston Otologic Implant, 316L SS *Gyrus ACMI (Olympus Medical), www.medical.olympusamerica.com*	Conditional 5	3	
Ronis Wire Piston Otologic Implant, 316L SS *Gyrus ACMI (Olympus Medical), www.medical.olympusamerica.com*	Conditional 5	3	
Shea Cup Piston Stapes Prosthesis *Platinum, Fluoroplastic, Otologic Implant Richards Medical Co., Memphis, TN*	Safe	1.5	35
Shea Malleus Attachment Piston *Teflon, Otologic Implant Richards Medical Co., Memphis, TN*	Safe	1.5	38
Shea SS and Teflon wire Prosthesis *Teflon, 316L SS, Otologic Implant Richards Medical Co., Memphis, TN*	Safe	1.5	38
Scheer FLPL Wire, Otologic Implant, 316L SS *Gyrus ACMI (Olympus Medical), www.medical.olympusamerica.com*	Conditional 5	3	
Scheer Piston, Teflon, 316L SS, Otologic Implant *Richards Medical Co., Memphis, TN*	Safe	1.5	33
Scheer Piston Stapes Prosthesis, 316L SS, *Fluoroplastic, Otologic Implant Richards Medical Co., Memphis, TN*	Safe	1.5	35
Schuk Wire Piston, Otologic Implant, 316L SS *Gyrus ACMI (Olympus Medical), www.medical.olympusamerica.com*	Conditional 5	3	
Schuknecht Gelfoam and Wire Prosthesis, *Armstrong style, 316L SS, Otologic Implant Richards Medical Co., Memphis, TN*	Safe	1.5	40
Schuknecht Piston Stapes Prosthesis *316L SS, Fluoroplastic, Otologic Implant Richards Medical Co., Memphis, TN*	Safe	1.5	35
Schuknecht Tef-wire Incus Attachment *ASTM-318-76 Grade 2 SS, Otologic Implant Storz, St. Louis, MO*	Safe	1.5	35
Schuknecht Tef-wire Malleus Attachment *ASTM-318-76 Grade 2 SS, Otologic Implant Storz, St. Louis, MO*	Safe	1.5	35

Object	Status	Field Strength (T)	Reference
Schuknecht Teflon Wire Piston *0.6-mm, Teflon, 316L SS, Otologic Implant* *Richards Medical Co., Memphis, TN*	Safe	1.5	38
Schuknecht Teflon Wire Piston *0.8-mm, Teflon, 316L SS, Otologic Implant* *Richards Medical Co., Memphis, TN*	Safe	1.5	38
Sheehy Incus Replacement *ASTM-318-76 Grade 2 SS, Otologic Implant* *Storz, St. Louis, MO*	Safe	1.5	35
Sheehy Incus Strut, 316L SS, Otologic Implant *Richards Medical Co., Memphis, TN*	Safe	1.5	38
Sheehy Stapes Replacement Strut *Otologic Implant, 316L SS* *Gyrus ACMI (Olympus Medical),* *www.medical.olympusamerica.com*	Conditional 5	3	
Sheehy-Type Incus Replacement Strut *Teflon, 316L SS, Otologic Implant* *Richards Medical Co., Memphis, TN*	Safe	1.5	35
Sheehy-Type Incus Replacement Strut *Otologic Implant, 316L SS* *Gyrus ACMI (Olympus Medical),* *www.medical.olympusamerica.com*	Conditional 5	3	
Shepherd Crook Piston Otologic Implant, 316L SS *Gyrus ACMI (Olympus Medical),* *www.medical.olympusamerica.com*	Conditional 5	3	
Shipp Modified Berger VT, Ventilation Tube *Gyrus ACMI (Olympus Medical),* *www.medical.olympusamerica.com*	Conditional 5	3	
Silverstein Malleus Clip, Ventilation Tube *Richards Medical Co., Memphis, TN*	Safe	1.5	38
SMart De La Cruz Piston *Otologic Implant, Nitinol/Fluoroplastic* *Gyrus ACMI (Olympus Medical),* *www.medical.olympusamerica.com*	Conditional 5	3	
SMart Malleus Piston, Otologic Implant, *Nitinol/Fluoroplastic* *Gyrus ACMI (Olympus Medical),* *www.medical.olympusamerica.com*	Conditional 5	3	
SMart Piston, Otologic Implant, Fluoroplastic/Nitinol *Gyrus ACMI (Olympus Medical),* *www.medical.olympusamerica.com*	Conditional 5	3	
SOUNDTEC Direct Drive Hearing System *SOUNDTEC, Inc., Oklahoma City, OK*	Unsafe 1	1.5	

Object	Status	Field Strength (T)	Reference
Spoon Bobbin Ventilation Tube *Richards Medical Co., Memphis, TN*	Safe	1.5	35
Spoon-Bobbin Vent Tube *Gyrus ACMI (Olympus Medical),* *www.medical.olympusamerica.com*	Conditional 5	3	
Spoon Bobbin Ventilation Tube *Otologic Implant, All Sizes* *Grace Medical, www.gracemedical.com*	Conditional 8	1.5, 3	
Stainless Steel/Fluoroplastic, Sanna-Type Piston *MRI information applies to Pistons* *SS/Teflon, P/N 410 600;* *Titanium/Teflon, P/N 409-XXX, 417-XXX;* *Platinum/Titanium, P/N 418-XXX, 419-XXX;* *Grace Medical, www.gracemedical.com*	Conditional 6	3	
Stainless Steel/Fluoroplastic, Sanna-Type Piston *MRI information applies to* *Platinum/Teflon, P/N 411-XXX, 412-XXX,* *415-XXX, 452-XXX, 453-XXX;* *Nitinol/Teflon, P/N 465-XXX, 466-XXX,* *467-XXX, 468-XXX, 469-XXX;* *Grace Medical, www.gracemedical.com*	Conditional 6	3	
Stainless Steel/Fluoroplastic, Sanna-Type Piston *MRI information applies to Buckets* *Titanium, CP2 & CP4* *P/N 420-XXX through 430-XXX* *OCR's, Middle Ear Implants* *Titanium CP2,* *other materials HA and Silicone* *ALTO 600 Series* *Titanium CP2* *Fixed Length 700 Series* *Grace Medical, www.gracemedical.com*	Conditional 6	3	
Stainless Steel Vent Tube & Stainless Steel Wire *VT-1400-0, Because the size of the metallic mass* *associated with this product, the MRI test findings apply to* *all of the following products from Micromedics, Inc.* *VT-0205-, Fluoroplastic with stainless steel wire* *VT-0702-, Silicone with stainless steel wire* *VT-1402-, Stainless Steel with Stainless Steel wire* *VT-1412-, Titanium with Stainless Steel wire* *VT-1505-, Polyethylene with Stainless Steel wire* *Micromedics, Inc., Eagan, MN*	Conditional 6	3	
Stapes, Fluoroplastic/Platinum, Piston, Otologic Implant *Microtek Medical, Inc., Memphis, TN*	Safe	1.5	36
Stapes, Fluoroplastic/SS Piston, Otologic Implant *Microtek Medical, Inc., Memphis, TN*	Safe	1.5	36

Object	Status	Field Strength (T)	Reference
Stapes Grommet, Replacement Strut *Otologic Implant, 316L SS* *Gyrus ACMI (Olympus Medical),* *www.medical.olympusamerica.com*	Conditional 5	3	
Stapes Prostheses, Bucket *Device Family, Stapes Prosthesis, Bucket;* *Family Product Number(s), 420-XXX, 421-XXX, 422-XXX,* *423-XXX, 424-XXX, 425-XXX, 426-XXX, 427-XXX,* *428-XXX, 429-XXX, 430-XXX, 431-XXX, 432-XXX;* *Device Material(s), Titanium, Nitinol* *Grace Medical, www.gracemedical.com*	Conditional 6	3	
Stapes Prostheses, Piston *Device Family, Stapes Prosthesis, Piston;* *Family Product Number(s), 409-XXX, 410-XXX, 411-XXX,* *412-XXX, 413-XXX, 415-XXX, 416-XXX, 417-XXX,* *418-XXX, 419-XXX, 440-XXX, 442-XXX, 450-XXX,* *451-XXX, 452-XXX, 453-XXX, 456-XXX, 460-XXX,* *461-XXX, 462-XXX, 464-XXX, 465-XXX, 466-XXX,* *467-XXX, 468-XXX, 469-XXX, 470-XXX, 471-XXX;* *Device Material(s), Titanium, Platinum, Stainless Steel,* *Nitinol, Fluroplastic* *Grace Medical, www.gracemedical.com*	Conditional 6	3	
Stapes Prostheses, Pistons *Device Family, Stapes Prostheses, Pistons;* *Family Product Number(s), 401-XXX, 402-XXX, 403-XXX,* *404-XXX, 405-XXX, 406-XXX, 408-XXX;* *Device Material(s), Fluoroplastic* *Grace Medical, www.gracemedical.com*	Safe	3	
Strasnick Prostheses, Device Family, *Strasnick Prosthesis;* *Family Product Number(s), 220-XXX, 270-XXX;* *Device Material(s), Titanium, Silicone* *Grace Medical, www.gracemedical.com*	Conditional 6	3	
SYNCHRONY Cochlear Implant *Med-El, www.medel.com*	Conditional 5	1.5, 3	
SYNCHRONY Pin Cochlear Implant *Med-El, www.medel.com*	Conditional 5	1.5, 3	
Tantalum Wire Loop, Otologic Implant *Gyrus ACMI (Olympus Medical),* *www.medical.olympusamerica.com*	Conditional 5	3	
Tantalum Wire loop, Stapes Prosthesis *Richards Medical Co., Memphis, TN*	Safe	1.5	35
Teflon Malleable Piston, Otologic Implant *Gyrus ACMI (Olympus Medical),* *www.medical.olympusamerica.com*	Conditional 5	3	

Object	Status	Field Strength (T)	Reference
Teflon Piston, Otologic Implant *Gyrus ACMI (Olympus Medical),* *www.medical.olympusamerica.com*	Conditional 5	3	
Teflon Wire Piston, Otologic Implant *Gyrus ACMI (Olympus Medical),* *www.medical.olympusamerica.com*	Conditional 5	3	
Tef-Platinum Piston, Platinum, Otologic Implant *Xomed-Treace Inc., A Bristol-Myers Squibb Co.*	Safe	1.5	35
Touma Modified Crook Piston *Otologic Implant, 316L SS* *Gyrus ACMI (Olympus Medical),* *www.medical.olympusamerica.com*	Conditional 5	3	
The Big Easy Piston, Stapes Prosthesis *Angel Medical Instruments, www.angelmedex.com*	Safe	1.5, 3	
Total Ossicular Replacement Prosthesis (TORP) *316L SS, Otologic Implant* *Richards Medical Co., Memphis, TN*	Safe	1.5	38
Trapeze Ribbon Loop Stapes Prosthesis *Platinum, Otologic Implant* *Richards Medical Co., Memphis, TN*	Safe	1.5	35
Trocar with Wire *Kurz Medical, www.kurzmed.com/en/products/mri-safety/*	Unsafe 1	1.5	
TTP Aerial Vario Titanium *Kurz Medical, www.kurzmed.com/en/products/mri-safety/*	Conditional 5	1.5, 3	
TTP Bell Vario Titanium *Kurz Medical, www.kurzmed.com/en/products/mri-safety/*	Conditional 5	1.5, 3	
TTP Tuebingen Type Aerial *Kurz Medical, www.kurzmed.com/en/products/mri-safety/*	Conditional 5	1.5, 3	
TTP Tuebingen Type Bell *Kurz Medical, www.kurzmed.com/en/products/mri-safety/*	Conditional 5	1.5, 3	
TTP VARIAC/VARIO System Partial *Kurz Medical, www.kurzmed.com/en/products/mri-safety/*	Conditional 5	1.5, 3	
TTP VARIAC/VARIO System Total *Kurz Medical, www.kurzmed.com/en/products/mri-safety/*	Conditional 5	1.5, 3	
Tuebingen Type Ventilation Tubes *with Wire, Gold, SS* *Kurz Medical, www.kurzmed.com/en/products/mri-safety/*	Unsafe 1	1.5	
Tuebingen Type Ventilation Tubes *with Wire, Silver, SS* *Kurz Medical, www.kurzmed.com/en/products/mri-safety/*	Unsafe 1	1.5	
Tuebingen Type Ventilation Tubes *with Wire, Titanium, SS* *Kurz Medical, www.kurzmed.com/en/products/mri-safety/*	Unsafe 1	1.5	

Object	Status	Field Strength (T)	Reference
UniBobbin VT, Ventilation Tube *Gyrus ACMI (Olympus Medical),* *www.medical.olympusamerica.com*	Conditional 5	3	
Venturi Plus VT, Ventilation Tube *Gyrus ACMI (Olympus Medical),* *www.medical.olympusamerica.com*	Conditional 5	3	
Venturi VT, Ventilation Tube *Gyrus ACMI (Olympus Medical),* *www.medical.olympusamerica.com*	Conditional 5	3	
Vibrant Soundbridge *Med-El, www.medel.com*	Unsafe 1	1.5	
Vibrant Soundbridge, VORP 502 Implant *Vibrating Ossicular Prosthesis* *MED-EL, www.medel.com*	Unsafe 1	1.5	
Vibrant Soundbridge, VORP 503 Implant *Vibrating Ossicular Prosthesis* *MED-EL, www.medel.com*	Conditional 5	1.5	
Vistafix Prosthesis *Cochlear Corporation, www.cochlear.com*	Conditional 5	1.5, 3	
Wehrs Incus Prosthesis, Otologic Implant *Gyrus ACMI (Olympus Medical),* *www.medical.olympusamerica.com*	Conditional 5	3	
Wildcat Ossicular Replacement Prosthesis *Grace Medical, www.gracemedical.com*	Conditional 6	3	
Williams Microclip, 316L SS, Otologic Implant *Richards Medical Co., Memphis, TN*	Safe	1.5	35
Williams Microclip, Wire clip, Otologic Implant, 316L SS *Gyrus ACMI (Olympus Medical),* *www.medical.olympusamerica.com*	Conditional 5	3	
Winkel Partial Plester Titanium *Otologic Implant* *Kurz Medical, www.kurzmed.com/en/products/mri-safety/*	Safe	3	
Xomed Baily Stapes Implant *Otologic Implant*	Safe	1.5	35
Xomed Ceravital Partial Ossicular Prosthesis *Otologic Implant*	Safe	1.5	
Xomed Stapes Prosthesis, Robinson-style, *Otologic Implant* *Richard's Co., Nashville, TN*	Safe	1.5	35
Xomed Stapes, ASTM-318-76 Grade 2 SS, *Otologic Implant* *Xomed-Treace Inc., A Bristol-Myers Squibb Co.*	Safe	1.5	35

Object	Status	Field Strength (T)	Reference

Patent Ductus Arteriosus (PDA), Atrial Septal Defect (ASD), Ventricular Septal Defect (VSD) Occluders, and Patent Foramen Ovale (PFO) Closure Devices

Object	Status	Field Strength (T)	Reference
Amplatzer Cardiac Plug, *(also known as ACP device)* *AGA Medical Corporation, www.sjm.com/aga-medical*	Conditional 6	3	
Amplatzer Cardiac Plug II *St. Jude Medical, www.sjm.com*	Conditional 6	3	
AMPLATZER Duct Occluder *St. Jude Medical, www.sjm.com*	Conditional 8	1.5, 3	
Amplatzer Duct Occluder II *AGA Medical Corporation, www.sjm.com/aga-medical*	Conditional 6	3	
Amplatzer Multifenestrated, Septal Occluder, *Cribriform* *AGA Medical Corporation, www.sjm.com/aga-medical*	Conditional 6	3	
AMPLATZER Multifenestrated Septal Occluder, *Cribriform* *St. Jude Medical, www.sjm.com*	Conditional 6	3	
Amplatzer Muscular VSD Occluder *AGA Medical Corporation, www.sjm.com/aga-medical*	Conditional 6	3	
AMPLATZER Muscular VSD Occluder *St. Jude Medical, www.sjm.com*	Conditional 6	3	
Amplatzer Muscular VSD PI Occluder *AGA Medical Corporation, www.sjm.com/aga-medical*	Conditional 6	3	
Amplatzer PFO Occluder *AGA Medical Corporation, www.sjm.com/aga-medical*	Conditional 6	3	
Amplatzer Post Infarction, *Muscular Ventricular Septal Device* *AGA Medical Corporation, www.sjm.com/aga-medical*	Conditional 6	3	
Amplatzer Septal Occluder *AGA Medical Corporation, www.sjm.com/aga-medical*	Conditional 6	3	
AMPLATZER Septal Occluder *St. Jude Medical, www.sjm.com*	Conditional 6	3	
Amplatzer Transcatheter Occlusion Device *AGA Medical Corporation, www.sjm.com/aga-medical*	Conditional 6	3	
Amplatzer Vascular Plug Device *AGA Medical Corporation, St. Jude Medical,* *www.sjm.com/aga-medical*	Conditional 6	3	
AMPLATZER Vascular Plug Device *St. Jude Medical, www.sjm.com*	Conditional 6	3	

Object	Status	Field Strength (T)	Reference
Amplatzer Vascular Plug 4, AVP4 device *AGA Medical Corporation, St. Jude Medical,* *www.sjm.com/aga-medical*	Conditional 8	1.5, 3	
Amsel Occluder Device *Amsel Medical Corporation, Cambridge, MA*	Conditional 6	3	
Atrial Septal Defect Occluder, Guardian Angel, 12-mm *Microvena Corporation, White Bear Lake, MN*	Safe	1.5	
Atrial Septal Defect Occluder, Guardian Angel, 40-mm *Microvena Corporation, White Bear Lake, MN*	Safe	1.5	
Atriasept Closure Device *Cardia, Inc., Eagan, MN*	Conditional 6	3	
Bard Clamshell Septal Umbrella, 17-mm, Occluder *C.R. Bard, Inc., www.crbard.com*	Safe	1.5	41
Bard Clamshell Septal Umbrella, 23-mm, Occluder *C.R. Bard, Inc., www.crbard.com*	Safe	1.5	41
Bard Clamshell Septal Umbrella, 28-mm, Occluder *C.R. Bard, Inc., www.crbard.com*	Safe	1.5	41
Bard Clamshell Septal Umbrella, 33-mm, Occluder *C.R. Bard, Inc., www.crbard.com*	Safe	1.5	41
Bard Clamshell Septal Umbrella, 40-mm, Occluder *C.R. Bard, Inc., Bellerica, MA*	Safe	1.5	41
BioSTAR Septal Repair Implant *NMT Medical, Inc., Boston, MA*	Safe	3	
BioTREK, Patent Foramen Ovale (PFO) *Closure device* *NMT Medical, Boston, MA*	Safe	3	
CardioSEAL Septal Occluder, 17-mm *NMT Medical, Inc., Boston, MA*	Safe	1.5	
CardioSEAL Septal Occluder, 23-mm *NMT Medical, Inc., Boston, MA*	Safe	1.5	
CardioSEAL Septal Occluder, 28-mm *NMT Medical, Inc., Boston, MA*	Safe	1.5	
CardioSEAL Septal Occluder, 33-mm *NMT Medical, Inc., Boston, MA*	Safe	1.5	
CardioSEAL Septal Occluder, 40-mm *NMT Medical, Inc., Boston, MA*	Safe	1.5	
CardioSEAL Septal Repair Implant *NMT Medical, Inc., Boston, MA*	Safe	3	107
CardioSEAL Septal Repair Implant *NMT Medical, Inc., Boston, MA*	Conditional 6	3	

Object	Status	Field Strength (T)	Reference
Celt ACD Vascular Closure Device *Vasorum, www.vasorum.ie*	Conditional 6	3	
Cocoon Septal Occluder *Vascular Innovations Co. Ltd, Nonthaburi, Thailand*	Conditional 6	3	
Figulla Flex II ASD Occluder *All Sizes* *Occlutech GmbH, www.occlutech.com*	Conditional 8	1.5, 3	
GORE CARDIOFORM Septal Occluder *W. L. Gore and Associates, Inc., www.wlgore.com*	Conditional 8	1.5, 3	
GORE HELEX Septal Occluder *W.L. Gore & Associates, www.goremedical.com*	Conditional 6	3	
HELEX ASD Closure Device *W. L. Gore and Associates, Inc., www.goremedical.com*	Conditional 5	3	
HELEX, ASD Closure Device *W. L. Gore and Associates, Inc., www.goremedical.com*	Conditional 5	3	
HELEX Septal Occluder *W.L. Gore and Associates, Inc., www.goremedical.com*	Conditional 5	3	
Intrasept Patent Foramen Ovale (PFO) Closure Device *Cardia Inc., Burnsville, MN*	Conditional 6	3	
Lock Clamshell Septal Occlusion Implant, *Size 17-mm* *C.R. Bard, Inc., www.crbard.com*	Conditional 5	1.5	41
Lock Clamshell Septal Occlusion Implant, *Size 23-mm* *C.R. Bard, Inc., www.crbard.com*	Conditional 5	1.5	41
Lock Clamshell Septal Occlusion Implant, *Size 28-mm* *C.R. Bard, Inc., www.crbard.com*	Conditional 5	1.5	41
Lock Clamshell Septal Occlusion Implant, *Size 33-mm* *C.R. Bard, Inc., www.crbard.com*	Conditional 5	1.5	41
Lock Clamshell Septal Occlusion Implant, *Size 40-mm* *C.R. Bard, Inc., www.crbard.com*	Conditional 5	1.5	41
Nexus Septal Occluder *W.L. Gore & Associates, www.goremedical.com*	Conditional 8	1.5, 3	
Nit-Occlud PDA-R Occluder *PFM s.r.l*	Conditional 6	3	
Nit-Occlud Spiral Coil *PFM Medical, Inc., Oceanside, CA*	Conditional 6	3	
Occulotech LAA Occluder *Occlutech, www.occlutech.com*	Conditional 8	1.5, 3	

Object	Status	Field Strength (T)	Reference
Occlutech PDA Occluder *Occlutech, www.occlutech.com*	Conditional 8	1.5, 3	
Perimembranous Ventricular Septal Defect *(PmVSD) Occluder* *Occlutech, www.occlutech.com*	Conditional 8	1.5, 3	
Post Myocardial Infarction Ventricular Septal Defect *(PIVSD) Occluder* *Occlutech, www.occlutech.com*	Conditional 8	1.5, 3	
Premere PFO Closure System *St. Jude Medical, www.sjm.com*	Conditional 5	3	
Rashkind PDA Occlusion Implant, Size 12-mm *C.R. Bard, Inc., www.crbard.com*	Conditional 5	1.5	41
Rashkind PDA Occlusion Implant, Size 17-mm *C.R. Bard, Inc., www.crbard.com*	Conditional 5	1.5	41
STARFlex Septal Repair Implant *NMT Medical, Inc., Boston, MA*	Safe	3	
Ultrasept PFO Occluder *Cardia, Inc., www.cardiainc.com*	Conditional 6	3	

Pellets and Bullets

Object	Status	Field Strength (T)	Reference
30 Caliber, 762 x 39, Copper Jacketed Round, *Armor Piercing, Norinco*	Unsafe 1	1.5	
BBs (Crosman)	Unsafe 1	1.5	
BBs (Daisy)	Unsafe 1	1.5	
Bullet, .357 inch, Aluminum, Lead *Pellets and Bullets* *Winchester*	Safe	1.5	42
Bullet, .357 inch, Bronze, Plastic *Pellets and Bullets* *Patton-Morgan*	Safe	1.5	42
Bullet, .357 inch, Copper, Lead *Pellets and Bullets* *Cascade*	Safe	1.5	42
Bullet, .357 inch, Copper, Lead *Pellets and Bullets* *Hornady*	Safe	1.5	42
Bullet, .357 inch, Copper, Lead *Pellets and Bullets* *Patton-Morgan*	Safe	1.5	42
Bullet, .357 inch, Lead *Pellets and Bullets* *Remington*	Safe	1.5	42

Object	Status	Field Strength (T)	Reference
Bullet, .357 inch, Nickel, Copper, Lead *Pellets and Bullets* *Winchester*	Safe	1.5	42
Bullet, .357 inch, Nylon, Lead *Pellets and Bullets* *Smith & Wesson*	Safe	1.5	42
Bullet, .357 inch, Steel, Lead *Pellets and Bullets* *Fiocchi*	Safe	1.5	42
Bullet, .380 inch, Copper, Nickel, Lead *Pellets and Bullets* *Winchester*	Unsafe 1	1.5	42
Bullet, .380 inch, Copper, Plastic, Lead *Pellets and Bullets* *Glaser*	Safe	1.5	42
Bullet, .44 inch, Teflon, Bronze *Pellets and Bullets* *North American Ordinance*	Safe	1.5	42
Bullet, .45 inch, Copper, Lead *Pellets and Bullets* *Samson*	Safe	1.5	42
Bullet, .45 inch, Steel, Lead *Pellets and Bullets* *Evansville Ordinance*	Unsafe 1	1.5	42
Bullet, 7.62 x 39-mm, Copper, Steel *Pellets and Bullets* *Norinco*	Unsafe 1	1.5	42
Bullet, 9-mm, Copper, Lead *Pellets and Bullets* *Norma*	Unsafe 1	1.5	42
Bullet, 9-mm, Copper, Lead *Pellets and Bullets* *Remington*	Safe	1.5	42
Shot, 00 Buckshot, Lead *Pellets and Bullets*	Safe	1.5	42
Shot, 12 gauge, Size: 00, Copper, Lead *Pellets and Bullets* *Federal*	Safe	1.5	42
Shot, 4, Lead *Pellets and Bullets*	Safe	1.5	42
Shot, 7 1/2, Lead *Pellets and Bullets*	Safe	1.5	42

Object	Status	Field Strength (T)	Reference

Penile Implants

Object	Status	Field Strength (T)	Reference
Penile Implant, AMS 700 *American Medical Systems Inc.,* *www.americanmedicalsystems.com*	Conditional 6	3	
Penile Implant, AMS 700 CXM *American Medical Systems Inc.,* *www.americanmedicalsystems.com*	Conditional 6	3	
Penile Implant, AMS 700 CX Inflatable *AMS, American Medical Systems,* *www.americanmedicalsystems.com*	Safe	1.5	43
Penile Implant, AMS 700 CXM *AMS, American Medical Systems,* *www.americanmedicalsystems.com*	Conditional 6	3	
Penile Implant, AMS 700 CXR *AMS, American Medical Systems,* *www.americanmedicalsystems.com*	Conditional 6	3	
Penile Implant, AMS 700 Inflate/Deflate Pump *AMS, American Medical Systems,* *www.americanmedicalsystems.com*	Conditional 6	3	
Penile Implant, AMS 700 LGX *American Medical Systems Inc.,* *www.americanmedicalsystems.com*	Conditional 6	3	
Penile Implant, AMS 700 Ultrex *AMS, American Medical Systems,* *www.americanmedicalsystems.com*	Conditional 6	3	
Penile Implant, AMS 700 Ultrex Plus *AMS, American Medical Systems,* *www.americanmedicalsystems.com*	Conditional 6	3	
Penile Implant, AMS 700 Ultrex Preconnected *AMS, American Medical Systems,* *www.americanmedicalsystems.com*	Conditional 6	3	
Penile Implant, AMS Ambicor *AMS, American Medical Systems,* *www.americanmedicalsystems.com*	Conditional 6	3	
Penile Implant, AMS Dynaflex *AMS, American Medical Systems,* *www.americanmedicalsystems.com*	Safe	1.5, 3	
Penile Implant, AMS Hydroflex *AMS, American Medical Systems,* *www.americanmedicalsystems.com*	Safe	1.5, 3	
Penile Implant, AMS Malleable 600 *AMS, American Medical Systems,* *www.americanmedicalsystems.com*	Safe	1.5, 3	

Object	Status	Field Strength (T)	Reference
Penile Implant, AMS Malleable 600M *AMS, American Medical Systems,* *www.americanmedicalsystems.com*	Safe	1.5, 3	
Penile Implant, AMS Malleable 650 *AMS, American Medical Systems,* *www.americanmedicalsystems.com*	Safe	1.5, 3	
Penile Implant, AMS Tactile Pump *AMS, American Medical Systems,* *www.americanmedicalsystems.com*	Conditional 6	3	
Penile Implant, DURA II Penile Prosthesis *AMS, American Medical Systems,* *www.americanmedicalsystems.com*	Safe	1.5, 3	
Penile Implant, Duraphase	Unsafe 1	1.5	
Penile Implant, Excel Inflatable Penile Prosthesis *Model 90-95XXSC, MP35N,* *Urethane, Silicone, Polysulfone* *Coloplast Corporation, www.coloplast.us/*	Conditional 6	3	
Penile Implant, Flex-Rod II (Firm) *Surgitek, Medical Engineering Corp., Racine, WI*	Safe	1.5	43
Penile Implant, Flexi-Flate *Surgitek, Medical Engineering Corp., Racine, WI*	Safe	1.5	43
Penile Implant, Flexi-Rod (Standard) *Surgitek, Medical Engineering Corp., Racine, WI*	Safe	1.5	43
Penile Implant, Genesis Malleable Penile Implant *Coloplast Corporation, www.coloplast.us/*	Conditional 6	3	
Penile Implant, Jonas *Dacomed Corp., Minneapolis, MN*	Safe	1.5	43
Penile Implant, Mentor Flexible *Mentor Corp, Minneapolis, MN*	Safe	1.5	43
Penile Implant, Mentor Inflatable *Mentor Corp., Minneapolis, MN*	Safe	1.5	43
Penile Implant, OmniPhase *Dacomed Corp., Minneapolis, MN*	Unsafe 1	1.5	43
Penile Implant, Osmond, External	Safe	1.5	
Penile Implant, Spectra *AMS, American Medical Systems,* *www.americanmedicalsystems.com*	Conditional 6	3	
Penile Implant, Spectra Concealable *American Medical Systems Inc.,* *www.americanmedicalsystems.com*	Conditional 6	3	
Penile Implant, Titan Inflatable Penile Prosthesis *Model 90-98XXIC* *Coloplast Corporation, www.coloplast.us/*	Conditional 6	3	

Object	Status	Field Strength (T)	Reference
Penile Implant, Titan Inflatable Penile Prosthesis *Model 90-98XXIC* *Coloplast Corporation, www.coloplast.us/*	Conditional 6	3	
Penile Implant, Titan Inflatable Penile Prosthesis *Model 90-98XXIC* *Coloplast Corporation, www.coloplast.us/*	Conditional 6	3	
Penile Implant, Titan Inflatable Penile Prosthesis *Model 90-98ICOTR* *Coloplast Corporation, www.coloplast.us/*	Conditional 6	3	
Penile Implant, Titan Inflatable Penile Prosthesis *Model 90-99SCOTR* *Coloplast Corporation, www.coloplast.us/*	Conditional 6	3	
Penile Implant, Uniflex 1000	Safe	1.5	

Pessaries

Object	Status	Field Strength (T)	Reference
95% Rigid Siliconem, Pessary *CooperSurgical, www.coopersurgical.com*	Safe	3	
Cube (with drainage holes) Pessary *CooperSurgical, www.coopersurgical.com*	Safe	3	
Cube with Drainm EvaCare Pessary, Silicone *Coloplast Corporation, www.coloplast.us/*	Safe	3	
Cube EvaCare Pessary, Silicone *Coloplast Corporation, www.coloplast.us/*	Safe	3	
Cube Pessary *CooperSurgical, www.coopersurgical.com*	Safe	3	
Cube Pessary, Silicone *Bioteque America, Inc., Fremont, CA*	Safe	3	
Cup Pessary EvaCare, Silicone *Coloplast Corporation, www.coloplast.us/*	Safe	3	
Cup Pessary, Silicone *Bioteque America, Inc., Fremont, CA*	Safe	3	
Dish Pessary with Support, EvaCare, Silicone *Coloplast Corporation, www.coloplast.us/*	Safe	3	
Dish Pessary, Silicone *Bioteque America, Inc., Fremont, CA*	Safe	3	
Donut, EvaCare Pessary, Silicone *Coloplast Corporation, www.coloplast.us/*	Safe	3	
Donut Pessary *CooperSurgical, www.coopersurgical.com*	Safe	3	
Donut Pessary, Silicone *Bioteque America, Inc., Fremont, CA*	Safe	3	
Gehrung with Support, EvaCare Pessary, Silicone *Coloplast Corporation, www.coloplast.us/*	Safe	3	

Object	Status	Field Strength (T)	Reference
Gelhorn Pessary, Silicone *Bioteque America, Inc., Fremont, CA*	Safe	3	
Gellhorn with Drain EvaCare Pessary, Silicone *Coloplast Corporation, www.coloplast.us/*	Safe	3	
Gellhorn/95% Rigid Pessary *CooperSurgical, www.coopersurgical.com*	Safe	3	
Gellhorn/Flexible - Short Stem Pessary *CooperSurgical, www.coopersurgical.com*	Safe	3	
Gellhorn/Flexible Pessary *CooperSurgical, www.coopersurgical.com*	Safe	3	
Gellhorn/Flexible Pessary *CooperSurgical, www.coopersurgical.com*	Safe	3	
Hodge with Support EvaCare Pessary, Silicone *Coloplast Corporation, www.coloplast.us/*	Safe	3	
Hodge EvaCare Pessary, Silicone *Coloplast Corporation, www.coloplast.us/*	Safe	3	
Incontinence Dish With Support/Folding Pessary *CooperSurgical, www.coopersurgical.com*	Safe	3	
Incontinence Dish/Folding Pessary *CooperSurgical, www.coopersurgical.com*	Safe	3	
Inflatoball Pessary *CooperSurgical, www.coopersurgical.com*	Safe	3	
Marland Pessary, Silicone *Bioteque America, Inc., Fremont, CA*	Safe	3	
Marland with Support EvaCare Pessary, Silicone *Coloplast Corporation, www.coloplast.us/*	Safe	3	
Marland EvaCare Pessary, Silicone *Coloplast Corporation, www.coloplast.us/*	Safe	3	
Oval with Support EvaCare Pessary, Silicone *Coloplast Corporation, www.coloplast.us/*	Safe	3	
Oval Pessary, Silicone *Bioteque America, Inc., Fremont, CA*	Safe	3	
Regular/Folding Pessary *CooperSurgical, www.coopersurgical.com*	Safe	3	
Rigid Acrylic Gelhorn Pessary *CooperSurgical, www.coopersurgical.com*	Safe	3	
Ring Pessary with Knob EvaCare Pessary, Silicone *Coloplast Corporation, www.coloplast.us/*	Safe	3	
Ring With Knob/Folding Pessary *CooperSurgical, www.coopersurgical.com*	Safe	3	

Object	Status	Field Strength (T)	Reference
Ring with Knob Pessary *also known as Knobbed Ring, Silicone* *Bioteque America, Inc., Fremont, CA*	Safe	3	
Ring With Nylon Pegs Pessary *CooperSurgical, www.coopersurgical.com*	Safe	3	
Ring With Support With Knob Pessary *CooperSurgical, www.coopersurgical.com*	Safe	3	
Ring With Support and Knob/Folding Pessary *CooperSurgical, www.coopersurgical.com*	Safe	3	
Ring with Support EvaCare Pessary, Silicone *Coloplast Corporation, www.coloplast.us/*	Safe	3	
Ring EvaCare Pessary, Silicone *Coloplast Corporation, www.coloplast.us/*	Safe	3	
Ring Pessary, Silicone *Bioteque America, Inc., Fremont, CA*	Safe	3	
Schatz/Folding Pessary *CooperSurgical, www.coopersurgical.com*	Safe	3	
Shaatz EvaCare Pessary, Silicone *Coloplast Corporation, www.coloplast.us/*	Safe	3	
Shaatz Pessary, Silicone *Bioteque America, Inc., Fremont, CA*	Safe	3	
Silicone Flexible Gelhorn Pessary *CooperSurgical, www.coopersurgical.com*	Safe	3	
Tandem-Cube Pessary *CooperSurgical, www.coopersurgical.com*	Safe	3	

Sutures

Object	Status	Field Strength (T)	Reference
Suture, 24k Gold Thread *Gold Thread, LLC, www.gold-thread.com*	Conditional 8	1.5, 3	
Suture, Biosyn, Needle removed, Glycomer 631 *United States Surgical, North Haven, CT*	Safe	1.5, 3	83
Suture, Bondek, Needle removed *Teleflex, www.teleflex.com*	Safe	1.5, 3	
Suture, Bondek Plus, Needle removed *Teleflex, www.teleflex.com*	Safe	1.5, 3	
Suture, Chromic gut, Needle removed, gut *United States Surgical, North Haven, CT*	Safe	1.5, 3	83
Suture, Deknatel 'cottony' II, Needle removed *Teleflex, www.teleflex.com*	Safe	1.5, 3	
Suture, Deknatel DEKLENE II, Needle removed *Teleflex, www.teleflex.com*	Safe	1.5, 3	
Suture, Deknatel DEKLENE MAXX, Needle removed *Teleflex, www.teleflex.com*	Safe	1.5, 3	

Object	Status	Field Strength (T)	Reference
Suture, Deknatel FORCE FIBER, Needle removed *Teleflex, www.teleflex.com*	Safe	1.5, 3	
Suture, Deknatel NextStitch, Needle removed *Teleflex, www.teleflex.com*	Safe	1.5, 3	
Suture, Deknatel NYLON, Needle removed *Teleflex, www.teleflex.com*	Safe	1.5, 3	
Suture, Deknatel PLEDGET, Needle removed *Teleflex, www.teleflex.com*	Safe	1.5, 3	
Suture, Deknatel POLYLENE, Needle removed *Teleflex, www.teleflex.com*	Safe	1.5, 3	
Suture, Deknatel SILK, Needle removed *Teleflex, www.teleflex.com*	Safe	1.5, 3	
Suture, Deknatel 'silky' II POLYDEK, Needle removed *Teleflex, www.teleflex.com*	Safe	1.5, 3	
Suture, Deknatel Surgical Suture, SS *Teleflex, www.teleflex.com*	Conditional 8	1.5, 3	
Suture, Deknatel TEVDEK II, Needle removed *Teleflex, www.teleflex.com*	Safe	1.5, 3	
Suture, GORE-TEX Suture, Needle Removed *W.L. Gore and Associates, www.goremedical.com*	Safe	1.5, 3	
Suture, Maxon, Needle removed *United States Surgical, North Haven, CT*	Safe	1.5, 3	83
Suture, Monodek, Needle removed *Teleflex, www.teleflex.com*	Safe	1.5, 3	
Suture, Monosof, Needle removed *United States Surgical, North Haven, CT*	Safe	1.5, 3	83
Suture, Novafil, Needle removed *United States Surgical, North Haven, CT*	Safe	1.5, 3	83
Suture, Plain gut, Needle removed *United States Surgical, North Haven, CT*	Safe	1.5, 3	83
Suture, Polyglytone, Needle removed *Teleflex, www.teleflex.com*	Safe	1.5, 3	
Suture, Polysorb, Needle removed *United States Surgical, North Haven, CT*	Safe	1.5, 3	83
Suture, PROLENE Suture with Beads and Collars *Ethicon, Inc., www.ethicon.com*	Conditional 6	3	
Suture, SecureStrand, Needle removed *United States Surgical, North Haven, CT*	Safe	1.5, 3	83
Suture, Sofsilk, Needle removed *United States Surgical, North Haven, CT*	Safe	1.5, 3	83
Suture, Spire'It Suture *Davol Inc., www.davol.com*	Conditional 6	3	

Object	Status	Field Strength (T)	Reference
Suture, Stainless Steel Suture, *Stainless Wire of Mani* *Mani, Inc., Japan*	Conditional 8	1.5, 3	
Suture, Surgical Stainless Steel Wire Suture *Ethicon, www.ethicon.com*	Conditional 8	1.5, 3	
Suture, Steel, Needle removed, 316L SS *United States Surgical, North Haven, CT*	Safe	1.5, 3	83
Suture, Steel Suture, Needle removed *Size 7 Metric, 316L SS Suture* *Covidien, www.covidien.com*	Conditional 6	3	
Suture, Surgilon, Needle removed *United States Surgical, North Haven, CT*	Safe	1.5, 3	83
Suture, Surgipro, Needle removed *United States Surgical, North Haven, CT*	Safe	1.5, 3	83

Vascular Access Ports, Infusion Pumps, and Catheters

Object	Status	Field Strength (T)	Reference
A Port Implantable Access System, Titanium *Therex Corporation, Walpole, MA*	Safe	1.5	44
Access Implantable, Titanium, Plastic *Celsa, Cedex, France*	Safe	1.5	44
ACCU-CHEK Insulin Pump, All Models *Roche Diagnostics, www.accu-chek.com*	Unsafe 1	1.5	
ACCU-CHEK Spirit Insulin Pump *Roche Diagnostics, www.accu-chek.com*	Unsafe 1	1.5	
Acuvance Jelco, FEP Radiopaque Intravenous *(I.V.) Catheter, Silicone* *Smiths Medical, www.smiths-medical.com*	Conditional 6	3	
Acuvance Plus, PUR Radiopaque Intravenous *(I.V.) Catheter, Silicone* *Smiths Medical, www.smiths-medical.com*	Conditional 6	3	
Acuvance Plus-W, PUR Radiopaque Intravenous *(I.V.) Catheter, Silicone* *Smiths Medical, www.smiths-medical.com*	Conditional 6	3	
AdvantIV, PUR Radiopaque Intravenous *(I.V.) Catheter, Silicone* *Smiths Medical, www.smiths-medical.com*	Conditional 6	3	
Ambulatory Infusion System, CADD - 1, *Ambulatory Infusion Pump* *Smiths Medical, www.smiths-medical.com*	Unsafe 1	1.5	
Ambulatory Infusion System, CADD - Legacy, *Ambulatory Infusion Pump* *Smiths Medical, www.smiths-medical.com*	Unsafe 1	1.5	

Object	Status	Field Strength (T)	Reference
Ambulatory Infusion System, CADD - Legacy 1, *Ambulatory Infusion Pump* *Smiths Medical, www.smiths-medical.com*	Unsafe 1	1.5	
Ambulatory Infusion System, CADD - Legacy PCA, *Ambulatory Infusion Pump* *Smiths Medical, www.smiths-medical.com*	Unsafe 1	1.5	
Ambulatory Infusion System, CADD - Legacy PLUS, *Ambulatory Infusion Pump* *Smiths Medical, www.smiths-medical.com*	Unsafe 1	1.5	
Ambulatory Infusion System, CADD - Micro, *Ambulatory Infusion Pump* *Smiths Medical, www.smiths-medical.com*	Unsafe 1	1.5	
Ambulatory Infusion System, CADD - MS 3, *Ambulatory Infusion Pump* *Smiths Medical, www.smiths-medical.com*	Unsafe 1	1.5	
Ambulatory Infusion System, CADD - PCA, *Ambulatory Infusion Pump* *Smiths Medical, www.smiths-medical.com*	Unsafe 1	1.5	
Ambulatory Infusion System, CADD - PLUS, *Ambulatory Infusion Pump* *Smiths Medical, www.smiths-medical.com*	Unsafe 1	1.5	
Ambulatory Infusion System, CADD - Prizm PCS II, *Ambulatory Infusion Pump* *Smiths Medical, www.smiths-medical.com*	Unsafe 1	1.5	
Ambulatory Infusion System, CADD - Prizm PCS, *Ambulatory Infusion Pump* *Smiths Medical, www.smiths-medical.com*	Unsafe 1	1.5	
Ambulatory Infusion System, CADD - Prizm VIP, *Ambulatory Infusion Pump* *Smiths Medical, www.smiths-medical.com*	Unsafe 1	1.5	
Ambulatory Infusion System, CADD - Solis, *Ambulatory Infusion Pump* *Smiths Medical, www.smiths-medical.com*	Unsafe 1	1.5	
Ambulatory Infusion System, CADD - TPN, *Ambulatory Infusion Pump* *Smiths Medical, www.smiths-medical.com*	Unsafe 1	1.5	
ambIT Infusion Pump *www.ambitpump.com*	Unsafe 1	1.5	
Atrial Flow Regulator, AFR *Occlutech Ltd., www.occlutech.com*	Conditional 5	1.5, 3	
Bardport Vascular Access Port *Bard Peripheral Vascular, www.bardpv.com*	Conditional 5	3	
BD Angiocath Autoguard IV Catheter *BD Medical, www.bd.com*	Conditional 5	3	

Object	Status	Field Strength (T)	Reference
BD Angiocath IV Catheter *BD Medical, www.bd.com*	Conditional 5	3	
BD Cathena IV Catheter *BD Medical, www.bd.com*	Conditional 6	3	
BD Cathena IV Catheter with Wings *BD Medical, www.bd.com*	Conditional 6	3	
BD Cathena IV Catheter with *BD Multiguard Technology* *BD Medical, www.bd.com*	Conditional 6	3	
BD Cathena IV Catheter with *BD Multiguard Technology with Wings* *BD Medical, www.bd.com*	Conditional 6	3	
BD Insyte IV Catheter *BD Medical, www.bd.com*	Conditional 5	3	
BD Insyte Autoguard IV Catheter *BD Medical, www.bd.com*	Conditional 5	3	
BD Insyte Autoguard BC IV Catheter *BD Medical, www.bd.com*	Conditional 5	3	
BD Nexiva Diffusics IV Catheter *BD Medical, www.bd.com*	Conditional 5	3	
BD Nexiva IV Catheter *BD Medical, www.bd.com*	Conditional 5	3	
Breeze Straight Luer Lock Centesis Drainage *Catheter All Sizes* *MedComp, www.medcompnet.com*	Safe	1.5, 3	
Broviac Catheter Single Lumen, Silicone, *Barium Sulfate* *Bard Access Systems, Salt Lake City, UT*	Safe	1.5	
Button Vascular Access Port *polysulfone polymer, Silicone* *Infusaid Inc., Norwood, MA and Angiodynamics, Inc.*	Safe	1.5	45
CathLink LP, Titanium *Bard Access Systems, www.bardaccess.com*	Safe	1.5	44
CathLink SP, Titanium *Bard Access Systems, www.bardaccess.com*	Safe	1.5	45
Cathlon FEP Intravenous (I.V.) Catheter, Silicone *Smiths Medical, www.smiths-medical.com*	Conditional 6	3	
Celsite Access Port (T401L), Vascular Access Port *B. Braun Medical, www.bbraun.com*	Conditional 8	1.5, 3	
Celsite Port and Catheter, Titanium *B. Braun Medical, www.bbraunusa.com*	Safe	1.5	45
Celsite Access Port, Vascular Access Port *B. Braun, www.bbraunusa.com*	Conditional 8	1.5, 3	

Object	Status	Field Strength (T)	Reference
Celsite PEEK Vascular Access Port *B. Braun, www.bbraun.com*	Conditional 8	1.5, 3	
Central Venous Port, Vascular Access Port *Covidien, www.covidien.com*	Conditional 6	1.5, 3	
Certainty Port, Implantable Vascular Access Port *MedComp, Harleysville, PA*	Conditional 6	3	
Chemosite Port I, Low Profile, *Single Lumen Vascular Access Port* *Covidien, www.covidien.com*	Conditional 6	3	
C-Port-DL Vascular Access Port *PHS Medical GmbH, www.phs-medical.de*	Conditional 6	3	
CODMAN 3000 Implantable Infusion Pump *Codman, www.depuysynthes.com*	Conditional 5	3	
Cool Line Catheter (REF CL-2295) *Zoll Circulation, www.zoll.com*	Conditional 8	1.5, 3	
Cozmo Pump, Insulin Pump *Smith Medical, www.smiths-medical.com*	Unsafe 1	1.5	
CT Rated Dual Port, Vascular Access Port *Medcomp, www.medcompnet.com*	Conditional 8	1.5, 3	
Dana Diabecare IISG Insulin Pump *Sooil, www.sooilusa.com*	Unsafe 1	1.5	
Deltec 3000, Large Volume Infusion Pump *Smiths Medical, www.smiths-medical.com*	Unsafe 1	1.5	
Deltec Micro 3100, Large Volume Infusion Pump *Smiths Medical, www.smiths-medical.com*	Unsafe 1	1.5	
Dignity Dual Port, Vascular Access Port *Medcomp, www.medcompnet.com*	Conditional 5	1.5, 3	
Dome Port, Vascular Access Port, Titanium *Davol Inc., Subsidiary of C.R. Bard, Inc.*	Safe	1.5	
Dual MacroPort, polysulfone polymer, Silicone *Infusaid Inc., Norwood, MA and Angiodynamics, Inc.*	Safe	1.5	44
Dual MicroPort, polysulfone polymer, Silicone *Infusaid Inc., Norwood, MA and Angiodynamics, Inc.*	Safe	1.5	44
Dual-Lumen PORT-A-CATH *Portal and Wing-Lock Connector, Vascular Access Port* *Smiths Medical, www.smiths-medical.com*	Safe	1.5	44
DuraCath Intraspinal Catheter *316L SS, Silicone* *Advanced Neuromodulation Systems, Plano, TX*	Conditional 6	3	
GRIPPER PLUS Needle, SS needle, 19 gauge *Smiths Medical, www.smiths-medical.com*	Conditional 5	3	
GRIPPER PLUS Safety Needle *Deltec, Inc., www.smiths-medical.com*	Conditional 5	3	

Object	Status	Field Strength (T)	Reference
GRIPPER PLUS Safety Needle *Smiths Medical, www.smiths-medical.com*	Safe	3	
Groshong Catheter	Conditional 5	1.5	
Groshong Catheter, dual lumen, 9.5 Fr. *Silicone, Barium Sulfate, Tungsten* *Bard Access Systems, www.bardaccess.com*	Safe	1.5	45
Groshong Catheter, single lumen, 8 Fr. *Silicone, Barium Sulfate, Tungsten* *Bard Access Systems, www.bardaccess.com*	Safe	1.5	45
Healthport ETI Spinal, Model ETI *Implantable Intracorporeal Access System* *Plan 1 Health s.r.l.*	Conditional 6	3	
Healthport PLP, Access Port *Plan 1 Health s.r.l.*	Conditional 6	3	
Healthport Focus Access Port *Plan 1 Health s.r.l.*	Conditional 6	3	
Heliosite Vascular Access Port *Vygon, www.vygon.com*	Conditional 6	3	
HeRO Vascular Access Device *HeRO Graft Component,* *HeRO Outflow Catheter Component* *GRAFTcath, Inc., Eden Prairie, MN*	Conditional 6	3	
Hickman Catheter, dual lumen, 10.0 Fr. *Silicone, barium sulfate* *Bard Access Systems, www.bardaccess.com*	Safe	1.5	45
Hickman Catheter, single lumen, 3.0 Fr. *Bard Access Systems, www.bardaccess.com*	Safe	1.5	45
Hickman Port, Pediatric, Vascular Access Port, *Titanium* *Davol, Inc., Subsidiary of C.R. Bard, Inc.,* *Salt Lake City, UT*	Safe	1.5	44
Hickman Port, Vascular Access Port, 316L SS *Davol Inc., Subsidiary of C.R. Bard, Inc.,* *Salt Lake City, UT*	Safe	1.5	44
Hickman Subcutaneous port, Vascular Access Port *SS, Titanium, Plastic* *Davol, Inc., Subsidiary of C.R. Bard, Inc.*	Safe	1.5	45
Hickman Subcutaneous port, Vascular Access Port *Venous Catheter, Titanium* *Davol Inc., Subsidiary of C.R. Bard, Inc.,* *Salt Lake City, UT*	Safe	1.5	44
HMP-Port, Vascular Access Port, Plastic *Horizon Medical Products, Atlanta, GA and* *Angiodynamics, Inc.*	Safe	1.5	44

Object	Status	Field Strength (T)	Reference
Implantable Infusion Pump, Model 3000-16 *Codman, www.depuysynthes.com*	Safe	1.5, 3	83
Implantable Infusion Pump, Model 3000-30 *Codman, www.depuysynthes.com*	Safe	1.5, 3	83
Implantable Infusion Pump, Model 3000-50 *Codman, www.depuysynthes.com*	Safe	1.5, 3	83
Implantofix II, Vascular Access Port, Polysulfone *Burron Medical Inc., Bethlehem, PA*	Safe	1.5	44
Infusaid, Model 400, Vascular Access Port *Infusaid Inc., Norwood, MA*	Safe	1.5	44
Infusaid, Model 600, Vascular Access Port *Infusaid Inc., Norwood, MA*	Safe	1.5	44
Infuse-A-Kit, Plastic *Infusaid, Norwood, MA and Angiodynamics, Inc.*	Safe	1.5	44
InfuseIT Pressure Infuser, 500 ml *Zefon International, Inc., m.zefon.com*	Conditional 7	3	
InfuseIT Pressure Infuser, 1000 ml *Zefon International, Inc., m.zefon.com*	Conditional 7	3	
InfuseIT Pressure Infuser, 3000 ml *Zefon International, Inc., m.zefon.com*	Conditional 7	3	
IVT1632, Vascular Access Port *With Connector Ring, INFU-KT* *ISOMed, www.fbmedical.fr*	Conditional 8	1.5, 3	
Jelco 2 FEP Radiopaque Intravenous *(I.V.) Catheter, Silicone* *Smiths Medica, www.smiths-medical.com*	Conditional 6	3	
Jelco FEP Intravenous (I.V.) Catheter, Silicone *Smiths Medical, www.smiths-medical.com*	Conditional 6	3	
Jelco-W FEP Radiopaque Intravenous *(I.V.) Catheter, Silicone* *Smiths Medical, www.smiths-medical.com*	Conditional 6	3	
Jet Port Plus Vascular Access Port *Clinical Plastic Products SA, Switzerland*	Conditional 6	3	
LifePort Plastic Port, Vascular Access Port *Angiodynamics, Inc., www.Angiodynamics.com*	Safe	1.5, 3	
LifePort Titanium Port, Vascular Access Port *Angiodynamics, Inc., www.Angiodynamics.com*	Conditional 6	3	
LifePort Vascular Access Port *AngioDynamics, www.angiodynamics.com*	Conditional 6	3	
LifePort Vascular Access System *attachable catheter and bayonet lock ring, plastic* *Strato Medical Group, Beverly, MA and Angiodynamics, Inc.*	Safe	1.5	44

Object	Status	Field Strength (T)	Reference
LifePort Vascular Access System *Strato Medical Group, Beverly, MA and* *Angiodynamics, Inc.*	Safe	1.5	44
LifePort Vortex LVTX 5213 *Dual Titanium Vascular Access Port* *Angiodynamics, Inc.*	Conditional 6	3	
Lifeport, Model 1013 Vascular Access Port, Titanium *Strato Medical Corp., Beverly, MA and* *Angiodynamics, Inc.*	Safe	1.5	44
LifePort, Model 6013 Vascular Access Port, Delrin *Strato Medical Corporation, Beverly, MA and* *Angiodynamics, Inc.*	Safe	1.5	44
Low Profile MRI Port Vascular Access Port, Delrin *Davol, Inc., Subsidiary of C.R. Bard, Inc.*	Safe	1.5	44
Low Profile MRI Port Vascular Access Port, Titanium *Davol, Inc. Subsidiary of C.R. Bard, Inc.*	Safe	1.5	45
Macroport Vascular Access Port, polysulfone, Titanium *Infusaid Inc., Norwood, MA and Angiodynamics, Inc.*	Safe	1.5	
Medcomp Power Injectable Port with CertainID *Vascular Access Port* *Medcomp, Medcompnet.com*	Conditional 5	1.5, 3	121
Mediport Vascular Access Port *Cormed*	Safe	1.5	
MedStream Programmable Infusion System *Catalog No. 91-4200US & 91-4201US* *Codman, www.depuysynthes.com*	Conditional 5	3	112
Medtronic MiniMed 2007 Implantable Insulin *Pump System* *Medtronic, Inc., www.medtronicdiabetes.com*	Unsafe 1	1.5	
MicroPort Vascular Access Port *Infusaid Inc., Norwood, MA and Angiodynamics, Inc.*	Safe	1.5	44
Medtronic MiniMed Paradigm REAL-Time *Insulin Pump Continuous Glucose Monitoring System* *Models 522, 722, and Revel Insulin Pumps* *Medtronic, Inc., www.medtronicdiabetes.com*	Unsafe 1	1.5	
Micro Needle Port *Central Venous Port, K-16002* *Nippon Covidien Ltd., www.covidien.co.jp*	Conditional 8	1.5, 3	
M.R.I. Hard-Base Implantable Port *Bard Peripheral Vascular, www.bardpv.com*	Conditional 5	3	
M.R.I. Implantable Port with Suture Plugs *Bard Access Systems, www.bardaccess.com*	Conditional 6	3	
M.R.I. isp Implanted PowerPort with Suture Rings *Bard Access Systems, www.bardaccess.com*	Conditional 6	3	

Object	Status	Field Strength (T)	Reference
M.R.I. Port Vascular Access Port *Davol, Inc., Subsidiary of C.R. Bard, Inc.*	Safe	1.5	44
M.R.I. PowerPort Vue, Vascular Access Port *Bard Access Systems, www.bardaccess.com*	Conditional 6	3	
M.R.I. Ultra SlimPort Implantable Port *Bard Peripheral Vascular, www.bardpv.com*	Conditional 5	3	
Multi-Lumen Acute Hemodialysis Catheter *Teleflex, Inc., www.teleflex.com*	Safe	1.5, 3	
Next Generation Chronic Hemodialysis Catheter *Covidien, www.covidien.com*	Safe	1.5, 3	
Non-Coring (Huber) Needle *Boston Scientific, www.bostonscientific.com*	Safe	1.5, 3	83
Norport-AC Vascular Access Port, Titanium *Norfolk Medical, www.norfolkmedical.com*	Safe	1.5	44
Norport-DL Vascular Access Port, 316L SS *Norfolk Medical, www.norfolkmedical.com*	Safe	1.5	44
Norport-LS Vascular Access Port, 316L SS *Norfolk Medical, www.norfolkmedical.com*	Safe	1.5	44
Norport-LS Vascular Access Port, Polysulfone *Norfolk Medical, www.norfolkmedical.com*	Safe	1.5	44
Norport-LS Vascular Access Port, Titanium *Norfolk Medical, www.norfolkmedical.com*	Safe	1.5	44
Norport-PT Vascular Access Port, Titanium *Norfolk Medical, www.norfolkmedical.com*	Safe	1.5	44
NorPort Single Lumen Port System, Vascular *Access Port* *Norfolk Medical, www.norfolkmedical.com*	Conditional 6	3	
Norport-SP Vascular Access Port *Norfolk Medical, www.norfolkmedical.com*	Safe	1.5	44
NuPort-LPA Vascular Access Port *PHS Medical GmbH, www.phs-medical.de*	Conditional 6	3	
OmegaPort Access System, Vascular Access Port *Norfolk Medical, www.norfolkmedical.com*	Safe	1.5	44
OmegaPort-SR Access System, Vascular Access Port *Norfolk Medical, www.norfolkmedical.com*	Safe	1.5	44
OneTouch Ping Insulin Pump *Animas Corporation, www.animas.com*	Unsafe 1	1.5	
Open-ended Catheter, single lumen, *6 Fr. (ChronoFlex)* *Davol, Inc., Subsidiary of C.R. Bard, Inc.*	Safe	1.5	45
Open-ended Catheter, single lumen, *8 Fr. (ChronoFlex)* *Davol, Inc., Subsidiary of C.R. Bard, Inc.*	Safe	1.5	45

Object	Status	Field Strength (T)	Reference
OptiPort Catheter, single lumen Silicone *Simms-Deltec, St. Paul, MN*	Safe	1.5	45
Optiva PUR Radiopaque Intravenous *(I.V.) Catheter, Silicone* *Smiths Medical, www.smiths-medical.com*	Conditional 6	3	
Optiva-W PUR Radiopaque Intravenous *(I.V.) Catheter, Silicone* *Smiths Medical, www.smiths-medical.com*	Conditional 6	3	
Optiva 2 PUR Radiopaque Intravenous *(I.V.) Catheter, Silicone* *Smiths Medical, www.smiths-medical.com*	Conditional 6	3	
P.A.S. PORT Elite with *PolyFlow Polyurethane Catheter* *Deltec, Inc., St. Paul, MN*	Safe	1.5, 3	83
Percutaneous Vascular Access System (PVAS) *DermaPort, Santa Clarita, CA*	Conditional 6	3	
Perfusafe 2 *Vygon, www.vygon.com*	Conditional 6	3	
PeriPort Vascular Access Port *Infusaid, Inc., Norwood, MA and Angiodynamics, Inc.*	Safe	1.5	44
Peritoneal Implantable Port *Bard Peripheral Vascular, www.bardpv.com*	Conditional 5	3	
Phantom Vascular Access Port *Norfolk Medical, www.norfolkmedical.com*	Safe	1.5	44
Plastic Port Vascular Access Port *Cardial, Saint-Etienne, France*	Safe	1.5	44
POLYSITE Implantable Vascular Access Port *Perouse Medical, www.perousemedical.com*	Conditional 6	3	
PORT-A-CATH GRIPPER Needle *Deltec, Inc., St. Paul, MN*	Safe	1.5, 3	83
PORT-A-CATH I, Standard Portal *with Ultra-Lock Connector* *Vascular Access Port* *Smiths Medical, www.smiths-medical.com*	Conditional 6	3	
PORT-A-CATH II Dual-Lumen *Low Profile with PolyFlow, Polyurethane Catheter* *Deltec, Inc., St. Paul, MN*	Safe	1.5, 3	83
PORT-A-CATH II Dual-Lumen with Silicone Catheter *Deltec, Inc., St. Paul, MN*	Safe	1.5, 3	83
PORT-A-CATH II Single-Lumen *Low Profile with PolyFlow, Polyurethane Catheter* *Deltec, Inc., St. Paul, MN*	Safe	1.5, 3	83

Object	Status	Field Strength (T)	Reference
PORT-A-CATH II Single-Lumen, *with PolyFlow Polyurethane Catheter* *Deltec, Inc., St. Paul, MN*	Safe	1.5, 3	83
PORT-A-CATH II Low Profile Intraspinal Portal *Smiths Medical, www.smiths-medical.com*	Conditional 6	3	
PORT-A-CATH Needle *Deltec, Inc., St. Paul, MN*	Conditional 5	1.5, 3	83
PORT-A-CATH Titanium Dual Lumen Portal, Titanium *Pharmacia Deltec, St. Paul, MN*	Safe	1.5	44
PORT-A-CATH Titanium Peritoneal Portal, Titanium *Pharmacia Deltec, St. Paul, MN*	Safe	1.5	44
PORT-A-CATH Titanium, Venous Low Profile Portal, *Titanium* *Pharmacia Deltec, St. Paul, MN*	Safe	1.5	44
PORT-A-CATH Titanium, Venous Portal, Titanium *Pharmacia Deltec, St. Paul, MN*	Safe	1.5	44
PORT-A-CATH, P.S.A. Port Portal, Titanium *Pharmacia Deltec, St. Paul, MN*	Safe	1.5	44
PORT-A-CATH, Epidural Portal and *Cath-Shield Connector* *Vascular Access Port* *Smiths Medical, www.smiths-medical.com*	Conditional 6	3	
PORT-A-CATH, Metal Hub 90 degree Bent Needle *Smiths Medical, www.smiths-medical.com*	Safe	3	
PORT-A-CATH, Metal Hub Straight Needle *Smiths Medical, www.smiths-medical.com*	Safe	3	
PORT-A-CATH, Peritoneal Portal with *Ultra-Lock Connector* *Smiths Medical, www.smiths-medical.com*	Conditional 6	3	
PORT-A-CATH, Plastic Hub 90-degree *Bent Needle* *Smiths Medical, www.smiths-medical.com*	Conditional 5	3	
PORT-A-CATH, Plastic Hub Straight Needle *Smiths Medical MD, Inc., St. Paul, MN*	Conditional 5	3	
Power Dual Tita Port *Clinical Plastic Products SA, Switzerland*	Conditional 6	3	
PowerPort ClearVUE isp with BiO Symbol, *Vascular Access Port* *Bard Access Systems, www.bardaccess.com*	Safe	1.5, 3	
PowerPort ClearVUE isp *with Polyurethane Catheter and* *Cathlock Vascular Access Port* *Bard Access Systems, www.bardaccess.com,* *www.bardbpv.com*	Safe	1.5, 3	

Object	Status	Field Strength (T)	Reference
PowerPort ClearVUE Slim Low Profile Port, *Vascular Access Port* *Bard Access Systems, www.bardaccess.com*	Safe	1.5, 3	
PowerPort Duo MRI Port *ChronoFlex Catheter and Cathlock, Vascular Access Port* *Bard Access Systems, www.bardaccess.com*	Safe	1.5, 3	
PowerPort Implantable Port With Suture Plugs *Implantable Vascular Access Port* *Bard Access Systems, www.bardaccess.com*	Conditional 6	3	
PowerPort M.R.I., Titanium *Bard Access Systems, www.bardaccess.com*	Conditional 5	3	
PowerPort Vascular Access Port, Titanium *Bard Access Systems, www.bardaccess.com*	Conditional 5	3	
PowerPort isp Implanted Port *Bard Access Systems, www.bardaccess.com*	Conditional 5	3	
PowerPort isp M.R.I. Implanted Port *Bard Access Systems, www.bardaccess.com*	Conditional 5	3	
PowerPort isp Implanted Port with Suture Plugs *Bard Access System, www.bardaccess.com*	Conditional 6	3	
PowerPort M.R.I. Implanted Port *Bard Access Systems, www.bardaccess.com*	Conditional 5	3	
PowerPort Slim Implantable Port with Suture Plugs *Implantable Vascular Access Port* *Bard Access Systems, www.bardaccess.com*	Conditional 6	3	
PowerPort Vue Titanium *Implantable Vascular Access Port* *Bard Access Systems, www.bardaccess.com*	Conditional 6	3	
Presternal Peritoneal Dialysis (PD) Catheter *Medtronic, Inc., www.Medtronic.com*	Conditional 5	1.5, 3	
ProFuse Dignity Infusion Port *Medcomp, Harleysville, PA*	Conditional 6	3	
Pro-Lock CT Safety Infusion Set *Medcomp, www.medcompnet.com*	Conditional 8	1.5, 3	
Prometra Programmable Pump *Flowonix Medical Inc, www.flowonix.com*	Conditional 5	1.5	
Prometra II Programmable Pump *Flowonix Medical Inc, www.flowonix.com*	Conditional 5	1.5	
ProtectIV FEP Radiopaque Intravenous (I.V.) Catheter, Silicone *Smiths Medical, www.smiths-medical.com*	Conditional 6	3	
ProtectIV Acuvance 2 PUR *Radiopaque Intravenous (I.V.) Catheter, Silicone* *Smiths Medical, www.smiths-medical.com*	Conditional 6	3	

Object	Status	Field Strength (T)	Reference
ProtectIV Plus PUR Radiopaque Intravenous *(I.V.) Catheter* *Smiths Medical, www.smiths-medical.com*	Conditional 6	3	
ProtectIV Plus-W PUR Radiopaque Intravenous *(I.V.) Catheter* *Smiths Medical, www.smiths-medical.com*	Conditional 6	3	
ProtectIV-W FEP Radiopaque Intravenous *(I.V.) Catheter* *Smiths Medical, www.smiths-medical.com*	Conditional 6	3	
Purple JPP-HP Vascular Access Port *Clinical Plastic Products SA, Switzerland*	Conditional 6	3	
Purple TJL-HP Vascular Access Port *Clinical Plastic Products SA, Switzerland*	Conditional 6	3	
qimoFlow+ *Perouse Medical, www.perousemedical.com*	Conditional 6	3	
Q-Port Vascular Access Port *Quinton Instrument Co., Seattle, WA*	Conditional 5	1.5	44
Quattro Catheter (REF IC-4593) *Zoll Circulation, www.zoll.com*	Conditional 8	1.5, 3	
Realize Injection Port, Access Port *Ethicon, www.ethicon.com*	Conditional 5	3	
RFID ProFuse Standard Port *Vascular Access Port* *Medcomp, www.medcompnet.com*	Conditional 5	3	
Rhapsody Vascular Access System *GrantAdler Corporation, Naperville, IL*	Conditional 6	3	
R-Port Premier Vascular Access Port, *Boston Scientific, www.bostonscientific.com*	Safe	1.5	83
Saf-T-Intima I.V. Catheter *18-G x 1.0 in.* *BD Medical, www.bd.com*	Conditional 6	3	
S.E.A. Vascular Access Port, Titanium *Harbor Medical Devices, Inc., Boston, MA*	Safe	1.5	44
Sophysa SOPH-A-PORT Mini S *Implantable Access Port* *Shire, www.shire.com*	Conditional 8	1.5, 3	
Sitimplant Titanium Vascular Access Port *Vygon, www.vygon.com*	Conditional 6	3	
SlimPort Dual Lumen Rosenblatt Implantable Port *Bard Peripheral Vascular, www.bardpv.com*	Conditional 5	3	
SlimPort Vascular Access Port *Bard Peripheral Vascular, www.bardpv.com*	Conditional 5	3	

Object	Status	Field Strength (T)	Reference
Smart Port CT-Injectable Port *AngioDynamics, www.angiodynamics.com*	Conditional 6	3	
Smart Port, Vascular Access Port *Angiodynamics, Inc., www.Angiodynamics.com*	Conditional 6	3	
Snap-Lock Vascular Access Port *Titanium, polysulfone polymer, Silicone* *Infusaid Inc., Norwood, MA and Angiodynamics, Inc.*	Safe	1.5	44
Solex Intravascular Heat Exchange Catheter *(Model SL-2593/8700-0671-01)* *Zoll Circulation, www.zoll.com*	Conditional 8	1.5, 3	
Solo MicroPump Insulin Pump *Medingo US, Inc., www.Medingo.com*	Unsafe 1	1.5	
SOPH-A-PORT Mini Spinal Implantable *Access Port* *Sophysa, www.sophysa.com*	Conditional 5	3	
Split-Cath III Double Lumen Catheter *All Sizes* *MedComp, www.medcompnet.com*	Safe	1.5, 3	
Standard M.R.I. Single Chamber System *Polysulfone Port, Titanium Connector, Silicone Catheter* *Cook Medical, www.cookmedical.com*	Conditional 6	3	
Standard Titanium Dual Chamber System *Titanium Port, Titanium Connector, Silicone Catheter* *Cook Medical, www.cookmedical.com*	Conditional 6	3	
Stealth Invisiport Vascular Access Port *Medical Murray, Inc., North Barrington, IL*	Conditional 6	3	
Synchromed, Model 8500-1 *Medtronic, Inc., www.medtronic.com/mri*	Conditional 5	1.5, 3	44
Tesio Catheter *Medcomp, Harleysville, PA*	Conditional 6	3	
Titanium Access Port, Product Code, 2200-X *Vascular Access Port* *Ethicon, www.ethicon.com*	Conditional 8	1.5, 3	
Titanium SlimPort Implantable Port *Bard Peripheral Vascular, www.bardpv.com*	Conditional 5	3	
Tita Jet Light Arterial II Vascular Access Port *Clinical Plastic Products SA, Switzerland*	Conditional 6	3	
Tita Jet Light Vascular Access Port *Clinical Plastic Products SA, Switzerland*	Conditional 6	3	
TitanPort Titanium Vascular Access Port *Norfolk Medical, www.norfolkmedical.com and* *Angiodynamics, Inc.*	Safe	1.5	

Object	Status	Field Strength (T)	Reference
TitanPort Vascular Access Port *AngioDynamics, www.angiodynamics.com*	Conditional 6	3	
T-Port HP, Power Injectable Port, *Vascular Access System* *PFM Medical, Inc., www.pfmmedicalusa.com*	Conditional 6	3	
T-Port Vascular Access Port *Clinical Plastic Products SA, Switzerland*	Conditional 6	3	
Triple Lumen *Arrow International, www.arrowintl.com*	Safe	1.5	
Triumph-1 Vascular Access Port, Titanium *AngioDynamics, www.angiodynamics.com*	Conditional 6	3	
Triumph-1 Plastic Port, Vascular Access Port *Angiodynamics, Inc., www.Angiodynamics.com*	Safe	1.5	
Uni-Shunt Catheter *Codman, www.Depuy.com*	Conditional 5	1.5, 3	
Vascular Access Catheter With Repair Kit	Safe	1.5	
Vasport Vascular Access Port, Titanium, *fluoropolymer* *Gish Biomedical, Inc., Santa Ana, CA*	Safe	1.5	44
Vaxcel Implantable Access System, *Plastic Low Profile Port* *Boston Scientific, www.bostonscientific.com*	Safe	1.5, 3	
Vaxcel Implantable Vascular Access System *with PASV Valve Technology, Titanium Mini Port* *With PASV valve* *Boston Scientific, www.bostonscientific.com*	Safe	1.5,3	
Vaxcel Implantable Vascular Access System *with PASV Valve Technology, Titanium Standard Port* *With PASV valve* *Boston Scientific, www.bostonscientific.com*	Safe	1.5, 3	
Vaxess, Titanium Mini-Port with Silicone catheter *Vascular Access Port, Titanium, Silicone* *Boston Scientific, www.bostonscientific.com*	Safe	1.5, 3	83
Vaxess, Titanium, Vascular Access Port, Titanium, *polyurethane* *Boston Scientific, www.bostonscientific.com*	Safe	1.5, 3	83
Vaxess Vascular Access Port, 19 gauge x 1/2", *90 degree hub* *Boston Scientific, www.bostonscientific.com*	Safe	1.5, 3	83
Vaxess Vascular Access Port *Boston Scientific, www.bostonscientific.com*	Safe	1.5, 3	83
ViaValve Safety I.V. Catheter, PUR Radiopaque *Smiths Medical ASD Inc., Southington, CT*	Conditional 6	3	

Object	Status	Field Strength (T)	Reference
Vital-Port, Dual, Vascular Access Port *Cook Medical, www.cookmedical.com*	Safe	1.5, 3	45
Vital-Port System, Dual Chamber, Titanium Petite *Vascular Access Port* *Cook Medical, Inc., www.cookmedical.com*	Conditional 5	3	
Vital-Port System, Dual Chamber, *Titanium Standard* *Vascular Access Port* *Cook Medical, Inc., www.cookmedical.com*	Conditional 5	3	
Vital-Port System, MRI Petite, *Vascular Access Port* *Cook Medical, Inc., www.cookmedical.com*	Conditional 5	3	
Vital-Port System, MRI Standard, *Vascular Access Port* *Cook Medical, Inc., www.cookmedical.com*	Conditional 5	3	
Vital-Port System, Titanium Mini, *Vascular Access Port* *Cook Medical, Inc., www.cookmedical.com*	Conditional 5	3	
Vital-Port System, Titanium Petite, *Vascular Access Port* *Cook Medical, Inc., www.cookmedical.com*	Conditional 5	3	
Vital-Port System, Titanium Petite Standard, *Vascular Access Port* *Cook Medical, Inc., www.cookmedical.com*	Conditional 5	3	
Vital-Port System, Titanium for *Peripheral Placement Mini* *Vascular Access Port* *Cook Medical, Inc., www.cookmedical.com*	Conditional 5	3	
Vital-Port Vascular Access Port *Cook Medical., www.cookmedical.com*	Safe	1.5	45
Vortex LP Plastic Port, Vascular Access Port *Angiodynamics, Inc., www.angiodynamics.com*	Safe	1.5, 3	
Vortex LP Titanium Port, Vascular Access Port *Angiodynamics, Inc., www.angiodynamics.com*	Conditional 6	3	
Vortex MP Port, Vascular Access Port *Angiodynamics, Inc., www.angiodynamics.com*	Conditional 6	3	
Vortex TR Plastic Port Vascular Access Port *Angiodynamics, Inc., www.angiodynamics.com*	Safe	1.5, 3	
Vortex TR Titanium Port Vascular Access Port *Angiodynamics, Inc., www.angiodynamics.com*	Conditional 5	3	
Vortex VX Port Vascular Access Port *Angiodynamics, Inc., www.angiodynamics.com*	Conditional 5	3	

Object	Status	Field Strength (T)	Reference
Vortex Port, Models LP, MP, TR, VX, *Vascular Access Port* *AngioDynamics, www.angiodynamics.com*	Conditional 5	3	
X-Port Duo Dual-Lumen Implantable Port *Bard Peripheral Vascular, www.bardpv.comá*	Conditional 5	3	
X-Port Implantable Port *Bard Peripheral Vascular, www.bardpv.com*	Conditional 5	3	
X-Port Inline Dual-Lumen Implantable Port *Bard Peripheral Vascular, www.bardpv.com*	Conditional 5	3	
X-Port Duo Dual-Lumen Implantable Port *Bard Peripheral Vascular, www.bardpv.com*	Conditional 5	3	

THE LIST

REFERENCES

1. New PFJ, et al. Potential hazards and artifacts of ferromagnetic and nonferromagnetic surgical and dental materials and devices in nuclear magnetic resonance imaging. Radiology 1983;147:139-148.

2. Becker RL, Norfray JF, Teitelbaum GP, et al. MR imaging in patients with intracranial aneurysm clips. AJNR 1988;9:885-889.

3. Shellock FG, Crues JV. High-field strength MR imaging and metallic biomedical implants: An *ex vivo* evaluation of deflection forces. Am J Roentgenol 1988;151:389-392.

4. Brown MA, Carden JA, Coleman RE, et al. Magnetic field effects on surgical ligation clips. Magn Reson Imaging 1987;5:443-453.

5. Dujovny M, et al. Aneurysm clip motion during magnetic resonance imaging: *In vivo* experimental study with metallurgical factor analysis. Neurosurgery 1985;17:543-548.

6. Barrafato D, Henkelman RM. Magnetic resonance imaging and surgical clips. Can J Surg 1984;27:509-512.

7. Moscatel M, Shellock FG, Morisoli S. Biopsy needles and devices: Assessment of ferromagnetism and artifacts during exposure to a 1.5 Tesla MR system. J Magn Reson Imaging 1995;5:369-372.

8. Shellock FG, Shellock VJ. Additional information pertaining to the MR-compatibility of biopsy needles and devices. J Magn Reson Imaging 1996;6:441.

9. Hathout G, Lufkin RB, Jabour B, et al. MR-guided aspiration cytology in the head and neck at high field strength. J Magn Reson Imaging 1992;2:93-94.

10. Fagan LL, Shellock FG, Brenner RJ, Rothman B. *Ex vivo* evaluation of ferromagnetism, heating, and artifacts of breast tissue expanders exposed to a 1.5 T MR system. J Magn Reson Imaging 1995;5:614-616.

11. Teitelbaum GP, et al. Ferromagnetism and MR imaging: Safety of carotid vascular clamps. Am J Neuroradiol 1990;11:267-272.

12. Gegauff A, Laurell KA, Thavendrarajah A, et al. A potential MRI hazard: Forces on dental magnet keepers. J Oral Rehabil 1990;17:403-410.

13. Shellock FG. *Ex vivo* assessment of deflection forces and artifacts associated with high-field strength MRI of "mini-magnet" dental prostheses. Magn Reson Imaging 1989;7 (Suppl 1):38.

14. Shellock FG, Slimp G. Halo vest for cervical spine fixation during MR imaging. Am J Roentgenol 1990;154:631-632.

15. Clayman DA, et al. Compatibility of cervical spine braces with MR imaging. A study of nine nonferrous devices. Am J Neuroradiol 1990;11:385-390.

16. Shellock FG. MR imaging and cervical fixation devices: Assessment of ferromagnetism, heating, and artifacts. Magn Reson Imaging 1996;14:1093-1098.

17. Soulen RL, Budinger TF, Higgins CB. Magnetic resonance imaging of prosthetic heart valves. Radiology 1985;154:705-707.

18. Shellock FG, Morisoli SM. *Ex vivo* evaluation of ferromagnetism, heating, and artifacts for heart valve prostheses exposed to a 1.5 Tesla MR system. J Magn Reson Imaging 1994;4:756-758.

19. Hassler M, Le Bas JF, Wolf JE, et al. Effects of magnetic fields used in MRI on 15 prosthetic heart valves. J Radiol 1986;67:661-666.

20. Frank H, Buxbaum P, Huber L, et al. *In vitro* behavior of mechanical heart valves in 1.5 T superconducting magnet. Eur J Radiol 1992;2:555-558.

21. Teitelbaum GP, et al. MR imaging artifacts, ferromagnetism, and magnetic torque of intravascular filters, stents, and coils. Radiology 1988;166:657-664.

22. Marshall MW, et al. Ferromagnetism and magnetic resonance artifacts of platinum embolization microcoils. Cardiovasc Intervent Radiol 1991;14:163-166.

23. Watanabe AT, Teitelbaum GP, Gomes AS, et al. MR imaging of the bird's nest filter. Radiology 1990;177:578-579.

24. Leibman CE, et al. MR imaging of inferior vena caval filter: Safety and artifacts. Am J Roentgenol 1988;150:1174-1176.

25. Shellock FG, Detrick MS, Brant-Zawadski M. MR-compatibility of the Guglielmi detachable coils. Radiology 1997;203:568-570.

26. Kiproff PM, et al. Magnetic resonance characteristics of the LGM vena cava filter: technical note. Cardiovasc Intervent Radiol 1991;14:254-255.

27. Teitelbaum GP, Raney M, Carvlin MJ, et al. Evaluation of ferromagnetism and magnetic resonance imaging artifacts of the Strecker tantalum vascular stent. Cardiovasc Intervent Radiol 1989;12:125-127.

28. Girard MJ, et al. Wallstent metallic biliary endoprosthesis: MR imaging characteristics. Radiology 1992;184:874-876.

29. Shellock FG, Myers SM, Schatz CJ. *Ex vivo* evaluation of ferromagnetism determined for metallic scleral "buckles" exposed to a 1.5 T MR scanner. Radiology 1992;185:288-289.

30. de Keizer RJ, Te Strake L. Intraocular lens implants (pseudophakoi) and steelwire sutures: A contraindication for MRI? Doc Ophthalmol 1984;61:281-284.

31. Albert DW, Olson KR, Parel JM, et al. Magnetic resonance imaging and retinal tacks. Arch Ophthalmol 1990;108:320-321.

32. Joondeph BC, Peyman GA, Mafee MF, et al. Magnetic resonance imaging and retinal tacks [Letter]. Arch Ophthalmol 1987;105:1479-1480.

33. Lyons CJ, Betz RR, Mesgarzadeh M, et al. The effect of magnetic resonance imaging on metal spine implants. Spine 1989;14:670-672.

34. Shellock FG, Mink JH, Curtin S, et al. MRI and orthopedic implants used for anterior cruciate ligament reconstruction: Assessment of ferromagnetism and artifacts. J Magn Reson Imaging 1992;2:225-228.

35. Shellock FG, Schatz CJ. High-field strength MR imaging and metallic otologic implants. Am J Neuroradiol 1991;12:279-281.

36. Nogueira M, Shellock FG. Otologic bioimplants: *Ex vivo* assessment of ferromagnetism and artifacts at 1.5 Tesla. Am J Roentgenol 1995;163:1472-1473.

37. Mattucci KF, et al. The effect of nuclear magnetic resonance imaging on metallic middle ear prostheses. Otolaryngol Head Neck Surg 1986;94:441-443.

38. Applebaum EL, Valvassori GE. Further studies on the effects of magnetic resonance fields on middle ear implants. Ann Otol Rhinol Laryngol 1990;99:801-804.

39. White DW. Interaction between magnetic fields and metallic ossicular prostheses. Am J Otol 1987;8:290-292.

40. Leon JA, Gabriele OF. Middle ear prosthesis: Significance in magnetic resonance imaging. Magn Reson Imaging 1987;5:405-406.

41. Shellock FG, Morisoli SM. *Ex vivo* evaluation of ferromagnetism and artifacts for cardiac occluders exposed to a 1.5 Tesla MR system. J Magn Reson Imaging 1994;4:213-215.

42. Teitelbaum GP, Yee CA, Van Horn DD, et al. Metallic ballistic fragments: MR imaging safety and artifacts. Radiology 1990;175:855-859.

43. Shellock FG, Crues JV, Sacks SA. High-field magnetic resonance imaging of penile prostheses: in vitro evaluation of deflection forces and imaging artifacts. In: Book of Abstracts, Society of Magnetic Resonance in Medicine. Berkeley, CA, Society of Magnetic Resonance in Medicine 1987;3:915.

44. Shellock FG, Nogueira M, Morisoli S. MR imaging and vascular access ports: *Ex vivo* evaluation of ferromagnetism, heating, and artifacts at 1.5 T. J Magn Reson Imaging 1995;4:481-484.

45. Shellock FG, Shellock VJ. Vascular access ports and catheters tested for ferromagnetism, heating, and artifacts associated with MR imaging. Magn Reson Imaging 1996;14:443-447.

46. Kanal E, Shaibani A. Firearm safety in the MR imaging environment. Radiology 1994;193:875-876.

47. Hess T, Stepanow B, Knopp MV. Safety of intrauterine contraceptive devices during MR imaging. Eur Radiol 1996;6:66-68.

48. Shellock FG, Shellock VJ. Evaluation of MR compatibility of 38 bioimplants and devices. Radiology 1995;197:174.

49. Shellock FG, Shellock VJ. Ceramic surgical instruments: ex vivo evaluation of compatibility with MR imaging. J Magn Reson Imaging 1996;6:954-956.

50. Shellock FG, Shellock VJ. Evaluation of cranial flap fixation clamps for compatibility with MR imaging. Radiology 1998;822-825.

51. Lufkin R, Jordan S, Lylcyk M. MR imaging with topographic EEG electrodes in place. Am J Neuroradiol 1988;9:953-954.

52. Marra S, et al. Effect of magnetic resonance imaging on implantable eyelid weights. Ann Otol Rhinol Laryngol 1995;104:448-452.

53. Zhang J, et al. Temperature changes in nickel-chromium intracranial depth electrodes during MR scanning. Am J Neuroradiol 1993;14:497-500.

54. Mark AS, Hricak H. Intrauterine contraceptive devices: MR imaging. Radiology 1987;162:311-314.

55. Go KG, et al. Interaction of metallic neurosurgical implants with magnetic resonance imaging at 1.5 Tesla as a cause of image distortion and of hazardous movement of the implant. Clin Neurosurg 1989;91:109-115.

56. Fransen P, Dooms G, Thauvoy. Safety of the adjustable pressure ventricular valve in magnetic resonance imaging: Problems and solutions. Neuroradiology 1992;34:508-509.

57. ECRI, Health devices alert. A new MRI complication? May 27, 1988.

58. To SYC, Lufkin RB, Chiu L. MR-compatible winged infusion set. Comput Med Imaging Graph 1989;13:469-472.

59. Shellock FG. MR-compatibility of an endoscope designed for use in interventional MRI procedures. Am J Roentgenol 1998;71:1297-1300.

60. Shellock FG, Shellock VJ. Cardiovascular catheters and accessories: *Ex vivo* testing of ferromagnetism, heating, and artifacts associated with MRI. J Magn Reson Imaging 1998;8:1338-1342.

61. Shellock FG, Shellock VJ. Metallic marking clips used after stereotactic breast biopsy: *Ex vivo* testing of ferromagnetism, heating, and artifacts associated with MRI. Am J Roentgenol 1999;172:1417-1419.

62. Shellock FG. MRI safety of instruments designed for interventional MRI: assessment of ferromagnetism, heating, and artifacts. Workshop on New Insights into Safety and Compatibility Issues Affecting In Vivo MR, Syllabus 1998; pp. 39.

63. Shellock FG, et al. Implantable spinal fusion stimulator: Assessment of MRI safety. J Magn Reson Imaging 2000;12:214-223.

64. Shellock FG, Shellock VJ. Stents: Evaluation of MRI safety. Am J Roentgenol 1999;173:543-546.

65. Teissl C, et al. Cochlear implants: *In vitro* investigation of electromagnetic interference at MR imaging-compatibility and safety aspects. Radiology 1998;208:700-708.

66. Teissl C, et al. Magnetic resonance imaging and cochlear implants: Compatibility and safety aspects. J Magn Reson Imaging 1999;9:26-38.

67. Ortler M, Kostron H, Felber S. Transcutaneous pressure-adjustable valves and magnetic resonance imaging: An ex vivo examination of the Codman-Medos programmable valve and the Sophy adjustable pressure valve. Neurosurgery 1997;40:1050-1057.

68. Shellock FG, Shellock VJ. MR-compatibility evaluation of the Spetzler titanium aneurysm clip. Radiology 1998;206:838-841.

69. Jost C, Kuman V. Are current cardiovascular stents MRI safe? J Invasive Cardiol 1998;10:477-479.

70. Shellock FG, Shellock VJ. MRI Safety of cardiovascular implants: Evaluation of ferromagnetism, heating, and artifacts. Radiology 2000;214:P19H.

71. Weishaupt D, et al. Ligating clips for three-dimensional MR angiography at 1.5 T: In vitro evaluation. Radiology 2000;214:902-907.

72. Hug J, et al. Coronary arterial stents: Safety and artifacts during MR imaging. Radiology 2000;216:781-787.

73. Taal BG, Muller SH, Boot H, Koop W. Potential risks and artifacts of magnetic resonance imaging of self-expandable esophageal stents. Gastrointestinal Endoscopy 1997;46;424-429.

74. Shellock FG. Metallic surgical instruments for interventional MRI procedures: Evaluation of MR safety. J Magn Reson Imaging 2001;13:152-157.

75. Edwards, M-B, Taylor KM, Shellock FG. Prosthetic heart valves: Evaluation of magnetic field interactions, heating, and artifacts at 1.5 Tesla. J Magn Reson Imaging 2000;12:363-369.

76. Shellock FG. New metallic implant used for permanent female contraception: Evaluation of MR safety. Am J Roentgenol 2002;178:1513-1516.

77. Shellock FG. Prosthetic heart valves and annuloplasty rings: Assessment of magnetic field interactions, heating, and artifacts at 1.5-Tesla. Journal of Cardiovascular Magnetic Resonance 2001;3:159-169.

78. Shellock FG. Metallic neurosurgical implants: evaluation of magnetic field interactions, heating, and artifacts at 1.5 Tesla. J Magn Reson Imaging 2001;14:295-299.

79. Rezai AR, Finelli D, Ruggieri P, Tkach J, Nyenhuis JA, Shellock FG. Neurostimulators: Potential for excessive heating of deep brain stimulation electrodes during MR imaging. J Magn Reson Imaging 2001;14:488-489.

80. Finelli DA, Rezai AR, Ruggieri P, Tkach J, Nyenhuis J, Hridlicka G, Sharan A, Stypulkowski PH, Shellock FG. MR-related heating of deep brain stimulation electrodes: An *in vitro* study of clinical imaging sequences. Am J Neuroradiol 2002;23:1795-1802.

81. Greatbatch W, Miller V, Shellock FG. Magnetic resonance safety testing of a newly-developed, fiber-optic cardiac pacing lead. J Magn Reson 2002;16:97-103.

82. Shellock FG, et al. Aneurysm clips: evaluation of magnetic field interactions and translational attraction using "long-bore" and "short-bore" 3.0-Tesla MR systems. Am J Neuroradiol 2003;24:463-471.

83. Shellock FG. Biomedical implants and devices: assessment of magnetic field interactions with a 3.0-Tesla MR system. J Magn Reson Imaging 2002;16:721-732.

84. Medtronic Heart Valves, Medtronic, Inc., Minneapolis, MN. Permission to publish 3-Tesla MR testing information for Medtronic Heart Valves, Medtronic LifeLine Technical Support, 877-526-7890, Medtronic, www.medtronic.com.

85. Shellock FG, Tkach JA, Ruggieri PM, Masaryk TJ. Cardiac pacemakers, ICDs, and loop recorder: Evaluation of translational attraction using conventional ("long-bore") and "short-bore" 1.5- and 3.0-Tesla MR systems. Journal of Cardiovascular Magnetic Resonance 2003;5:387-397.

86. Product Information, Style 133 Family of Breast Tissue Expanders with Magna-Site Injection Sites, McGhan Medical/INAMED Aesthetics, Santa Barbara, CA.

87. Shellock FG, Gounis M, Wakhloo A, Detachable coil for cerebral aneurysms: *In vitro* evaluation of magnet field interactions, heating, and artifacts at 3-Tesla. American Journal of Neuroradiology 2005;26:363-366.

88. Shellock FG. Forder J. Drug eluting coronary stent: *In vitro* evaluation of magnet resonance safety at 3-Tesla. Journal of Cardiovascular Magnetic Resonance 2005;7:415-419.

89. Shellock FG, et al. Implantable microstimulator: Magnetic resonance safety at 1.5-Tesla. Investigative Radiology 2004;39:591-594.

90. Shellock FG. MR safety and the Reveal Insertable Loop Recorder. Signals, No. 49, Issue 3, pp. 8, 2004

91. Reveal Plus Insertable Loop Recorder, http://www.medtronic.com/ physician/reveal/mri.html, Medtronic, Inc.

92. Kinetra Dual Program Neurostimulator for Deep Brain Simulation, 7428, Medtronic, Inc., Kinetra MRI labeling. www.Medtronic.com

93. RF BION Microstimulator, Alfred E. Mann Foundation, Valencia, CA; www.aemf.org

94. Codman, a Johnson and Johnson Company; Cerebrospinal Fluid Shunt Valves and Accessories, www.depuy.com

95. Codman, a Johnson and Johnson Company; Cerebrospinal Fluid Shunt Valves and Accessories, www.depuysynthes.com

96. Medtronic Neurosurgery. Cerebrospinal Fluid Shunt Valves and Accessories, www.medtronic.com

97. Sophysa, www.sophysa.com

98. MED-EL Corporation, www.medel.com

99. Medtronic Neurological Technical Services Department, Technical Note. MRI Guidelines for Neurological Products, Issue No. NTN 04-03 Rev 2, July, 2005. Important Note: Before scanning a patient with this implant or device, obtain the latest MRI safety information by contacting Medtronic, www.Medtronic.com.

100. Henderson J, Tkach J, Phillips M, Baker K, Shellock FG, Rezai A. Permanent neurological deficit related to magnetic resonance imaging in a patient with implanted deep brain stimulation electrodes for Parkinson's disease: Case report. Neurosurgery 2005;57:E1063.

101. Rezai AR, Baker K, Tkach J, Phillips M, Hrdlicka G, Sharan A, Nyenhuis J, Ruggieri P, Henderson J, Shellock FG. Is magnetic resonance imaging safe for patients with neurostimulation systems used for deep brain stimulation (DBS)? Neurosurgery 2005;57:1056-1062.

102. Shellock FG. MR Safety at 3-Tesla: Bare Metal and Drug Eluting Coronary Artery Stents. Signals No. 53, Issue 2, pp. 26-27, 2005.

103. Shellock FG. MR Safety and Cerebral Spinal Fluid Shunt (CSF) Valves. Signals, No. 51, Issue 4, pp. 10, 2004.

104. Shellock FG, Habibi R, Knebel J. Programmable CSF shunt valve: *In vitro* assessment of MRI safety at 3-Tesla. American Journal of Neuroradiology 2006;27:661-665.

105. Ceballos EM, Parrish RK. Plain film imaging of Baerveldt glaucoma drainage implants. American Journal of Neuroradiology 2002;23;935-937.

106. Martin AD, et al. Safety evaluation of titanium middle ear prostheses at 3.0 Tesla. Otolaryngol Head Neck Surg 2005;132:537-42.

107. Shellock FG, Valencerina S. Septal repair implants: Evaluation of MRI safety at 3-Tesla. Magnetic Resonance Imaging 2005;23:1021-1025.

108. Nehra A, Moran CJ, Cross DT, Derdeyn CP. MR safety and imaging of Neuroform Stents at 3-T. Am J Neuoradiol 2004;25:1476-1478.

109. Westerway SC, et al. Implanon implant detection with ultrasound and magnetic resonance imaging. Aust NZ Obstet Gynaecol 2003;43:346-350.

110. Shellock FG, Wilson SF, Mauge CP. Magnetically programmable shunt valve: MRI at 3-Tesla. Magnetic Resonance Imaging 2007;25:1116-21.

111. Zieman M, Kanal E. Copper T 380A IUD and magnetic resonance imaging. Contraception 2007;75:93-5.

112. Shellock FG, Crivelli R, Venugopalan R. Programmable infusion pump and catheter: Evaluation using 3-Tesla MRI. Neuromodulation 2008;11:163-170.

113. Shellock FG, Valencerina S. Ventricular assist implant (AB5000): *In Vitro* assessment of MRI issues at 3-Tesla. Journal of Cardiovascular Magnetic Resonance 2008;10:23-30.

114. Diaz FL, Tweardy L, Shellock FG. Cervical external immobilization devices: Evaluation of magnetic resonance imaging issues at 3.0 Tesla. Spine 2010;35:411-5.

115. Nyenhuis J, Duan L. An evaluation of MRI safety and compatibility of a silver-impregnated antimicrobial wound dressing. J Am Coll Radiol 2009;6:500-5.

116. Shellock FG. Valencerina S. In vitro evaluation of MR imaging issues at 3-T for aneurysm clips made from MP35N: Findings and information applied to 155 additional aneurysm clips. Am J Neuroradiol 2010;31:615-619.

117. Geffen N, et al. Is the Ex-PRESS glaucoma shunt magnetic resonance imaging safe? J Glaucoma 2009;70:532-6.

118. Gill KR, Pooley RA, Wallace MB. Magnetic resonance imaging compatibility of endoclips. Gastrointest Endosc 2009;70:532-6.

119. Shellock FG, et al. Assessment of MRI issues for a 3-T "immune" programmable CSF shunt valve. Am J Roentgenol 2011;197:202-207.

120. Karacozoff AM, Shellock FG. In vitro assessment of a fiducial marker for lung lesions: MRI issues at 3 T. Am J Roentgenol 2013;200:1234-7.

121. Titterington B, Shellock FG. Evaluation of MRI issues for an access port with a radiofrequency identification (RFID) tag. Magn Reson Imaging 2013;31:1439-44.

122. Audet-Griffin A, Pakbaz S, Shellock FG. Evaluation of MRI issues for a new, liquid embolic device. Journal of Interventional Neuroradiology 2014; 2014;6:624-629.

123. Shellock FG, Giangarra CJ. Assessment of 3-Tesla MRI issues for a bioabsorbable, coronary artery scaffold with metallic markers. Magnetic Resonance Imaging 2014;32:163-7.

124. Titterington B, Shellock FG. A new vascular coupling device: Assessment of MRI issues at 3-Tesla. Magn Reson Imaging 2014;32:585-9.

125. Linnemeyer H, Shellock FG, Ahn CY. In vitro assessment of MRI issues at 3-Tesla for a breast tissue expander with a remote port. Magn Reson Imaging 2014;32:297-302.

126. Shellock FG, Audet-Griffin A. Evaluation of magnetic resonance imaging issues for a wirelessly-powered lead used for epidural, spinal cord stimulation. Neuromodulation 2014;17:334-339.

127. Saeedi M, Thomas A, Shellock FG. Evaluation of MRI issues at 3-Tesla for a transcatheter aortic valve replacement (TAVR) bioprosthesis. Magnetic Resonance Imaging 2015;33:497-501.

128. Shellock FG, Cronenweth C. Assessment of MRI issues at 3-Tesla for a new metallic tissue marker. International Journal of Breast Cancer. 2015;823759.

129. Moghtader D, Hans-Joachim Crawack HJ, Shellock FG. Assessment of MRI issues for a new cerebral spinal fluid shunt, gravity assisted valve (GAV). Magnetic Resonance Imaging 2017;44:8-14.

130. Victoria, T, Johnson AM, Adzick AS, Hedrick HL, Shellock FG. Evaluation of MRI issues for an occlusive balloon used for fetoscopic endoluminal tracheal occlusion (FETO). Fetal Diagnosis and Therapy (In Press)

APPENDIX I

Criteria for Significant Risk Investigations of Magnetic Resonance Diagnostic Devices

Guidance for Industry and Food and Drug Administration Staff

Document issued on: June 13, 2014

This document supersedes "Guidance for Industry and FDA Staff – Criteria for Significant Risk Investigations of Magnetic Resonance Diagnostic Devices" issued on July 14, 2003.

On June 13, 2014 this document was edited to amend a table on specific absorption rate (SAR) and make minor formatting and contact updates. For questions regarding this document, contact Jana Delfino, Ph.D., at 301-796-6503, or by e-mail at jana.delfino@fda.hhs.gov.

U.S. Department of Health and Human Services
Food and Drug Administration
Center for Devices and Radiological Health
Magnetic Resonance and Electronic Products Branch
Division of Radiological Health
Office of In Vitro Diagnostics and Radiological Health

This guidance represents the Food and Drug Administration's (FDA's) current thinking on this topic. It does not create or confer any rights for or on any person and does not operate to bind FDA or the public. You can use an alternative approach if the approach satisfies the requirements of the applicable statutes and regulations. If you want to discuss an alternative approach, contact the FDA staff responsible for implementing this guidance. If you cannot identify the appropriate FDA staff, call the appropriate number listed on the title page of this guidance.

PREFACE

Public Comment

Written comments and suggestions may be submitted at any time for Agency consideration to Division of Dockets Management, Food and Drug Administration, 5630 Fishers Lane, Room 1061, (HFA-305), Rockville, MD, 20852. When submitting comments, please refer to the exact title of this guidance document. Comments may not be acted upon by the Agency until the document is next revised or updated.

Additional Copies

Additional copies are available from the Internet. You may also send an e-mail request to CDRH-Guidance@fda.hhs.gov to receive a copy of the guidance. Please use the document number 793 to identify the guidance you are requesting.

INTRODUCTION

This guidance describes the device operation conditions for magnetic resonance diagnostic devices that FDA considers significant risk for the purposes of determining whether a clinical study requires Agency approval of an Investigation Device Exemption (IDE). Magnetic resonance diagnostic devices are class II devices described under 21 CFR 892.1000. The product codes for these devices are:

LNH Magnetic Resonance Imaging System

LNI Magnetic Resonance Spectroscopic System

This guidance supersedes **Guidance for Magnetic Resonance Diagnostic Devices – Criteria for Significant Risk Investigations**, issued September 29, 1997. We have revised our recommendation for the main static magnetic field strength, increasing it to 8 Tesla for most populations. This is based on ongoing experience in the field and numerous literature reviews (1, 2).

FDA's guidance documents, including this guidance, do not establish legally enforceable responsibilities. Instead, guidances describe the Agency's current thinking on a topic and should be viewed only as recommendations, unless specific regulatory or statutory requirements are cited. The use of the word *should* in Agency guidances means that something is suggested or recommended, but not required.

STUDIES OF MAGNETIC RESONANCE
DIAGNOSTIC DEVICES

If a clinical study is needed to demonstrate substantial equivalence, (i.e. conducted prior to obtaining 510(k) clearance of the device), the study must be conducted under the IDE regulation (21 CFR Part 812). FDA believes that a magnetic resonance diagnostic device used under any one of the operating conditions listed below is a significant risk device as defined in 21 CFR 812.3(m)(4) and, therefore, that studies involving such a device do not qualify for the abbreviated IDE requirements of 21 CFR 812.2(b). In addition to the requirement of having an FDA-approved IDE, sponsors of significant risk studies must comply with the regulations governing institutional review boards (21 CFR Part 56) and informed consent (21 CFR Part 50).

SIGNIFICANT RISK MAGNETIC RESONANCE DIAGNOSTIC DEVICES

You should consider the following operating conditions when assessing whether a study may be considered significant risk:

- main static magnetic field
- specific absorption rate (SAR)
- gradient fields rate of change
- sound pressure level

Generally, FDA deems magnetic resonance diagnostic devices significant risk when used under any of the operating conditions described below.

Main Static Magnetic Field

Population	*Main static magnetic field greater than (Tesla)*
adults, children, and infants aged > 1 month	8
neonates i.e. infants aged 1 month or less	4

Specific Absorption Rate (SAR)

Site	Dose	Time (min) equal to or greater than:	SAR (W/kg)
whole body	averaged over	15	>4
head	averaged over	10	>3.2

If you have questions about significant risk criteria related to local SAR, you may wish to contact FDA.

Gradient Fields Rate of Change

Any time rate of change of gradient fields (dB/dt) sufficient to produce severe discomfort or painful nerve stimulation

Sound Pressure Level

Peak unweighted sound pressure level greater than 140 dB.

A-weighted root mean square (rms) sound pressure level greater than 99 dBA with hearing protection in place.

These criteria apply only to device operating conditions. Other aspects of the study may involve significant risks and the study, therefore, may require IDE approval regardless of operating conditions. See the guidance entitled "Significant Risk and Nonsignificant Risk Medical Device Studies" (http://www.fda.gov/downloads/regulatoryinformation/guidances/ucm126 418.pdf) for further discussion.

After FDA determines that the device is substantially equivalent, clinical studies conducted in accordance with the indications reviewed in the 510(k), including clinical design validation studies conducted in accordance with the quality systems regulation, are exempt from the investigational device exemptions (IDE) requirements. However, such studies must be performed in conformance with 21 CFR 56 and 21 CFR 50.

(1) Kangarlu A, Burgess RE, Zu H, et al. Cognitive, cardiac and physiological studies in ultra high field magnetic resonance imaging. Magnetic Resonance Imaging, 1999;17:1407-1416.

(2) Schenck John F, Safety of strong, static magnetic fields. Journal of Magnetic Resonance Imaging, 2000;12:2-19.

APPENDIX II

WEBSITES FOR MRI SAFETY, BIOEFFECTS, AND PATIENT MANAGEMENT

There are two websites devoted to MRI safety, bioeffects, and patient management: www.MRIsafety.com and www.IMRSER.org

www.MRIsafety.com

The international information resource for MRI safety, bioeffects, and patient management.

This website provides up-to-date information for healthcare providers and patients seeking answers to questions on MRI safety-related topics. The latest information is also provided for screening patients with implants, materials, and medical devices. *This website is updated on a regular basis by Frank G. Shellock, Ph.D.*

Key Features

- <u>The List:</u> A searchable database that contains information for thousands of implants, devices, and other objects tested for MRI issues.
- <u>Safety Information:</u> Concise information that pertains to the latest recommendations and guidelines for patient care and management in the MRI environment.
- <u>Screening Forms:</u> Information and forms for screening patients and other individuals available to imaging facilities in a "downloadable" PDF format.

www.IMRSER.org

The web site of the Institute for Magnetic Resonance Safety, Education, and Research (IMRSER)

The Institute for Magnetic Resonance Safety, Education, and Research (IMRSER) was formed in response to the growing need for information on matters pertaining to magnetic resonance (MR) safety. The IMRSER is the first independent, multidisciplinary, professional organization devoted to promoting awareness, understanding, and communication of MRI safety issues through education and research.

The functions and activities of the IMRSER involve development of MR safety guidelines and dissemination of this information to the MR community. This is accomplished through the efforts of the two Advisory Boards: the Medical, Scientific, and Technology Advisory Board and the Corporate Advisory Board.

The Medical, Scientific, and Technology Advisory Board consists of recognized leaders in the field of MR including diagnostic radiologists, clinicians, research scientists, physicists, MRI technologists, MRI facility managers, and other allied healthcare professionals involved in MR technology and safety. The members of the Medical, Scientific, and Technology Advisory Board represent academic, private, research, and institutional MR facilities utilizing scanners operating at static magnetic field strengths ranging from 0.2-Tesla (including dedicated-extremity and interventional MR systems) to 7-Tesla. In addition, the Food and Drug Administration has assigned a Federal Liaison to the IMRSER.

The Corporate Advisory Board is comprised of representatives from the medical industry including MR system manufacturers, contrast agent pharmaceutical companies, RF coil manufacturers, MR accessory vendors, medical product manufacturers, and other related corporate organizations.

The Institute for Magnetic Resonance Safety, Education, and Research develops MR safety guidelines utilizing the pertinent peer-reviewed literature and by relying on each board member's extensive clinical, research, or other appropriate experience. Notably, documents developed by the IMRSER consider and incorporate MR safety guidelines and recommendations created by the International Society for Magnetic Resonance in Medicine (ISMRM), the American College of Radiology (ACR), the Food and Drug Administration (FDA), the National Electrical Manufacturers Association (NEMA), the Medical Devices Agency (MDA), the International Electrotechnical Commission (IEC), the International Commission on Non-Ionizing Radiation Protection (ICNIRP), and other organizations.

The MR Safety Papers section of this website includes a wide selection of peer-reviewed articles that are available to site visitors as PDF files, posted with permission from the respective journals.

APPENDIX III

WEBSITES FOR BIOMEDICAL COMPANIES

3M Healthcare -	www.3m.com
Abbott Vascular Devices -	www.abbottvascular.com
Abiomed, Inc. -	www.abiomed.com
Acclarent, Inc. -	www.acclarent.com
Advanced Bionics Corporation -	www.bionicear.com
Adtech Medical Instrument Corporation –	www.adtechmedical.com
Aesculap, Inc. -	www.aesculap.com
Alcon Laboratories Inc.-	www.alcon.com
Allium Medical Solutions -	www.allium-medical.com
Alpha-Bio Tec Ltd. -	www.alpha-bio.net
Alphatec Spine -	www.alphatecspine.com
Alsius Corporation -	www.alsius.com
Ambu -	www.ambu.com
Ampco Safety Tools -	www.ampcosafetytools.com
American Medical Systems -	www.americanmedicalsystems.com
Angiodynamics, Inc. -	www.angiodynamics.com
Animas Corporation -	www.animascorp.com
Ansul-	www.ansul.com
Arbor Surgical Technologies, Inc. -	www.arborsurgical.com
Argon Medical -	www.argonmedical.com
Arthrex -	www.arthrex.com
Applied Medical -	www.appliedmed.com
Ascension Orthopedics, Inc. -	www.ascensionortho.com
Aspire Medical -	www.aspiremedical.com
AtriCure, Inc. -	www.atricure.com
Atritech, Inc. -	www.atritech.com
Atrium Medical Corporation -	www.atriummed.com
ATS Medical -	www.atsmedical.com
B. Braun Medical -	www.bbraunusa.com
Baxa Corporation -	www.baxa.com
Baxter International, Inc. -	www.baxter.com
Becton, Dickinson, and Co. -	www.bd.com
Biomerix Corporation -	www.biomerix.com

Biomet, Inc. -	www.biomet.com
Bioness, Inc. -	www.bioness.com
Bioplate, Inc. -	www.bioplate.com
Biopro, Inc. -	www.bioproimplants.com
Biosensors International -	www.biosensorsintl.com
BioTex, Inc.-	www.biotexmedical.com
Biotronik -	www.biotronik.com
Blackstone Medical, Inc. -	www.blackstonemedical.com
Bolton Medical, Inc. -	www.boltonmedical.com
Boston Scientific Corporation -	www.bostonscientific.com
Bracco Diagnostics Inc. -	www.bracco.com
Bronchus Technologies, Inc. -	www.bronchus.com
Calypso Medical Technologies -	www.calypsomedical.com
Cameron Health -	www.cameronhealth.com
Capella Medical Devices, Ltd. -	www.cappella-med.com
Cardia, Inc. -	www.cardia.com
Cardiac Dimensions -	www.cardiacdimensions.com
Cardica -	www.cardica.com
Cardinal Health -	www.cardinal.com
CardioKinetix Inc. -	www.cardiokinetix.com
CardioMEMS, Inc. -	www.cardiomems.com
CareFusion -	www.carefusion.com
Cayanne Medical -	www.cayennemedical.com
Centinal Spine -	www.centinalspine.com
Coaxia, Inc. -	www.coaxia.com
Codman, a Johnson and Johnson Company -	www.depuysynthes.com
Coherex Medical -	www.coherex.com
Coloplast Corporation -	www.coloplast.com
Conceptus, Inc. -	www.conceptus.com
ConforMIS, Inc. -	www.conformis.com
ConvaTec Wound Therapeutics -	www.convatec.com
Cook Medical -	www.cookmedical.com
Corassist Medical -	www.corassist.com
Cordis -	www.cordis.com
Corvia Medical-	www.corviamedical.com
Covidien -	www.covidien.com
C.R. Bard, Inc. -	www.crbard.com
Cyberkinetics Neurotechnology Systems, Inc. -	www.cyberkineticsinc.com
Cyberonics, Inc. -	www.cyberonics.com
Datascope Corporation -	www.datascope.com

DePuy Synthes. -	www.depuysynthes.com
DeRoyal Technologies -	www.deroyal.com
DexCom, Inc. –	www.dexcom.com
Edwards Lifeciences -	www.edwards.com
Endologix, Inc. -	www.endologix.com
EnteroMedics, Inc. -	www.enteromedics.com
ev3, a Covidien Company -	www.ev3.net
Ethicon -	www.ethicon.com
Evalve, Inc. -	www.evalveinc.com
Facet-Link, Inc. -	www.facet-link.com
Ferno -	www.ferno.com
Finetech Medical Ltd. -	www.finetech-medical.co.uk
Flowonix Medical, Inc. -	www.flowonix.com
Gendron, Inc. -	www.gendroninc.com
General Electric Healthcare -	www.gehealthcare.com
Genstar Technologies -	www.genstartech.com
GI Dynamics, Inc. -	www.gidynamics.com
Glaukos Corporation -	www.glaukos.com
GrantAdler Corporation -	www.grantadler.com
GT Urological -	www.gturological.com
Health Beacons Inc. -	www.healthbeacons.com
Hisamitsu Pharmaceutical Co., Inc. -	www.hisamitsu.co.jp/english
Hitachi Medical Systems America -	www. hitachimed.com
Hobbs Medical -	www.hobbsmedical.com
Hollister Inc. -	www.hollister.com
Hood Laboratories -	www.hoodlabs.com
IDEV Technologies, Inc. -	www.idevtechnologies.com
Integra Lifesciences Corporation -	www.integralife.com
Interrad Medical, Inc. -	www.interradmedical.com
Intrinsic Therapeutics, Inc. -	www.intrinsic-therapeutics.com
Intuitive Surgical, Inc. -	www.intuitivesurgical.com
Invatec -	www.invatec.com
iRhythm Technologies, Inc. -	www.irhythmtech.com
Ivantis -	www.ivantisinc.com
JenaValve Technology -	www.jenavalve.com
Kaneka Corporation -	www.kaneka.co.jp
KCI USA, Inc. -	www.kci1.com
KFx Medical Corporation -	www.kfxmedical.com
Kimberly-Clark Health Care -	www.kimberly-clark.com
Kips Bay Medical, Inc. -	www.kipsbaymedical.com

Labcor Laboratorios Ltda. -	www.labcor.com
LeMaitre Vascular -	www.lemaitre.com
LivaNova-	www.livanova.com
LMA North America -	www.lmana.com
LSI Solutions, Inc. -	www.lsisolutions.com
Magmedix -	www.magmedix.com
Mallinckrodt Pharmaceuticals -	www.mallinckrodt.com
Medcomp -	www.medcompnet.com
MED-EL -	www.medel.com
Medivance, Inc. -	www.medivance.com
Medline Industries, Inc. -	www.medline.com
Medtronic, Inc. -	www.medtronic.com
Mentor Corporation -	www.mentorcorp.com
Micardia Corporation -	www.micardiac.com
Micell Technologies -	www.micell.com
Microline Surgical -	www.microlinesurgical.com
Microvention -	www.microvention.com
MiniMed, Inc. -	www.minimed.com
Minrad, Inc. -	www.minrad.com
Moximed, Inc. -	www.moximed.com
Molynlycke Health Care -	www.molynlycke.com
Mylan Technologies Inc. -	www.mylantech.com
Neovasc, Inc.-	www.neovasc.com
Newmatic Medical -	www.newmaticmedical.com
NGK Metals Corporation -	www.ngkmetals.com
NuVasive, Inc. -	www.nuvasive.com
Obalon-	www.obalon.com
Occlutech Ltd.-	www.occlutech.com
Olympus Medical -	www. medical.olympusamerica.com
Optonol Ltd. -	www.optonol.com
OrbusNeich Medical, Inc. -	www.orbusneich.com
Orthofix -	www.orthofix.com
Ossur Americas -	www.ossur.com
Otto Bock HealthCare -	www.ottobockus.com
Paradigm Spine -	www.paradigmspine.com
PMT Corporation -	www.pmtcorp.com
Praxair Healthcare Services -	www.praxair.com
ProStrakan -	www.prostrakan.com
Pulmonx -	www.pulmonx.com
Pulsar Vascular -	www.pulsarvascular.com

Radianse, Inc. -	www.radianse.com
Rex Medical -	www.rexmedical.com
Rhythmlink International, LLC -	www.rhythmlink.com
SAM Medical Products -	www.sammedical.com
Second Sight Medical Products, Inc. -	www.2-sight.com
Shelhigh Inc. -	www.shelhigh.com
Sicel Technologies, Inc. -	www.siceltech.com
Siemens Medical Solutions -	www.siemens.com
Sientra -	www.sientra.com
Smith & Nephew, Inc. -	www.smith-nephew.com
Smiths Medical -	www.smiths-medical.com
Sorin Group -	www.sorin.com
Spiration Inc. -	www.spiration.com
St. Jude Medical, Inc. -	www.sjm.com
Stentys -	www.stentys.com
Stryker Instruments -	www.stryker.com
SuperDimension -	www.superdimension.com
Svelte Medical Systems, Inc. -	www.sveltemedical.com
Teleflex Medical -	www.teleflex.com
TaeWoong Medical Co., Ltd. -	www.stent.net
The Viking Corporation -	www.vikingcorp.com
Theragenics Corporation -	www.theraseed.com
Torax Medical -	www.toraxmedical.com
TriVascular, Inc. -	www.trivascular.com
Uromedica Inc. -	www.uromedica-inc.com
Valcare Medical Ltd. -	www.valcaremedical.com
Varian Medical Systems -	www.varian.com
Vascular Dynamics -	www.vasculardynamics.com
Vascular Graft Solutions LTD -	www.graftsolutions.com
Vascutek Ltd. -	www.vascutek.com
Vesocclude Medical -	www.vesoccludemedical.com
Vygon Ltd. -	www.vygonus.com
Western Enterprises -	www.westernenterprises.com
W.L. Gore and Associates, Inc. -	www.wlgore.com
Wright Medical Technology -	www.wmt.com
Xeridiem -	www.xeridiem.com
Xlumena -	www.xlumena.com
Zimmer -	www.zimmer.com

APPENDIX IV

Establishing Safety and Compatibility of Passive Implants in the Magnetic Resonance (MR) Environment

Document issued on December 11, 2014.

This document supersedes Establishing Safety and Compatibility of Passive Implants in Magnetic Resonance (MR) Environment, August 21, 2008.

This document may be obtained from the Food and Drug Administration's website, as follows:

http://www.fda.gov/ucm/groups/fdagov-public/@fdagov-meddev-gen/documents/document/ucm107708.pdf

Frank G. Shellock, Ph.D. is a physiologist with more than 30 years of experience conducting laboratory and clinical investigations in the field of magnetic resonance imaging. He is an Adjunct Clinical Professor of Radiology and Medicine at the Keck School of Medicine, University of Southern California, Adjunct Professor of Clinical Physical Therapy, Division of Biokinesiology and Physical Therapy, School of Dentistry, University of Southern 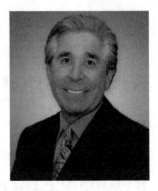 California, the Director of MRI Studies at the Biomimetic Microelectronic Systems, National Science Foundation (NSF) - Engineering Research Center, University of Southern California, and the Founder of the Institute for Magnetic Resonance Safety, Education, and Research (www.IMRSER.org). As a commitment to the field of MRI safety, bioeffects, and patient management, he created and maintains the internationally popular web site, www.MRIsafety.com.

Dr. Shellock has authored or co-authored more than 250 publications in the peer-reviewed literature. He co-authored the MRI safety section of the Cardiovascular MR Self-Assessment Program (CMR-SAP) for the American College of Cardiology and three of his medical textbooks are best sellers - **Reference Manual for Magnetic Resonance Safety, Implants and Devices**; **Magnetic Resonance Procedures: Health Effects and Safety**; and **Kinematic MRI of the Joints: Functional Anatomy, Kinesiology, and Clinical Applications**. His most recent medical textbook includes contributions from more than forty internationally respected authors and is entitled, **MRI Bioeffects, Safety, and Patient Management**.

Dr. Shellock is a member of the Sub-Committee on MRI safety issues for the American Society for Testing and Materials (ASTM) International. Additionally, he serves in advisory roles to government, industry, and other policy-making organizations. Over the years, he has been involved with the MRI Safety Committees for both the American College of Radiology and the International Society for Magnetic Resonance in Medicine. The Joint Commission appointed Dr. Shellock to the Diagnostic Ionizing Radiation and Magnetic Resonance Expert Panel, where he served from 2012 to 2015. He is an Associate Editor for the Journal of Magnetic Resonance Imaging and a Reviewing Editor for several medical and scientific journals including Radiology, Investigative

Radiology, Magnetic Resonance in Medicine, Magnetic Resonance Imaging, the American Journal of Roentgenology, the Journal of Cardiovascular Magnetic Resonance, Circulation, Neuroradiology, the European Heart Journal, Neurosurgery, and the Journal of the American College of Cardiology.

Dr. Shellock's memberships in professional societies include the American College of Radiology, the International Society for Magnetic Resonance in Medicine (ISMRM), the Radiological Society of North America, and the Hawaiian Radiological Society. He is a member and Fellow of the American College of Radiology, International Society for Magnetic Resonance in Medicine, the American College of Cardiology, and the American College of Sportsmedicine.

In 1994, Dr. Shellock received the *Kressel and Crues Educational Award* for exceptional educational contributions to the Section for Magnetic Resonance Technologists (SMRT). The American College of Radiology awarded him a Distinguished Committee Service Award for years of dedicated service to the *Practice Guidelines and Technical Standards Committee – Body MRI.*

Dr. Shellock is a recipient of a National Research Service Award from the National Institutes of Health, National Heart, Lung, and Blood Institute and has received numerous grants from governmental agencies, private organizations, and medical device companies. He participates in research to define safety for implants and devices including cardiac pacemakers, implantable cardioverter defibrillators, neurostimulation systems, and other electronically-activated devices.

Dr. Shellock has lectured both nationally and internationally and has provided plenary lectures to numerous organizations including the Radiological Society of North America, the International Society for Magnetic Resonance in Medicine, the American College of Radiology, the American Roentgen Ray Society, the American Society of Neuroradiology, the Environmental Protection Agency, the Oklahoma Heart Institute, the Head and Neck Radiology Society, the Center for Devices and Radiological Health (FDA), the Magnetic Resonance Managers Society, the American Heart Association, the American College of Cardiology, the American Society of Neuroimaging, the Society for Cardiovascular Magnetic Resonance, the Heart Rhythm Society, the Association for Medical Imaging Management, the Radiology Business Management Association, the Finnish Radiological Society, the International Congress of Radiology, the Japanese Society of Neuroradiology, the British Chapter of the International Society for

Magnetic Resonance in Medicine, the Royal Australian and New Zealand College of Radiologists, the Institute of Physics and Engineering in Medicine, the Karolinska Institute, Cape Peninsula University of Technology and the University of Johannesburg in South Africa.

Dr. Shellock's company, Shellock R & D Services, Inc./Magnetic Resonance Safety Testing Services, specializes in the assessment of MRI issues for implants and devices, as well as the evaluation of electromagnetic field-related bioeffects:

(www.MagneticResonanceSafetyTesting.com).